Complete Japanese Traditional (Kampo) Medicine

Kampo Medical Literature Editorial Committee,
The Japan Society for Oriental Medicine
Editors

Complete Japanese Traditional (Kampo) Medicine

Springer

Editor
Kampo Medical Literature Editorial Committee
The Japan Society for Oriental Medicine
Minato-ku, Tokyo, Japan

ISBN 978-981-96-7142-7 ISBN 978-981-96-7143-4 (eBook)
https://doi.org/10.1007/978-981-96-7143-4

Translation from the Japanese language edition: "Kampo Igaku Daizen" by Kampo Medical Literature Editorial Committee, The Japan Society for Oriental Medicine, © The Japanese Society for Oriental Medicine 2022. Published by Seifudo Shoten. All Rights Reserved.

This Springer imprint is published by the registered company Springer Nature Singapore Pte Ltd.
The registered company address is: 152 Beach Road, #21-01/04 Gateway East, Singapore 189721, Singapore

Foreword

Publication of the English Edition of the *Complete Japanese Traditional (Kampo) Medicine*

Additional Step Forward towards Internationalization of Japanese Traditional (Kampo) Medicine

As the JSOM Director in charge of the Editing Committee on Kampo Medicinal literature, I wish to explain what this publication intends to achieve in terms of advancing internationalization.

The predecessor to this *Complete Japanese Traditional (Kampo) Medicine* was *Introduction to KAMPO Japanese Traditional Medicine* published in 2002. It was created about two decades ago as the first step to standardizing Japanese Traditional (Kampo) Medicine. What led to its publication were changes ongoing at the time in Japan. An extraordinary coincidence was that the WHO started working on a chapter on Traditional Medicine in producing its International Classification of Diseases (ICD-11) 11th Edition. In order to substantiate the description of Japanese Traditional (Kampo) Medicine, the publication of the English version of the above-mentioned *Introduction to KAMPO* became an urgent task. In 2004, this was accomplished in the form of the English edition, *Introduction to KAMPO—Japanese Traditional Medicine*. Produced in two years, this edition constituted the full English translation of the Japanese text. Though it may have seemed a simple process at first, probably a huge obstacle arose. That is to say, the task of rendering the terminology of *Japanese Traditional (Kampo) Medicine* appropriately into English terminology. At a time when there was no clear agreement on the English equivalent for *Japanese Traditional (Kampo)* terminology, translation into English must have posed immense difficulty. The predecessor played the pioneering role in this volume, which led the way in uncharted territory. Since that time, the environment surrounding Traditional Medicine in the world has undergone a huge change. The establishment of ISO/TC 249, which began in 2010 (later named Traditional Chinese Medicine), created a context for the promotion of the standardization of Traditional Medicine. While providing this context, it became an arena for securing rights and interests, thereby amplifying the necessity for internationalization. In other words, we needed to clearly define what Japanese Traditional (Kampo) Medicine was from global perspective, and to present it clearly to the wider world.

The *Introduction to KAMPO* was a pioneering work but lacked consistency in this respect. Its contents urgently required an overhaul. Before undertaking this revision, however, first and foremost we had to resolve the issue of terminology. After interviewing our members on several occasions, the Committee for Terminology and Disease Names in 2014 completed the *Glossary of Japanese Traditional (Kampo) Medicine Terminology* (English version). The Editing Committee for Dictionary of Kampo Medicine took over the project and added the meaning and commentary on the terms listed. The work was extremely difficult, requiring collation with the English terminology used in the chapter on Traditional Medicine in WHO's ICD-11. The fruit of the labor was *The Dictionary of Kampo Medicine (Basic terms)* published in 2020. Work was then begun on preparing an English version of the *Complete Japanese Traditional (Kampo) Medicine* based on this consolidation of terminology. However, because writing a textbook in English directly for Japanese speakers presents many issues, a Japanese version had to be prepared first and this then had to be translated into English. In this way, the publication we are presenting here was accomplished. Now, since the Japanese text was to be translated into English and the speed of completion was key, we decided to use as a source text *Introduction of KAMPO and Textbook of Traditional Japanese Medicine* prepared by the MHLW Research Group led by Dr. Makoto Arai, because this had been partly translated into English already. This is how the Japanese text came about, but its core purpose was to serve as the original text for the English edition. The preparation of an English edition then became our pressing task, also it would serve as reference source for the joint journal of JSOM and the Japan Society of Medical and Pharmaceutical Sciences for Traditional Medicine—*Traditional & Kampo Medicine*. The role of the Director, responsible for the English edition, was transferred to Dr. Tetsuro Oikawa.

I wish to conclude by expressing my sincere gratitude to all the authors who so willingly offered their time for our endeavor, Dr. Yosuke Amano (The Chair of the Editing Committee for Dictionary of Kampo Medicine, who continued in his role in the new committee) and Dr. Makoto Arai (Vice Chair of the same committee), all those who were involved in supervising the chapters (Dr. Masayuki Kashima, Dr. Yoshihide Yakazu, Dr. Masamitsu Nakajima, Dr. Toshiaki Makino, and Dr. Toshihiro Togo) alongside all committee members who undertook the peer review. My heartfelt thanks go to all members of the JSOM Secretariat, Stephen Brown who edited the English, and members of ASCA Corporation who were responsible for the translation. Last but not least, let me convey my sincere gratitude to the Japanese publisher, Seifusha Co., Ltd., which undertook the task of publication despite all current difficulties due to the pandemic and gave us numerous constructive suggestions on how to proceed with our seminal task.

Takao Namiki

Director of the Editing Committee on Kampo
Medicinal Literature, Japan Society
for Oriental Medicine (JSOM),
(Former Director of the Editing Committee
for Dictionary of Kampo Medicine;
Member of the Committee for Terminology and Disease Names)
Tokyo, Japan
June 2021

Preface

Globally, the harmonization of Traditional Medicine and Western Medicine are moving forward. In June 2020, the WHO introduced a new chapter on Traditional Medicine in its International Classification of Diseases 11th Revision (ICD-11). The initiative was taken in the wake of data gathering in developing countries. However, it signifies the recognition of the role that Traditional Medicine plays in today's world. What we need now is closer definition and description of details about Traditional Medicine from the perspectives of Western medicine.

The Japanese government healthcare system had positioned Kampo medicines alongside Western medicines. Since 1961 when the national health insurance system was instituted, crude drugs were treated as raw material for decoction and Kampo medicines for medical use have been licensed with effective indications, with a strong requirement for evidence along Western Medicine lines for them to be granted government approval. Japan approves the use of both Kampo and Western medicines for patients receiving treatment under the national health insurance system. This is rare in the world. Thus Japan is in poll position for the harmonization of Kampo Medicine and Western Medicine to take place.

The 2001 Model Core Curriculum for Medical Education issued by Japan's Ministry of Education, Culture, Sports, Science and Technology (MEXT) stated "ability to outline Wakan-yaku can be acquired." After two revisions, the wording of the 2016 version became "the ability to outline the characteristic nature of Kampo Medicine and the indications and pharmacodynamic actions of principal Wakan-yaku (Japanese Kampo medicines)" with the addition of "Medicine" in the phrasing for the first time. This is a significant development. It means the recognition of the medical practice that underlies the Kampo medicines. In 2002, the Japan Society for Oriental Medicine (JSOM) published its first ever textbook on Kampo Medicine, *Nyumon Kampo Igaku* (meaning Kampo medicine for beginners). An edition for students followed, and then another for specialists. We have thus been promoting discussions and standardization of learning content.

Our latest endeavor is to revise the textbook, *Nyumon Kampo Igaku*, for the first time in two decades. What is the importance of studying Kampo Medicine? What is its relevance to healthcare in the 2020s?

In Japan, Kampo medicines are used in almost all clinical departments. According to a 2011 survey, there were as many as 558 cases of doctors prescribing Kampo medicines out of 627 cases (89%). Many academic societies have published guidelines for treatment including descriptions of Kampo medicines. There are 118 such publications to date.

The problem, however, is that there is a trend sometimes in recent publications to regard as satisfactory the knowledge merely of one Kampo medicine to treat a disease or symptom. Such an approach would simply add a Kampo medicine to the list of prescribable drugs, making the physician into a slightly more agile prescriber of medication. Kampo medicines should not be used in the framework of Western medicine prescription in such a way. When a Kampo medicine is to be prescribed, Kampo Medicine diagnosis should be applied, with selection and identification of more than one Kampo medicines as appropriate. This is desirable because we need the knowledge and training basis of Traditional Medicine that reviews the disease state if the prescribed medication cannot deliver the effectiveness expected.

Notably, Japan is facing a rapid unfolding of its hyper-aging society. Incidence of geriatric disease increases with aging. This means that if just the Western Medicine approach is adopted, the number of drug prescriptions will keep rising. Healthcare in Japan has become heavily dependent on the dispensing of medication. What the aging society really needs, however, is a healthcare approach for the elderly that makes use of the body's own healing mechanisms, relying less on medication. Indeed, to this end, the study of traditional medicines and their conceptual appreciation and application are necessary.

My own understanding of Kampo Medicine is that it is a discipline that tries to work out what the most appropriate treatment is for a patient in his or her current state and prevailing conditions. In treating a patient, the practitioner needs to deploy the five senses to the utmost limit. Because the practitioner can choose the useful Kampo medicines (or treatment techniques) based on appropriate consultation practice, the consultation itself leads to improved diagnostic ability of the practitioner. If the patient's condition improves as a result of the treatment administered, this leads to greater confidence and delight in daily practice. Kampo Medicine has this built-in cycle of positivity. A new student of Kampo Medicine may only manage to understand and learn about all the patterns (Kampo Medicine diagnoses), but once he or she gets to grips with yin-yang and deficiency and excess categorization, he or she can readily see how not only the Kampo medicines but also the Western medicines, diet, and lifestyle aspects come into play in patient treatment. My hope is that every healthcare practitioner will use the study of Kampo Medicine so as to improve skills and knowledge to deliver an even better quality of healthcare to patients.

Tokyo, Japan Takashi Ito

Preface to the English Edition

As explained in detail by our former Director, Dr. Namiki, we are now pleased to have published the English version of *Complete Japanese Traditional (Kampo) Medicine*. As we were editing this book, the wave of internationalization of traditional medicine grew even stronger, and it became crucial to make it more clear that this is the traditional medicine of Japan. For this reason, we have decided to title the book *Complete Japanese Traditional (Kampo) Medicine*.

Once again, we would like to express our deepest gratitude to all those involved in the editing and publication of this book, and we hope that readers around the world will become more aware of our country's traditional medicine.

Director of the Editing Committee on Kampo Medicinal Literature, Japan Society for Oriental Medicine (JSOM)
Tetsuro Oikawa
Tokyo, Japan
October 2024

Kampo Medical Literature Editorial Committee

Editors

Tetsuro Oikawa	Center for Kampo Medicine, Tokyo Medical University Hospital (Tokyo, Japan)
Tatsuhiko Suzuki	Faculty of Pharmaceutical Sciences, Teikyo Heisei University (Tokyo, Japan)
Tomoko Suzuki	Department of Oriental Medicine, Saitama Medical University (Iruma-gun, Japan)

Authors

Hideki Adachi	Adachi Clinic (Tokyo, Japan)
Seigou Akao	Nagoya Toyo Clinic (Nagoya, Japan)
Tetsuo Akiba	Akiba Clinic of Traditional Medicine (Sanmu, Japan)
Yosuke Amano	Nihon Isen (Tokyo, Japan)
Makoto Arai	Department of Kampo Medicine, Tokai University School of Medicine/Department of General Internal Medicine, St. Marianna University School of Medicine (Kawasaki, Japan)
Toshiyuki Atsumi	Department of Pharmaceutical Sciences, School of Pharmaceutical Sciences, Kyushu University of Medical Science (Nobeoka, Japan)
Masashi Beppu	Department of General Medicine, Division of Comprehensive Patient Care, Graduate School of Medical and Dental Sciences, Institute of Science Tokyo (Tokyo, Japan)
Makoto Fujimoto	Department of Japanese Oriental Medicine, Graduate School of Medicine and Pharmaceutical Sciences(School of Medicine), University of Toyama (Toyama, Japan)
Motoko Fukuzawa	Omotesando Fukuzawa Clinic (Tokyo, Japan)
Hirozo Goto	Hokusei Hospital (Toyama, Japan)
Toshihiko Hanawa	Kitasato University Kitasato Institute Hospital (Tokyo, Japan)
Akito Hisanaga	Department of Psychiatry, Hospital Bando (Bando, Japan)
Hironobu Iguchi	Sawa Memorial Hamamatsu Hospital (Hamamatsu, Japan)
Tatsuya Ishige	Kobushi ENT Clinic (Yashio, Japan)
Go Ito	Oriental Medicine Therapy Center of Kitasato Institute Hospital, Kitasato University (Tokyo, Japan)
Takashi Ito	Akashi Clinic Kanda (Tokyo, Japan)
Mosaburo Kainuma	Department of Japanese oriental Medicine, Graduate School of Medicine and Pharmaceutical Sciences, Toyama University Hospital (Toyama, Japan)
Toru Kaneko	Kaneko Otolaryngology Clinic (Utsunomiya, Japan)
Masayuki Kashima	Department of General Internal Medicine, Japanese Red Cross Kumamoto Hospital (Kumamoto, Japan)
Tatsuro Katsuno	Sumida Kampo Clinic, Chiba University (Tokyo, Japan)
Kazuyoshi Kawazoe	Division of Natural Medicine and Therapeutics, Department of Clinical Pharmacy, School of Pharmacy, Showa Medical University (Tokyo, Japan)
Akira Kinebuchi	Aoyama Kinebuchi Clinic (Tokyo, Japan)
Toshiaki Kogure	Maebashi Fueki Clinic (Maebashi, Japan)
Hiroshi Kosoto	The Association of East-Asian Medicine (Tokyo, Japan)
Takaaki Kosuge	Kosuge Clinic Yokohama Suzaku Kampo Medical Center (Yokohama, Japan)
Kenshu Lai	Kampo Lai Clinic (Tokyo, Japan)

Toshiaki Makino	Department of Pharmacognosy, Graduate School of Pharmaceutical Sciences, Nagoya City University (Nagoya, Japan)
Kazuo Mitani	Nara Medical University/Mitani Family Clinic (Sakai, Japan)
Tadamichi Mitsuma	Department of Kampo Medicine, Aizu Medical Center Hospital, Fukushima Medical University (Aizuwakamatsu, Japan)
Yoshiharu Motoo	Department of Internal Medicine, Fukui Saiseikai Hospital (Fukui, Japan)
Masafumi Murai	Department of Kampo Medicine, Social Medical Corporation Teijinkai Shinsapporo Hibarigaoka Hospital (Sapporo, Japan)
Shin-ichi Muramatsu	Division of Oriental Medicine, Center for Community Medicine, Jichi Medical University (Shimotsuke, Japan)
Masamitsu Nakajima	Division of Kampo Medicine and Pharmacognosy, Faculty of Pharmaceutical Sciences, Hiroshima International University/Division of Kampo Medicine, National Hospital Organization Kure Medical Center (Higashi-hiroshima, Japan)
Takao Namiki	International University of Health and Welfare Narita Hospital (Narita, Japan)
Masaru Natsuaki	Department of Dermatology, Hyogo Medical University (Nishinomiya, Japan)
Shinji Nishida	Nishida Clinic (Sakai, Japan)
Tatsuya Nogami	Department of Kampo Medicine, Tokai University School of Medicine (Isehara, Japan)
Hiroshi Odaguchi	Kitasato University Kitasato Institute Hospital (Tokyo, Japan)
Hirokuni Okumi	Ihoukai Medical Association Okumi Clinic (Osaka, Japan)
Akira Saito	Wako-ent Clinic/Saitama Medical University (Wako, Japan)
Hiroshi Sato	Isomura Clinic (Tokyo, Japan)
Takashi Seki	The Integrative Medicine Center, Fuji Toranomon Orthopedic Hospital (Gotenba, Japan)
Yuki Sekiguchi	Yokohama Motomachi Women's Clinic LUNA (Yokohama, Japan)
Yutaka Shimada	Osawano Clinic (Toyama, Japan)
Eiichi Tahara	Department of Kampo Medicine, Aizu Medical Center, Fukushima Medical University (Aizuwakamatsu, Japan)
Masanori Takashi	Acupuncture & Moxibustion NAS Clinic (Chigasaki, Japan)
Mayumi Tamada	Institute of Oriental Medicine Tokyo Women's Medical University (Tokyo, Japan)
Koichiro Tatsumi	Department of Respirology, Graduate School of Medicine, Chiba University (Chiba, Japan)
Katsutoshi Terasawa	Professor emeritus Toyama University, M.D., Ph.D. (Toyama, Japan)
Yoshiharu Tobina	Onchido Yakazu Clinic (Tokyo, Japan)
Toshihiro Togo	Visiting professor, Meiji University of Integrative Medicine (Nantan, Japan)
Kazushi Uneda	Department of Kampo Medicine, Aizu Medical Center, Fukushima Medical University (Aizuwakamatsu, Japan)
Takahisa Ushiroyama	Osaka Medical and Pharmaceutical University Health Science Clinic (Takatsuki, Japan)
Keido Yakazu	Onchido Yakazu Clinic (Tokyo, Japan)
Yoshihide Yakazu	Onchido Yakazu Clinic (Tokyo, Japan)
Shuji Yakubo	Department of Medicine, The Nippon Dental University School of Life Dentistry (Tokyo, Japan)
Hideaki Yamaguchi	K Children's Clinic (Nagoya, Japan)
Hitoshi Yamashita	Graduate School of Health Sciences, Morinomiya University of Medical Sciences (Osaka, Japan)
Hiromichi Yasui	Japan Institute of TCM Research (Yokkaichi, Japan)
Makoto Yoshitomi	Yusuhara Public Hospital (Takaoka-gun, Japan)
Ikuro Wakayama	Kansai University of Health Sciences (Sennan-gun, Japan)
Kako Watanabe	Obiyama Central Hospital (Kumamoto, Japan)
Koji Watanabe	Watanabe Sanfujinka (Hiki-gun, Japan)

Other Authors of Chapter 8

Atsushi Chino	Department of Japanese-Oriental (Kampo) Medicine, Chiba Central Medical Center (Chiba, Japan)
Yukari Gono	Department of General Medicine, Kitasato University School of Medicine (Sagamihara, Japan)
Tomoyuki Hayasaki	Kampo Clinic, Keiyukai Yoshida Hospital (Asahikawa, Japan)
Hiroaki Hikiami	Shikino care center (Takaoka, Japan)
Yoshiro Hirasaki	Department of Japanese-Oriental Medicine, Graduate School of Medicine, Chiba University (Chiba, Japan)
Takayuki Hoshino	Kitasato University Kitasato Institute Hospital (Tokyo, Japan)
Hiromitsu Hotta	Michitose Clinic (Tokyo, Japan)
Yoshihiro Imazu	Shiba Daimon Imazu Clinic (Tokyo, Japan)
Yuji Kasahara	Kasahara Clinic (Nagareyama, Japan)
Hideo Kimura	Department of Kampo Medicine, Sakurajyuji Hospital, Fukuoka City (Fukuoka, Japan)
Keiko Matsuura	Nanasai Clinic (Tokyo, Japan)
Kiyoshi Minamizawa	Department of Oriental Medicine, Kameda Medical Center (Kamogawa, Japan)
Hiroki Mizobe	Iwate Medical University (Morioka, Japan)
Kazuhiro Muroga	Operacity Clinic (Tokyo, Japan)
Ko Nishimura	Hane Pediatric Clinic (Toba, Japan)
Hideki Okamoto	Akashi Clinic Kanda (Tokyo, Japan)
Kaori Sawai	Sapporo Maternity Women's Hospital (Sapporo, Japan)
Naotoshi Shibahara	Kampo Education and Training Center, Institute of Natural Medicine, University of Toyama (Toyama, Japan)
Takahiro Shintani	Yasuraginaika (Saitama, Japan)
Kunihiko Suzuki	K. Clinic HIROO (Tokyo, Japan)
Kosuke Tajima	Tokyo Women's Medical University, Adachi Medical Center (Tokyo, Japan)
Yukiko Ueda	Fukuzaitaku Clinic (Tokorozawa, Japan)
Shinji Ueno	Kouseikai Nishikata Hospital (Tochigi, Japan)
Takahiro Yamada	Kinkikai Clinic (Tokyo, Japan)

Chapter 9 Authors in Addition to the Editorial Committee

Katsunori Miyake	Research and Education Center for Plant Resources, Tokyo University of Pharmacy and Life Sciences (Hachioji, Japan)
Tadahiro Yahagi	Laboratory of Pharmacognosy, School of Pharmacy, Nihon University (Funabashi, Japan)

Translation Editor

The Kampo Medical Literature Editorial Committee would like to thank Dr. Brown for his contributions.

Stephen Seiji BROWN	Seattle Institute of East Asian Medicine (SIEAM)

Contents

Part I

Kampo Medicines Treatment

General Theory of Kampo Medicine

1

Takashi Ito, Katsutoshi Terasawa, Hiroshi Kosoto, Yoshihide Yakazu, Hiromichi Yasui, Tetsuo Akiba, Tatsuro Katsuno, Masayuki Kashima, Koji Watanabe, Keido Yakazu, Makoto Yoshitomi, Masamitsu Nakajima, Akira Kinebuchi, Hiroshi Sato, and Eiichi Tahara

1 Kampo Medicine as Part of Modern Medicine

Takashi Ito

1.1 Kampo Medicine in the World

1.1.1 Introduction

Kampo medicine is a unique traditional Japanese medicine which was adopted around the fifth and sixth centuries and underwent unique changes due to the Japanese climate and dietary habits. It attaches great importance to the *"Shokanron* 傷寒論 (*Treatise on Cold Damage*)," one of the three great classics of Chinese medicine, and mainly applies its prescriptions for both acute and chronic medical care.

Traditional East Asian medicine, which traces its roots back to ancient Chinese medicine, developed in countries of East Asia. This medicine developed differently in China, Korea, and Japan and has different characteristics. It is called "traditional Chinese medicine" in China, "traditional Korean medicine" in South Korea, and "Kampo medicine" in Japan. The characteristics of Kampo medicine, or the Japanese-style traditional medicine, will be explained below.

1.1.2 Abdominal Examination as the Primary Diagnosis in Kampo Medicine

Yoshimasu Todo (1702–1773), a doctor of Kampo medicine who led the Koho School in the Edo period, proposed the theory that all diseases were caused by one poison (*Manbyo ichidoku*). Yoshimasu refused to apply the yin and yang and five-element theory to medicine. He relied primarily on "abdominal diagnosis"—a diagnosis based on findings such as tension and tenderness in the abdomen—to decide on a prescription. Abdominal diagnosis was relatively easier to master than pulse diagnosis and was advantageous in training.

T. Ito
Akashi Clinic Kanda, Tokyo, Japan

K. Terasawa
Toyama University, Toyama, Japan

H. Kosoto
The Association of East-Asian Medicine, Tokyo, Japan

Y. Yakazu (✉) · K. Yakazu
Onchido Yakazu Clinic, Tokyo, Japan
e-mail: office@jsom.or.jp

H. Yasui
Japan Institute of TCM Research, Yokkaichi, Japan

T. Akiba
Akiba Clinic of Traditional Medicine, Sanmu, Japan

T. Katsuno
Sumida Kampo Clinic, Chiba University, Tokyo, Japan

M. Kashima
Department of General Internal Medicine, Japanese Red Cross Kumamoto Hospital, Kumamoto, Japan

K. Watanabe
Watanabe Sanfujinka, Hiki, Japan

M. Yoshitomi
Yusuhara Public Hospital, Takaoka, Japan

M. Nakajima
Division of Kampo Medicine and Pharmacognosy, Faculty of Pharmaceutical Sciences, Hiroshima International University, Higashihiroshima, Japan

Division of Kampo Medicine, National Hospital Organization Kure Medical Center, Higashihiroshima, Japan

A. Kinebuchi
Aoyama Kinebuchi Clinic, Tokyo, Japan

H. Sato
Isomura Clinic, Tokyo, Japan

E. Tahara
Department of Kampo Medicine, Aizu Medical Center, Fukushima Medical University, Aizuwakamatsu, Japan

Kampo Medical Literature Editorial Committee, The Japan Society for Oriental Medicine (ed.), *Complete Japanese Traditional (Kampo) Medicine*, https://doi.org/10.1007/978-981-96-7143-4_1

1.1.3 Acupuncture and Moxibustion Specialists Distinguished from Medical Doctors

In Japan, there is a national system to certify specialists in acupuncture and moxibustion, which is unlike China and South Korea. These specialists usually obtain certification for both acupuncture and moxibustion simultaneously and are generally called acupuncture and moxibustion practitioners. As of 2018, approximately 120,000 specialists were practicing this medicine. Meanwhile, medical doctors were roughly estimated to be 330,000 (same year). Doctors are allowed to practice acupuncture and moxibustion as part of their medical practice, but few doctors actually practice these therapies. These are mostly being practiced by specialists in acupuncture and moxibustion.

A unique invention in Japanese acupuncture was inserting needles using the acupuncture tube. The well-known method was invented by Sugiyama Waichi (1610–1694). It minimizes the pain of insertion and is widely used in the world today. Recently, skin stimulation including stroking or scraping with special needles is attracting attention and is being used for pediatric and adult chronic diseases. Painlessness and less stimulation are noticeable characteristics of Japanese acupuncture (See Chap. 7, Sect. 1.1).

1.1.4 Consistent Composition of Crude Drugs in Formulas

In Japan, a prescription was fixed traditionally without modifying the amount of crude drugs for the purpose of having sufficient clinical effects with a small dose. This is because the crude drugs imported from China were expensive, and frequently used formulas could be prepared in advance. The tradition of choosing to treat not with crude drugs but with formulas is extremely useful at present in studying and applying many Japanese Kampo extract formulas and their formulation methods. In contrast, academic papers on traditional Chinese medicine (TCM) disclose that one prescription was used for many cases, but with crude drugs modified according to individual cases. Therefore, the prescription was actually modified and was not uniform.

1.1.5 Contribution to the Restoration of Traditional Chinese Medicine (Preserving Skills and Classics and Bringing Them Back to China)

Most people do not know that Kampo practitioners in Japan contributed to preserving, discovering, and studying the classics of traditional Chinese medicine. They helped restore traditional Chinese medicine through documents of traditional medicine written under the influence of modern science. In China, like in Japan, there was an era when traditional medicine was suppressed. In the Qing Dynasty, the imperial ordinance was issued to abolish the section of acupuncture and moxibustion at the medical office in the Palace (*taiyiyuan*) in 1822. After that, acupuncture and moxibustion were in adverse circumstances among civilians and were driven to the verge of disappearance at the start of the Republic of China. In Japan, the Imperial Diet made a resolution that Kampo medicine would no longer be recognized as medicine in 1895. China (Republic of China) followed this resolution and established an act to abolish traditional Chinese medicine in 1929. However, advocates of traditional Chinese medicine started a campaign calling for its preservation and finally managed to organize a traditional Chinese medicine committee in the Ministry of Health in 1937. Thus, traditional Chinese medicine was saved from extinction.

In Japan, Chinese medical classics were directly imported from China after the Japanese official delegates were sent to China during the Sui Dynasty (600–618). Our predecessors were eager to preserve them, analyze their contents, and discover new facts. Many years of this effort bore fruit. At the end of the Edo period, research on traditional medicine reached a peak. Precious Japanese documents and texts were exported back to China in and after the Meiji period. According to a survey in 2006, 296 kinds of texts on traditional Chinese medicine were taken back to China, and 751 kinds of texts on traditional Japanese medicine were sent to China. At present, there are approximately 4000 sets, or at least tens of thousands of texts on ancient Chinese medicine which Japan has possessed in Japan. This is an extensive collection. In addition, the Japanese books on traditional medicine, which were written and influenced by modern science, contributed greatly to the advent of "new" traditional medicine in the People's Republic of China (PRC). This came to light with the publication of Japanese medical texts in China. The most influential Japanese medical book in and after the Meiji period was "*Kokan'igaku* 皇漢医学 (*Traditional medicine originated in China and developed uniquely in Japan*)" written by Yumoto Kyushin (1876–1941), which has been reprinted a total of nine times including the period after establishment of PRC. Sixteen kinds of new translations on acupuncture and moxibustion were published in the PRC, which were originally written by Sorei Yangiya (1906–1959), Bunshi Shirota (1900–1974), Yoshio Nagahama (1915–1961), Kobe Akabane (1895–1983), Shohaku Homma (1904–1962), and Yoshio Manaka (1911–1989).

1.1.6 Integration with Modern Medicine

Use of Western and Traditional Medicines in the National Insurance System

Kampo medicine has been changing and influenced by the thinking of different periods. In modern times, Kampo medicine was integrated into Western medicine. In 1895, the Imperial Diet decided to integrate Japanese medicine into Western medicine. The practice of Kampo medicine almost disappeared. It was recognized after World War II (1945) that it could compensate for weaknesses of Western medicine, such as side effects. In 1961, when the national insurance program for universal health coverage was launched, crude drugs were recognized as materials for producing Kampo formulas. The formulas gradually increased, from initially six kinds in 1967 up to 148 kinds at present. Now more than 80% of medical doctors prescribe Kampo formulas in an ordinary clinical setting. Japan is the only country that has integrated Kampo medicine with Western medicine and is leading the world.

Introduction of Kampo Medicine to Medical Education and Certification of Kampo Specialists (See Chap. 1, Sect. 4.1)

The Japan Society for Oriental Medicine published *"Nyumonkampoigaku* 入門漢方医学 *(Introduction of Kampo Medicine),"* in 2002, followed by other books. Their purpose was to clarify the details of education in traditional medicine with the intention of integration with Western medicine. The Committee for Certification of Specialists in the Japan Society for Oriental Medicine started training Kampo specialists in 1989. The Society has approximately 2000 experts as of 2021, which accounts for only 0.7% of the total number of medical doctors. As pre-graduation education, the Medical Core Curriculum requires the students to "be able to explain the outline of Kampo medicine" in 2001. Almost all university departments of medicine were providing lectures on Kampo medicine; however, the curriculum was not standardized. In 2020, the Japan Council for Kampo Medical Education (composed of instructors in charge of the education of Kampo medicine in the university departments of medicine nationwide) published a standard text for pre-graduation education.

Consideration of Medical Safety

The Ministry of Health, Labor and Welfare (MHLW) maintains a policy of not separating Kampo formulas from Western formulas and publishes information about the side effects of Kampo as well as Western formulas on their Web pages regularly. This means that Japan is prominent in medical safety management. In the acupuncture and moxibustion industry, the Japan Society of Acupuncture and Moxibustion has worked out its safety measures and published Safety Guidelines for Japanese Acupuncture and Moxibustion Practice [1]. The Committee for Medical Safety in the Japan Society for Oriental Medicine is conducting investigations on medical safety.

1.1.7 Features of Achievements of Modern Kampo Medicine

Writings by Otsuka Aimed at Integration with Western Medicine

The *"Shokanron* 傷寒論 *(Treatise on Cold Damage),"* a classic of ancient Chinese medicine, describes treatments for acute febrile diseases. The detailed analysis of this text enlightened Japanese researchers and made them compile theories about the treatment of infectious and various chronic diseases. Otsuka Keisetsu (1999–1989) was one of the members of the school that valued the formulas of the Koho School taken from the *"Shokanron* 傷寒論 *(Treatise on Cold Damage)"* and *"Kinkiyouryaku* □□□□ *(Synopsis of the Golden Chamber)."* Otsuka compiled the theories of his predecessors with the aim of integrating Kampo with modern Western medicine. His writings had a great influence on the education and clinical practice of Kampo medicine today. The idea of yin/yang, deficiency/excess, and qi/blood[TM1]/fluid[TM1] of Kampo medicine is based on statements in the *"Shokanron* 傷寒論 *(Treatise on Cold Damage)"* because of the great influence of the Koho School. The five elements and the zang-fu organs theory are studied to explain the formulas of later eras (formula of Gosei School) as well as theories of acupuncture and moxibustion.

Attempt to Objectivize Traditional Medical Diagnostic Systems

There were many attempts to objectify diagnostic systems of traditional medicine. A typical example was an attempt by a group led by Terasawa Katsutoshi, who used a stochastic method to create a diagnostic standard (static blood[TM1] score) by giving each detected symptom points according to the severity of blood[TM1] stasis in traditional medicine. He thus proved that there was a correlation between the score and blood viscosity. Particularly, patients suffering from serious blood[TM1] stasis with not less than 20 points (score) experienced a significant increase in blood viscosity and a decline in erythrocyte deformability. It was reported that administration of Keishibukuryogan (formulas to treat blood[TM1] stasis) not only improved the symptoms but also decreased the blood[TM1] stasis score and improved these indexes.

Informing the Evidence Related to Kampo Formulas

In traditional medicine, analysis of a large number of cases has not yet been conducted as in Western medicine, where many cases have been statistically analyzed. This kind of analysis supports the validity and becomes an important basis for using Kampo medicine today and has a great influence on clinical application. The Committee of Evidence-based Medicine (EBM) in the Japan Society for Oriental Medicine is engaged in the verification of evidence related to Kampo formulas and is publishing results on its Web pages [2]. To search for crude drugs or ingredients of a Kampo formula in a clinical report, etc., check the URL of the relevant prescription on Standards of Reporting Kampo Products (STORK) [3]. This website also shows various treatment guidelines, including recommendations for using Kampo formulas [4]. Traditional diagnosis is the most important component of Kampo medicine. It is also important, however, to organize and provide evidence and information.

This section is a reproduction of "Characteristics of Kampo" on the website of The Japan Liaison of Oriental Medicine (JLOM), with some additions and corrections [5].

1.2 Distinctive Features of Japanese Kampo Medicine

Katsutoshi Terasawa

1.2.1 Medical Theory Proposed by Yoshimasu Todo

A system of knowledge amalgamated as Kampo medicine, as described in this chapter, actually comprises a broad spectrum of knowledge obtained from historical and inevitable cultural development. Its defining backbone is the medical theory by Yoshimasu Todo (1702–1773). Yoshimasu denied all theories of traditional Chinese medicine, including yin and yang theory, five elements theory, zang-fu, and meridians and collaterals. Instead, he proposed a unique medical theory on the basis of the so-called existential empiricism or structuralism-based recognition method. Yoshimasu's basic principles were as follows:

1. The physician must be able to cure the patient on the basis of exact observation without speculation or conjecture (such a physician is called *Shitsui*疾医).
2. An ideal physician is Bian Que of ancient times. Ancient literatures should be learned that show "a world in the raw" with no speculation, conjecture, or modification.
3. Existing Chinese medicine, in which diseases are classified into many categories and diagnosed, then various measures are discussed, is filled with speculation and conjecture. In reality, all diseases develop from only one poison, transform in the body, and merely are manifested in the form of various signs and symptoms. Accordingly, this poison can be eliminated with another poison—a drug. Thus, the phrase "All kinds of disease are caused by one poison (Manbyo Ichidoku theory)" was born.
4. Kampo formulas closer to their ancient prototypes are preferable, because those ancient formulas were devised by Shitsui and actually have been and are very effective. Accordingly, it is recommended that treatment basically be based on the *"Shokanron* 傷寒論 *(Treatise on Cold Damage)"* and *"Kinkiyouryaku* 金匱要略 *(Synopsis of the Golden Chamber)"* first established by Zhang Zhong Jing. Since many speculations, conjectures, and annotations were later added to these classics, the ancient original forms must be selected carefully. The most important thing is that each formulation should be administered after being matched to a specific form of poison, or "pattern." This is called a formula corresponding to the pattern identification (*Hoshosotai*).
5. Since a poison is attacked with another poison, a violent reaction/response occurs in the healing process. This is called a paradoxical healing response (*Mengen*). The physicians of old said that "if administration of a medicine does not induce *Mengen*, the disease will not cure." Kampo doctors should not fear *Mengen*; otherwise, they will not become good Kampo doctors (*Shitsui*).
6. The use of some poisons may cause the patient's death. However, the death is not due to the poison (drug). Precisely, life or death is decided by God, not by human beings. Thus, the physician should realize that they cannot predict life or death and devote to doing their best for the treatment of disease. There is a saying "We can only do what is humanly possible and leave the rest to fate."
7. Kampo formulations, whether ancient formulations or subsequent formulations, must be directly tested via repeated trials in clinical settings to evaluate the form of illness (pattern) and efficacy. Such is the case with crude drugs. Then only the formulations and crude drugs for which the efficacy has been established are used in clinical practices. This process is called a direct trial experiment (*Shinshi Jikken*). Doctors can satisfactorily use even subsequent formulations, which are not ancient, if proven to be effective in *Shinshi Jikken*.
8. Unless the true form of poison is identified without any speculation or conjecture, the optimal formulations cannot be selected. For that purpose, the entity of poison must be grasped by abdominal examination, which is clinically the most important medical examination. Tension, stiffness, muscle contracture, and palpitation that manifest in the abdominal region must be closely and carefully palpated. The next important examination is to check for the signs appearing on the body surface. Detailed observation and careful auscultation should be carried out for spontaneous sweating, heat sensation in the upper half of the body and coldness in the lower half of the body, redness, swelling, and edema, in addition to inquiry about the frequencies of urination and defecation, as well as the properties of urine and stool. Skills concerning pattern diagnosis necessary for formula selection must be learned and acquired by the physician himself or herself in clinical practices and cannot be conferred to offspring or transmitted in writing.

Behind this approach, there are "tacit knowledge" and "explicit knowledge," which were proposed by Ikujiro Nonaka (Japanese economic scholar). Clinical knowledge to determine the form of illness, or pattern, manifesting in and on a patient corresponds to the former. This cannot be expressed in language, in contrast to the latter, which can be expressed. This is stated in a sentence "Skills concerning pattern diagnosis necessary for formula selection must be learned and acquired by the physician himself or herself in clinical practice and cannot be conferred to offspring or transmitted in writing" in the eighth principle. Needless to say, the "tacit knowledge" which cannot be expressed in language might be explained logically with yin and yang and five elements theory. However, "Language cannot express all the subtleties of a matter, and the methodology of categorizing all things into five elements cannot approach the truth of the whole." Therefore, the greatest problem in the logical analysis based on element reductionism (as in pattern identification and treatment in TCM) is that the logic cannot reach the starting point of "tacit knowledge" retrospectively. What is the methodology that enables one to grasp "tacit knowledge" itself as a whole? Yoshimasu Todo proposed abdominal signs or body surface findings that are tangible physical findings as a mediator for grasping the whole picture. He does not discuss why such abdominal signs appear. Based on system control theory, it is considered that problem resolution is sought by an appropriate formulation (a black box), adapting the black box form to grasp illness on the basis of structuralism. The reason abdominal examination is particularly emphasized and valued in Kampo medicine is that abdominal signs obtained by abdominal examination provide very precise information for the recognition of the black box form of illness.

The second great achievement of Yoshimasu Todo is to have established the "independence of formulas," which actually resulted in the work *"Ruijuho* 類聚方 *(Classified Collection of Prescriptions)"* (1). Until then, Kampo formulas had been perceived to be used for particular classified diseases. Yoshimasu disregarded the classified diseases and instead regarded formulas as being appropriately utilized depending on the pathological condition (the form of poison), insisting on his "Manbyo Ichidoku theory." A concrete example of this methodology developed by Yoshimasu can be seen in saikokeishito, which is used without reserve in Kampo practice for a wide variety of diseases, such as frequent headache, chronic hepatitis, chronic pancreatitis, spinal canal stenosis, irritable bowel syndrome, and subacute-phase common cold. For its use, it is essential that the presence of the pathological condition fit the saikokeishito, or saikokeishito pattern. This is confirmed in parallel with the signs of proneness to have a tendency of qi counter flow, the tendency of spontaneous sweating, fullness, and discomfort in the chest and hypochondrium (*Kyokyokuman*), tension of the abdominal points (中脘CV-12), tension of the rectus abdominis, and feeling nervousness or irritability.

1.2.2 Yoshimasu's Medical Theory and the Subsequent Development

The development of Kampo medicine is based on Yoshimasu's medical theories. Merely following his theories as a golden rule, however, might force beginners in Kampo medicine to navigate without a compass. Thus, subsequent generations of practitioners have adopted, when necessary, some or all of the yin and yang, qi, blood[TM1], fluid[TM1], and five zang organs theory repudiated by Yoshimasu. In this regard, the most influential were the medical theories Manase Dosan (1507–93) wrote about, which were the medical mainstream back then. As described in the preceding chapter, Manase added his unique interpretation of Chinese Jin-Yuan medicine. His medical textbook titled *"Keitekishu* 啓迪集 *(Collection of Manase's Medical Ideology and Experience (Keiteki Collection))"* (the preface was written in 1574) contains the idealism-based, intricate, and detailed theory of Chinese medicine in an extremely simplified form and points the direction to seek the form of illness fit for a certain formula. In brief, it reminds one of a prototype of a formula corresponding to pattern identification. This tendency is particularly notable in "*Chufumon* (the wind-impact field)" and "*Shokanmon* (the cold damage diseases field)." What is noteworthy here is that Manase Dosan and derivative schools used yin and yang and the five elements theory as a compass for formula selection adjunctively, whether they were obviously conscious of it or not. Specific examples can be seen in "*Igakutenshoki* 医学天正記 *(Clinical Records of Tensho Period*, published in 1627)," the clinical notes of Manase Gensaku (1549–1631), the adoptive heir of Manase Dosan. He did not use a logic-based framework of element reductionism for reaching a particular formula but instead described a direct approach to the appropriate formula. The school based on Yoshimasu's methodology was called the Koho School, whereas the school started by Manase was called the Gosei School. In the mid-eighteenth century when Yoshimasu was active, these two schools were dramatically opposed to each other. From the viewpoint of medical practice and education of the younger generation, however, they came to realize that integrated use of the methodologies of both schools would be fruitful. Thus, a new school that applied eclectic medical methods was established chiefly by physicians of the Edo Igakukan (medical school of the Shogunate government). This was called the Setchu School. Asada Sohaku (1815–1894), a leader of the Setchu School, wrote "*Futsugoyakushitsuhokankuketsu* 勿誤薬室方函口訣 *(Oral Transmission of Futsugo Pharmacy)*, a collection of more than 600 prescriptions from long medical experience." In this text, formulas are listed in the order of the Japanese alphabet. This text may have succeeded in Yoshimasu's policy of "independence of formulas," that he proposed by setting formulas free from their restriction to disease names. The characteristics of Kampo medicine arose from the above-mentioned history with the schools of Kampo medicine—the Gosei, Koho, and Setchu—which were born and developed in Japan. By the Taisho and early Showa periods (early twentieth century), there were four Kampo schools:

1. A school promoted by Wada Keijuro (1872–1916), Yumoto Kyushin (1876–1941), and Otsuka Keisetsu

(1900–80), moving toward the rediscovery of Koho → Kokan medical school (included in the Koho School)

2. A lineage traced by Okuda Kenzo (1884–1961), Wada Masatsugu, Fujihira Ken (1914–1997), Ogura Shigenari, and others → Koho School
3. A lineage from Mori Dohaku and Yakazu Kaku to Yakazu Domei (1905–2002) → Gosei School
4. A lineage from Niizuma Sogoro and Hosono Shiro (1899–1988) to Sakaguchi Hiroshi (1921–2003) → Setchu School

The decisive feature of the Edo period, however, is cooperative systems of exchange among schools due to the "union for a common purpose" begun in the 1930s. The period between 1931 and 1941 is considered to have been the early development stage for the current "Kampo medicine." After the war (1945), the "Union for a common purpose" transformed into the Japan Society for Oriental Medicine (established in 1950) and the Association of East-Asian Medicine (restarted in 1954). Since "Kampo medicine" developed in this way in the modern era, its current distinctive features are as follows: (1) The basic principle is a formula corresponding to pattern identification. (Treatment by pattern identification). (2) Every school values abdominal examination. (3) Pulse examination varies among schools: six position pulse diagnosis is likely to be used in both the Setchu and Gosei Schools, but not in the Koho School. (4) Unlike TCM, which uses dialectic-assisted treatment comprising pattern determination by element reduction-based reasoning, Kampo medicine favors a direct grasp of tacit knowledge based on findings from a structuralist view using yin and yang, qi, blood[TM1], fluid[TM1], and five zang organs theory. (5) Accordingly, current pattern names in Kampo medicine do not use disease names such as Blood[TM1] impediment and Liver[TM1] yang deficiency pattern. Instead of classification of diseases, it uses formula names which serve to cure patients' patterns such as the kakkonto pattern and saikokeishito pattern. (6) Yoshimasu's medical theory excludes idealism and seeks a clue among tangible signs and symptoms. The current Kampo medicine also makes continuous efforts to establish pattern diagnoses with the aid of diagnostic tools used in Western medicine (including diagnostic imaging and pathological diagnosis). (7) In actual clinical settings, appropriate and safe combinations of Kampo medicines and Western drugs are being administered according to the situation. (8) Objective evaluation of clinical efficacy and monitoring of adverse drug reactions are routinely conducted if necessary through blood tests and other laboratory tests.

Even though the above-mentioned common characteristics are shared, each Kampo school has different representative formulas for routine use. This is well understood by the Japanese Ministry of Health, Labor, and Welfare, whose acceptance and understanding are implied by the resources on the Kampo extract products listed in the National Health Insurance (NHI) drug tariff (Table 1.1).

In addition, formulations other than the classical formulas, or Zhong Jing's formulas (derived from *"Shokanron* 傷

Table 1.1 Classified sources of Kampo extract products listed in the NHI-covered drug

(a) Sources are "*Shokanron* 傷寒論 (*treatise on cold damage*)" and "*Kinkiyouryaku* 金匱要略 (*synopsis of the Golden Chamber*)" Routine formulas used in the Koho School are as follows: (69 formulas)
Inchinkoto (茵蔯蒿湯), inchingoreisan (茵蔯五苓散), unkeito (温経湯), eppikajutsuto (越婢加朮 湯), ogikenchuto (黄耆建中湯), ogonto (黄芩湯), orento (黄連湯), kakkonto (葛根湯), kanzoto (甘草湯), kambakutaisoto (甘麦大棗湯), kikyoto (桔梗湯), kyukikyogaito (芎帰膠艾湯), keishikaogito (桂枝加黄耆湯), keishikakakkonto (桂枝加葛根湯), keishikakobokukyoninto (桂枝加厚朴杏仁湯), keishito (桂枝湯), keishikashakuyakuto (桂枝加芍薬湯),keishikashakuyakudaioto (桂枝加芍薬大黄湯), keishikaryukotsuboreito (桂枝加竜骨牡蛎湯), keishishakuyakuchimoto (桂枝芍薬知母湯), keishininjinto (桂枝人参湯),keishibukuryogan (桂枝茯苓丸), keimakakuhanto (桂麻各半湯), goshuyuto (呉茱萸湯), goreisan (五苓散), saikokaryukotsuboreito (柴胡加竜骨牡蛎湯), saikokeishito (柴胡桂枝湯), saikokeishikankyoto (柴胡桂枝乾姜湯), san'oshashinto (三黄瀉心 湯), sansoninto (酸棗仁湯), sammotsuogonto (三物黄芩湯), shigyakusan (四逆散), shishihakuhito (梔子柏皮湯), shakanzoto (炙甘草湯), shakuyakukanzoto (芍薬甘草湯), shokenchuto (小建中湯), shosaikoto (小柴胡湯), shoseiryuto (小青竜湯), shohangekabukuryoto (小半夏加茯苓湯), shimbuto (真武湯), daiokanzoto (大黄甘草湯), daiobotampito (大黄牡丹皮湯), daikenchuto (大建中湯), daisaikoto (大柴胡湯), daijokito (大承気湯), choijokito (調胃承気湯), choreito (猪苓湯), tokakujokito (桃核承気湯), tokikenchuto (当帰建中湯), tokishigyakukagoshuyushokyoto (当帰四逆 加呉茱萸生姜湯), tokishakuyakusan (当帰芍薬散), ninjinto (人参湯), hainosankyuto (排膿散及湯), bakumondoto (麦門冬湯), hachimijiogan (八味地黄丸), hangekobokuto (半夏厚朴湯), hangeshashinto (半夏瀉心湯), byakkokaninjinto (白虎加人参湯), bukuryoin (茯苓飲), boiogito (防已黄耆湯), maoto (麻黄湯), maobushisaishinto (麻黄附子細辛湯), makyokansekito (麻杏甘石湯), makyoyokukanto (麻杏薏甘湯), mashiningan (麻子仁丸), mokuboito (木防已湯), ryokankyomishingeninto (苓甘姜味辛夏仁湯), ryokyojutsukanto (苓姜朮甘湯), and ryokeijutsukanto (苓桂朮甘湯)
(b) Sources are *"Gedaihiyoho* 外台秘要方(*Arcane Essentials from the Imperial Library*)*"* and *"Senkinho* 千金方 (*prescriptions worth a thousand gold*)*"* (*sixth to eighth century*) Routine formulas being used in Kampo schools are (four formulas):
Orengedokuto (黄連解毒湯), shimpito (神秘湯), choyoto (腸癰湯), and tokito (当帰湯)

(continued)

Table 1.1 (continued)

(c) Sources are “*Wazaikyokuho* 和剤局方(*prescriptions of Bureau of Welfare Pharmacy (abbreviated)*),” “*Mambyokaishun* 万病回春 (*restoring health from myriad of diseases*), “*Saiseiho* 済生方(*Yan's prescriptions for saving lives*), “*Joka*(*Nyoka*)*satsuyo* 女科撮要(*outline of gynecology*),” and others Routine formulas being used in Gosei and Sechu schools are (48 formulas):
Anchusan (安中散), ireito (胃苓湯), unseiin (温清飲), kamikihito (加味帰脾湯), kamishoyosan (加味逍遥散), kihito (帰脾湯), kyukichoketsuin (芎帰調血飲),keihito (啓脾湯), kososan (香蘇散), gokoto (五虎湯), goshakusan (五積散), goshajinkigan (牛車腎気丸), gorinsan (五淋散), jiinkokato (滋陰降火湯),jiinshihoto (滋陰至宝湯), shikunshito (四君子湯), shimotsuto (四物湯), juzentaihoto (十全大補湯), junchoto (潤腸湯), shofusan (消風散), shomakakkonto (升麻葛根湯), shin'iseihaito (辛夷清肺湯), jinsoin (参蘇飲), seijobofuto (清上防風湯), seishoekkito (清暑益気湯), seishinrenshiin (清心蓮子飲), seihaito (清肺湯), senkyuchachosan (川芎茶調散), sokeikakketsuto (疎経活血湯), daibofuto (大防風湯), chikujountanto (竹茹温胆湯), chotosan (釣藤散), tsudosan (通導散), tokiinshi (当帰飲子), nijutsuto (二朮湯), nichinto (二陳湯), nyoshinsan (女神散), ninjin'yoeito (人参養栄湯), hangebyakujutsutemmato (半夏白朮天麻湯), bushirichuto (附子理中湯), heiisan (平胃散), bofutsushosan (防風通聖散), hochuekkito (補中益気湯), yokuininto (薏苡仁湯), yokukansan (抑肝散), rikkunshito (六君子湯), ryutanshakanto (竜胆瀉肝湯), and rokumigan (六味丸)
(d) Emperical formulas in Japan. These formulas have been created in Japan and are commonly used in Kampo schools (21 formulas):
Otsujito (乙字湯), kakkonkajutsubuto (葛根加朮附湯), kakkontokasenkyushin'i (葛根湯加川芎辛夷), kumibinroto (九味檳榔湯), keigairengyoto (荊芥連翹湯), keishikajutsubuto (桂枝加朮附湯), keishikaryojutsubuto (桂枝加苓朮附湯), keishibukuryogankayokuinin (桂枝茯苓丸加薏苡仁), saikanto (柴陥湯), saikoseikanto (柴胡清肝湯), saibokuto (柴朴湯), saireito (柴苓湯), shichimotsukokato (七物降下湯), jumihaidokuto (十味敗毒湯), shosaikotokakikyosekko (小柴胡湯加桔梗石膏), jizusoippo (治頭瘡一方), jidabokuippo (治打撲一方), choreitogoshimotsuto (猪苓湯合四物湯), bukuryoingohangekobokuto (茯苓飲合半夏厚朴湯), yokukansankachimpihange (抑肝散加陳皮半夏), and rikkosan (立効散)

Table 1.2 Handling of the formulas other than Zhong Jing's (derived from “*Shokanron* 傷寒論 *(Treatise on Cold Damage)*” or “*Kinkiyouryaku* 金匱要略 *(Synopsis of the Golden Chamber)*”) Typical examples are:

Group 1: The formulas recognized as analogs to Zhong Jing's, based on formula versus pattern
Orengedokuto (黄連解毒湯) → regarded as an analog of san'oshashinto (三黄瀉心湯) Shimpito (神秘湯) → regarded as fit to a dual pattern of makyokansekito (麻杏甘石湯) pattern plus fullness and discomfort in chest and hypochondrium pattern Tokikenchuto (当帰建中湯) → regarded as an analog of shokenchuto (小建中湯) Goshajinkigan (牛車腎気丸) & rokumigan (六味丸) → regarded as an analog of hachimigan (八味丸) Gokoto (五虎湯) → regarded as an analog of makyokansekito (麻杏甘石湯) Kamishoyosan (加味逍遥散) → use based on abdominal pattern such as Kyokyo Kuman (fullness and discomfort in chest and hypochondrium)
Group 2: Application of five zang organs theory
Yokukansan (抑肝散) kihito (帰脾湯) and kamikihito (加味帰脾湯), hangebyakujutsutemmato (半夏白朮天麻湯)
Group 3: Application of qi, blood[TM1], fluid[TM1] theory
Rikkunshito (六君子湯), shikunshito (四君子湯), juzentaihoto (十全大補湯), ninjin'yoeito (人参養栄 湯), shimotsuto (四物湯), and goshakusan (五積散)

寒論 (*Treatise on Cold Damage*)” or “*Kinkiyouryaku* 金匱要略 (*Synopsis of the Golden Chamber*)”) listed in Table 1.1 are recognized as analogs of the classical formulas and frequently used for pattern-based treatment. Five zang and qi, blood[TM1], and fluid[TM1] theory are also adopted if needed (Table 1.2).

1.2.3 Summary

The characteristics of Kampo medicine have been discussed above. The fundamental difference between the current Western medicine and Kampo medicine paradigms may be an underlying thought: the former is based on element reductionism, while the latter is based on structuralism. From a structuralist perspective, disease-fighting reactions and responses expressed at random in a living body can be grasped as a whole as orderly patterns in mutual relationships. A similar relationship is found between Chinese medicine and Kampo medicine. Namely, the five-element theory represents reduction into five elements. The yin and yang theory represents reduction into dualism. The qi, blood[TM1], fluid[TM1] principle represents reduction into a triumvirate. Just as the biochemical reductionism of modern science cannot fully explain the totality of human beings, whose minds and bodies are as one (*Shinshin Ichinyo*), and exist in a dynamic symbiosis, element reductionism in TCM fails to accurately express conditions of illness as it is. Pattern diagnosis based on structuralism is “tacit knowledge,” and essentially all tacit knowledge cannot be transformed into “explicit knowledge.” As Yoshimasu insisted, tacit knowledge should be acquired on one's own. Nevertheless, “acquiring a tacit knowledge of patterns on your own” should not take the place of education. Accordingly, yin and yang, deficiency excess, qi, blood[TM1], fluid[TM1], and the five zang organs theory are used as an expedient—a compass indicating the rough direction. In addition, the mission assigned to doctors who take the lead in Kampo medicine is to carefully and precisely describe aspects of tacit knowledge in the raw and explicit knowledge, as far as possible. Describing is one of the ways of understanding tacit knowledge. Describing is a kind of work to transform tacit knowledge into explicit knowledge.

2 History of Kampo Medicine

2.1 Diversity in Japanese Kampo Medicine and Japonization from a Perspective of Medical History

Hiroshi Kosoto

2.1.1 What is "Kampo Medicine"?

Kampo medicine has a long history. Traditional medicine originating in ancient China spread from the Korean Peninsula to Japan and other East-Asian countries, resulting in peculiar developments.

"Kam" of "Kampo" means "China." Primarily the Kanji or Chinese character "*Kam*/*Kan* (漢)" (Han in Chinese) is the name of a dynasty or era (the Western Han Dynasty [202 BC–9 AD] and the Eastern Han Dynasty [25 AD–220 AD]). Since ancient times, Japanese people have used "*Kam*" as a pronoun of China and also used "*To* (唐)" (Tang in Chinese) as another pronoun of China. Furthermore, to express things in Chinese, we used to employ the Kanji "|*Kam*/*Kan*" or "*To*," whereas Chinese people employed the Kanji "*Wa* (和,倭)" or "*Koku* (国)" to express things in Japanese. Examples are "*Kanji* (漢字)" versus "*Kokuji* (国字)," "*Kanbun* (漢文)" versus "|*Kokubun* (国文)" or "*Wabun* (和文)," "*Kango* (漢語)" versus "*Kokugo* (国語)" or "*Wago* (和語)," and "*Kanseki* (漢籍)" versus "*Kokusho* (国書)." Kampo is not exceptional and is used versus "*Waho* (和方)" and "*Rampo* (蘭方)."

What is "*Ho*/*Po* (方)"? "*Ho*/*Po*" means a means, measure(s), method(s), or skill(s) and may refer to "*Hogi* (方技)," "*Hojutsu* (方術)" and "*Iho* (医方)."

Many occupations require special skills. Among them, medicine has been thought to need the highest skills and techniques, because it treats human life. Accordingly, "*Hogi*" and "*Hojutsu*" have been used as words to specifically refer to medical techniques since the Former Han Dynasty. In "*Kanjogeimonshi* 漢書芸文志," "*Hogi*" is used as a generic name for medical books, divided into four categories: *Ikei*, *Keiho*, *Bochu*, and *Shinsen* (医経・経方・房中・神仙). In "*Kanjoheiteiki* 漢書平帝紀," the words "*Shihen*, *Hojutsu*, and *Honzo* (史篇・方術・本草)" appear. "*Gokanjo* 後漢書 (*History of the Later Han Dynasty*)" contains the history of medical techniques and physicians, "*Hojutsuden* (方術伝)." "*Hojutsu*" or "*Hogi*" includes acupuncture and moxibustion. The most famous medical text, however, is "*Koteidaikei* 黄帝内経 (*Yellow Emperor's Inner Classic*)."

The word "*Iho*" often appears and includes acupuncture and moxibustion in books following the historical book "*Shiki* 史記 (*Records of the Grand Historian*)," which particularly refers to secret medical techniques as "*Kimpo* (禁方)" (*Kobuki-Hensoden* [孝武紀・扁倉伝]).

Thus, "*Kampo* (漢方)" means Han medical techniques expressed as "*Kampogi* (漢方技)," "*Kampojutsu* (漢方術)," or "*Kan'iho* (漢医方)," and is a synonym for "Chinese medical techniques," as is understood. More accurately, Kampo is the term referred to by the Japanese for the medical techniques introduced in China. As far as I know, the term "*Kampo*" was first used in a book authored by Sohaku Asada around the end of the Edo period or the early Meiji period. He seems to have employed "*Kampo*" as *Koho*, namely *Chochukei-ho*, which means medical care principles conducted by *Zhang Zhongjing* (張仲景, *Chochukei* in Japanese). Some people believe Kampo is limited to pharmacotherapy because "*Ho*" reminds them of "*Hozai*" or "*Hoyaku* (both formulation[s])." In fact, however, it should be emphasized that "*Ho*" primarily means "medicine."

In China, it was not necessary that they call their own medicine "*Kampo*." Rather, since the introduction of Western medicine, their own medicine has been called "*Kokui* (国医)" and after the establishment of the People's Republic of China, "*Chuigaku* (中医学)," the abbreviation of "*Chugoku Igaku* (中国医学)" has been and is adopted. Given these circumstances, Japanized traditional Chinese medicine can be called "Kampo medicine."

Some people maintain that Japanese Kampo medicine was established in the early stage of the Showa period (1926–1989) and should be limited to the Koho School advocating "formula pattern-based treatment (方証相対*hoshosotai*)" adhered to "*Shokanron* 傷寒論 (*Treatise on Cold Damage*)." However, their thoughts do not cover the entire Japanese traditional Kampo medicine, so they cannot consider its diversity. Japanese Kampo medicine ascends to "*Ishimpo* 医心方(*Prescriptions from the Heart of Medicine*)" in the Heian period and had been cultivated via the Kamakura, Nambokucho, and Muromachi periods through the Edo period. Japanese Kampo medicine cannot be discussed by somebody who has never surveyed the books authored by the Japanese physicians listed in "*Kinseikampoigakushoshusei* 近世漢方医学書集成 (*A Complete Collection of Kampo Medicine Books in the Early Modern Period*)" (chiefly compiled by Keisetsu Otsuka and Domei Yakazu in 1979–84). The compilation itself is the message of the recent pioneers who established Showa Kampo medicine.

2.1.2 Traditional Medicine in China

Traditional medicine in China has about 3000 years of history, which is twice as long as that in Japan.

In China, its intrinsic medicine began to be formed under accumulated vast experience and knowledge in the Yin and Zhou Dynasties and through the Spring and Autumn and Warring States periods. The process of formation in the pre-Qin (先秦) period can be imaged from classics written in ancient Chinese (inscriptions on bone and tortoise shell) including "*Shurai* 周礼 (*The Rites of Zhou*)," "*Ryoshishunju*

呂氏春秋 (*Master Lü's Spring and Autumn Annals*)," "*Enanji* 淮南子 (*Book of Master Huai Nan*)," "*Shiki* 史記(*Records of the Grand Historian*)," and "*Kanjogeimonshi* 漢書芸文志" and from newly excavated medical history-related materials such as *Changsha Mawangdui* Han Tomb (長沙馬王堆漢墓).

In the Han Dynasty, Chinese medicine was systematized and consolidated. Three great medical classics descending from the Han period are "*Koteidaikei* 黄帝内経 (*Yellow Emperor's Inner Classic*)," "*Shinnohonzokyo* 神農本草経 (*Shennong's Classic of Materia Medica*)," and "*Shokanron* 傷寒論 (*Treatise on Cold Damage*)". These are still most highly appreciated as fundamental textbooks of Kampo medicine in Japan as well as in China. The source of Kampo medicine is in these classics. In other words, we cannot understand Kampo medicine without understanding these classics. Accordingly, a large number of books for annotation and research on "*Koteidaikei* 黄帝内経 (*Yellow Emperor's Inner Classic*)," "*Shokanron* 傷寒論 (*Treatise on Cold Damage*)," and *Honzo* (本草; Chinese materia medica; mainly *Honzokomoku* 本草綱目 (*Compendium of Materia Medica*) after the early modern period) have been published in Japan as well.

Koteidaikei 黄帝内経 *(Yellow Emperor's Inner Classic)*

This is also known as "*Ikei* (医経)," a medical book that describes general doctrines of medicine and physiotherapies (acupuncture and moxibustion). This corpus that collects medical literatures in the Spring and Autumn periods followed by the Warring States period consists of these texts: "*Somon* 素問 (*Basic Questions*)," "*Reisu* 霊枢 (*Spiritual Pivot*)," "*Taiso* 太素 (*Yellow Emperor's Inner Classic: Grand Basis*)" and "*Kouteidaikeimeido*黄帝内経明堂 (*Yellow Emperor's Inner Classic: Bright Hall*)." "*Somon* 素問 (*Basic Questions*)" and "*Reisu* 霊枢 (*Spiritual Pivot*)" focus on basic theories while " *Taiso* 太素 (*Yellow Emperor's Inner Classic: Grand Basis*)" and "*Kouteidaikeimeido*黄帝内経明堂 (*Yellow Emperor's Inner Classic: Bright Hall*)" deal with clinical medicine, although there is a consistent philosophical doctrine through the corpus: China-specific yin and yang five-element theory. There is no need to explain the yin and yang theory in detail. In the medical field, however, yin and yang are assigned to deficiency and excess; cold and heat; interior and exterior; chronic and acute; and solid and hollow viscera, respectively. Based on the assignment, physiology and pathology are explained. In the five-element theory, five major elements of the universe (wood[TM1], fire[TM1], earth[TM1], metal[TM1], and water[TM1]) are assigned to five zang organs(liver[TM1], heart[TM1], spleen[TM1], lung[TM1], and kidney[TM1]), five fu organs(gallbladder[TM1], small intestine[TM1], stomach[TM1], large intestine[TM1], and bladder[TM1]), five sense organs (eye, tongue, lip, nose, and ear), five tissues (muscle, blood vessel, skin [肌肉], hair [皮毛], and bone), and five emotions (anger, joy, thought, melancholy, and fear). Each set of five follows the principles of five elements in the way of productive/engendering (相生, *Sojo*) (wood[TM1]→fire[TM1]→earth[TM1]→metal[TM1]→water[TM1]→wood[TM1]) and conflicting/restraining (相克, *Sokoku*) relationships (wood[TM1]←fire[TM1]←earth[TM1]←metal[TM1]←water[TM1]←wood[TM1]) to keep physiological functions. A well-balanced status is regarded as healthy, whereas an imbalanced status due to a pathogen or disturbed qi (Ki) is a disease. Accordingly, diagnosis is to determine which region and how the region is imbalanced, and treatment is to restore the imbalance by means of a drug(s) and/or acupuncture/moxibustion technique(s). Based on these concepts, it is said that the merits of Kampo medicine comprise viewing the whole, not a local or regional site, and thereby aiming at the restoration of spontaneous healing capability rather than attacking and eliminating the pathogen and/or lesion.

Shinnohonzokyo 神農本草経 *(Shennong's Classic of Materia Medica)*

This is a book of pharmacology/pharmacognosy (薬物学), the source of so-called *BenCao*, that describes individual Kampo formulas and their effects as well as characteristics. *Shen Nong* (神農, God of Agriculture) is one of the three legendary emperors (along with *Huang Di* [黄帝] and *Fu Xi* [伏羲].) and has been called the father of Chinese medicine. The book contains a total of 365 entries of animal, plant, and mineral crude drugs divided into three classes: the first (上品, *johon*), second (中品, *chuhon*), and third (下品, *gehon*) classes. This is referred to as the three-class classification of *BenCao*. The first-class (also called上薬, *joyaku*) crude drugs are life-nourishing medicines (養命薬) that are non-toxic and should be taken for a long-term period. The second-class crude drugs are medicines nourishing physical strength (養性薬) that are toxic or non-toxic and therefore should be taken carefully. The third-class crude drugs are therapeutic medicines (治病薬) that are toxic and thus should not be taken for a long-term period. These are the basic rules for medication. The concept of drugs in Western medicine corresponds to the third class. The *BenCao* medicines are in a broader range of concepts than Western drugs. The fundamental principles for use are that health should be kept with intake of the first- or second-class medicines, whereas taking the third-class medicines is a last resort that is not so favorable. In addition, another characteristic feature of traditional Chinese *BenCao* is valuing their combination. For composition of a formula, component crude drugs are selected according to a certain rule of proportion, as each drug has a specific role (sovereign [君, first-class medicines exhibiting the main efficacy of the formula], subject [臣, second-class medicines assisting the sovereign drug], vassal [佐, third-class medicines assisting the subject drug(s) or suppressing adverse/side effects of the formula], or servant [使, third-class medicines suppressing or neutralizing adverse/side effects of the formula]). There are also combination principles in which the combination of two crude drugs (A and B) alters efficacy in a way that causes seven emotions (七情, *shichijo*): single use of A or B [単行, *tanko*], mutual support between A and B [相須, *sosu*], B assisting A [相使, *soshi*], mutual repulsion between A and B [相反, *sohan*], A repulsing B [相悪, *soaku*], mutual killing [相殺, *sosatsu*], and B neutralizing A (with remaining B efficacy) [相畏, *soi*]. *Sohan* and *Soaku* mean contraindications. Based on these concepts, it is considered that Chinese crude drugs in single use are merely materials and that actual treatment needs formulation comprising several crude drugs. Thus formulas have extensively developed in China. Crude drugs as materials were sometimes processed to modulate efficacy. The medicinal processing is referred to as Xiu Zhi (修治, *shuji*) or Pao Zhi (炮炙, *hosha*). Furthermore, dosage form varies from pill (丸, *gan*), powder (散, *san*), decoction (湯, *to*), alcoholic tincture (酒漬, *shuseki*), and oil decoction (膏煎, *kosen*), which were devised in formulation, depending on efficacy and usage. The drug efficacy or effects described in *BenCao* are still good references for ingredient-related and pharmacological studies in pharmacognosy. In ancient China, it's not an exaggeration that everything in nature is regarded as medicinal. Chinese pharmacology/pharmacognosy has thus gradually developed into natural history. In pharmacological books prepared in contemporary ancient Europe, plants are classified from a morphological viewpoint, contrasted with a perspective of efficacy for humans in China. A comparison in plant classification between Europe and China reveals an intrinsic difference in thinking patterns between the West and Orient: non-human-oriented or human-oriented.

Following the "*Shinnohonzokyo* 神農本草経(*Shennong's Classic of Materia Medica*)," "*Meiibetsuroku* 名医別録 (*Miscellaneous Records of Famous Physicians*)" newly listing 365 crude drugs, was published as an additional *Bencao* book at the end of the Han Dynasty. Thereafter, "*Honzokeishitchu* 本草経集注 (*Variorum of Shennong's Classic of Materia Medica*); 730 items)" revised by *Tao Hongjing* (陶弘景) around 500 CE in the Liang Dynasty, "*Shinshuhonzo* 新修本草 (*Newly Revised Pharmacopoeia*); 830 items)" in 659, "*Kaihohonzo* 開宝本草 (*Materia Medica of the Kaibao Reign;* 984 items)" in 974, "*kayuhonzo* 嘉祐本草 (*Materia Medica of the Jiayou Reign; 1084 items*)" in1061, "*Shoruihonzo* 証類本草 (*Classified Materia Medica*;1774 items)" in 1108, "*Honzohiniseiyo* 本草品彙精要 (*Collected Essentials of Materia Medica*; 1815 items)" in 1505 in the Ming period, and "*Honzokomoku* 本草綱目 (*Compendium of Materia Medica*; 1892 items)" in 1590 were compiled.

Shokanron 傷寒論 *(Treatise on Cold Damage)*

This is a book of therapeutic medicine using drug formulations, each well composed of multiple crude drugs, for various pathological conditions. The source was one book consisting of "*kinkiyoryaku* 金匱要略 (*Synopsis of the Golden Chamber*)" for various diseases and "*Shokanron* 傷寒論 (*Treatise on Cold Damage*)" for cold damage disease. The author is said to be *Zhang Zhongjing* (張仲景) who was a governor of Changsha (長沙) at the end of the Later Han Dynasty. *ShangHan* (傷寒) means cold-damaged acute febrile disease like typhoid fever. Its pathological conditions are divided into six stages of disease progression or transformation in "*Shokanron* 傷寒論 (*Treatise on Cold Damage*)." These six stages are three yin and three yang stages; for each stage, appropriate formulas are set up. For example, kakkonto is one of the appropriate formulations for the first stage and shosaikoto, for the third stage. Therefore, accurate differentiation of the stage of disease, or absence of diagnostic mistakes, will always lead to effective formulas. This mechanism by which diagnosis is directly linked to treatment is extensively interpreted by Japanese Kampo physicians, resulting in the creation of the concept of "pattern (証, *sho*). "*Sho*" is thought to be applicable to every type of disease. This concept was the goal of Koho School, the mainstream of Japanese Kampo medicine in the late Edo period. In other words, the conception that Kampo medicine does not employ the treatment based on the name of a disease but uses so-called *hoshosotai* or *sho*-based treatment (随証治療) is derived from here.

Medieval to Modern Times

Many medical books that had been authored before the Tang Dynasty were principally all in the line of the previously mentioned three medical classics. Representative medical books in the Tang Dynasty included "*Senkinho* 千金方 (*Prescriptions Worth a Thousand Gold*)" by *Sun Simiao* (孫思邈) in 650–660 and "*Gedaihiyoho* 外台秘要方 (*Arcane Essentials from the Imperial Library*)" by *Wang Tao* in 752.

In the Song Dynasty, a considerable amount of medical books and formularies were published, including "*Taiheiseikeiho* 太平聖恵方 (*Taiping Benevolence Prescriptions*)" by *Wang Huaiyin* et al. in 992, "*Seisaisoroku* 聖済総録 (*General Record of Sagely Benefaction*)" compiled by imperial command, and "*Wazaikyokuho* 和剤局方 (*Prescriptions of Bureau of Welfare Pharmacy (abbreviated)*)." Particularly, "*Taiheikeiminwazaikyokuho* 太平恵民和剤局方 (*Prescriptions of Bureau of Taiping People's Welfare Pharmacy*)" authored by *Chen Shiwen* (陳師文) et al. in 1170–210 contains the Kampo formulas being well used even today.

In the Jin and Yuan Dynasties, innovative medical theories were developed and extended by four famous doctors from four different schools of medicine: *Liu Wansu* (劉完素, ca 1120–1200), *Zhang Congzheng* (張従正, 1156–1228), *Li Dongyuan* (李東垣, 1180–1251), and *Zhu Zhengheng* (朱震亨, 1281–1358). *Liu* created bofutsuseisan; *Li*, hochuekkito; and *Zhu*, jiinkokato. The Jin-Yuan medical theories were passed down from generation to generation, forming the theoretical platform of today's Chinese medicine.

Complying with the trend of Jin-Yuan medicine, many medical books were also published in the Ming and Qing Dynasties. The representative materia medica of the Ming Dynasty is "*Honzokomoku* 本草綱目 (*Compendium of Materia Medica*)," authored by *Li Si Chen* (李時珍) in 1578, and the representative formulary is "*Mambyokaishun* 万病回春 (*Restoring Health from Myriad of Diseases*)" which was authored by *Gong Ting-xian* (龔廷賢) in 1587 and which has greatly influenced Japanese medicine. In the Qing Dynasty, a new medical theory of febrile disease theory (温病学) was developed and has supported the theoretical platform of today's Chinese medicine.

After the People's Republic of China was established via the Republic of China, previous theories in traditional medicine were integrated and organized under governmental direction, resulting in today's theoretical system of traditional Chinese medicine.

2.1.3 Development of Japanese Kampo Medicine

Prior to the Nara Period

Continental medical culture was introduced into Japan in the same way as other continental cultures, mainly via the Korean Peninsula until around the sixth century. The first record of introduced medical books dates back to 562 CE (slightly after the introduction of Buddhism), when a Chinese physician monk named *Zhi Cong* (智聡, *Chiso*) brought "*Yakusho* (薬書)," *Meidozu* (明堂図)," and others to Japan via Korea. *Meidozu* may be a diagram of acupuncture points in the body.

Since the seventh century, copious amounts of medical culture had become directly imported from China with the start of the formal exchange with China that was mediated by Japanese envoys to the Tang and Sui Dynasties. The physician Enichi (恵日) and the student Fukuin (福因) played a major role in such exchanges. Eventually, the *Ritsuryo* system was introduced, and the *Taiho Ritsuryo* (Taiho code) was enforced in 701 for administrative reorganization. A medical law known as the Ishitsuryo (医疾令) stipulates the medical system. By the Ishitsuryo, the Chinese medical textbooks from the Han to the Six Dynasties period, including "*Myakukyo* 脈経 (*The Pulse Classic*)" written by *Wang Shuhe* (王叔和) in the late third century, "*Kootsukyo* 甲乙経 (*Systematic Classic of Acupuncture and Moxibustion*)" by *Huangfu Mi* (皇甫謐) in the late third century, "*Honzokeishitchu* 本草経集注 (*Variorum of Shennong's Classic of Materia Medica*)," "*Shohinho* 小品方 (*Prescriptions from Small Articles*)" by *Chen Yanzhi* (陳延之) in the late fifth century, "*Shukenho* 集験方 (*Collection of Proven Prescriptions*)," "*Somon* 素問 (*Basic Questions*)," and "*Shingyo* 針経 ((*Yellow Emperor's*) *Classic of Acupuncture*)" were prescribed as textbooks. This Japanese stipulation exactly follows that in the early Tang system, as the then-Chinese system is imitated. The needling canon "*Shingyo* 針経 ((*Yellow Emperor's*) *Classic of Acupuncture*)" is the old name of "*Reisu* 霊枢 (*Spiritual Pivot*)," and the canon combined with "*Somon* 素問 (*Basic Questions*)" composes "*Koteidaikei* 黄帝内経 (*Yellow Emperor's Inner Classic*)." "*Somon* 素問 (*Basic Questions*)" plus "*Reisu* 霊枢 (*Spiritual Pivot*)" plus "*Meido* 明堂 (*Bright Hall*)" were integrated and recompiled into "*Kootsukyo* 甲乙経 (*Systematic Classic of Acupuncture and Moxibustion*)," a clinical acupuncture text. "*Koteidaikei* 黄帝内経 (*Yellow Emperor's Inner Classic*)" plus "*Shokanron* 傷寒論 (*Treatise on Cold Damage*)" plus other classics were integrated and recompiled into "*Myakukyo* 脈経 (*The Pulse Classic*)," the canon of the pulse.

"*Honzokeishitchu* 本草経集注 (*Variorum of Shennong's Classic of Materia Medica*)" is a revision of the "*Shinnohonzokyo* 神農本草経 (*Shennong's Classic of Materia Medica*)." "*Shohinho* 小品方 (*Prescriptions from Small Articles*)" *and* "*Shukenho* 集験方 (*Collection of Proven Prescriptions*)" are formulary-focusing medical books based on the "*Shokanron* 傷寒論 (*Treatise on Cold Damage*)." Any of these books are in the line of the three great classics.

Heian Period

In the Heian period, Japan-specific medical books were compiled with elevated cultural

consciousness, including "*Daidoruijuho* 大同類聚方 (*Classified Assembly of Prescriptions of the Daido Period*)" and "*Kinranho* 金蘭方 (*Prescriptions of Gold and Eupatorium*)," which are said to have been selected by Hirosada Izumo in 808 and his son Minetsugu Fujiwara before 870, respectively, under the then emperor's command. But the two existent books are considered forged documents.

Sending official envoys to the Tang Dynasty was finally canceled after 838. By that year, most of the main medical books had been imported into Japan. The inventory "*Nihonkoku Kenzaisho Mokuroku* 日本国見在書目録 (*Inventory of Chinese Medical Texts in Japan*)" (Fujiwara Sukeyo; around 898) contains 166 Han-made discrete medical books with a total of 1309 volumes, implying a great appetite of Japanese people for Chinese medical culture.

In 984, making the best use of these introduced medical books, Yasunori Tanba, of the eighth generation offspring of naturalized Chinese, compiled *"Ishimpo* 医心方 (*Prescriptions from the Heart of Medicine*)*,"* the earliest extant Japanese medical corpus, consisting of 30 volumes. Almost all of the content consists of citations from 200 different Chinese books. In this meaning, the Japanese medical corpus is really a Chinese medical corpus; nevertheless, there are reflections of the climate and tastes from processes of selection of food and drug, and elimination of the Five Elements Theory and the Pulse Theory. Whereas in China the classical texts are only preserved in Song Dynasty printed books, the existent medical book is an old copy prepared soon after the creation and provides precious materials for the research of medical books originating in the six dynasties to the Sui and Tang Dynasties.

Kamakura and Nanbokucho Periods

In the early Kamakura period, medical books published in the Song Dynasties were remarkably introduced from China, because an innovative development in printing technology was made in the Song period so that a large amount of printed, not hand-copied, medical classics became widely spread. This trend was epoch-making in terms of the popularization of medical knowledge. In addition, as aforementioned, the huge medical corpuses "*Taiheiseikeiho* 太平聖恵方 (*Taiping Benevolence Prescriptions*)" and "*Seisaisoroku* 聖済総録 (*General Record of Sagely Benefaction*)" as well as the government-designated formulary "*Taiheikeiminwazaikyokuho* 太平恵民和剤局方 (*Prescriptions of Bureau of Taiping People's Welfare Pharmacy*)" were compiled and published. In the early Southern Song period as well, medical books were issued one after another. These printed books streamed in through Japan-Song trade, a part of which is evident in the descending old-edition medical books at the Kanazawa-Bunko Museum in Kanagawa Prefecture.

In the time of samurai, new medicine-responsible persons shifted from doctors working at the imperial court to monk physicians working at Zen temples, while the main target of medical care also shifted from nobles to common people. Representative medical corpuses include "*Ton'isho* 頓医抄 (*Excerpts for Novice Doctors*); completed in 1303)" and "*Man'ampo* 万安方 (*Prescriptions for Complete Safety*); completed in 1315)" authored by a monk-physician of Seizen Kajiwara and "*Fukudenho* 福田方 (*Prescriptions for Good Fortune*)" by Yurin around 1363. Unlike the previous Japanese medical books that were just exact excerpts from Chinese medical classics, "*Ton'isho* 頓医抄 (*Excerpts for Novice Doctors*)" and "*Fukudenho* 福田方 (*Prescriptions for Good Fortune*)" were both translated from *Kanbun* to *Wabun* for easy understanding via extensive utilization of newly introduced medical books and were sprinkled with authors' unique viewpoints.

Muromachi Period

Between Japan and China's Ming Dynasty, the Kango trade (using a tally or trading license) started in the Muromachi period. Physicians who had studied for several years in Ming came home and became the leaders of the medical circle, including Shokei Takeda (at the end of the Nanbokucho period), Gekko, Sanki Tashiro, Joun Saka, Akichika Nakarai, and Ian Yoshida.

The then up-to-date Ming's medicine was based on the innovative medical theory newly created in the Jin and Yuan Dynasties. In brief, Jin-Yuan medicine officially aimed at integrating the aforementioned theories of the three great medical classics but actually resulted in opening a new window on Chinese medicine. The successors of the four aforementioned famous physicians (*Liu Wansu*, *Zhang Congzheng*, *Li Dongyuan*, and *Zhu Zhengheng*) in the Jin and Yuan periods took the initiative in respective schools characterized by therapeutic policy. Especially Li and Zhu medicine (focusing on complementing nutrition [補養]) became popular in the name of Li-Zhu medicine also in Japan.

Physicians in the educated class of the Muromachi period earnestly sought to learn and spread the new Li-Zhu medicine. In 1528, at the peak of the trend, a printed medical book was first published in Japan. The book is *"Ishotaizen* 医書大全 (*Complete Collection of Medical Books*)*"* that was compiled by Soritsu Yu in Ming and published there in 1446, then reprinted and translated by Sozui Asaino (in Sakai, Japan) at his own expense. In Japan, medical books were printed and published 500 years behind China. Furthermore, 70 years later, the technique of printing with movable types was introduced in Korea, owing to troops dispatched to Korea by Hideyoshi Toyotomi. By using that technique, a great number of medical and pharmaceutical books (published mainly in the Jin, Yuan, and Ming periods) were printed and widely distributed in Japan. These are so-called old-type printed versions. Japanese medical book-publishing culture started here.

Azuchi-Momoyama Period

One of the skilled physicians from the end of the Muromachi period to the Azuchi-momoyama period is Dosan Manase (1507–94). He is a remarkable doctor and contributor who established the then-Chinese medicine in Japan. Dosan Manase learned medicine from Sanki Tashiro and founded a medical school named Keitekiin in Kyoto. In parallel, he consolidated and grouped medical books issued in the Song, Jin-Yuan, and Ming Dynasties, then wrote many medical books, such as *"Keitekishu* 啓迪集 (*Collection of Manase's Medical Ideology and Experience* (*Keiteki Collection*))*,"* to enlighten and educate medical students. His medical theory was based on Jin-Yuan medicine, especially the doctrine by *Zhu Zhengheng*, through Ming's medical books. Manase's medicine grounded on the yin and yang five elements theory and using experiential formulas flexibly was handed down to succeeding physicians, including Gensaku Manase. These followers actively adopted medical books (such as *Mambyokaishun* 万病回春 (*Restoring Health from Myriad of Diseases*)) published in the later Ming period and flourished until the middle to end of the Edo period, via a peak in the early Edo period. This school is called Gosei School versus Koho School that emerged later.

Gosei (Shimpo) School

There are a variety of Goseiho schools, depending on the adopted Chinese medical book. Among them, the most influential was Li-Zhu medicine, or two physicians: *Li Dongyuan* and *Zhu Zhengheng*.

Katsuki Gyuzan (1656–1740) was a Confucian physician who authored *"Gyuzanhoko* 牛山方考 *(Gyuzan's Investigation of Prescriptions),"* *"Gyuzankatto* 牛山活套 *(Gyuzan's Guide to Conventional Remedies),"* *"Rojinhitsuyoyashinaigusa* 老人必用養草 *(Essentials of Healthcare for the Elderly),"* and others and is a typical member of the Gosei School in the middle of the Edo period. However, Gyuzan did not blindly believe Chinese medical books; he developed a theory of his own after digesting knowledge.

After Dosan Manase, Japanese Kampo medicine appears to have focused on the use of drug prescriptions that is regarded as the fundamental basis of medicine. In other words, it is said that Japan valued practice, whereas China respected theory (the view of Shutei Nakagawa in *"Ihoshinkoben* 医方新古弁 *(Old and New Schools of Medicine)"*). *"Shuhokiku* 衆方規矩 *(Principles for a Multitude of Prescriptions*) by Dosan Manase in 1636, *"Ihokuketsushu* 医方口訣集 *(Collection of Oral Transmissions of Medical Prescriptions)"* written by Doju Nagasawa, supplemented by Sanryu Nakayama, and annotated by Yushoshi Kitayama in 1681, and "*Kokonhoi* 古今方彙 *(Collection of Ancient and Contemporary Prescriptions*)" by Tsugen Koga in 1747 are included in extended Dosan medicine. Until the middle of the Edo period, Chinese medical books were well read, including *"Igakuseiden* 医学正伝 *(Orthodox Transmission of Medicine)"* by *Gutan* (虞摶) in 1515, *"Igakunyumon* 医学入門 *(Introduction to Medicine)"* by *Li Chan* (李梴) in1575, "*Mambyokaishun* 万病回春 *(Restoring Health from Myriad of Diseases*)" by *Gong Ting-xian* in 1587, and *"Juseihogen* 寿世保元 *(Longevity and Life Preservation)"* by *Gong Ting-xian* in 1615. Furthermore, among *"Shodenwakumon* 正伝或問 *(Enquiry into Orthodox Transmission of Medicine)"* that is only a part of the *"Igakuseiden* 医学正伝 *(Orthodox Transmission of Medicine)"* published as one book, *"Ihotaiseiron* 医方大成論 *(Complete Compendium of Medical Reasoning)"* that is the extracted medical theory of the *"Ishotaizen* 医書大全 *(Complete Collection of Medical Books),"* *"Jushikeihakki*十四経発揮 *(Elucidation of Fourteen Meridians)"* written by *Katsu Ju* (滑寿) in 1341, "*NankeiHongi* 難経本義 *(Original Meaning of Classic of Difficult Issues*)" also by *Katsu Ju* in 1361, *"Unkirono* 運気論奥 *(Discussion of Mysteries of Theory of Five Circuits and Six Qi)"* by *Ryu Onjo* (劉温舒) in 1099, *"Ikeisokaishu* 医経溯洄集 *(Revisiting the Medical Classics)"* by *Ori* (王履) in the end of the Yuan Dynasty or the beginning of the Ming Dynasty, *"Kyokuhohakki* 局方発揮 *(Elucidation of Dispensary Formulas)"* by *Shu Shinko* (or *Zhu Zhengheng* in Chinese) in 1347, *"Kakuchiyoron* 格致余論 *(Treatise of Inquiry on the Properties of Things)"* also by *Shu Shinko* in 1347, "*Honzojorei* 本草序例 *(Introduction to Classic of Materia Medica*) that is only a part of the *"Shoruihonzo* 証類本草 *(Classified Materia Medica)"* and was published as one book, and "*Somongenkigembyoshiki* 素問玄機原病式 *(Investigation of Pathogenesis and Profound Mechanisms of Diseases in Basic Questions*)" by *Liu Wansu* around 1154, seven physicians' books were selected and well sold as "Seven physicians' book series." Eminent Kampo physicians included Gensaku Manase (1549–1631) who authored *"Igakutenshoki* 医学天正記 *(Clinical Records of Tensho Period),"* *"Ihomeikan* 医法明鑑 *(A Clear Mirror of Medical Principles),"* *"Enjusatsuyo* 延寿撮要 *(Essential Guide for Health Care and Longevity),"* etc., Genya Okamoto (1587–1645) who wrote *"Kadenyoyakushu* 家伝預薬集 *(Collection of Traditional Prepared Formulas),"* *"Gen'yahoko* 玄冶方考 *(Gen'ya's Study of Prescriptions),"* "*Tokashu* 灯下集 *(Collection of Drug Properties by the Lamp*)," etc., Kengi Furubayashi (1779–1657) who wrote *"Nikkichutoho* 日記中棟方 *(Selected Treatment for Common Diseases),"* *"Myoyakusokkoho* 妙薬速効方 *(Excellent Formulas for Emergencies),"* etc., Doju Nagasawa (–1637) who wrote *"Ihokuketsushu* 医方口訣集 *(Collection of Oral Transmissions of Medical Prescriptions),"* "*Zohonodoku* 増補能毒 *(Supplement to Drug Properties*)," etc., Yushoshi Kitayama *"Kitayamaian* 北山医案 *(Case Records of Kitayama Yushoshi),"* *"Ihokojoken* 医方考縄愆 *(Annonation Textbook of Investigations of Medical Prescriptions*)," etc., and Sanryu Nakayama (1614–84) who wrote *"Shishozakki* 遂生雑記 *(Miscellaneous Notes on Foodstuffs for Longevity),"* and "*Byokayoran* 病家要覧 *(Essential Compendium for Patients*), etc. In addition to aforementioned Gyuzan Katsuki, there were Kensai Kato (1669–1724) who is the author of *"Iryotebikigusa* 医療手引草 *(Handbook for Clinical Practice),"* "*Hengyokurokuhachihonzo* 片玉六八本草 *(Minimumal 6x8 Materia Medica*)," *"Hoteki* 方的 *(Targetted Formulas),"* etc., Gensen Tsuda (1737–1809) who authored *"Kangakuchitai* 勧学治体 *(Recommendations for Medical*

Educational System)," *"Sekizanigon* 積山遺言 *(Medical Proverbs by Sekizan (Tsuda Gensen))"*, etc., Shunpo Kitao (1658–1741) who wrote *"Teijidan* 提耳談 *(Detailed Guidance about Diseases),"* *"Tosoan Kaho kukai/kuge* 当壯庵家方口解 *(Instruction on the Toso'an Family Prescriptions),"* *"Sokanidan* 桑韓医談 *(Medical Dialogue between Japan and Korea),"* etc., Futei Fukui (1725–92) who wrote *"Surankanshukenho* 崇蘭館集験方 *(Collected Prescriptions from the Surankan school),"* *"Hodokubenkai* 方読弁解 *(Oral Tradition about Collection of Ancient and Modern Formulas),"* *"Hinkomyakukai* 瀕湖脈解 *(Elucidation of Binhu's(Li Shi Zhen's) Pulse Diagnosis),"* etc., Tokaku Wada (1744–1803) who is an author of *"Shosozatsuwa*蕉窓雑話 *(Record of Wada Tokaku's Teaching on Medicine),"* *"Shosohoikai* 蕉窓方意解 *(Guide to Wada Tokaku's Favorite Prescriptions),"* *"Dosui sagen* 導水瑣言 *(Trivial Book on EdemaTreatment),"* etc., and Kien Takashina (1773–1843) who wrote *"KyukokanIfu* 求古館医譜 *(Principles of Kyukokan),"* *"Kyukokanhofu* 求古館方譜 *(Prescriptions of Kyukokan),"* *"Denka Rekikenho* 伝家歴験方 *(Family Empirical Formulary),"* etc. Ippo Okamoto (1654–1716) translated and annotated a large number of Chinese medical books, including *"Igakusanzobenkai* 医学三蔵弁解 *(Explanation of Three Organ Systems),"* "*Ikeisokaishuwagosho* 医経溯洄集倭語鈔 (Japanese Commentary on Revisiting the Medical Classics)," and *"Jushikeirakuhakkiwage*十四経絡発揮和解 *(Japanese Interpretation of Elucidation of Fourteen Meridians)"*; in addition, he wrote medical books for enlightenment.

Koho School

In the latter half of the seventeenth century, while it was after the middle of the Edo period, a Kampo school adhering to the *"Shokanron* 傷寒論 *(Treatise on Cold Damage)"* for an ideal medicine was in the majority of the then Japanese Kampo circle. This school advocating the spirit of the *"Shokanron* 傷寒論 *(Treatise on Cold Damage)"* compiled in the Han Dynasty was called Koho School. In China, *"Shokanron* 傷寒論 *(Treatise on Cold Damage)"* was reevaluated in the Song Dynasty, and its spirit was pursued by a group of reversionistic physicians in the Ming to Qing Dynasty. Some of them analyzed *"Shokanron* 傷寒論 *(Treatise on Cold Damage)"* in their own way and divided its content into two parts: what meets their view (was admitted as the original classic described by *Zhang Zhongjing*) and what does not meet their view (was not admitted via regarding as additional inserts by descendants such as *Wang Shuhe*). They may be said to have been rather radical. Japanese Koho School members were inspired by them. Inspired Japanese physicians included Gen'i Nagoya (1628–96; *"Igaku Gutoku* 医学愚得 *(Humble Opinion about Inner Classic),"* *"Ihomonyo* 医方問余 *(Medical Principles and Prescriptions),"* *"Kaiaittoku* 怪痾一得 *(Clinical records of strange diseases),"* *"Kinkiyoryakuchukai* 金匱要略註解 *(Annotation and Interpretation of Synopsis of the Golden Chamber),"* *"Epposhokumotsuhonzo* 閲甫食物本草 *(Eppo's Food as Materia Medica)* and many others), Konzan Goto (1659–1733; *"Shisetsuhikki* 師説筆記 *(Notes of Goto Konzan's Lectures),"* *"Konzansenseiisetsu* 艮山先生医説 *(Goto Konzan's Lectures about Medicine),"* etc.), Shuan [or Shutoku] Kagawa (1683–1755; *"Ijisetsuyaku* 医事説約 *(Ippondo's Prescriptions for Various Diseases),"* *"Ippondokoyoigen* 一本堂行余医言 *(Ippondo Advanced Studies of Medical Texts),"* *"Ippondoyakusen* 一本堂薬選 *(Ippondo's Selection of Crude Drugs),"* etc.), Kitetsu Naito (1701–35; *"Ikeikaiwakuron* 医経解惑論 *(Solving the Questions of Medical Classics),"* *"Shokanzatsubyoronruihen* 傷寒雑病論類編 *(Reconstruction of Treatise on Cold Damage and Miscellaneous Diseases,)"* Toyo Yamawaki (1705–62; *"Zoshi* 蔵志 *(Records of Dissection),"* *"Yojuinisoku* 養寿院医則 *(Yojuin's Rules of Medicine),"* *"Yojuinhokan* 養寿院方函 *(Yojuin's Prescptions),"* etc.), Todo Yoshimasu (1702–73; *"Ijiwakumon* 医事或問 *(Questions and Answers on Medical Topics),"* *"Idan* 医断 *(Proposition of Medicine),"* *"Ihobunryoko* 医方分量考 *(Investigation of Weight Units for Medical Prescriptions),"* *"Kenshuroku* 建殊録 *(Case Reports of Distinction (by Yoshimasu Todo)),"* *"Koshoigen* 古書医言 *(Medical Citations from the Classics),"* *"Hoki* 方機 *(Flexibility of Formulation),"* *"Hokyoku* 方極 *(Pearl of Formulas),"* *"Yakucho* 薬徴 *Effect and Indications of Medicinal Herbs),"* *"Ruijuho* 類聚方*(Classified Collection of Prescriptions),"* and many others), Nagatomi Dokushoan 1732–66; *"Tohoko* 吐方考 (Investigation of Emetic Formulas)," *"Manyuzakki* 漫遊雑記 *(Miscellaneous Notes of Journeys),"* *"Hokohiroku* 葆光秘録 *(Secret Records of Wisdom),"* etc.), Murai Kinzan (1733–1815; *"Idonisennenganmokuhen* 医道二千年眼目篇 *(Focus on 2000-year-old Medical Principles),"* *"Yakucho Zokuhen* 薬徴続編 *(Supplement to Effect and Indications of Medicinal Herbs),"* *"Yakuryoko* 薬量考 *(Investigation of Medicinal Dosages),"* *"Ruijuhogi* 類聚方議 *(Discussion of Classified Collection of Prescriptions),"* *"Wahoichimanho* 和方一万方 *(Ten Thousand Japanese Prescriptions),"* etc.), and Kamei Nammei (1741–1814; *"Kokonsaiirohauta* 古今斎以呂波歌 *(Kokonsai's Iroha (Japanese ABC) Poems),"* *"Nammei Mondo* 南冥問答 *(Questions and Answers with Kamei Nammei),"* etc.). They had different standpoints. Among them, Todo Yoshimasu was a Kampo physician with a remarkable perspective.

Todo Yoshimasu proposed a conception that all diseases are derived from one poison, and a variety of pathologic conditions occur depending on the location of the poison (*Manbyo ichidoku setsu*). Claiming that since all drugs are poison, the physician should attack the causative poison with drug poisons, he instituted aggressive therapies. Todo asserted that even if a therapy failed to cure a patient, it is the patient's fate (*Tenmei setsu*), which should not be attributed to the physician. His assertion evoked controversy in the then-medical circle. Todo denied the concepts of Chinese natural philosophy including the yin and yang and five elements theory. He thoroughly dissected the sentences of *"Shokanron* 傷寒論 *(Treatise on Cold Damage)"* to compile "*Ruijuho*" in 1764 followed by *"Yakucho* □□ *(Effect and Indications of Medicinal Herbs)"*

in 1785. Thus Todo Yoshimas became the most outstanding person at Koho School. At this time point, it may be said that a Japanese-taste concept or cause of *sho* was formed. His straightaway medical theory swept through the physicians' world in the late Edo period, resulting in a great influence on today's Japanese Kampo medicine. His son Nangai succeeded Todo and sought to revise the father's radical conception by explaining pathology and treatment with the qi, blood[TM1], and fluid[TM1] doctrine. Nangai's medical conception also underlies contemporary Kampo medicine. Yodo Odai (1799–1870; *"Hogizasshi* 方伎雑誌 *(Miscellaneous Notes about Medicine),"* *"Ruijuhokogi* 類聚方広義 *(Expanded Interpretation for Classified Collection of Prescriptions),"* and *"Iyo* 医余 *(Exegesis of Medical Principles),"* etc.), who was well known at Edo at the end of the Edo Shogunate, adhered to Todo's medical concept and bridged between the Edo and today's Kampo medicine.

Setchu School

While Chinese people respected logic or abstract concepts, Japanese people valued practical and concrete images. These tendencies were true in medicine. Since Koho School physicians were apt to become extremists, a group of flexible physicians appeared who took first account of effective formulas and incorporated clinically good points of medical

. This group was called Setchu School, comprising aforementioned Wada Tokaku, Ogino Gengai (1737–1806; *"Shirakuhen* 刺絡編 *(Text of Shiraku (Pricking Collaterals)),"* *"Tohohen* 吐法編 *(Treatise on Emetic Methods),"* etc.),Nakagami Kinkei (1744–1833; *"Seiseidoitan* 生々堂医譚 *(Seiseido's Discussion on Medicine),"* *"Seiseidoyojoron* 生々堂養生論 *(Seiseido's Treatise on Health Cultivation),"* *"Seiseidoshokanyakugen* 生々堂傷寒約言 *(Seiseido's Essential Points on Treatise on Cold Damage),"* *"Seiseidozakki* 生々堂雑記 *(Seiseido's Miscellaneous Essays on Medicine),"* etc.), Hara Nan'yo (1752–1820; *"Keiketsuikai* 経穴彙解 *(Terminology and Interpretation of Meridian Points),"* *"Kikihoki* 寄奇方記 *(Comments on Uncommon Formulas),"* *"Shokanronyawa* 傷寒論夜話 *(Notes on Treatise on Cold Damage),"* *"Sokeiguki* 叢桂偶記 *(Medical Essays of Sokeitei),"* *"Sokeiteiijishogen* 叢桂亭医事小言 *(Medical Lectures of Sokeitei),"* "*Toridegusa* 砦草 (*Notes for the Medic in the Field*), etc.), and Katakura Kakuryo (1751–1822; *"Shokankeibi*傷寒啓微 *(Revealing Mysteries in the Treatise on Cold Damage),"* *"Sankahatsumo* 産科発蒙 *(Edification on Obstetrics),"* *"Seikendochiken* 静倹堂治験 *(Clinical Record of Seikendo),"* *"Seinosatan* 青嚢瑣探 *(Preliminary Research of Blue Bag Manuscript),"* *"Bairai Shinsho* 黴癘新書 *(New Book of Syphilis),"* *"Hoeisuchi* 保嬰須知 *(Essential Knowledge for Pediatricians),"* etc.). Even today, the clinical technique by Tokaku Wada is highly appreciated. Quite a few people tried to take the middle course between Rampo and Kampo medicine. Among them, one leader was Seishu Hanaoka (1760–1835; *"Shunrinkengansambenran* 春林軒丸散便覧 *(Shunrinken's Prescriptions of Pills and Powders),"* *"Seishusenseichikenroku* 青洲先生治験録 *(Clinical record of Hanaoka Seishu),"* and many others)" from Kishu. He is well known as the first surgeon on earth to have successfully achieved extraction of breast cancer by use of an anesthetic of crude drugs developed by himself. One of his successors is Homma Soken (*"Naika Hiroku* 内科秘録 *(Secret Records of Internal Medicine),"* *"Yokahiroku* 瘍科秘録 *(Secret Record of Treatment of Sores),"* etc.) In the Kampo circle of the early Meiji period, Asada Sohaku (1815–94; *"Futsugoyakushitsuhokan* 勿誤薬室方函 *(Prescriptions of Futsugo Pharmacy)"* *"Futsugoyakushitsuhokankuketsu* 勿誤薬室方函口訣 *(Oral Transmission of Futsugo Pharmacy),"* *"Igakutenkei* 医学典刑 *(Standard Text of Medicine),"* *"Kissoshoei* 橘窓書影 *(Kisso Chronological Case Records),"* *"Kohoyakugi* 古方薬議 *(Discussion of Crude Drugs in Classical Prescriptions),"* *"Myakuhoshigen* 脈法私言 *(Confidential Pulse Methodology),"* *"Shokanronshi* 傷寒論識 *(Insight into Treatise on Cold Damage),"* *"Zatsubyoronshi (ronshiki)* 雑病論識 *(Insight into Treatise on Miscellaneous Diseases),"* *"Kokokumeiiden* 皇国名医伝 *(Biography of Famous Japanese Physicians),"* *"Sentetsuiwa* 先哲医話 *(Collected Essays of Excellent Physicians of the Past),"* *"Igakuchikan* 医学智環 *(Circle of Medical Knowledge),"* and many others) amazingly flourished as a Sechu school physician. Sohaku played the lead in the last stage as a Kampo magnate from the end of the Edo period to the Meiji period. There are many lessons to be learned from his clinical achievement.

Kosho School

In the late Edo period, a new Kampo group of Kosho school emerged under criticism and reflection on the past selfish interpretation of literature and thrived at the end of the Edo period. The Kosho school succeeded the academic tradition of historical investigation in the Qing Dynasty and introduced it into the medical field to seek facts through objective analysis of Kampo classics. Motoyasu Taki (1755–1810; *"Shokanronshugi*傷寒論輯義 *(Interpretation of Treatise on Cold Damage),"* *"Kinkiyoryakushugi* 金匱要略輯義 *(Commentary on the Synopsis of the Golden Chamber),"* *"Somonshi* 素問識 *(Knowledge of Basic Questions),"* *"Reisushi* 霊枢識 *(Insight into Spiritual Pivot),"*

"*Henjakusokoden* 扁鵲倉公伝彙考 (*Investigation of Collected Works of Bianque and Cang-gong*)," "*Myakugakushuyo* 脈学輯要 (*Collected Esentials of Pulse Studies*)," "*Isho* 医賸 (*Additional Medical Commentary*)," etc.), one of his sons Mototsugu Taki (1789–1827; "*Isekiko* 医籍考 (*Comprehensive Annotated Bibliography of Chinese Medical Texts*)," "*Nangyo Sosho*難経疏証 (*Commentary on Classic of Difficult Issues*)," etc.), another son Motokata Taki (1795–1857; "*Shokanronjutsugi* 傷寒論述義 (*Treatise on Cold Damage Annotated for Meaning*)," "*Kinkiyoryakujutsugi* 金匱要略述義 (*Commentary on the Synopsis of the Golden Chamber*)," "*Somonshoshi* 素問紹識 (*Sequel to Insight on Basic Questions*)," "*Yakujitsugi* 薬治通義 (*Comprehensive Principles of Drug Therapeutics*)," "*Shokankoyo*傷寒広要 (*Expanded Essentials of Treatise on Cold Damage*)," "*Zatsubyokoyo* 雑病広要 (*Expanded Essentials of Miscellaneous Diseases*)," etc.) and others of Edo Igakukan (medical school) were representative physicians of the Kosho school of Kampo medicine. Furthermore, there were many medical scholars such as Ranken Izawa (1777–1829; "*Ranken'iwa* 蘭軒医話 (*Ranken's Medical Talks*)," "*Ranken'idan* 蘭軒医談 (*Ranken's Medical Discourses*)," etc.), *Chusai Shibue* (1805–58; "*Reisukogi* 霊枢講義 (*Lectures on Spiritual Pivot*)," etc.), Hoso Kojima (1797–1848; "*Kaseiguki* 河清寓記 (*A Bobliography of Rare Books*)," etc.), Tatsuyuki Mori (1807–85); "*Honzokeikochu* 本草経攷注 (*Annotation and Interpretation on Shennong's Classic of Materia Medica*)," "*Shokanronkochu*傷寒論攷注 (*Research and annotation of Treatise on Cold Damage*)," "*Somonkochu* 素問攷注 (*Annotation and Interpretation of Basic Questions*)," and many others), and Narihiro Yamada (1807–81; "*Igakukansui* 医学管錐 (*Deep Inquiry into Old Medical Commentaries*)" and many others). Achievements of these Kosho school physicians were introduced to China, the Kampo originator, after the Meiji Restoration and even today are highly appreciated. Although it tends to be considered that scholars of historical investigation exclusively search literature, there were actually quite a few excellent clinicians such as Narihiro Yamada.

Materia Medica

Of the Chinese books of herbalism, "*Honzokeishitchu* 本草経集注 (*Variorum of Shennong's Classic of Materia Medica*)" was first introduced into Japan in the Asuka period; "*Shinshuhonzo* 新修本草 (*Newly Revised Pharmacopoeia*)," in the Nara period. In the late Heian period, "*Shoruihonzo* 証類本草 (*Classified Materia Medica*)" came over and was in use as the standard book of materia medica through the Kamakura-Muromachi period. In the early Edo period, the import of "*Honzokomoku* 本草綱目 (*Compendium of Materia Medica*)" had immeasurable effects as the fundamental literature of materia medica. Japanese herbal books in the Edo period include "*Yakushonodoku* 薬性能毒 (*Medicinal Properties, Efficiency, and Toxicity*)" written by Dosan Manase at the end of the sixteenth century, "*Epposhokumotsuhonzo* 閲甫食物本草 (*Eppo's Food as Materia Medica*)" (Gen'i Nagoya,1669), "*Hozubiyohonzo* 庖厨備用本草 (*Materia Medica from a Japanese Household Recipe*)" (Gensho Mukai, 1671), "*Honzobengi* 本草弁疑 (*Correction of Misunderstandings about Materia Medica*)" (Genri Endo, 1681), "*Honchoshokukan* 本朝食鑑 (*The Japanese Encyclopedia of Foods*)" (Hitsudai Hitomi, 1692), "*Koekihonzotaisei* 広益本草大成 (*Complete Compendium of Materia Medica of Wide Benefit*)" (Ippo Okamoto, 1698), "*Yamatohonzo* 大和本草 (*Japanese Materia Medica*)" (Ekiken Kaibara, 1708), "*Yoyakusuchi* 用薬須知 (*Essential Knowledge for Using Medicines*)" (Gentatsu Matsuoka, 1726), "*Yakurohonzo* 薬籠本草 (*Medicine Basket Materia Medica*)" (Gyuzan Katsuki, 1727), "*Ippondo Yakusen*" (Shuan Kagawa, 1731–38), "*Yakucho* □□ (*Effect and Indications of Medicinal Herbs*)"

(Todo Yoshimasu, 1771), "*Honzokomokukeimo* 本草綱目啓蒙 (*Elucidation of Compendium of Materia Medica*)" (Ranzan Ono, 1803–05), and "*Kohoyakuhinko* 古方薬品考 (*Investigation of Crude Drugs in Classical Prescriptions*) (Naokata Naito, 1840).

Attention should be paid to abdominal examination (腹診[術] *fukushin*[*jutsu*]) as a Kampo diagnostic method uniquely improved and developed in Japan. *Fukushin*, which is essential for Japanese Kampo medicine, sprouted in the Nanbokucho period and propagated through the Edo period. However, since it is complex and remains to be fully clarified, it is not further referred to here.

Conclusion

Gosei, Koho, Sechu, and Kosho schools as well as the materia medica field have been outlined. These schools and fields cannot be clearly discriminated. The Gosei School is thought to be based on Jin-Yuan medicine; however, Jin-Yuan medicine did not neglect *Chochukei's Koho*. The Koho School, even Todo Yoshimasu, used medicines other than those described in the "*Shokanron* 傷寒論 (*Treatise on Cold Damage*)" and "*Kinkiyouryaku* □□□□ *Synopsis of the Golden Chamber*)." The Sechu school is a generic name for groups of physicians who accepted *Iho* from various schools, while the Kosho school refers to a group of physicians who introduced a method of studying old documents into desk research. Since sechu and classicist schools are defined from different viewpoints, the two are difficult to discriminate. Some maintain that there was no exchange between schools in the Edo period, which is not correct. Actually, there were occasional exchanges even between Rampo (Western medicine) and Kampo families. For another example, there was an intimate exchange even between Yodo Odai regarded as a true Koho physician, and Sohaku Asada belonging to a Sechu or Kosho school. Some critics limit Japanese Kampo medicine to a particular school that emphasizes the formula corresponding to pattern identification and avoids referring to etiology. Such a view, however, was merely established in the early Showa period. Japanese Kampo medicine is not comprehensible from such a limited perspective. Rather, in the Edo period, especially after the Genroku era, Japanese Kampo medicine covered a far broader field including Rangaku (the study of Dutch) and natural history than traditional Chinese medicine in the Qing Dynasty. Comparison in the level of knowledge alone on traditional medicine reveals that today's Kampo circle is far inferior to that in the Edo period.

Meiji Period to Prewar Showa Period

Yoshihide Yakazu and Hiromichi Yasui

2.1.4 Decline of Kampo Medicine

As the Meiji period unfolded, Kampo medicine headed steadily into decline. One of the reasons for this perhaps was that the Japanese people who had just been liberated from the national policy of isolation became mesmerized by the apparent splendor of Western civilization and took to idolizing all things Western in the prevailing trend of the times. However, the most salient reason for the decline of Kampo medicine was the adoption by the Meiji Government of German medicine as the model for Japan's medical system. After this move, Kampo medicine no longer had a standing in the mainstream of medical practice in Japan.

Dawning of the Meiji Period: Advent of Tribulation for Kampo Medicine

With the Edo period coming to its close, Japan took a new course of direction. In 1868 came the Meiji Restoration. The new government embarked on the pursuit of Westernization, on the prioritization of national prosperity and strong defense, and on the economic policy of free-market capitalism. It pushed these national policies forcefully in order to catch up with the developed countries of Europe and America. In terms of medicine and healthcare, what was needed was modern medicine with its armory of preventive medicine that could cope with the communal way of life required in the armed forces, schools, and factories. This is why the government headed toward establishing a medical system on the German model.

Medical License Examination: Resistance by Kampo Medicine Practitioners

The Meiji Government promoted modern public health policies. In 1874, its new medical system was promulgated to the three metropolitan areas[1] and in the following year of 1875,[2] it instituted the Medical License Examination that tested candidates in seven subject areas[3] similar to those of Western medical practice (Yoho). In other words, unless you studied Western medicine and obtained a medical license thereby, you could not become qualified as a doctor. To rival this, the "Six Wise Men of Kampo Medicine" led by Sohaku Asada set out the six subject areas of Kampo medicine. Despite their effort, the requirement of passing the Medical License Examination (now the National Medical Practitioners Qualifying Examination) based on Yoho ("Western medicine") was promulgated in 1876 to all prefectures across Japan.

In response, the Kampo medicine practitioners of the day united under the banner of the "political restoration of Kampo medicine." Narihiro Yamada became the first leader of Onchisha (Association to Preserve Traditional Knowledge), a society formed in 1879 by Sohaku Asada, Tatsuyuki Mori, and other practitioners. The society fought for the survival of Kampo medicine in mainstream medical practice.

The society's activities later led to the publication of journals such as "*Onchiidan* 温知医談 (*Medical Dialogue of Onchi-sha*)" (1879 to 1889), "*Wakanirinshinshi* 和漢医林新誌 (*News of Japanese Medical Literature*)" (1881 to 1887), "*Keikoiho* 継興医報 (*Successive Medical Reports*)" (1893 to 1897), and other periodicals, as well as the establishment of Kampo medicine clinics such as the Wakan Igaku Koshujo (Tokyo Onchi Gakko school, 1883) and Onchi Byoin hospital (1884). However, with the successive deaths of the eminent leaders of Onchisha in the passage of time, members left the society in droves as they sensed a lost cause. In 1887, Onchisha had no option but to disband.

Rejection of the Kampo Practitioner Petition: Demise of Kampo Medicine

Then Kampo medicine practitioners pinned their last hopes on the Imperial Diet, and Kokkan Azai, the third president of Onchisha united some 3000-strong former members and colleagues across the country to form Teikoku Ikai (Imperial Medical Association) in 1890 in order to file a petition to fight for their cause in the Diet assembly. Sadly, in the eighth National Assembly of the Imperial Diet held in 1895, the petition for the continuation of the recognition of Kampo

[1]The three prefectures of Tokyo, Kyoto, and Osaka

[2]The Medical License Examination had been stipulated in Article 37 of the Medical System Regulations but it was in 1875, the following year, that it was put into actual practice.

[3]In "*Shokoshishi* 松香私志 (*Memoire of Nagayo Sensai*)," a book written by Baron Sensai Nagayo, who was the Director of the Bureau of Medicine that created and established the Medical System Regulations, the seven subjects listed were physics, chemistry, anatomy, physiology, pathology, internal medicine and surgery, and pharmacy. We have followed this listing here, but until 1876, physics and chemistry were classed together as one subject area to form six subject areas altogether.

medicine practitioners was turned down with a very narrow margin[4] of 27 votes, bringing to a close the five-year-long battle in the Imperial Diet over the continuation of Kampo medicine. After this, only existing Kampo medicine practitioners were entitled to their own qualifications during their lifetime. Their apprentices had to pass the examinations of Western medicine in order to be Kampo medical practitioners.

In 1900, Kokkan Azai wrote "*Kokubobun* 告墓文 (*Reports and Decisions for the Graves of Azai's Family Line*)" and declared the demise of Kampo medicine to his ancestors in the grave, apologizing for his inadequacies and powerlessness. Kampo medicine thus was unable to ride the huge waves of Westernization that surged across Japan at the time. In legislative terms, Kampo medicine lost its status as a legitimate medical practice.

Decline of Kampo Medicine and Two Rescue Measures

Nevertheless, this did not mean that Kampo's medicine was utterly discredited. At the time, the government was attempting to improve the practice of Western medicine in Japan. At its forefront was Sensai Nagayo (1838–1902), who was the creator of the new Medical System.[5] Nagayo did not totally reject Kampo medicine.

For fear of the social confusion that may result in the wake of the amendment of the Medical Practitioners' Law, the Meiji Government consulted Nagayo, asking "Would this not put Kampo medicine practitioners into difficulty?"[6] He responded by proposing two concessionary rescue measures. The first of these was to allow Kampo medicine practitioners who were already practicing to continue in their practice. The second was to allow Kampo medicine practitioners to offer treatment and engage in research in Kampo medicine so long as they hold a license in Western medicine. Thanks to these measures, doctors who had graduated from university schools of medicine came to reappraise the practice of Kampo medicine, and started new treatment and research activities, albeit at a later date.

After passing the middle of the Meiji Era, the Kampo medicine practitioners who had been granted lifetime license to practice Kampo medicine as a transitional provision of the new medical license system gradually died due to old age, and with some exceptions, most of the Kampo medicine practices were left with nobody to succeed and carry on. The reason for this is that the medical apprentices could no longer become Kampo medicine practitioners because the medical license was only given to practitioners of Western medicine. This led to a rapid decline in Kampo medicine and even in academic terms, Kampo medicine virtually faced extinction. The course of events is outlined in Table 1.3..

2.1.5 Restoration of Kampo Medicine

Though Kampo medicine was sidelined from legitimate medical practice in Japan in 1895, this was not to say that it totally disappeared. Despite being few in number, longstanding Kampo medicine practitioners who traced their practice history back to the Edo period continued in their treatments and passed down their knowledge and skills. Doctors and pharmacists of Kampo medicine who were master practitioners, although few and far between, handed down to their apprentices the fine details of Kampo medicine. Slowly but surely, Kampo medicine resumed on its road to recovery. We shall describe below the Kampo medicine practitioners who contributed to the restoration of Kampo medicine during the period spanning the Meiji and Showa periods.

[4]The amended bill put forward by the Kampo medicine practitioners was defeated, 78 votes in favor and 105 votes against the bill.

[5]Legislation that was issued to the three metropolitan prefectures in order to introduce a "modern medical and public health system" into Japan at the beginning of the Meiji period. It contained legislation affecting the entire administration of public health, including the healthcare system and medical education. Later, the scope of this legislation was extended to take effect in all other prefectures across Japan.

[6]Original wording: Would the enforcement of the medical practitioner regulations pose difficulties or not to Kampo medicine practitioners?

Table 1.3. Conflict between Western Medicine and Chinese Medicine in the Meiji Era

Western medicine Meiji Government	1874: Promulgation of medical system to the three metropolitan prefectures 1875: Medical license examination established testing in 7 subjects of the Western system	1876: Requirement of passing medical license examination under the Western system notified to all prefectural governments	1883: Medical qualification system enacted 1884: Medical license examination regulations and medical license regulations enforced	1895: The eighth Imperial diet rejected the Kampo medical practitioner continuation petition; passing a Western medicine examination becomes mandatory in order to qualify as a doctor
Kampo medicine Onchisha & others	1875: Six wise men of Kampo medicine including Sohaku Asada fought back with 6 subjects of Kampo medicine	1879: Onchisha formed and Kampo medicine continuation petition filed repeatedly but rejected	1883: Wakan Igaku Koshujo established 1884: Onchi Byoin hospital opened; Sohaku Asada became the first director	1887: Onchisha disbanded 1890: Kokkan Azai and colleagues formed Teikoku Ikai and fought through the diet

Meiji Period Koho School: Keijuro Wada, Proponent of the Superiority of Kampo Medicine

The movement for the restoration of Kampo medicine was first advocated by Keijuro Wada (1872–1916). In his infancy, he witnessed the curing of a relative's intractable disease by a Kampo medicine practitioner. He was deeply moved by this experience and went on to study both Kampo and Western medicine. He became a doctor and started his medical practice, specializing solely in Kampo medicine. He was an admirer of Yoshimasu Todo. He interpreted the medical art of the Todo School using medical concepts of the day and applied it to clinical practice. In 1910, he wrote a book called "*Ikai'notettsui* 医界之鉄椎 (*Iron Hammer to the Medical World*)," in which he expounded the excellence of Kampo medicine in therapeutics.

Enlightened by this book, physicians started to study Kampo medicine. They gradually grew in number and bolstered the movement for the restoration of Kampo medicine.

Showa Period Koho School (1): Kyushin Yumoto, Promoter of Integration with Western Medicine

Kyushin Yumoto (1876–1941) read Wada's "*Ikai'notettsui* 医界之鉄椎 (*Iron Hammer to the Medical World*)" and decided to study Kampo medicine. Basically, he followed the teachings of Todo Yoshimasu and Yodo Odai and practiced medicine following "*Shokanron* 傷寒論 (*Treatise on Cold Damage*)" and "*Kinkiyouryaku* □□□□ (*Synopsis of the Golden Chamber.*)"

Not automatically advocating the negation of Western medicine, he held a long-cherished desire to start the fusion and integration of the two practices of medicine. Thus he wrote a book called "*Kokan'igaku* 皇漢医学 (*Traditional medicine originated in China and developed uniquely in Japan*)" (1927–28), which cast fresh limelight on Kampo medicine as the Showa period started. His line of thoughts and desires was pursued later by one of his pupils, Keisetsu Otsuka.

Showa Period Koho School (2): Kenzo Okuda, Traditionally Trained Practitioner

Kenzo Okuda (1884–1961) grew up in a family of doctors who had studied under the Yoshimasu school. After graduating from the Japan Medical College, later renamed Nippon Medical School, he received a wide range of Kampo medicine education and training from his father, mostly based on "*Shokanron* 傷寒論 (*Treatise on Cold Damage*)" and "*Kinkiyouryaku* □□□□ *Synopsis of the Golden Chamber*)" and enhanced by studies of "*Daikei* 内経 (*Yellow Emperor's Inner Classic*)," "*Nangyo* 難経 (*Classic of Difficult Issues*)," *Honzokomoku* 本草綱目 (*Compendium of Materia Medica*), *OnekiRon* 温疫論 (*Treatise on Pestilence*), and "*Jushikeihakki* 十四経発揮 (*Elucidation of Fourteen Meridians*)." Among his publications are "*Kokan'igakuyoho kaisetsu* 皇漢医学要方解説 (*Explanation of Important Prescriptions from Kokan Igaku Traditional Medicine*)" and "*Shokanronkogai* 傷寒論梗概 (*Outline of Treatise on Cold Damage*)." After his death, his pupils published "*Shokanronkogi* 傷寒論講義 (*Lecture on Treatise on Cold Damage*)" (his lecture notes on "*Shokanron* 傷寒論 (*Treatise on Cold Damage*)"). Okuda was close to Kyushin Yumoto who belonged to the same Koho School and he wrote the Afterword for Yumoto's book, *Kokan'igaku*. Some say that Yumoto had regarded Okuda as his successor.

In contrast to Wada and Yumoto, Okuda's medical practice did not run along the course of integration with Western medicine but was descended from the Koho School that originated from Todo Yoshimasu. This in fact resulted in relaying the essence of Koho to posterity, with many pupils emanating, mostly doctors who graduated from Chiba University School of Medicine. Okuda is one of the very few Koho Kampo medicine practitioners who had received traditional education and training and who continued in the heritage of a rare Kampo medicine family that had survived undisrupted even into the Meiji period. Ken Fujihira, Yoshio Nagahama, Kiyoo Ito, Shigenari Ogura and other doctors succeeded and followed in his footsteps.

Showa Gosei School: Dohaku Mori, Founder of Ikkando Igaku (Ikkando Medicine)

Dohaku Mori (1867–1931) studied Kampo medicine under Kaishin Yusa. He became widely known as an excellent Kampo medicine practitioner and practiced his own unique clinical treatment. His pupil, Kaku Yakazu, outlined his medical practice in the book "*Kampoikkandoigaku* 漢方一貫堂医学 (*Kampo Medicine in Ikkando School*)" (1964), but this describes only one of the styles that Mori adopted in his late years. For more details, refer to the section on Kampo Ikkando Igaku (See Chap. 1 column [Kampo Ikkando medicine]). His pupils Kaku Yakazu, then Domei Yakazu, Yudo Yakazu, Kiichi (Zuisho) Nakajima, Nobuyasu Ishino, and other practitioners succeeded him and followed in his footsteps.

Asada Setchu School: Kimura Hakusho

Sohaku Asada (1814–1894) was said to be one of the two great doctors[7] of the late Edo period. He had many pupils, among whom were Hakusho Kimura (Tokyo), Kosho Nakano (Osaka), and Sogoro Niizuma (Kyoto) who became well known for continuing in Kampo medicine therapies and passing down the Asada School Kampo medicine to succeeding practitioners from the Meiji period through the Taisho period onto the Showa period and beyond.

[7] The other renowned doctor was Yodo Odai (1799–1870).

Hakusho Kimura (1866–1931) started his practice in Tokyo and opened the Saiseijuku school to educate pupils. Among them were doctors who had graduated from university medical schools and those who came to play important roles in the later period of the restoration of Kampo medicine. His successor was his adoptive heir Chokyu Kimura. In Osaka, Kosho Nakano was succeeded by Komon Morita, and in Kyoto, Sogoro Niizuma passed on his baton to Shiro Hosono.

2.1.6 Beginning of Restoration Period Leading to the Present Day

Before and after the World War II, research organizations and educational institutions of Kampo medicine were established, and activities promoting the revival and restoration of Kampo medicine were strongly promoted. In the Kanto region, Kenzo Okuda, Keisetsu Otsuka, and Domei Yakazu, and in the Kansai region, Shiro Hosono, led these activities. The impetus for the big revival movement came from the concerted effort made by practitioners to present a united front transcending the divides of different schools of Kampo medicine.

United Movement Transcending Schools and Occupational Roles in Practice: Kaiko Gakuen

As mentioned in the previous section, Kampo medicine came to be divided into different schools that were practiced by some of its members, but there had been no mutual collaboration among Kampo medicine practitioners of different schools. The second-generation practitioners who were concerned about this lack of coordination among different schools rose to present a united front so that they could create momentum for a new movement. In 1935, Kaiko Gakuen was established by seven leading lights: Keisetsu Otsuka of the Koho School, Chokyu Kimura of the Setchu School, Domei and Yudo Yakazu of the Gosei School, and the pharmacist Totaro Shimizu, the acupuncture and moxibustion practitioner Sorei Yanagiya[8] and the medical historian Yasuhide Ishihara. (Kaiko Gakuen later became the Association of East-Asian Medicine.) This collaborative effort became instrumental in resolving the issues among different schools of practice.

Kaiko Gakuen opened its doors in 1936 and held lectures on Kampo medicine. In the following year, it relocated to Takushoku University and continued there as the Takushoku University Kampo Medicine Course until 1949, though with disruption during the Pacific War. A total of about 900 students took the course and educated ensuing leaders of Kampo medicine and acupuncture/moxibustion. The Association of East-Asian Medicine was founded out of Kaiko Gakuen with the purpose of reviving traditional East-Asian medicine. The first issue of its journal *East-Asian Medicine*[9] was published in 1939.

Textbook for Doctors of Western Medicine: *"Kamposhinryonojissai* 漢方診療の実際 *(Standard Practice of Kampo Medicine)"*

This second generation of Kampo medicine practitioners then set about in collaboration, writing a textbook of Kampo medicine so that they could bolster the restoration movement. The authors comprised the three leaders of all the schools of the time, Chokyu Kimura of the Setchu School, Keisetsu Otsuka of the Koho School, and Domei Yakazu of the Gosei School, together with the pharmacist Totaro Shimizu. This textbook featured an unprecedented aim, that is, it was intended for the busy clinician, who would use it to study and learn Kampo medicine without any prior knowledge, in a short space of time, and without great difficulty. This can be regarded as the very first textbook on Kampo medicine for doctors of Western medicine. This textbook entitled *"Kamposhinryonojissai* 漢方診療の実際 (*Standard Practice of Kampo Medicine*)*"* was published in 1941.

As its foreword claimed, the textbook started right from page one by discussing the various theories of disease treatment. The Kampo medicine terminologies were mostly understandable with common sense. It was a radical book in that it could be readily understood in most parts if you had knowledge of Western medicine. The availability of this textbook meant that doctors who had only studied Western medicine could use Kampo medicine also. This book came to be widely read and was reprinted numerous times.[10] The National Health Insurance reimbursement listing of Kampo medication that began later, starting in 1976, became possible thanks to this groundwork. The methodology adopted by this book is also responsible for the phenomenal increase in the use of Kampo medication.

From the Postwar Time Until Today

Tetsuo Akiba and Tatsuro Katsuno

2.1.7 Summary from the Postwar Period Until the Present Time

Japanese Kampo medicine was greatly affected by the World War II lasting until 1945. Of promising young Kampo physicians, Chokyu Kimura and Keisaburo Mori were killed in the war, and Yudo Yakazu died from a disease at the front, not at

[8]For information about Sorei Yanagiya and the history of acupuncture and moxibustion, see History of Acupuncture (Refer to Chap. 6, Sect. 4).

[9]*East-Asian Medicine* merged in 1941 during World War II with the journal *Idononihon* 医道の日本 (*The Japanese Journal of Acupuncture & Manual Therapies*) and became the journal *Kampo and Kanyaku*. It resumed publication as *Kampo no Rinsho* (*Journal of Kampo Medicine*) in 1954 and is in publication to date.

[10]In 1969, the book's title was renamed to *Kampo Shinryo Iten* (Medical Dictionary of Kampo Practice) and is still in print.

home, after the war. Just before the end of the war, Shizuka Ayukawa and Kazuo Yumoto deceased in succession. And in 1946, Hisashi Koide was sadly missed in the postwar confusion.

Although the youth of abilities who were to lead the next generation were lost, Kampo medicine began to step on the road to restoration with the postwar reconstruction in Japan.

The first challenge was a request (to prohibit acupuncture and moxibustion) that was submitted to the then Japanese Ministry of Health and Welfare by the General Headquarters (GHQ) of Allied military forces in September 1947. This surprise request drove a large-scale protesting movement among acupuncturists and moxibustionists concerned throughout Japan, resulting in the successful rejection of the request, partly owing to the efforts of Dr. Hidetsurumaru Ishikawa (Kyoto Imperial University Professor Emeritus) and Dr. Takeshi Itakura (former Director of the Eastern Therapeutics Institute [東亜治療研究所, Toa Chiryo Kenkyusho]). However, it is beyond question that the prejudice of the allied nations toward Oriental medicine threatened the Kampo physicians engaging in the treatment with Kampo medicines (湯液) other than acupuncture and moxibustion.

While the postwar confusion settled down and economic recovery began, public interest had been increasingly given to Kampo medicine. Drug poisoning and health hazards due to environmental contamination were also headlined frequently, possibly because people became aware of the negative aspects of industrialization and associated economic growth. In the period of 1955–1964, there was a Kampo boom in which Kampo medicine and related matters were picked up in the media almost every day.

Meanwhile, the National Health Insurance system for the whole nation was established in 1961 and thereafter has allowed the people living in Japan to receive medical treatment equally at inexpensive costs. In the early days, most patients were not insured, and Kampo medicines were not often used in clinical practice, although insured medical care had been legally allowed using the crude drugs listed in the drug tariff, or drug price list. Kampo therapy was greatly changed in the qualitative as well as quantitative perspectives in 1976 when a large number of Kampo medicines were added to the drug tariff [6]. In parallel, medical education in universities and medical schools was also reformed enough to convert Kampo therapy—from a special therapeutic means by limited specialists to a universal therapeutic means by general practitioners [7]. This change was obvious, as indicated by the fact that the physicians who prescribe Kampo medicines in routine work accounted for 89% today in 2011.

A 75-year history of Kampo medicine after the war will be described here, focusing on the treatment with Kampo medicines (湯液), in the realms of academy, medical care and education systems, and social trend of thoughts.

2.1.8 Trends in the Academic World

Restart Toward Modern Kampo

The Kampo world that had collapsed by the unprecedented defeat of Japan began to do its own activities.

At the big turning point of the postwar period, Professor Yaeji Ito (Department of Ophthalmology, Chiba Medical College [Now Chiba University School of Medicine]) published an article entitled "Foreign cultures that affected Meiji medicine" in the April issue of *"Nippon Rekishi* 日本歴史 *(The History of Japan)"* in 1947. He pointed out the irrationality in the medicine and medical care systems in the early Meiji Era that excluded Kampo medicine, emphasizing the necessity of their reconstruction. He offered a non-credit course for Oriental medicine to open the door for participants outside the college as part of the reconstruction.

In 1948, novel movements were generated, including the publication of the book *"Wakanyakuyoshokubutsu* 和漢薬用植物 *(Medicinal Plants of Japan)"* by Tatsuo Kariyone and Yushiro Kimura. The first joint memorial service for the Kampo physicians who died during wartime was held by the Association of East-Ajian Medicine (東亜医学協会, Toa Igaku Kyokai), which set up the preparatory committee comprising Keisetsu Otsuka, Domei Yakazu, and Rin'ichi Kiga. This was a symbolic event for restart after the war. In the same year, Tokyo Kampo Medical Society (東京漢方医学会、Tokyo Kampo Igakkai) (Tomekichi Muto and Kenzo Okuda) and Yokohama Onchiikai (温知医会, Onchi Medicinal Society) (Itsuma Takagi and Kazuo Tatsuno) were established to initiate energetic activities.

The year 1949 became the commemorative year for Japan Kampo medicine slipped out of the postwar disorder to firmly advance toward the future. More specifically, in those days, arrangements remarkably progressed for the establishment of the Japan Society for Oriental Medicine (JSOM) as the core organization for the academic activities of Kampo medicine professionals. On March 15, Kazuo Tatsuno, Keisetsu Otsuka, Domei Yakazu, Yoshio Nagahama, Masaaki Maruyama, and Ken Fujihira gathered and formed a Kampo study group to hold monthly meetings. At the October meeting, agreements were made about the formation of the arrangement committee for the first JSOM meeting. Kazuo Tatsuno was elected as manager for the arrangement of general affairs. On November 17, the arrangement committee to hold the first JSOM meeting was established, and the charter was formulated with the use of the Tatsuno's house as the tentative office. The committee comprised 11 members: Shiro Hosono, Keisetsu Otsuka, Masatsugu Wada, Kazuo Tatsuno, Yoshio Nagahama, Domei Yakazu, Jyun Yamazaki,

Masaaki Maruyama, Yoshio Manaka, Ken Fujihira, and Yukihiro Morita.

In the same year, Totaro Shimizu issued the book "*Nippon Yakugakushi* 日本薬学史 (*History of Japanese Pharmacology*)," and Yaeji Ito (Prof. of Chiba University) submitted to the Ministry of Education an application for the establishment of a national research institute for Oriental medicine. In addition, the ninth Kampo medicine course was revived at Koryo (former, Takusyoku) University, with listed lecturers including Kazuo Tatsuno, Keisetsu Otsuka, Domei Yakazu, Totaro Shimizu, and Sorei Yanagiya.

The Japan Society for Oriental Medicine (JSOM)

With the advent of 1950, the organizing committee for the tentative JSOM was held to prepare and send the charter to the persons concerned. On March 12, the JSOM inaugural meeting was held in the meeting room of Kitasato Memorial Medical Library, Keio University School of Medicine. The name of the society was finally fixed after a brisk discussion. In the election of the president, nominated candidates declined one after another because of health or age problems, resulting in vacancies for the post. Then, the new organization was launched with Kazuo Tatsuno (responsible for general affairs) as the chief executive. The number of JSOM members at the inauguration was 93; 38 members were honorary who participated in response to requests from the secretariat, while 60 were regular who had paid the membership fee.

Since its inauguration, JSOM has aimed to join the Japanese Association of Medical Sciences (JAMS) as one of the member societies. In July 1953, 4 years after the inauguration, JSOM submitted to JAMS the first entry application, which was rejected by 26 votes to 3 votes at the Liaison Committee of JAMS held in the meeting room of the Japan Medical Association on August 27. The second application submitted in 1961 was also rejected by 31 votes to 14 votes. However, under President Kunio Matsuda, the fourth application in 1991 received a two-thirds favorable vote to pass: JSOM was approved as the 87th affiliated specialist medical society. One of the goals at the inauguration of JSOM was achieved 41 years later.

Since then, another important goal for JSOM as a society of clinical medicine has been the establishment of a specialist system similar to that in other medical societies. JSOM had sought to frame its specialist system, in parallel to the submission of entry application to JAMS. In 1990, the specialist system was accredited. However, once JSOM became a member of the Japanese Board of Medical Specialties, Kampo specialists have been and are authorized as sophisticated-field specialists after the accreditation of base-field specialists. In 2005, the Ministry of Health, Labor, and Welfare approved JSOM as a specialist qualification organization that can publicize the Kampo specialist. The number of JSOM members increased from 98 at the start to 1035 in 1970, 9751 in 1990, and 8407 in 2020, favorably with some margin of error. In 2020, 2067 new Kampo specialists were registered, and high-level Kampo therapy has been carried out in practice.

Medical and Pharmaceutical Society for WAKAN-YAKU

The Medical and Pharmaceutical Society for WAKAN-YAKU was born in 1984 from "the WAKAN-YAKU symposium," which was first organized in 1967 by Yuichi Yamamura and others, evolving to resolve. Its objectives were to discuss up-to-date information about the resources, quality control, mechanisms of action, and clinical studies of WAKAN-YAKU from the scientific perspective and to bridge basic and clinical medicine. A notable point was that the Society claims to quest for the harmony of natural science (based on elemental reductionism) and traditional medicine and pharmacy (being a complex and multicomponent system). For that purpose, medical and pharmaceutical scientists as well as medical doctors and pharmacists, all studying WAKAN-YAKU in various forms, should assemble to exchange information. Curiously, this concept was consistent with the historical background, in which therapeutic measures of non-Western medicine had been highly rated all over the world, although since the 1980s medical care costs had been elevated annually. Traditional medicine was highlighted globally in the 1990s. The society may have been the first to propose the value of academic WAKAN-YAKU research.

Association of East-Asian Medicine

Since the prewar periods, the Association of East-Asian Medicine has existed as an association of Kampo medicine and has been widely known as the publisher of a monthly issued magazine "*Kampotokan-yaku* 漢方と漢薬(*Journal of Kampo Medicine and Crude Drugs*)." The magazine was started in May 1934, changed its name to "*Shoyaku Chiryo* 生薬治療 (*Japanese Journal of Pharmacognosy*)" in 1944, and was published until volume 125 (publication suspended) as the official magazine for the Japanese Society of Kampo Medicine (日本漢方医学会). "*Kampotokan-yaku* 漢方と漢薬 (*Journal of Kampo Medicine and Crude Drug*)" was a product of collective efforts for Kampo medicine by Kampo medicine professionals concerned in then Japan. The articles of choice appeared in the magazine every month, not only enough to imply the vigor in the newborn Japan's Kampo circle, but also to give vivid and evergreen impressions even now in the twenty-first century. Naturally, the call for the resumption of publication of "*Kampotokan-yaku* 漢方と漢薬 (*Journal of Kampo Medicine and Crude Drug*)" occurred among the Kampo professionals.

Although magazines related to Oriental medicine had been perpetually published since soon after the war, regrettably many had been immediately suspended, and some had been eventually stopped. Such difficulty in continuous publication was believed to be unconquerable. Ultimately in 1953, there was no monthly magazine related to Kampo in Japan. This misfortune inspired a desire for an ideal monthly magazine that contains significant content (presenting typical Japanese Kampo papers and the latest related national and international news as well as providing a good impression). The desire was also a matter of honor for Japan.

Preceding cases of suspended publication were investigated in detail. As a result, the best way to assure continuous publication of the magazine was found: a publisher coterie of six persons led by Domei Yakazu was selected and was regarded as responsible for the publication, while the publication funding was secured; the Association of East-Asian Medicine, which had issued *"Kampotokan-yaku* 漢方と漢薬 *(Journal of Kampo Medicine and Crude Drug,)"* served as the publisher; Rin'ichi Kiga of *"Kampotokan-yaku* 漢方と漢薬 *(Journal of Kampo Medicine and Crude Drug)"* was recommended as the editor. Finally on September 1, 1954, "*KamponoRinsho* 漢方の臨床 (*Journal of Kampo Medicine*)" vol.1, No.1 was released. Since then, this journal has been continuously and uneventfully issued, did reach Vol. 67 in 2020, and is highly evaluated as a typical Oriental medicine magazine in Japan.

Other Academic Activities

Japan Kampo Society: Founded in 1968 as the Western Japan Kampo Society by the Hiroshima Kampo Society (広島漢方研究会), the Kampo Society (かんぽう会), the Kinki Kampo Society (近畿漢方研究会), the Kagoshima Kampo Society (鹿児島漢方研究会), and the Kyushu Kampo Society (九州漢方研究会), its first inaugural meeting and academic conference were held in the same year. Renamed as the Japan Kampo Society and supported by nine Kampo societies, the society holds general meetings annually and issues its journal, *"Kinki* 金匱 *(Golden Chamber (abbreviated))."* Since 2002, the Japan Kampo Society also annually holds the Forum on Chronic and Intractable Diseases.

International academic activities have also been actively pursued; the International Society of Oriental Medicine (ISOM) was established in 1975 as an international academic society joined mainly by traditional medicine clinicians and researchers in Japan, Korea, and Taiwan, which holds its society meetings once in 2–3 years. In 2009, the International Society for Japanese Kampo Medicine (ISJKM) was established in London (now headquartered in Germany) to promote academic exchange among practitioners and researchers of Japanese Kampo throughout the world, holding its academic meetings on a periodic basis.

2.1.9 Establishment of Education and Research Bases

It is evident that education and research facilities play an important role in Kampo medicine to develop wisdom. Major facilities are picked up here in the order of establishment, and their activities are briefly summarized.

Oriental Medicine Research Center of Kitasato Institute (now Kitasato University Oriental Medicine Research Center)

The center was established in 1972 as the first comprehensive research institute for Oriental medicine in Japan. The first Director was Keisetsu Otsuka. On March 8, 1986, the center became the first Japanese institution to be designated as a WHO Collaborating Center for Traditional Medicine. Since then pioneering activities have been carried out.

Toyama Medical and Pharmaceutical University and Research Institute for WAKAN-YAKU (now Institute of Natural Medicine, University of Toyama)

The university and research institute were founded in 1975 and 1978, respectively, in the place of Toyama abundant in pharmaceutical industries with a long history and tradition. A Department of Japanese Oriental (Kampo) Medicine (和漢診療学講座) was originated here with the inaugural professor of Katsutoshi Terasawa. The Institute has been designated as a WHO Collaborating Center for Traditional Medicine.

Kinki University Research Institute of Oriental Medicine

The institute started as a Kampo-specialized research institution under the direct control of Kinki University in Osakasayama, Osaka, in 1975, when Kinki University Hospital was also opened. The first professor for the Department of Oriental Medicine was Shigeru Arichi. The Research Institute consisted of the basic research division (in which Oriental medicine [Kampo] is earnestly studied) and the clinical practice division (in which clinical treatment is conducted), aiming to contribute to the improvement and enhancement of medical care.

Hyogo Prefectural Institute of Oriental Medicine and Affiliated Clinic

In 1976, the Oriental Medicine Laboratory was established at Hyogo Prefectural Amagasaki Hospital, which started Kampo and acupuncture therapies, followed by the establishment of the Institute of Oriental Medicine (inaugural head physician of Katsuhiko Matsumoto) in 1977. In 1981, the Department of Oriental Medicine was established at Amagasaki Hospital to provide Kampo therapy under health insurance, and not only clinical but also basic research was conducted at the institute. This was the first time that a general hospital, not a university hospital, had an outpatient clinic specializing in Kampo therapy and an institute of Oriental medicine. After transfer to Hyogo Prefectural Amagasaki General Medical Center, the Institute of Oriental Medicine and its affiliated clinics were abolished in June 2015 and reorganized as the Department of Chinese Medicine and the Acupuncture and Moxibustion Therapy Clinic.

Ehime Prefectural Central Hospital Institute of Oriental Medicine

The institute was established in 1989 by the inaugural director, Hidehiko Mitsufuji. Since then, clinical practice and research work of Oriental medicine (acupuncture, moxibustion, and Kampo) have been carried out under a unique policy that patients to be treated are "those who have had long-lasting health problems (agony and agony-derived anxiety), which have not been resolved by any medical treatment at hand," or "those with chronic health impairment." With the relocation of the new hospital in 2013, the institute was reorganized to establish two new departments (i.e., the Department of Kampo Medicine and Acupuncture and Moxibustion Therapy Clinic).

Institute of Oriental Medicine, Tokyo Women's Medical University School of Medicine

The institute was opened in 1992 with Hiroshi Obata named inaugural director and provided with a health improvement facility and a clinical facility for acupuncture and moxibustion. Its aim is to practice Kampo which bridges Oriental medicine and Western medicine.

2.1.10 Transition of the Medical System and Its Background

The medical system that is the core of social security systems was greatly changed soon after the war: the National Health Insurance system was implemented in 1961. Since then, Kampo therapy had gradually grown up to create a Kampo boom, which started in 1976 and lasted for some time.

Realization of the National Health Insurance System

The most remarkable event in Japan's medical and medical care systems after World War II was the realization of a National Health Insurance system. For Japanese public medical insurance, the basic scheme was formulated at the end of the Taisho period and was increasingly expanded in the Showa period, though to limited populations. The universal health insurance system benefiting the Japanese people started in 1961. Amazingly, 20 kinds of crude drugs were included in the drug tariff 2 years before, in 1959, which indicates that insured treatment with Kampo decoction (湯剤) using crude drugs (of limited kinds) has become possible.

Already prior to the start of the universal system, insurance benefits for Kampo therapy were frequently paid via consultation with the insurer. In 1941, a request from the Japanese Society of Kampo Medicine(日本漢方医学会)that the then insurance system should be revised for the future because the official prices for drugs as well as acupuncture and moxibustion did not satisfy necessary expenses.

The crude drugs added to the drug price list increased to 43 kinds in 1965 and jumped to approximately 200 kinds—sufficient for daily clinical practice—in 2020 today.

Appearance of Extracts

There was a trend that calls heightened for new and easy-to-handle dosage forms enabling oral dosing, not decoction. Reportedly Tadanao Nakayama, the author of *"Kampoigakunoshinkenkyu 漢方医学の新研究 (New Investigation of Kampo Medicine),"* insisted on the development of Kampo extract powder (エキス末) instead of decoction before the war.

As the inaugural Director of the Eastern Therapeutics Institute (東亜治療研究所) set up in the Fraternity Memorial Hospital (同愛記念病院) in 1943, Takeshi Itakura tried to confirm the efficacy of an experimentally prepared Kampo extract formulation on tuberculous pleurisy in a comparative clinical trial. The trial, reported to have proceeded to the clinical administration stage, was discontinued by the defeat of Japan. However, undoubtedly his studies somehow contributed to the manufacture and research of Kampo extract products that have been developed since soon after the war.

Among private medical institutions, Seikoen Hosono Clinic (Director, Shiro Hosono) of Kyoto created practical Kampo formulations soon after the war, with great expectation for a bright future of extract formulations. More specifically, as a Kampo institution based on modern medicine, the clinic originally developed and prepared a lot of extract products in a convenient form that matched the lifestyle desired by urban residents. Furthermore, the clinic was truly ahead of the extract formulations era that began more than 20 years later, in 1976. This foresight has been highly praised. It is also noted that Seikoen Hosono Clinic produced not a few Kampo physicians.

In 1957, the Ministry of Health and Welfare approved the Kampo extract powder at a time when there was no distinction between medical use and over-the-counter (OTC) Kampo extract powder. Ten years later in 1967, four kinds of ethical Kampo extract products were first listed in the drug tariff. These Kampo products were initially used only by a few Kampo physicians but have been increasingly called for by ordinary people.

Drug Tariff Listing of Kampo Medicines

The situation changed completely in 1976 when as many as 42 kinds of Kampo extract products were listed in the drug tariff under a classification of "ethical Kampo products." This led general physicians unfamiliar with Kampo medicines to the wide use of Kampo products and also researchers in various fields to the evaluation of the efficacy of those products. Kampo medicines became officially evaluated as drugs.

Thereafter, the number of tariff-listed Kampo products has increased progressively, reaching 148 prescriptions and a total of more than 800 products in 2000.

The number of crude drugs that were first listed in the drug tariff in 1960 also increased to approximately 200 at the present time. These drugs are totally or partially covered by public health insurance under the Western medicine system. The possible reason is that the efficacy and safety of ethical Kampo products have become recognized as solid evidence and accepted among a large number of medical doctors who rely on Western medicine.

Drug Tariff Deletion Problem

Increases in medical care and welfare costs have been noticed by the Japanese government since 1965 and became abruptly manifest in 1973 when free medical care for the elderly was introduced. Soon later in 1976, massive Kampo extract formulations were included in the drug tariff, as mentioned above. Under these integrated situations, the government attributed the cost increase partly to the increase in extract formulations. Concretely, as reported in 1983, the then subordinate officer Yoshimura announced that stomachic digestant (健胃消化剤), combination cold remedies (総合感冒薬), cataplasm (パップ剤) and Kampo products would be removed from the drug tariff. This proposal may have derived from the speculation that Kampo extract formulations were exempted from clinical trials usually required before the tariff listing because of their long-year use as therapeutics in Japan. It must have been considered that the conditions were unfair for Kampo products as compared with Western new drugs that must pass through strict clinical studies. In addition, there was an institutional principle that since some of the OTC Kampo medicines available in pharmacies after the Meiji period were practically as efficacious as ethical Kampo medicines, such medicines should not be covered by health insurance. These two reasons were repeatedly informed to medical care professionals and the pharmaceutical industry association, which were forced to take measures each time.

Japanese Association of Clinical Kampo Physicians (日本臨床漢方医会)

The tariff deletion problem of Kampo products resurfaced in 1993. In the same year, when the Council on Medical Insurance announced "how to provide the drugs analogous to OTC drugs" in the form of a proposal, the movement toward deletion became more evident in the review of fiscal 1997 insurance benefits. To stop non-coverage by insurance, it is necessary to take political measures. However, for the academic association, JAOM to conduct political activities was difficult. Thus a profit organization of the Japanese Association of Clinical Kampo Physicians was set up in November 1997 to act instead of JAOM. In only 1 week, about 240 promoters gathered, and 2 weeks later more than 1000 members joined, showing how many people are concerned about the crisis of insured Kampo clinical practice.

Adverse Effects Problem for Shosaikoto (小柴胡湯)

On March 1, 1996, the Ministry of Health and Welfare announced the occurrence of interstitial pneumonia in 88 patients who had taken shosaikoto since 1994, resulting in death of 10 patients. Shosaikoto has been mainly used for the "improvement of hepatic dysfunction and chronic gastrointestinal disturbance in chronic hepatitis." The use of this Kampo medicine has already been reported to induce the onset of interstitial pneumonia in patients with chronic hepatitis. In April 1991, the package insert contained a sentence regarding the possible onset of interstitial pneumonia in the section on adverse effects of precautions. In December 1992, precaution against interstitial pneumonia was mentioned more above in the section on "general precaution." Since March 1992, indications for interferon α and β have been extended to chronic active hepatitis type C. Because their combined use with shosaikoto had been reported to cause interstitial pneumonia in several patients, the use of interferon α and shosaikoto was contraindicated in January 1994. Nevertheless, during the subsequent 2 years, the disease newly occurred in 88 patients, of whom 10 died. This led to the announcement mentioned above.

Usually, therapeutic drugs entail more or less adverse effects or reactions. However, the announcement regarding Shosaikoto provoked sharp reactions from Japanese people as well as the media, far beyond the anticipation of the people concerned. This incident suddenly awakened the consciousness of medical care professionals, who clearly realized the fact that they had been content with a myth that Kampo medicines are safe therapeutics.

This issue and the tariff deletion problem had the same root: ethical Kampo products, represented by shosaikoto, had been listed in the drug tariff without undergoing fundamental clinical trials. This historical fact may have amplified the severe public reactions in Japan after the announcement of accumulative data on adverse drug reactions.

Clinical Evidence of Kampo Therapy

The historical element common to the tariff deletion and Shosaikoto adverse effects problems was obviously the tariff listing of Kampo medicines without efficacy evidence in clinical trials. In other words, clinical evidence of Kampo medicines as therapeutic drugs was demanded. This demand is clearly understood in consideration of the fact that therapeutics able to be covered by the existing insurance are not called for deletion from the tariff due to increased medical care costs or adverse drug reactions (of which the incidences are within medical common sense). Kampo medicine professionals were required to make collective efforts to present the results (i.e., evidence) demonstrating the efficacy of Kampo medicines in clinical studies.

Individual research institutions started conducting clinical studies actively. In 1991, the then Ministry of Health and Welfare notified the reevaluation of eight items of ethical Kampo extract formulation: orengedokuto, keisikashakuyakuto, shakuyakukanzoto, shosaikoto, shoseiryuto, daiokanzoto, byakkokaninjinto, and rikkunshito. Sequentially, placebo-controlled, double-blind comparative clinical studies of these Kampo medicines are being conducted.

Activities of JAOM Evidence-Based Medicine Committee [8]

In 2001, the Evidence-based Medicine (EBM) Committee was constituted in JAOM. The aim was to show that already pervading clinical treatment with Kampo medicines is "EBM" by demonstrating the efficacy of Kampo therapy, which has been asked for by people living in Japan.

Prior to the setup of the EBM Committee, many clinical studies had been conducted, and most of their results had been reported in overseas as well as domestic medical journals. Therefore, the initial objective of the committee was to compile a large body of evidence in a book via categorizing by defined clinical field, evaluating, and summarizing the results. Of 3014 reports published between 1986 and 2001, 833 reports were divided into the defined categories, and each report was reviewed to finally select robust evidence reports, totaling 93. These 93 papers were then submitted to the JAOM board of directors, and the final EBM Committee report was submitted to the Ministry of Health and Welfare and other agencies concerned in 2005. Thereafter, revisions have been continuously made. In 2020 today, structured abstracts and evaluations with signs of reviewers are published both in English and Japanese on the JAOM website and are free and accessible for everybody everywhere in the world.

As a result of these efforts, clinical evidence of Kampo therapy became widely recognized, and the Kampo products being used also became appreciated as drugs with established efficacy.

Establishment of the Japan Liaison of Oriental Medicine (JLOM)

The movement surrounding Japan's traditional medicine did not stay in Japan but became involved in waves of the latest globalization in the traditional medicine of China and other East-Asian countries. This was a historical trend. Since the 1990s, while expectations for complementary and alternative medicine have been heightened in the United States and Europe, worldwide expectations have been elevated for traditional medicine. China and Korea took a national policy of promoting the overseas presence of their own traditional medicine. In Japan, however, there was no administrative agency supervising traditional medicine in an academic manner. Thus as an international negotiator, the Japan Liaison of Oriental Medicine (JLOM) was born in 2005 from the association of four Japanese medical societies (i.e., Japan Society for Oriental Medicine, Medical and Pharmaceutical Society for WAKAN-YAKU, Japanese Society of Pharmacognosy, and Japan Society of Acupuncture and Moxibustion) and two WHO cooperative centers (i.e., Kitasato University Oriental Medicine Research Center and Department of Japanese Oriental Medicine, University of Toyama).

JLOM became responsible for establishing a national support system for Japanese traditional medicine, classifying traditional medicine in the 11th revision of the International Classification of Diseases (ICD-11), and cooperating in international standardization of raw materials and equipment related to traditional medicine (ISO/TC249). As of December 2020, JLOM was newly joined by six organizations (i.e., Japan Dental Society of Oriental Medicine, Japan Traditional Acupuncture and Moxibustion Society, Japan Acupuncture & Moxibustion Association, Japan College Association of Oriental Medicine, All Nippon Acupuncture & Moxibustion Massage Association, and Japan Society of Acupuncture Course in Universities). In this way, the foundation for international negotiations has finally been laid for Japan's traditional medicine, and a system for dealing with the difficulties that arise in the age of internationalization solidified.

The International Classification of Diseases (ICD) is a classification of diseases, injuries, and causes of death established by WHO. In Japan, the ICD is used as a classification standard for official statistics (vital statistics and patient surveys) and medical record management. The 11th revision of the International Classification of Diseases (ICD-11) was adopted by the WHO General Assembly in May 2019, and a new section on traditional medicine was introduced as a supplementary chapter. It is of great historical significance that the classification of pathological conditions in traditional East-Asian medicine, including Japanese traditional medicine, was recognized by WHO for the first time. Consequently, however, the differences and standardization of Japanese, Chinese, and Korean traditional medicine classifications drew attention.

ISO/TC249 is a technical committee established within the International Organization for Standardization (ISO) in 2009 to establish international standards for herbal medicines and preparations, acupuncture and moxibustion equipment (needles, moxa, etc.), diagnostic equipment used in traditional medicine, and related medical information with the aim of promoting international distribution in East-Asian traditional medicine. Five working groups have been set up, focusing on the quality and safety of raw materials and traditional processing, the quality and safety of manufactured TCM products, the quality and safety of acupuncture needles, the quality and safety of medical devices other than acupuncture needles, and terminology and informatics. It is essential to ensure that standards are based on scientific evidence and historical facts so that the future development of traditional Japanese medicine will not be hindered.

2.1.11 Revolution in the Medical Education System

Kampo Education in Universities

After the war, a Kampo-related regular course was first set up in Toyama Medical and Pharmaceutical University (now University of Toyama Faculty of Medicine) among medical universities and faculties/schools of medicine. Toyama Medical and Pharmaceutical University was founded in 1975, and 4 years later in 1979, Wakan Clinic (和漢診療室、wakan-shinryoshitsu) was opened in the University Hospital. The inaugural head of the clinic was Katsutoshi Terasawa, who was invited from Chiba University. In 1983, the name of "Wakan Clinic" was changed to Wakan Shinryobu (和漢診療部), then to Department of Japanese Oriental Medicine (和漢診療科) in 2004.

In 1990, the professorship was placed in the University Hospital Wakan Shinryobu (first professor Katsutoshi Terasawa). In 1993, the Department of Japanese Oriental Medicine was set up in the Faculty of Medicine. Thereafter in 2005, the University was integrated with another university and a college and turned its name to the University of Toyama. Toyama is traditionally famous for the pharmaceutical industry and is characterized by promoting research and education of Kampo medicine, providing many persons with talent or skills to the world.

Model Core Curriculum [7]

The medical education model core curriculum issued in 2001 by the Ministry of Education, Culture, Sports, Science, and Technology was epoch-making in emphasizing the necessity that any schools/faculties of medicine and medical universities should offer medical students a core curriculum in which "ability to outline WAKAN-YAKU can be acquired" in an appropriate period until graduation. This led all of the 80 schools/faculties of medicine and medical universities in Japan to provide a proper education for Kampo medicines. The knowledge of Kampo medicines excluded by the Cabinet more than 140 years before was revived in medical education after a long absence.

In the 2011 revision, a revision of the "ability to outline the characteristics and use of WAKAN-YAKU (Kampo medicines) can be acquired" was made. More than 10 years after the issue, the number of medical doctors experiencing lectures on Kampo medicine in universities has gradually increased in clinical settings. Ethical Kampo products, like Western drugs, have been smoothly accepted in clinical practice as therapeutics. However, Kampo lecture hours in universities are still insufficient, and recently an increasing number of relevant persons have emphasized the importance of Kampo in postgraduate education.

In the field of pharmaceutical sciences as well, especially pharmacy, education of Kampo medicines and Kampo medicine is essential, as is described as "crude drugs and Kampo medicines in modern medical care" in the 2002 core curriculum of a pharmaceutical education model. As a result, learning a broader range of knowledge became needed in addition to conventional pharmacognosy, medical botany, and natural product chemistry. This consequence is reasonable, given that Kampo medicines and crude drugs are pharmaceutical products being used in medical practice. In 2006, pharmaceutical education for training pharmacists extended from 4 to 6 years, and greater emphasis has been placed on pharmaceutical health care including Kampo in pharmaceutical education.

In addition, the dental education model core curriculum revised in 2016 states, "Understand basics of the drug (including WAKAN-YAKU) actions." In 2017, the nursing education model core curriculum also stated, "Be able to explain the actions, mechanisms, indications, adverse events, and nursing assistance of WAKAN-YAKU (Kampo medicines)." Thus, an era has arrived in which the necessity of understanding Kampo medicines has been widely advocated as part of the educational curriculum in medical fields (see section D, "Transition and current status of Kampo education" of this chapter for details).

Problems in the Prescription of Kampo Medicines

Although the widespread use of ethical Kampo products has been almost half a century, so-called abuse or disorder occurs in prescription. Kampo medicines are originally decoction, of which formulas were defined in a traditional "manner" and did not deviate largely. However, with the appearance of simple and convenient extract formulations, the combined use of more than two formulations (of which the necessity is doubtful) has occurred without difficulty. This situation will last until new "manners" for the prescription of extract formulations are established and spread. Novel development or innovation is expected to utilize Kampo extract formulations—therapeutics derived from precious natural resources—efficiently and effectively.

2.1.12 Change in Social Thinking

In retrospect in postwar history, the driving force that has pushed forward Kampo medicine is obviously the expectation of Japanese people for Kampo medicines. Facing disasters of environmental pollution and drug poisoning in the rapid economic growth period starting in around 1960, the people promptly found out the fragility of an industrialized society and sought to restore the deteriorating natural environment. Such a movement of mind was very common to the Japanese, consistent with the spirit of keeping healthy by combining natural products (crude drugs).

As a result of the so-called governmental screening of budget requests abruptly carried out in 2009, a designated working group was reported to have reached a conclusion that "OTC drug analogs should be excluded from the coverage of the National Health Insurance." This action was regarded as a novel "exclusion of Kampo medicines from the reimbursement," and ignited the aspiration of people for Kampo therapy, as evidenced by a total of 924,808 signatures collected in a short period of about 2 weeks. People did not want to purchase Kampo medicines according to the instructions of a guidebook but did clearly express their desire to take Kampo medicines as the drugs prescribed on the basis of established diagnoses by experienced physicians. And they also have confidence that Kampo therapy will be a medical treatment able to better protect their health in the future perspective of higher quality medical care in Japan. We must keenly realize our obligation to fulfill their expectations as Kampo specialists.

Column

Prominent Kampo Physicians

Manase Dosan

Yoshihide Yakazu and Masayuki Kashima

Late Muromachi Period to Azuchi-Momoyama Period

In the Muromachi period, Japan had increasing relationships with Ming (China)[11]. Japanese physicians who studied in China[12] and their disciples took the lead in the medical association ~~field~~ in Japan. In those days, the nation's medical systems were collapsing due to many wars. However, this situation was greatly improved by Manase Dosan. He introduced available Chinese medicine to Japan and established its practice.

Manase, the Pioneer

Manase systematized the theories of the traditional Chinese medicine of the Ming Dynasty. Running the Keiteki-in School for medical education, he was well treated by men of power in the warring period, including Oda Nobunaga and Toyotomi Hideyoshi.

Born in Kyoto, Studied Under a Famous Physician in Kanto District, and Returned to Kyoto

Manase was born in Yanagihara, Kamigyo-ku, Kyoto, in 1507 and studied at Shokoku-ji Temple, one of the five most important Rinzai temples of Kyoto. At the age of 23, he traveled to study at Ashikaga School in Tochigi Prefecture, where he learned profoundly. He also studied medicine under the tutelage of famous physicians in the Kanto District, including Tashiro Dodo and Sanki.[13] When he was 39 years old, he returned to Kyoto and started a medical practice.

Being highly honored as a good physician, he examined Emperor Ogimachi and men of power in the warring period, including Ashikaga Yoshiaki and Mori Motonari. He also provided medical care for Oda Nobunaga, Toyotomi Hideyoshi, and others, winning their confidence. He also had good relationships with Sen No Rikyu and other intellectuals.

"*Keitekishu*"啓迪集 (Collected Teachings)

Manase was active in the sixteenth century, and this period was characterized by the spread of book culture to the general public, which had previously been limited to the nobility and temples. In those days, the majority of books available in Japan were comprised of Japanese manuscripts that had been handed down from the earlier Heian and Kamakura periods, as well as Chinese books (literature written in classical Chinese) exported from China and Korea. Despite this, books written in Japanese by Manase Dosan gained popularity.

Manase wrote many books. He drew from a broad range of medical texts published in the Ming Dynasty, especially those of the Zhu Danxi[14] School, and he systematized their contents using medical principles unique to Japan. His most renowned book, *Keitekishu* 啓迪集 (*preface provided by himself in 1574*), is a great compilation of Manase's medicine. He also wrote formula compendia *Shuho Kiku* 衆方規矩[15] and *Shussho Haizai*出証配剤, the former being com-

[11]The Ming Dynasty (1368–1662) lasted for about 300 years. This corresponds to the Muromachi period to the first half of the Edo period in Japan. As such, Ming medicine represents the precursor to modern Chinese medicine, and it also led to the Gosei School of Japanese Kampo medicine.

[12]These include Takeda Shokei, Gekko (priest physician), Tashiro Sanki, and Nakarai Akichika. However, all relevant literary materials were based solely on Japanese traditions, thus representing something groundbreaking. It appears, therefore, that not so many actually studied abroad.

[13]Although some authors identify Dodo as Tashiro Sanki, this is incorrect. The two persons differed in identity; a likely story is, "Dodo studied abroad in China and returned back to Japan with knowledge in medicine of the Jin and Yüan Dynasties, and Tashiro studied and spread it."

[14]Zhu Danxi, one of the four great authorities of the medicine of the Jin and Yüan Dynasties (see page 13).

[15]At present, it is almost denied that the *Shuho Kiku* was written by the first Manase. In the Manase School, the name Manase Dosan was succeeded over generations by the head. It is conjectured that this book was dictated by Okamoto Genya (1587–1645), the third Manase, who was a disciple of Manase Gensaku (the second Manase), and edited by Okamoto's disciple (Endo et al., Research on *Shuho Kiku* (in Japanese), Kampo Med. 56(3)435–444, 2005).

monly distributed in Japan in the Edo period. Other books he wrote include the medicine books *Yakusho Nodoku* 薬性能毒 and *Gikinhonzo* 宜禁本草; the health maintenance books *Yojo Haikai* 養生俳諧 and *Koso Myoron* 黄素妙論; and the acupuncture/moxibustion book *Shinkyu Shuyo* 鍼灸集要. The specialized book *Kareishoniho* 遐齢小児方 (pediatric formulas) is known as Japan's first pediatric textbook. None had been so familiar with such a broad range of medical knowledge before Manase.

Gosei School and *Sassho Benchi*

The aforementioned *Keitekishu* 啓迪集 is also known as *Sassho Benchi Keitekishu* 察証弁治啓迪集. The term *sassho benchi* means, "Carefully observe the pattern and determine the appropriate treatment," or "Individual patient conditions should be diagnosed in detail to determine appropriate treatments."

This concept emphasized practical aspects, such as drug use, rather than abstract theorizations, thus establishing a methodology based on direct observations of signs and symptoms. It developed into the Gosei School, which was based on Ming medicine.

Note that the term "*bensho ronchi*" is used in Chinese medicine, conveying nearly the same meaning as Manase's "*sassho benchi*." It is surprising that Manase used this term in Japan much earlier than in China.

Open, Step-by-Step Education

Manase not only systematized the latest knowledge about Chinese medicine using his own theoretical basis "*sassho benchi*," but also endeavored to provide systematic education. Manase's education is characterized by openness to the public and step-by-step progress.

Books written by Tashiro Sanki, the master of Manase, contained many terms and phrases based on strange Chinese characters of his own creation that could only be understood by his disciples. Hence, his books held mysteries that could not be understood without knowing the special writing rules. Manase, on the other hand, made easy-to-understand descriptions without abstruse terms, and his writings were openly available to the public.

However, this did not mean limitless publication but was to be learned step-by-step according to the level of the student. Specifically, his education took place in nine steps, from the introductory book *Kirigami* 切紙 to the highest-level *Keitekishu* 啓迪集. His disciples were not allowed to learn the content of each step until clearing the previous step. This highly systematized and manualized educational approach produced many prominent disciples, including Manase Gensaku.

Yoshimasu Todo

Yoshihide Yakazu and Masayuki Kashima

Middle Edo Period/Koho School

Until the first third of the Edo period, the Gosei School (led by Manase Dosan and others) was the mainstream. In the second third, casual handbooks appeared and began to be criticized. In addition, there was a rapid increase in patients with syphilis and smallpox in this period, which were very difficult to treat with the medicines available. Furthermore, in those days, there was a boom of *Shanghanlun* 傷寒論 research in China, which reached the cities of Edo and Kyoto in Japan in the last half of the seventeenth century. A reformation campaign of "return to the old" was being conducted in schools of Confucianism. This influenced the medical world and spurred research of the *Shanghanlun* 傷寒論 as the starting point for classical medicine.

In this context, starting in the mid-Edo period, the Koho School emerged as a new school of medicine in which traditional medical principles were denied. Otherwise, the *Shanghanlun* 傷寒論 was most valued as the source of ideal medicine. This new trend extended into the mainstream of Kampo medicine[16].

A Revolutionist

Being a great authority of the Koho School, which involved various views, Yoshimasu Todo did not restore the principles of the *Shanghanlun* 傷寒論. Instead, he refuted traditional medical principles and established a completely new methodology by "identifying the principles of treatment" as described in the *Shanghanlun* 傷寒論 (detailed below).

Yoshimasu Todo was born in Aki Province (present-day Hiroshima Prefecture) in 1702 and was named Tamenori. His penname was initially Toan and then changed to Todo. After deciding to become a physician at 19 years of age, he devoted himself to researching the formulas of the *Shanghanlun* 傷寒論 and *Jingui Yaolüe* 金匱要略 for their high efficacy. He came to doubt the Yin-Yang and the five elements theory while studying classic texts. In his 30s, he worked to build his own medical system based on the *Shanghanlun* 傷寒論 and "*Jingui Yaolüe* 金匱要略 (detailed below). Thereafter, he ambitiously moved to Kyoto and started his practice at 37 years of age. Although he initially lived in poverty, his practice grew, and the number of disciples increased. He eventually became a leading physician of the mid-Edo period.

[16] In modern Japanese Kampo medicine, the mainstream approach focuses on the Koho School. Pathophysiological analysis, however, is not placed in a black box but includes the "qi, blood, fluid" concept. Nevertheless, this was not basically introduced as a concept for pathophysiological analysis but as a system to categorize groups of symptom combinations and choices of formulas for their indications. Furthermore, presently in Kampo medicine, formulas of the Gosei School and principles of Chinese medicine are included. Thus, the barriers between schools have been eliminated.

"All Diseases Single Poison Theory" and Formulas Corresponding to Pattern Identification

Yoshimasu proposed the "all diseases single poison theory," that all diseases stem from one toxin. Additionally, he insisted, "All medicines are poisons, and poisons should be controlled with poisons." Thus he administered his treatments using potent medicines. He used a mercury drug with high side effects[17] in his practice. Some patients died from treatment with the drug due to its high toxicity. Yoshimasu claimed, however, that "physicians who treat disease with poisonous drugs are not liable for the outcome, whether the patient lives or dies, because it is destiny" (the Theory of Destiny)." He thus stirred up a great debate.

Yoshimasu denied the Yin-Yang and the five elements theory and placed the pathophysiological aspects of disease into a "black box" without analyzing them. Accordingly, he introduced a completely new system of "choosing formulas suitable to combinations of signs and symptoms" (detailed below), thus establishing the concept of "*hosho sotai*" (formula corresponding to pattern identification).[18] Thereafter, the mainstream of Kampo medicine increasingly relied on this concept of "*hosho sotai*," rather than the conventional theoretical basis of the Manase School.

"Ruijuho 類聚方*"* and *"Yakucho* 薬徵*"*

Disciple Tsuru Genitsu organized Yoshimasu's medical theories and published them in a book titled "*Idan*" later in 1759, which produced a sensation. This is because this book included the aforementioned medical theories (medical principles) unique to Yoshimasu Todo. This medical system that denied the Yin-Yang and five elements theory and used the "all diseases single poison theory," to control poison (pathogen) with poison (medicine) was introduced to the general public at large. This created a dispute between the pros and cons in the medical world.

Additionally, Yoshimasu edited *Ruijuho* 類聚方 in 1751, disassembling the contents of the *Shanghanlun* 傷寒論 and *Jingui Yaolüe* 金匱要略. He re-edited the passages concerning the 220 formulas mentioned therein and described their indications. This completely new methodology based on "selected rules of medical treatment" was successful in clinical practice and thus became the rule (criteria/model) for the use of classical formulas.

Yoshimasu made the greatest effort to write *Yakucho*. Likewise with *Ruijuho* 類聚方, Yoshimasu selected formulas from among those described in *Shanghanlun* 傷寒論 and *Jingui Yaolüe* 金匱要略 to find ingredients in common use in both books and identified common efficacies from the descriptions in these classics. Examples include saiko (Bupleurum root) for fullness and discomfort in the chest and hypochondrium, calcium sulfate for severe thirst, and ginseng for epigastric stuffiness and resistance. This style of describing the effects of ingredients differed markedly from that in herbal medicine texts and is characterized by direct correspondence to signs. Among the books by Yoshimasu, *Yakucho* 薬徵 may be said to have had the greatest impact on later history. Asada Sohaku's *Koho Yakugi* 古方薬議 is said to have been written with hints from *Yakucho* 薬徵.

Importance of Abdominal Examination

Yoshimasu set the goal of curing a disease with "poisons" using potent drugs to eliminate toxins. Accordingly, he described the identity of these toxins as "what is invisible and silent." On the other hand, he specified "what is visible" to be "that which can be observed by abdominal examination." Accordingly, he considered that abdominal examination was the best way to understand the existence of "poison" as a visible reality. For this reason, he placed importance on abdominal examination, based on which he administered his treatments. He states in the abdominal sign section of *Idan* as follows: "The abdomen is the essential part of the body for life, all diseases have root causes here."

Asada Sohaku

Yoshihide Yakazu, Masayuki Kashima, and Koji Watanabe

End of Edo Period to Meiji Restoration

Asada Sohaku was active in the days of dramatic historical changes, from the end of the Edo period to the Meiji Restoration (beginning of the Meiji Era). Being highly skilled in clinical practice, Asada earned trust not only from the Shogunate in Edo but also from the Meiji Government. Based on its medical policy, however, the Meiji Government formulated an act to abolish Kampo physicians in 1875. The Examination for Practicing Medicine (present National Examination for Medical Practitioners) exclusively concerned Western medicine, and all physicians had to be knowledgeable of Western medicine.

Kampo physicians organized themselves to protest this medical policy; their aim was "political renaissance of Kampo medicine." Under the leadership of Yamada Gyoko, Asada Sohaku, Mori Risshi, and others, Onchisha (an association of Kampo physicians) was formed to drive the Kampo survival campaign, but their aim was not realized.

Last Prominent Figure in Kampo Medicine in Meiji Era

At the end of the Edo period, Odai Yodo and Asada Sohaku were the two great physicians in the capital of Edo. Asada was allowed to attend the Shogun when he was 41 years old (promoted from a town doctor). At age 47, he had an

[17] In those days, syphilis was prevalent not only in Japan but also in the rest of the world, and mercury drugs were the standard treatment; no antibiotics were available.

[18] This means that there should be a one-to-one correspondence between Kampo medicine formulas and Kampo medicinal diagnoses (patterns).

audience with the 14th Shogun Iemochi. He was then appointed as a "*goten-i* (medical doctor employed by the Shogun). At age 52, he earned the trust of *Oo*ku (Shogun's harem in Edo Castle) to take the position of *Hogen* (deputy chief physician serving the Shogunate). In those days, the status of physicians serving in high positions for the Shogunate was usually patrimonial. With his clinical expertise, Asada promoted himself from a town doctor to the *Hogen*.

His position was secure even after the historical change from the Edo Shogunate to the Meiji Government. Asada, the last Kampo physician for the Crown Prince, served Emperor Taisho[19] in his childhood and was called "the last prominent figure in the Meiji Era."

As a digression, there is a well-known brand name, "ASADA-AME," a sweet that was named after Asada. Studying under Asada, Horiuchi Isaburo (the founder of ASADA-AME Co., Ltd.) had the starch syrup formula transferred from Asada. In 1887, he launched it with the name "*Okusuri Sarashi Mizuame*" (bleached starch syrup medicine), but it did not sell as expected. Then, he relaunched the product with the new name "ASADA-AME" in 1889. This was a great commercial success and made it a long seller, even to the present day.

Studied Old Formulas in Kyoto and Learned About *Koshogaku* (Evidential Textual Research) in Edo

Asada Sohaku was born in 1815 at Chikuma-gun, Shinshu (presently Matsumoto, Nagano Prefecture), as the third-generation medical practitioner succeeding his grandfather. His first name was Tadatami, then Koretsune. He was officially given the courtesy name Shikishi and nicknamed Sohaku.[20] He pennamed himself Ritsuen after his native land.

When he was 18 years old, Asada traveled to Kyoto to study, where he interacted with many people studying and discussing the *Shaghanlun* 傷寒論. His cohorts included students of the private school of Nakanishi Shinsai (a leading disciple of Yoshimasu Todo and a great authority on the interpretation of *Shaghanlun*), as well as students of the school of Kawagoe Kozan (a leading disciple of Nakanishi Shinsai who established his own school) and students of Yoshimasu's school who learned directly from Yoshimasu. In effect, Asada absorbed the concepts of various schools through Yoshimasu.

When he was 22 years old, Asada started a medical practice in Edo and then met the Shogunate medical officer Motoyasu Soen[21]. Motoyasu introduced him to the three great physicians in the medical world in Edo in those days, i.e., Taki Genken, Kojima Gakko, and Kitamura Naohiro, who belonged to the Koshogaku (evidential textual research) School. Thus, Asada had increasing relationships with significant persons affiliated with the Edo Medical House.

Settchu School: A Compromise Between Classical Formulas and Koshogaku Schools

Asada belonged to the Setchu School of Kampo medicine and like many other Kampo physicians, placed the highest importance on the *Shaghanlun* 傷寒論. Furthermore, he had personal relationships with the physicians of the Edo Medical House, mainly those interested in *Koshogaku*, thus broadening his view from classical formulas to *Koshogaku*.

"Treatment should be based essentially classical old formulas[22], but the use of formulas of the Gosei School may be considered in some cases," Asada stated on the starting page of "Ritsuen's Teachings on Medicine" in his book *Kisso Shoei* 橘窓書影. He did not theoretically rely on the formulas of the Gosei School (using the theoretical basis for traditional Chinese medicine like Dosan).

Sohaku established a new system of medical practice with a broad scope, combining the theories of schools of Kyoto and Edo to make the best use of classical formulas and Koshogaku.

"Futsugo Yakushitsu Hokan" and *"Futsugo Yakushitsu Hokan Kuketsu"*

Asada wrote a great many books concerning medical science and practice, as well as medical history and even literature. In particular, two formula books, i.e., *Futsugo Yakushitsu Hokan* 勿誤薬室方函 and *Futsugo Yakushitsu Hokan Kuketsu* 勿誤薬室方函口訣 were valued as standard commentaries of Kampo formulas, which are very influential in modern Kampo medicine in Japan.

Futsugo Yakushitsu Hokan, a compendium of common formulas, is a direct source of modern Japanese Kampo formulas. Regarding Kampo extract preparations for ethical use, formulas are not always identical to those described in their original sources; some are based on crude drug compositions in the *Futsugo Yakushitsu Hokan* compendium. For example, *Anchusan* does not contain processed ginger but contains amomum seed. *Otsujito* does not contain ginger root or jujube fruit but contains angelica root. These formulas are based on crude drug compositions described in *Futsugo Yakushitsu Hokan* 勿誤薬室方函.

Accordingly, *Futsugo Yakushitsu Hokan Kuketsu* 勿誤薬室方函口訣, a text of notes of oral instructions, concisely

[19] Appointed as the attending physician for Emperor Taisho upon his nativity, Asada rescued the Emperor soon after birth, when he became critically ill with repeated convulsions by administering the Kampo medicine *Somato*.

[20] The name "Sohaku" was given by Motoyasu Soen.

[21] The name "Sohaku" was given by Motoyasu Soen.

[22] The Chinese character "法" was used in place of "方" in the original book.

stated prescribing goals for 579 common formulas, including classical formulas, formulas of the Gosei School, and traditional Japanese Kampo formulas, and is widely applied in modern times.

Asada also wrote a drug commentary book titled *Koho Yakugi* 古方薬議 (book of classical formulas). Although it is said to have been written based on concepts from Todo's *Yakucho* 薬徵, it does not exclusively focus on signs as in Todo's book[23], but has descriptions based partially on traditional medical theories. Calcium sulfate, for example, was described as "spicy in taste, cold in nature, capable of clearing heat," to explain the drug's essential indication. Perhaps, he was greatly influenced by Koshogaku.

These texts of Asada led to the reestablishment of Japanese Kampo medicine in the Showa Era that followed.

Kampo Medicine (*Keishikaryojyutsubuto*) Administered to the French Minister

Suffering low back pain, the French minister in Japan, Léon Roches, was treated by a famous physician of Western medicine but did not get any results. His condition was diagnosed as rheumatism by the physician and got increasingly worse with treatment. Eventually, the pain intensified to deprive the minister of sleep at night and made him unable to do his work satisfactorily. For this reason, the Shogunate directed Asada to treat the minister in 1865. Visiting the minister's house in Yokohama, Asada located the cause of disease in the spine by pulse examination. He asked the minister, "Did you experience bruises when you were young?" The minister answered, "I experienced many falls from my horse on battlefields 18 years ago." Then, Asada examined the patient's spine thoroughly and found two depressions. He diagnosed the painful condition as sequelae to bruises due to falls from the horse. He prescribed *Keishikaryojyutsubuto*, and the long-persisting lower back pain ceased completely in one week. Thereafter, Asada was bestowed with two watches and three carpets from the French Emperor Napoleon III[24]. He was highly praised in a French newspaper as "The great physician of Japan." His clinical skills became known to those outside Japan.

Kampo Ikkando Medicine

Yoshihide Yakazu and Keido Yakazu

The Origin of the Name Ikkando

Mori Dohaku (1867–1931), a Kampo physician who was active in the Meiji to Early Showa Periods in Japan, ran a clinic named *Ikkando Ryoin*. Ikkando was named after "Yusa Ikkando," the drug store of Yusa Kaishin[25], the master of Dohaku Mori. The word *Ikkan* originates from the phrase "consistency in one's way (吾道一貫)" in the Analects of Confucius. This indicates Mori's Dohaku steely resolve that he would go his own way to restore the fortunes of Kampo medicine, which had dramatically declined in his time.

Ikkando Medicine

Mori Dohaku's therapeutic philosophy in his late years was described by his student Yakazu Kaku, who published a book titled Kampo Ikkando Medicine in 1964[26]. This book mainly featured the "Classification of Constitutions by the Three Major Patterns" (blood™ stasis constitution, organ toxin constitution, and detoxicative constitution) and relevant treatments known as "*Goho*" (the five basic formulas *Tsudosan*, *Bofutsushosan*, *Saikoseikansan*, *Keigairengyoto*, and *Ryutanshakanto*). For this reason, the three major patterns and the five basic formulas (*Sandaisho Goho*) are often collectively called Ikkando medicine. However, this is nothing more than the therapeutic philosophy of Mori Dohaku in his late years, and the common use of the *Goho* is largely attributed to the historical context of those days (described below).

In fact, Mori Dohaku used not only the *Goho,* but also a broad range of other formulas. This is because Ikkando's "codex of standard medicine" was "*Kokonhoi*古今方彙 (*Collection of Ancient and Contemporary Prescriptions*)"[27]. Accordingly, he increased the therapeutic efficacy of his formulas by breaking the barrier between the *Koho* School formulas and *Gosei* School formulas and using them in combination with acupuncture and moxibustion. This is in marked contrast with Yumoto Kyushin (1876–1941), a Kampo physician in the same era as with Dohaku Mori, mainly using classic formulas with "*Shokanron* 傷寒論 (*Treatise on Cold Damage*)" as the bible for his practice.

The Three Major Patterns and the Five Formulas

The "Classification of Constitutions by the Three Major Patterns" was a unique therapeutic philosophy based on

[23]Yoshimasu described calcium sulfate as the "main treatment for severe thirst."

[24]The gifts from the French Emperor did not reach Asada because they were usurped by a government officer.

[25]Yusa Kaishin was an obstetrician in Miyagi Prefecture. Formerly, his given name was said to be Taishin. At present, his given name is written in kanji characters as "快慎" (on the posthumous Buddhist name monument) or "快真" (on the epitaph).

[26]Actually, based on the dictation by Yakazu Kaku, his younger brother Yakazu Yudo classified symptoms into three major patterns, and Yakazu Domei systematized this classification.

[27]A compendium of formulas edited by Koga Tsugen (1745). While the majority of formulas are listed in the Japanese text "*Manbyokaishun* 万病回春 (*Restoring Health from Myriad of Diseases*)," a large number (1229) of formulas are listed from 63 Chinese medical books. Since so many formulas, including classic formulas and *Gosei* School formulas, were classified by type of disease, this text gained greater popularity among general practitioners than "*Shuhokiku* 衆方規矩 (*Principles for a Multitude of Prescriptions*)."

"constitutional classification." In those days, there were two diseases that could not be cured in any way. They were tuberculosis and cerebral stroke (cerebrovascular disorder). To prevent these diseases, Mori Dohaku worked to establish a therapeutic philosophy involving some aspects of preventive medicine, which he outlined as follows:

Blood[TM1] stasis constitution

- Cause: Static blood[TM1]
- Focuses of prevention: Cerebral stroke, gastric ulcers, hemorrhoids, gynecopathy
- Treatments: *Tsudosan*[28] (actually, other formulas were also used, including *Kyukichoketsuindaiichikagen*, *Botanpisan*, and *Saikosokanto*, as well as the classic formulas *Tokishakuyakusan*, *Keishibukuryogan*, *Tokakujokito*, *Daiobotanpito*, *Geoketsugan*, *Daioshachugan*, and *Teitogan*)

Organ Toxin Constitution

- Causes: Food toxicity (accumulation of metabolic waste products) and fluid toxicity[29].
- Focuses on prevention: Lifestyle-related diseases such as arteriosclerosis, cerebral stroke, and kidney disease
- Treatment: *Bofutsushosan*

Detoxicative Pattern Constitution

- Cause: "The toxicity as mentioned herein is defined as toxicity eliminated with an antidote (*Shimotsuorengedokuto*), rather than as organ toxicity" and is deemed a heat toxicity requiring the use of a heat-clearing drug[30].
- Focuses on prevention: Infectious diseases such as tuberculosis and syphilis
- Treatment: Formulas, mainly *Shimotsuorengedokuto*[31]

These formulas are prescribed by combining the heat-clearing medicine *Orengedokuto* with *Shimotsuto*, which is used to ensure *kyufuku* (prolonged use of medicine). Other formulas are available based on this formula: *Saikoseikanto*, enriched with effects of clearing heat and detoxification and enriching yin qi; *Keigairengyoto*, enriched with effects of dispersing pathogenic wind and promoting pus discharge; and *Ryutanshakanto*, enriched with effects of *seikan shaka* (clearing liver heat) and fluid regulation.

In clinical practice, *Saikoseikansan* is used for children who are susceptible to bronchitis, tonsillitis, pharyngitis, rhinitis, and otitis media. *Keigairengyoto* is used for adolescents who are susceptible to tuberculosis, chronic sinusitis, otitis media, and neurosis. *Ryutanshakanto* is used for adults who are susceptible to sexually transmitted diseases such as gonorrhea, cystitis, and female urogenital disease.

These constitution classes and treatments are still now used for various diseases. For example, drugs in use for detoxification constitution can be applied to allergic diseases such as atopic dermatitis.

Waves of Prosperity and Living Environmental Changes due to the Pacific War

Concerning the historical context, the end of World War I was followed by unprecedented waves of prosperity, which changed the dietary habits of the Japanese people. They were encouraged to adopt diets of high nutritional density (particularly meat eating). Accordingly, the number of patients with cerebral stroke increased. Therefore, the number of patients with an organ toxin constitution increased. It can be guessed, therefore, that Mori Dohaku often prescribed *Bofutsushosankagen* in his later years.

However, after the death of Mori Dohaku and the start of World War II (Pacific War), food shortages led to a lack of nutrition in the public. In that situation, with people's mental stress and fatigue, warming and tonifying Kampo medicines became increasingly indicated. Therefore, his disciples were no longer able to use the Goho formulas, which are based on the concept of *kanryokoge* (heat clearing and purgative method). Although this situation persisted for some time after the end of the war, the Goho formulas became useful again at last in the ensuing period of rapid growth.

Hence, the pathological conditions varied depending on the daily life environment and dietary habits. Accordingly, the patterns vary, and the choice of treatments (formulas) varies. This represents the principles and general rules of Kampo medicine.

As described above, the "*Sandaisho Goho*" is nothing more than the therapeutic philosophy of Mori Dohaku in his later years, which was established owing much to the historical context. Additionally, it is quite interesting that this philosophy of treatment is unique to Japan, as it was established based on clinical experience rather than theoretical conceptualization.

Treatment of Spanish Flu

Beginning in 1918 during World War I, the pandemic of Spanish influenza (commonly known as Spanish flu) is his-

[28] Mori Dohaku used this formula for crush syndrome in victims of injuries from collapsing houses, etc., following the Great Kanto Earthquake. The use of this formula thus became established in Kampo medicine.

[29] Four organ toxicities were defined: food toxicity, wind toxicity, fluid toxicity, and syphilis.

[30] A constitution characterized by susceptibility to external stimulation and likely to develop inflammatory reactions. In terms of modern medicine, this condition is often characterized by chronic inflammation.

[31] This is similar to *Unseiin* but is more accurately described as *Shimotsutogoorengedokutoka-rengyo-saiko-kanzo*.

torically prominent for the vast damage it caused. In those days, when neither antibiotics nor antivirals had been discovered, a great many people in the world were killed by the pandemic. At that time, Mori Dohaku classified his patients into three types and treated them. He saved many lives by administering *Kososan-ka-hange-byakujyutsu-bukuryo* for the gastrointestinal type, administering *Shoseiryuto-ka-kyonin*-sekko (calcium sulfate) for the pneumonia type, and administering *Shomakakkonto-ka-byakushi-senkyu*-saishin for the encephalopathy type. These were prescriptions from Mori Dohaku's clinical practice and hence may be said to represent Ikkando medicine in its broad sense.

Extract Preparations Based on Ikkando's Formulas

- *Saikoseikanto*
- *Ryutanshakanto* (some Kampo extract preparations for ethical use have other sources)
- *Keigairengyoto*

3 Differences Between Kampo Medicine, Traditional Chinese Medicine, and Traditional Korean Medicine

Masayuki Kashima and Makoto Yoshitomi

3.1 Introduction

Traditional medicines that originated in ancient China spread from East Asia to Southeast Asia over their long spans of history. In each region, these medical practices evolved and developed in their own way. In Japan, the traditional medicine that emanated from ancient China is referred to generically as "Kampo," but it refers particularly to the practices that have developed in a uniquely Japanese way. In China, the name used in the same sense is traditional Chinese medicine (TCM), and in Korea, traditional Korean medicine. Each of these medical practices has its own distinctive features, but they have a lot in common. This includes the basic interpretations of classical scholarship that the medicines are based on, the terminology employed to describe basic concepts, the types of key formulas, and the diseases treated. This is because traditional medicines originating in ancient China have a long history of roughly two millennia, and despite there being some differences in detail between regions and historical periods, the existing traditional medicines of East Asia directly trace their practices to the mid to late Ming Dynasty (sixteenth to seventeenth century). Kampo medicine stands out among the traditional medicines of East Asia as one that has undergone a remarkable transformation especially in its concepts.

In this chapter, we set out to examine the salient differences between Kampo medicine and traditional Chinese and traditional Korean medicines. Because the main trends of Kampo medicine in Japan have undergone changes along with the tide of each historical era, the Kampo medicine referred to here is that which has been in mainstream practice after 1925 (Showa Period).

3.2 Differences Between Kampo Medicine and Traditional Chinese Medicine (TCM)

3.2.1 Ideas and Perspectives

The medicine that originated in ancient China believes that both nature, which is the macrocosm, and the human body, which is a microcosm, are formed of qi, the fundamental constituents of the universe. A system of qi circulation analogous to nature is believed to exist in the human body. Both these systems are thought to be governed by the laws of movements of qi. In nature, qi follows these laws of movement, creating movement and change constantly, as in the comings and goings of day and night or of the seasons. The qi in the body reacts in synchrony with nature. Through eating or breathing, both qi of nature and qi of the body constantly interchange with each other, inside and outside the human frame. In short, vital phenomena are viewed quintessentially as these movements and changes in qi. From this perspective of qi, good health is attaining a dynamic balance of qi inside and outside the body while maintaining a certain stable constancy. Disease is the state when this balance breaks down. This explains why Chinese medicine since ancient times has attempted to understand and explain human physiology and pathophysiology by applying the laws of qi movement.

Although on a continuum with this cosmology, TCM that is currently taught in Chinese universities does not directly refer to this but merely keeps to the application of theories that emerge from this perspective. What is different about Kampo medicine is that, despite acknowledging this cosmology to a certain degree, it deems the impact of laws of qi movement on the human body to be difficult to pinpoint accurately. Therefore, it mainly attempts to classify the physiological manifestations that can be assessed objectively and to work out the relationships between the classified manifestations and their therapies.

3.2.2 Academic Context

Principles of Yin and Yang and the Five Elements

The principles of Yin and Yang and the five elements form the basis of the philosophy of ancient China. These provide the principal rationales for the laws of nature and movements of qi, which govern nature and the human body. The principle of Yin and Yang notably is the cornerstone that is adopted by all traditional medicines of East Asia. In TCM, it is not only used in classification but is widely used as the most fundamental concept in explaining the mechanisms by which the laws operate. In Kampo medicine, however, although Yin and Yang are used for classification purposes, only the barest minimum reference is made to it in explanations of mechanisms. As to the principle of the five elements, Kampo medicine introduces it only as a method of classification and restricts its application to clinical practice. Differences exist in the extent to which this principle is used as an explanatory means for concepts among different traditional medicines outside Japan. That is, TCM and other medicines that originated from ancient China, according to the different stances they adopt.

Diagnostic System

In both TCM and Kampo medicine, diagnosis is the determination of the "pattern"—the diagnostic concept of the disease state (pathophysiology) unique to the traditional medicines of East Asia. Having said that, there is a huge difference in meaning between what this "pattern" means in Kampo medicine and in TCM. Pattern in TCM means the analysis of the pathophysiology, in short, what is causing the disease and how essential qi is changing in which system of the body. By contrast, pattern in Kampo medicine is the classification of indications of therapies, the classification of the patterns of vital reaction such as fever, and the combination of this with a corresponding method of therapy. This becomes most obvious in the consultation over medication formulas.

Regarding the key elements in clinical practice (what are called clinical pearls in Western medicine), TCM and traditional Korean medicine use the term *gejue* in generic reference to notes in Chinese verse. In Kampo medicine the term *kuketsu*, meaning (oral) traditional keys of treatment, is used. In TCM and traditional Korean medicine, *gejue* is only used as additional learning material for novice students. By contrast, in Kampo medicine, creating *kuketsu* is considered to be a significant requisite of being a good practitioner. This is regarded as evidence of clinical excellence; that is to say, a good practitioner has to have the knowledge of many useful *kuketsu* about symptoms that a particular therapy can be indicated for or about special characteristics of patients [9].

Perception of the Cause of Disease and of Pathogenic Qi

TCM believes that diseases result from the impedance of smooth and stable qi movement that synchronizes with the changes of qi in the natural world. Etiology is classified into the internal cause (extreme emotional disturbance), which is a disordered movement of internal qi; external cause (six-excesses external pathogen), which is the inability of the body to deal with or adapt to changes of qi in nature; and causes that are neither internal nor external (e.g., external injury, intemperance). Etiology is considered to be the most important element in analyzing pathophysiology. By contrast, Kampo medicine places emphasis on the vital reaction pattern presented at the time rather than analyzing and discussing the cause of the disease. In TCM and traditional Korean medicine, appropriate therapies are chosen by meticulously classifying the type of pathogenic qi which is the disease-inducing factor, and the position of this pathogenic qi in the body as well as its behavior. In Kampo medicine, the disease-inducing pathogenic qi is simply recognized in terms of qi stagnation, fluid[TM1] retention (fluid[TM1] toxicity), blood[TM1] stasis, or coldness. The location of the pathogenic qi within the body is merely perceived as whether it is superficial or deep inside the body. No close analysis is made in this regard, and no detailed explanation is made on the type, mechanism of its emergence, or the consequential pathophysiology of the pathogenic qi.

Deficiency and Excess

TCM refers to deficiency and excess in terms of pathophysiology. If yang becomes excessive (yang excess pattern) in terms of yin and yang interaction, yin becomes used up and reduced (yin deficiency pattern). The occurrence of excess results in relative deficiency, and therefore both deficiency and excess arise simultaneously in pathophysiology. In terms of the struggle between healthy qi and pathogenic qi, deficiency means the shortage of healthy qi since it is mobilized to fight against pathogenic qi, and excess means that pathogenic qi is rampant. In this sense, TCM assumes that both deficiency and excess coexist. By contrast, Kampo medicine uses the concept of deficiency and excess as a classification of phenomena, treating deficiency as a state of inadequacy of disease-combating response or the patient's inadequate physical strength or frailty of constitution that makes it difficult to generate a disease-combating response. Excess meanwhile means a state in which the body is mounting a powerful disease-combating response or that a patient's physical strength or good constitution can generate a powerful disease-combating response. In Kampo medicine, deficiency and excess are regarded as the two poles of the same continuum of disease-combating response or of physical and constitutional strength. Therefore, there is no question of both deficiency and excess coexisting within an individual. Therefore, when it is not possible to identify either deficiency or excess, the state is described as medium (between excess and deficiency). In other words, with regard to the concepts of deficiency and excess, Kampo medicine uses the term excess to describe the state when a powerful purgative that makes the body dissipate energy is usable or necessary, and conversely, the term deficiency describes the state when the body cannot tolerate or does not require a powerful purgative. In this sense, this is a classification for the indications of therapies.

Cold and Heat

TCM classifies cold and heat in both the body and in pathogenic qi. Meanwhile, Kampo medicine classifies cold and heat in the human body but basically does not analyze cold and heat in pathogenic qi. Therefore, TCM uses the expression exterior cold pattern to describe the disease state of fever in the early stage of cold infection in winter with strong chills because TCM focuses on the existence of pathogenic qi with the characteristic of a cold. By contrast, Kampo medicine uses the expression exterior heat pattern because it focuses on the body's reaction of running a high temperature.

Constituents of the Body

TCM considers the constituents of the body to be qi, blood[TM1], fluid[TM1]. Qi is further divided into defensive qi, nutritive qi, original qi, yang qi, and others, with essence and spirit also assumed to exist. TCM discusses their physiological actions, their production, and their metabolisms. Kampo medicine, on the other hand, accepts the existence of qi, blood[TM1], fluid[TM1]. These, however, are only used to classify symptoms, and there is no discussion of their production, metabolisms, etc. As regards pathophysiology, TCM lists qi disorders as qi deficiency, qi stagnation, qi counterflow and qi sinking, and blood[TM1] disorders as blood deficiency, blood stasis (See Chap. 2, Column A7), blood[TM1] heat, and blood[TM1] cold, and lists fluid[TM1] disorders as yin deficiency, dampness, and phlegm-fluid[TM1] retention. These are analyzed as conditions and mechanisms that may arise in individual parts of the human body. Kampo medicine, meanwhile, only goes so far as to classify qi disorders into qi deficiency, qi stagnation (qi depression), and qi counterflow and blood[TM1] disorders into blood[TM1] deficiency and blood stasis, and fluid[TM1] disorders as fluid[TM1] retention (fluid[TM1] toxicity). Thus, they are treated more as classification headings for symptoms. Basically, Kampo medicine does not set out to provide explanations of mechanisms or analyze pathophysiology. It instead describes the individual indications of the formulas that would deal with these conditions.

Zang-Fu Organs

TCM discusses the states of disease of each of the five zang organs and six fu organs caused by pathogenic qi and abnormalities of qi, blood[TM1], and fluid[TM1], which affect these organs. It also analyzes the causes of the disorders and the consequential pathophysiology. By contrast, present-day Kampo medicine does not consider organs like the heart[TM1] and lung[TM1] as original concepts of East-Asian medicine but in most instances regards these organs identically as does modern medicine. Even with the spleen[TM1], liver[TM1], and kidney[TM1], where the original concepts of East-Asian medicine apply, Kampo medicine does not analyze the abnormalities of each constituent. It only describes the conditions simply as states of excess/deficiency, such as spleen[TM1] deficiency or kidney[TM1] deficiency. Kampo medicine treats the six fu organs in the same way as the organs with the same name in modern medicine and does not apply any original concepts to them.

External Contraction Disorders

TCM analyzes external contraction diseases, which are acute infections, into two major systems of cold damage and warm disorder, depending on the type of the invading external pathogen. Kampo medicine, however, does not analyze pathogenic qi and instead attempts to deal with all external contraction disorders using cold damage methodology. Both TCM and Kampo medicine adopt the *"Shokanron 傷寒論 (Treatise on Cold Damage)"* as a basic text for cold damage. As regards the classification of the three yins and the three yangs of the *"Shokanron 傷寒論 (Treatise on Cold Damage),"* TCM uses the term "six-stage patterns identification" and lists the meridians and collaterals as well as zang-fu organs that correspond to each stage. Kampo medicine differs from this in its use of the term *rokubyoi* (meaning six-stage patterns) and considers these stages only as a description of the pattern of reaction against a disease. Furthermore, TCM uses "six-stage pattern identification" just for external contraction disorders with a few exceptions, whereas Kampo medicine tends to apply its six-stage patterns more widely to internal damage disorders, not just to external contraction disorders.

Four Examinations

With respect to the four examinations, TCM considers pulse diagnosis and tongue diagnosis to be of special importance. In the questioning examination of patients, it places particular importance on identifying the cause or mechanism of disease. Kampo medicine, meanwhile, places importance on abdominal examination, which developed independently in Kampo medicine practice, and in questioning examination, Kampo medicine places importance on checking for the characteristic symptoms that are likely to appear in the responder, which correspond to specific formula indications.

Treatment Plan

With respect to treatment plans, TCM carries out treatment according to the disease mechanism, which is how a disease operates. This means that treatment is quite often changed, especially to make seasonal adjustments. Kampo medicine, however, places priority on giving treatment according to presenting symptoms.

Medication Formulas

Compared to TCM, Kampo medicine generally uses about one-third the quantity of crude drugs. It treats one formula as an individual unit and only uses a relatively limited range of modifications. TCM, by contrast, places more importance on diagnosis and treatment plans rather than on the formulation unit. TCM favors a more tailor-made formulation combining crude drugs that would apply to the state of the disease.

Kampo medicine uses a large number of formulas that are sourced from "*Shokanron* 傷寒論 (*Treatise on Cold Damage*)," "*Kinkiyouryaku* □□□□ *Synopsis of the Golden Chamber*)" "*Taiheikeiminwazaikyokuho* 太平恵民和剤局方 (*Prescriptions of Bureau of Taiping People's Welfare Pharmacy*)" and "*Mambyokaishun* 万病回春 (*Restoring Health from Myriad of Diseases*)." Notably, Kampo medicine is well stocked with proven applications of 148 formulas adopted as prescription Kampo formulations that have been successfully used to treat various diseases. Meanwhile, TCM has recently developed a large number of galenical preparations called "traditional Chinese medicinal products."

Crude Drugs

Kampo medicine mostly uses crude drugs that are listed in Imperial Materia Medica texts

or in the "*Honzokomoku* 本草綱目 (*Compendium of Materia Medica*)." By contrast, TCM in recent years often uses crude drugs that are only used in specific regions and not listed in either the Imperial Materia Medica books or the "*Honzokomoku* 本草綱目 (*Compendium of Materia Medica*)."

In Japan, China, and Korea, although a crude drug may go under the same name, there are many that differ in the original plant that the drug is derived from or the part of the plant that is used. There are also some crude drugs that go under a different name in Japan, China, and Korea, although they are of the same origin (See Chap. 4, Sect. 1).

TCM and traditional Korean medicine often use crude drug preparations by pharmacists, whereas Kampo medicine resorts to them as little as possible.

Meridians, Acupuncture Point Selection, and Manual Techniques

TCM often takes the approach of combining *Tuina* (massage) and acupuncture and moxibustion to treat meridians and points. Meanwhile, *Tuina*, which is called *Anma* in Japan, is usually performed independently of acupuncture and moxibustion.

In the application of points in acupuncture and moxibustion, TCM uses combinations of points based on their actions on the constituent elements of the body (called point functions), based on the analysis of the pathophysiology. Kampo medicine, on the other hand, in traditional practice often uses a combination of points known through oral traditions (*kuketsu*), or five-element point combinations of Meridian Therapy. Also, direct local treatments are often applied wherever there are symptoms, outside the scope of traditional theory, for purposes of pain relief and alleviation of muscular tension. Acupuncturists in Japan use relatively fine-gauge needles and apply mild stimuli. In some cases, the needle only contacts the skin to apply stimulus instead of being inserted into acupuncture points.

In moxibustion, TCM uses either stick moxibustion or needle-head acupuncture. In Kampo medicine, direct moxibustion is commonly applied.

3.2.3 Daoyin and Diet Therapy

In TCM Daoyin (traditional exercise) is called qigong and is regarded as a major domain in medicine. Kampo medicine basically does not regard Daoyin as part of medical therapy.

Traditional medicines originating in ancient China have used diet therapy as a fundamental part of preventive medicine and health enhancement. Diet therapy considers food as medicine that can be used on an everyday basis. As such, special food items have been incorporated as part of meals according to the physical condition and time of year using the same theories that are used in prescribing crude drug formulas. TCM has a branch known as medicinal cooking, which is used for treatment, prevention, and health enhancement by actively including crude drugs in what patients eat. In traditional Korean medicine, the same practice is basically followed, but the focus is primarily on what food items are eaten in combination. The Sasang typology of Korea uses its own independent theories in stipulating the food item that should be eaten or not eaten depending on the person's physical constitution.

Kampo medicine, on the other hand, rarely refers to diet therapy currently as part of medicine proper. It only goes so far as to recommend eating fresh foods in season and incorporates the dietary habit of using the same type of seasonings that are used in preparing crude drugs. Nevertheless, there is also a school of Kampo medicine that practices diet therapy based on whole grains and vegetarianism that was developed in Japan in the Taisho and Showa periods (from around 1910 to the late 1980s). This system is based on its own original yin and yang principle, which is totally different from the traditional yin and yang principle.

3.2.4 Social Context

In China and Korea, the license for medical practitioners is different for doctors of Western medicine and practitioners of TCM and traditional Korean medicine. The universities that provide medical education and their respective curricula are independent of each other. Most notably, practitioners of traditional Korean medicine are strictly prohibited by law from undertaking diagnosis and treatment in Western medicine.

Meanwhile, in Japan, no distinction is made between the medical license for Western medicine and Kampo medicine, and there is only one medical license. Education and training are mainly concerned with Western medicine. In recent years, Japanese medical schools have started to offer several hours of lectures on Kampo medicine within the official curriculum. With respect to acupuncture, moxibustion, and *anma* massage, there is a separate national qualification for practitioners. Medical doctors are allowed to practice acupuncture and moxibustion or *anma* massage as part of their medical practice, but these are not officially recognized for reimbursement under the national medical insurance system. Within the provision of the Japanese National Health Insurance system, doctors can offer these therapies by commissioning acupuncture and moxibustion practitioners and *anma* practitioners by granting the right to claim insurance reimbursement for seven conditions of musculoskeletal pain. In Japan, doctors are almost totally fixed to the market mechanism of the National Health Insurance system. Doctors, in principle, are prohibited from engaging simultaneously in treatment that is covered by the health insurance system as well as treatment that is not covered under the system. Therefore, the practice of acupuncture and moxibustion and of *anma* is extremely limited for doctors.

3.3 Differences Between Kampo Medicine and Traditional Korean Medicine

3.3.1 Traditional Korean Medicine

The mainstream of traditional Korean medicine developed using the *Dongeuibogam* (Heo Jun, 1610), the medical compendium that is a comprehensive compilation of the knowledge and practice of traditional Chinese medicine until the Ming Dynasty, starting from the Ly Dynasty era. Traditional Korean medicine is not greatly different from TCM, which is based on traditional Chinese medicine ideology, in terms of its philosophy, theory, and clinical practice. In Japan, Dosan Manase of the Gosei School adopted almost the same concepts as Heo Jun, who was his contemporary. If any differences are to be specified, they are that *Dongeuibogam* strongly reflects Taoist philosophy and that it includes crude drugs and therapeutic methods originating in the Korean Peninsula.

At the end of the Ly Dynasty, Lee Je-ma wrote *The Principal of Life Preservation in Oriental Medicine* (1894) and advocated the Sasang typology. Because of its distinctiveness, it was reappraised in university education and is applied both to medical education and clinical practice. Sasang typology classifies human subjects into four types of physical constitution based on the five elements theory, which is not the same as the five elements theory that is used in ordinary medical practice. Its particular feature is to advocate the use of formulation and diet therapy tailored to different constitutions.

4 History and Present Status of Kampo Education

Masamitsu Nakajima

This section introduces the history and outline of education for Kampo medicine in general, followed by current education for medical doctors, pharmacists, nurses, and practitioners of acupuncture and moxibustion (Table 1.4).

In Japan, the Medical Qualification System was established by law in 1883, and Kampo medicine was excluded from medical education. On the other hand, since this system did not prohibit Kampo medicine, medical doctors were able to practice it. Nevertheless, it declined greatly after the Meiji Government-designated German medicine as legitimate instead of Kampo medicine. It barely continued to be practiced by a limited number of doctors and pharmacists. In these circumstances, most doctors who studied only Western medicine and graduated from a university school of medicine seldom used Kampo formulas, even though they were allowed to use them. After about half a century, thanks to the steadfast efforts of our predecessors, Kampo medicine gradually became recognized anew. Several nationwide research groups and academic societies were established, including the Association of East-Asian Medicine in 1938, the Japan Society for Oriental Medicine (JSOM) in 1950, and the Japan Kampo Society in 1967. Moreover, clinical training and research in Kampo medicine were promoted extensively. At that time, Kampo formulas were not covered by the national insurance program, and the university schools of medicine did not provide sufficient education for Kampo medicine. As a result, most doctors had no knowledge about Kampo medicine and no experience in prescribing Kampo formulas. Nevertheless, a small number of Kampo practitioners and pharmacists continued to prescribe them. In 1957, Kampo extract formulas were sold over the counter and used also as ethical drugs. They were easier to prescribe than decoctions and became known for their usefulness. The ethical Kampo formulas were included in the National Health Insurance drug price list in 1976, which enabled their administration to patients in the national insurance program. Since the number of formulas in the list increased to 148, there are more chances to prescribe. Be that as it may, only a few university schools of medicine provided students with short courses in Kampo medicine, and those interested had to study by themselves after graduation.

Table 1.4 Major education systems of Kampo medicine after the Meiji Restoration [10–13]

Year	Medical education	Pharmacy education	Acupuncture and moxibustion education	Nursing education
1867	Meiji Restoration			
1988			National certificate	
1989	Certification of Kampo specialist (JSOM)			
2000		Certification of pharmacists versed in Kampo and crude drugs		
2001	Model Core Curriculum for Medical Education (MEXT)			
2002		Model Core Curriculum for Pharmacy Education (MEXT)		
2005	JSOM-certified Kampo specialist (MHLW)			
2011	First revision of Model Core Curriculum for Medical Education			
2013		Revised Model Core Curriculum for Pharmacy Education		
2016	Second revision of Model Core Curriculum for Medical Education			
2017				Model Core Curriculum for Nursing Education (MEXT)

4.1 Education of Kampo Medicine for Medical Doctors

4.1.1 Pre-graduation Education

As our predecessors spread the usefulness of Kampo medicine, medical doctors not specialized in Kampo medicine began to use Kampo formulas widely in their practice of Western medicine to obtain better outcomes. Along with this, the number of scientific reports on Kampo's research increased. The circumstances around Kampo medicine changed, demanding more Kampo education prior to graduation. In March 2001, the Ministry of Education, Culture, Sports, Science and Technology (MEXT) published the "Model Core Curriculum for Medical Education," [10, 11] which for the first time included the aim to acquire the "ability to summarize WAKAN-YAKU (Kampo formulas)." Ten years later, in March 2011, the statement was revised to the "ability to explain the characteristics and current uses of WAKAN-YAKU and Kampo formulas" [12]. This was revised again in 2016 so that the "ability to summarize the characteristics of Kampo medicine and the indications and mechanisms of action of WAKAN-YAKU (Kampo formulas) can be acquired." Thus, the acquisition of knowledge about Kampo medicine was set as a pre-graduation aim in Japanese medical education. At present, all university schools of medicine are teaching Kampo medicine according to the Model Core Curriculum for Medical Education.

4.1.2 Post-graduation Education

JSOM is devoted to post-graduation education/training and holds many training sessions and study meetings to impart a higher level of expertise to Kampo specialists. These opportunities have contributed to the education of non-specialists in Kampo medicine, and now about 90% of them are prescribing Kampo formulas clinically. Recently, in some universities, there have been increasing opportunities for Kampo education and training, such as clinical apprenticeships for undergraduates and faculty training for Kampo education. The increase in education/training opportunities will increase the number of Kampo specialists and develop a more solid education base for Kampo medicine.

As the present status of Kampo medicine in Japanese medical education suggests, students study both Kampo medicine (traditional medicine) and Western medicine. A medical doctor diagnoses patients from the viewpoints of both Kampo medicine and Western medicine and prescribes a formula that suits them. In other words, even a Kampo specialist has studied and knows Western medicine. It is a remarkable feature that Japanese doctors and specialists can combine Western medicine and traditional medicine.

4.1.3 Certification of Kampo Specialists

Many doctors prescribe Kampo formulas at present. Of course, all doctors who prescribe Kampo formulas are not Kampo specialists. There are experienced experts with much knowledge who have been apprenticed to a skilled leader or teacher and primarily use Kampo formulas and others who have met certain requirements and have been certified as a Kampo specialist. Many of these certified doctors may have experience and expertise; many of those who have had an apprenticeship may be certified specialists. They are not incompatible.

In Japan, the certification of Kampo specialists was introduced by JSOM in 1989. It is a system recognized by the Council of Society Board Certification. In August 2005, the Ministry of Health, Labour and Welfare (MHLW) permitted the advertisement of a "JSOM-certified Kampo specialist." [13] According to this system, doctors who meet certain requirements will be recognized as specialists by JSOM. The specialist shall master Kampo medicine and practice its unique procedure in accordance with patients' symptoms and physical state while mastering Western medicine and being certified as its specialist. The member shall be a board-certified member or specialist of an academic society of any main clinical field (internal medicine, general surgery, pediatrics, etc.) designated by the Japanese Medical Specialty Board, meet certain requirements, such as acquisition of credits, and have a clinical training of Kampo at a JSOM-designated facility for at least 3 years. The member shall pass the preliminary screening for detailed clinical case reports and performance in the educational core curriculum and the certification test (written and oral) (for those who have passed the preliminary screening). Certification shall be renewed every 5 years after acquisition. Apart from the JSOM-certified Kampo specialist, another certification started in 2006 is intended to get more doctors interested in becoming specialists in Kampo medicine. This certification cannot be used for advertisement but will be granted to doctors other than board-certified members or specialists of any basic clinical fields designated by the Japanese Medical Specialty Board.

4.2 Education of Kampo Medicine for Pharmacists

In Japan, pharmacists as well as doctors can continue treatment by providing and changing Kampo formulas as they monitor patients' condition. Pharmacists can open a pharmacy and practice Kampo medicine by themselves. At the pharmacy, they can sell OTC Kampo drugs without a prescription from doctors. As mentioned earlier, Kampo education was not provided at schools of medicine for a long period after 1883. During this period, individual doctors and pharmacists took responsibility for carrying on the practice of Kampo medicine. Even after the schools of medicine stopped teaching Kampo medicine, the schools of pharmacy continued classes on pharmaceutical botany and pharmacognosy. Not that many schools of pharmacy went deeply into clinical Kampo medicine, but quite a few schools of pharmacy attached more importance to Kampo education than the schools of medicine. To take an example, according to a survey on education at the schools of medicine/pharmacy/dentistry in 1987, 8% of the schools of medicine and 56% of the schools of pharmacy were engaged in Kampo education. In 2002, one year after medical education, the Model Core Curriculum for Pharmacy Education stipulated its general purpose of "mastering basic knowledge about the theory of Kampo medicine, typical prescriptions and indications of Kampo formulas, and assessment of efficacy to understand crude and Kampo drugs to be used in modern medicine," in its section on "crude drugs and Kampo medicines in modern medical care." Many pharmacists dispense prescriptions under the direction of doctors and are familiar with Kampo formulas. Pharmacists, however, have fewer opportunities of practicing Kampo medicine and treating patients than doctors. Their main role is operating Kampo pharmacies and selling OTC Kampo formulas. Though not many, there are pharmacists with extensive knowledge and experience who provide effective treatment to patients by mainly prescribing Kampo formulas at their pharmacy. In 2006, pharmacy education for pharmacists shifted from a 4-year to a 6-year program, with more focus on clinical pharmacy, including Kampo formulas. In 2013, the curriculum was revised to state the "use of Kampo formulas in the practice of medicine," with a more practical general purpose of "mastering the basics of Kampo medicine, including its theory, general concept of diseases, typical indications, side effects, and precautions."

Regarding certification of pharmacists, joint certification between the Japan Pharmacists Education Center and the Japanese Society of Pharmacognosy inaugurated certification of pharmacists versed in Kampo and crude drugs in 2000. Certification is granted based on evaluation by training and testing to check for minimum ability and aptitude for a specialized field. Certified Kampo pharmacists have a proven ability but are not necessarily experienced.

4.3 Education of Kampo Medicine for Nurses

In 2017, Kampo education was added to the Model Core Curriculum for Nursing Education. It aimed at acquiring the "ability to explain the efficacy, mechanism of action, indications, and adverse effects of major WAKAN-YAKU (Kampo formulas) and nursing aid in Kampo medicine." According to a survey reported in 2016 on the "status quo and awareness of Kampo education at 4-year schools of nursing nationwide, 71% of the schools recognized the necessity of Kampo education. Many schools of nursing have yet to offer an intensive course in Kampo medicine. Investigation is ongoing into the effective incorporation of Kampo medicine in nursing education.

4.4 Education of Practitioners of Acupuncture and Moxibustion

The last topic is the education of practitioners of acupuncture and moxibustion in modern times. In 1874, the medical system regulation defined acupuncture as a folk remedy. In 1880, training in acupuncture and massage for the visually impaired started at private schools, which were replaced later by public schools. Training in acupuncture and massage was provided by public schools for the blind, and this saved acupuncture from extinction and contributed partly to the preservation of acupuncture and massage until today. After many revisions, the Regulation for the Control of Acupuncture and Moxibustion Businesses was established in 1911. This required practitioners of acupuncture and moxibustion to undergo clinical training and pass an examination or to graduate from one of the schools designated by the head of local government. The regulation led to the development of acupuncture schools. Also, designated schools of acupuncture and moxibustion for sighted people were founded. After World War II, in 1947, the Law of License for Practicing Massage, Acupuncture, Moxibustion, and Non-surgical Orthopedics was enacted. This law granted license to those who have graduated from a designated school or training facility and passed an examination administered by a prefectural governor. After that, the institution of education by apprenticeship disappeared. This has been replaced by vocational schools that teach acupuncture, moxibustion, and massage. In 1988, regulation for acupuncture, moxibustion, massage, and shiatsu was revised drastically. Students were required to study acupuncture and moxibustion in a 3-year course after graduating from senior high school and to pass a national examination. In 1993, the first national examination was conducted. Since 1990, the government relaxed the regulations, which accelerated the establishment of new acupuncture schools. There are 4-year courses for undergraduates and also for graduates (See Chap. 6, Sect. 2).

5 Medical Ethics for Kampo Medicine in Japan

Akira Kinebuchi and Hiroshi Sato

5.1 Introduction

Recently, medical ethics has increasingly attracted attention. In Kampo medicine, improvement of medical safety has become a pressing issue after a case of interstitial pneumonia was presumably induced by Shosaikoto. The basic principles of medical ethics have already been established, though they have undergone changes in each era of modern medicine. It goes without saying that the ethical principles of modern medicine should be applied to Kampo medicine. It is often difficult, however, to apply these principles to Kampo medicine without modification.

This section indicates several issues of medical ethics in the practice of Kampo medicine.

5.2 Different Understanding of Recognition of Diseases Between a Patient and a Practitioner or Between Practitioners

People recognize the importance of informed consent (IC) in modern medicine more than ever. In many cases, a certain consensus is reached about a disease and a drug to treat it between a patient and a practitioner or between practitioners, which means that modern medicine has succeeded in providing an appropriate explanation and fulfilling its duty to obtain IC.

Meanwhile, Kampo medicine has rarely provided medical treatment based on IC until recently. Even if a practitioner attempts an explanation, patients often have little or no Kampo medical information (yin-yang, deficiency excess, qi/blood[TM1]/fluid[TM1], zang-fu organs, etc.). In addition, each medical doctor sometimes made different Kampo diagnoses. Some diagnose a condition as kidney[TM1] deficiency, while others diagnose it as spleen[TM1] deficiency. It may be possible to set a standard for diagnosis methods. However, setting diagnostic standards to choose prescriptions is difficult to unify, at least at this moment.

Now that patients may request an explanation for the grounds for prescribing a formula, the practitioners should be ready to provide it.

5.3 Limitations of Kampo Medicine and Principle of Respecting Autonomy

Patients with advanced cancer sometimes request nonsurgical treatment with Kampo products.

The principle of respecting autonomy is one of the basic principles of medical ethics. Some practitioners may respect patients' decisions and start treatment using Kampo products. In such a case, the practitioners should be careful, because the patients are likely to accept abundant incorrect information on the internet without question. The practitioners should ask them why they refuse modern medicine and should explain in detail the merits and demerits of modern Western medicine, the limitations of Kampo medicine, and the different roles of Kampo and Western medicines in treatment so that the patients may be able to make their final decision.

5.4 The Necessity of Recognition as Experimental Medicine

There are many outpatients who have already used evidence-based Kampo drugs or consulted other Kampo practitioners only to have unfavorable prognoses. These patients should be treated by changing the combination or weighing of patient information. Customization of treatment to suit individual patients' needs has an experimental aspect and can be called an experimental treatment. The Declaration of Helsinki states "Unproven Interventions in Clinical Practice" (see note for details). The statement refers to IC as an essential prerequisite. The practitioners of Kampo medicine, particularly experts, should be aware that they are practicing experimental medicine.

Table 1.5 Ten points to realize medical safety

1. Disseminating a safety-oriented culture which unites and makes the most of individual efforts
2. Involving patients and communicating with them to deepen mutual understanding and enhance safety
3. Sharing experiences and learning lessons
4. Setting, observing, and checking rules and procedures
5. Creating an organization which allows a cross-sectional exchange of opinions
6. Being proactive in grasping and checking important points
7. Paying attention to one's own health care, which is a minimum requirement for healthcare professional
8. Preventing an accident by using technology and taking measures
9. Checking patient names and medicines again for appropriate dose and dosage
10. Maintaining a good environment for patient care and creating a good working environment

5.5 Conclusion

This section indicated several issues, including the different understanding of morbidity between a patient and a medical doctor or between doctors, limitations of Kampo medicine, whether or not to respect the autonomy of patients, and the experimental Kampo approach, particularly by experts. The prerequisite common to these issues is IC, which will surely be more important in future Kampo medicine. We hope that this section will be a good starting point for discussion.

Note

Declaration of Helsinki as a standard of ethical principles for medical research involving human subjects.

37 Unproven Interventions in Clinical Practice

In the treatment of an individual patient, where proven interventions do not exist or other known interventions have been ineffective, the physician, after seeking expert advice, with informed consent from the patient or a legally authorized representative, may use an unproven intervention if, in the physician's judgment, it offers hope of saving life, reestablishing health, or alleviating suffering. This intervention should subsequently be made the object of research designed to evaluate its safety and efficacy. In all cases, new information must be recorded and, where appropriate, made publicly available.

6 Medical Safety of Kampo Medicine

Eiichi Tahara

6.1 What is Medical Safety?

The Ministry of Health, Labour and Welfare (MHLW) in Japan proposes ten points to realize safe medicine (Table 1.5). Medical safety can be summarized as "sharing information among different clinical departments and with patients and establishing a safety-oriented culture through the improvement of risk-preventive measures for the security of people, including healthcare professionals, and the introduction of preventive technology and strategy, particularly about the handling of medicines and maintenance of a good working environment." In the process toward medical safety, it is necessary to review incidents in the past, understand the procedure and environment up to the present, propose the points to be improved, and develop far-reaching enlightenment activities.

6.1.1 Activities of the Medical Safety Committee of the Japan Society for Oriental Medicine

The Medical Safety Committee was devised and inaugurated by Hiroshi Sato, then President, on July 2, 2017. Since then, the committee has focused its activity on the medical safety of Kampo formulas. From a short-term perspective, the committee is engaged in examining and analyzing the side effects of Kampo formulas and medical accidents (side effects of Kampo formulas, near misses, medical safety incidents at pharmacies), countermeasures, and enlightenment. This section will introduce such committee activity. Kampo medicine refers to both decoction and acupuncture and moxibustion. Regarding the medical safety of acupuncture and moxibustion, the Japan Society of Acupuncture and Moxibustion has the Safety Guidelines for Japanese Acupuncture and Moxibustion Practice (See Chap. 7, Sect. 3).

6.1.2 Side Effects of Kampo Formulas

The Medical Safety Committee chose three major side effects of Kampo formulas, (pseudoaldosteronism, drug-induced liver injury, and drug-induced pneumonia) and collected and reported data from academic papers, etc. from the past that are recognized as most appropriate at present [14]. In addition, the committee refers to Kampo drug-induced mesenteric phlebosclerosis, which is attracting attention these days. Pseudoaldosteronism is likely to be caused when more than 2.5 g per day of glycyrrhiza (*kanzo*) is used. The incidence rates are reported to be 1.7%, 3.3%, and 11.1% when the daily dose is 2.0 g, 4.0 g, and 6.0 g, respectively [15]. See other sections (See Chap. 3, Sect. 3.1.7, Chap. 4, Sect. 3.3.3)

Liver injury may be due to toxicity or allergic reaction. Reportedly, DLST results are likely to be false positives, which means it is difficult to diagnose Kampo drug-induced liver injury based on positive DLST. Many cases of Kampo drug-induced liver injury are reportedly caused by scutellaria root (*ogon*), and particular attention should be paid to using formulas containing it. For early detection of Kampo drug-induced liver injury, it is essential to conduct blood tests regularly. Reportedly, incidence rates are 0.10% for Kampo formulas in general and 0.5 to 1.0% for Scutellaria root-containing formulas at Kitasato University and the University of Toyama [16]. For diagnosis, blood testing should be conducted one to 2 months after administration.

The incidence rate of Kampo drug-induced pneumonia is not known but can be estimated to be extremely low, or 4 per 100,000 people a year (0.004%), extrapolating from a report of shosaikoto-induced pneumonia. Though the details are not disclosed, another report revealed that many Kampo formulas that were suspected of causing the disease contained scutellaria root. For details, refer to the study on the survey report [14]

The incidence rate of mesenteric phlebosclerosis is not known. A nationwide fact-finding survey involving 222 cases is available [17]. Survey patients included 78 males and 144 females (ratio of 1:1.8) aged 26–89 (63.8 on average). The rate of male patients was fewer than that of female outpatients. The typical symptoms were abdominal pain, diarrhea, and abdominal distention. Among 147 patients (87.0%) with experience with Kampo formulas, 119 patients (81.0%) used Kampo formulas containing gardenia fruit (*sanshishi*) for 13.6 years on average, with 92.6% and 69.5% of them for at least 5 years and 10 years, respectively. The risk seemed to increase as the administration continued for a long duration.

6.1.3 Report of Kampo Drug-Related Near Misses at General Hospitals [18]: The Importance of Information Sharing with Different Healthcare Professionals

We collected and analyzed Kampo drug-related near misses. We accessed the open database of the Japan Council for Quality Health Care Japanese site: http://www.med-safe.jp/index.html and analyzed data on medical safety information (for general hospitals) and Kampo drug-related near misses at the pharmacy. There were 626 Kampo drug-related cases. Medical accidents included drug-induced liver injury. The near misses included wrong dose/dosage at prescription due to failure to check for extract packet content, wrong dispensing due to similar formula number, appearance, and name, and wrong administration due to failure to check for formula name and hasty deduction from Chinese characters and manufacturer's name (Table 1.6). Such near misses were often reported by other healthcare professionals and patients as well as pharmacists responsible for dispensing and their colleagues. The near-miss report should be shared not only among the pharmacists but also with other healthcare professionals to enhance medical safety.

Medical safety incidents at pharmacies (based on analysis of inquiries by pharmacists) [19] (Fig. 1.1)

According to the analysis of 2200 Kampo formulas related to near misses at pharmacies, inquiries by pharmacists revealed wrong formula names, doses, and dosages in prescriptions, prevention of side effects, etc. Separation of dispensaries from medical practice proved to be somehow effective in preventing medical accidents. On the other hand, it was also revealed that pharmacists frequently made dispensary mistakes, including wrong formula names and doses. In fact, there were Kampo formulas with similar names, which caused mix-ups.

6.1.4 Other Medical Safety-Related Matters

Safe use of Kampo formulas for the elderly and polypharmacy is attracting attention these days. For the elderly, refer to the symptoms of the elderly (See Chap. 5, Sect. 8.2.4). Polypharmacy in Kampo medicine relates to the administration of formulas without treatment by pattern identification. Inadvertent addition of extract formulas, such as duplication or addition of glycyrrhiza and other crude drugs, will increase side effects [20]. (See Chap. 4, Sect. 3.3.3)

6.1.5 Conclusion

The Medical Safety Committee has the function of investigating side effects and near misses of Kampo formulas regularly to update information, accumulating side effects in the database, creating manuals and guidelines, and enlightening people about Kampo medical safety through its website and by hosting symposiums.

Non-Kampo specialists often prescribe Kampo drugs only on the basis of the Western diagnosis. From the viewpoint of medical safety, Kampo medicine should be promoted to be appropriately based on its theory (treatment by pattern identification).

Table 1.6 Classification of 623 near misses

Timing	No. of near misses	Classification of near misses	No. of near misses	Special circumstances of Kampo formulas
1.1.1.1. Prescription	28	Wrong dose	12	Wrong single/daily dose
				Failure to check for "packet number" or "weight unit"
				Failure to check for weight per packet
				Wrong pediatric dose
		Wrong dosage	5	Preconception about "3 times a day" and "after meal"
		Confused/wrong drug name	5	Similar formula name
				Predictive conversion of prescription system
		Missed prescription	3	
		Others	3	Combined use of Western and Kampo drugs
1.1.2. Dispensing	94	Confused/wrong drug name	46	Similar number/appearance of drugs
				Similar formula name
				Preconception about Kampo drug being Daikenchuto
		Count/measurement error	17	Preconception about "unit-dose packet" and "3 times a day"
				Wrong pediatric dose
		Wrong formula	12	Preconception about formulas in numerical order or storing place
		Inquiry failure	6	Failure to check for unit dose
		Missed dispensing	3	
		Other	10	Failure to check for simple suspension, resulting in grinding
1.1.1.3. Administration	419	Missed administration	233	Failure to check for formula name
				Missed administration before meal
				Preconception about two drugs in a packet
				Failure to check for administration method
		Wrong dose	73	Preconception about unit-dose packet
		Wrong timing	37	
		Wrong patient	33	Dissolution of a drug in hot water
		Failure to check instructions	16	Administration of a prohibited drug that caused side effects
		Wrong administration route	7	Enteral administration
		Wrong formula	6	Failure to check for formula name
		Other	14	
4. Administration (patient side)	67	Missed dose	42	Missed dose before meal
		Wrong timing/date	16	
		Wrong unit dose	5	Preconception based on experience
		Other	4	
1.5. Returning/adding drugs	7	Confused/wrong formula name	7	Similar formula no./appearance
				Preconception about Kampo formula name in Chinese characters
6. Checking drugs that patients bring	6	Confused/wrong formula name	4	Similar formula name
				Similar formula no./appearance
		Wrong dose	1	Failure to check for "packet" or "gram"
		Wrong dosage	1	
7. Other	2		2	Lack of understanding of Kampo formulas as "medicines"

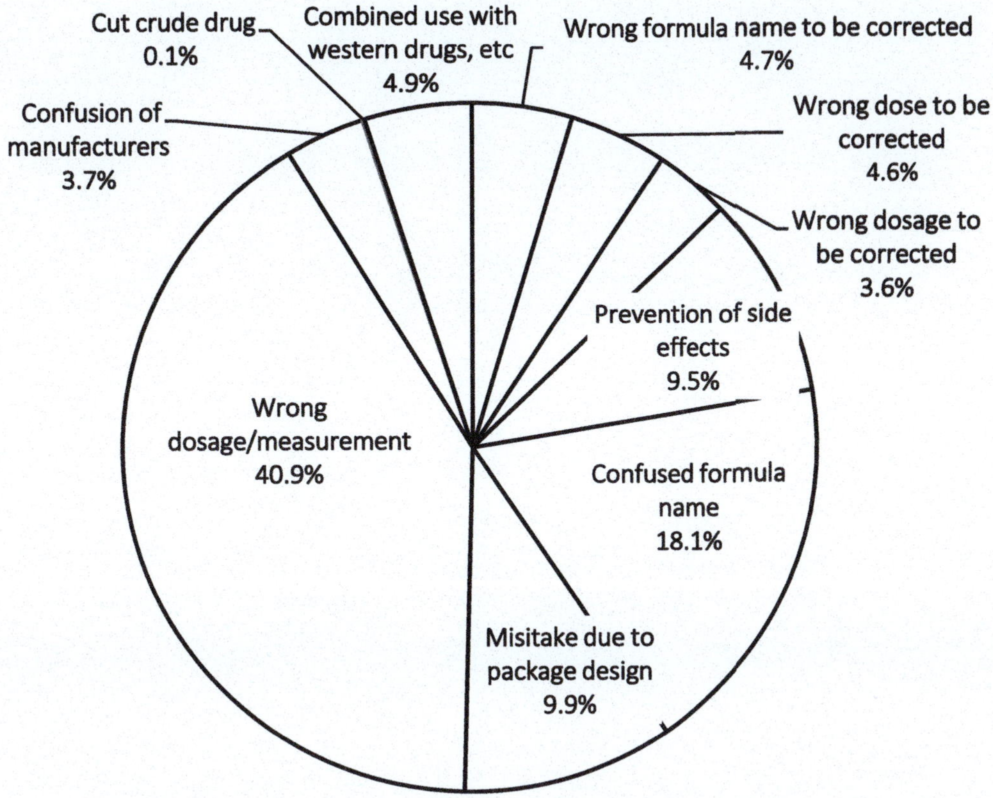

Fig. 1.1 Classification of incidents [19]

References

1. SAKAMOTO Ayumi (Supervising Editor), Committee for Safe Acupuncture, Academic & Research Department, The Japan Society of Acupuncture and Moxibustion. Safety Guidelines for Japanese Acupuncture and Moxibustion Practice, 2020 edition. Ishiyaku Pub, Inc., 2020. https://safety.jsam.jp/pg157.html (See 2021-4-20)
2. Committee for EBM of The Japan Society for Oriental Medicine. http://www.jsom.or.jp/medical/ebm/index.html (See 2021-4-18)
3. National Institutes of Biomedical Innovation, Health and Nutrition. STORK (Standards of Reporting Kampo Products). http://mpdb.nibiohn.go.jp/stork/ (See 2021-4-18).
4. The Japan Society for Oriental Medicine. Clinical Practice Guidelines Containing Kampo Products in Japan 2019 KCPG2019, http://www.jsom.or.jp/medical/ebm/cpg/index.html (See 2021-4-18).
5. The Japan Liaison of Oriental Medicine. http://jlom.umin.jp/page4.html (See 2021-2-8)
6. Akiba T. Nihon Toyo Igaku Zasshi. Jpn J Orient Med. 2010;61(7):881–8.
7. Medical Education Program Research and Development Project Committee. A model core curriculum in medical education, ed. Sato T Chairman, 40; 2001
8. JAOM-EBM Committee ed. Evidence reports of Kampo treatment 2010 – 345 RCT. [Internet]. http://www.jsom.or.jp/medical/ebm/er/index.html
9. Matsuda K. Tradition and development of Japanese Kampo medicine. Kampo Med. 2002;56(6):595–604.
10. Imazu Y, SungJoon K, Odaguchi H, Yanagisawa H, Sakiyama T. Present Kampo education at 80 university schools of medicine. Kampo Med. 2012;63:121–30.
11. Model Core Curriculum for Medical Education 2016 revised edition. (MHLW), P776, https://www.mext.go.jp/component/b_menu/shingi/toushin/__icsFiles/afieldfile/2017/06/28/1383961_01.pdf. Last access on 4 Apr 2021
12. Japan Society for Oriental Medicine (JSOM). JSOM and another certifications for Kampo specialists. http://www.jsom.or.jp/medical/specialist/system.html. Last access on 4 Apr 2021
13. Model Core Curriculum for Pharmacy Education 2013 revised edition (MHLW), P71–72. https://www.mext.go.jp/component/a_menu/education/detail/__icsFiles/afieldfile/2015/02/12/1355030_02.pdf. Last access on 4 Apr 2021
14. Chino A, et al. Representative side effects caused by Kampo prescriptions: Pseudoaldosteronism, drug-induced liver injury and drug-induced lung injury: the report from the medical safety Committee of the Japan Society for Oriental Medicine (2019). Kampo Med. 2020;71(3):262–7.
15. Mantani N, Oka H, Sahashi Y, et al. Relationship between incidence of Pseudoaldosteronism and daily dose of Glycyrrhiza: review of the literature. Kampo Med. 2015;66(3):197–202. (abstract in English)
16. Mantani N. Kampo drug-induced liver injury: its diagnosis, incidence, and clinical practice. Kampo Med. 2015;66(4):342–51. (abstract in English)
17. Shimizu S. A report on national survey of mesenteric phlebosclerosis cases. A shared research report on research for overcoming intractable diseases by using Health and Labour Sciences Research Grant. "A comprehensive research into homology and difference in epidemiology, pathology, diagnosis and treatment of rare and intractable intestinal diseases" represented by Toshifumi Hibi). Comprehensive research report 2013, 2014, p 91–93.
18. Sekine M, Makino T, Tanaka K, et al. Medical safety committee report (2020): medical accidents information and minor incidents from medical institutions related to Kampo products. Kampo Med. 2021;72(2):182–203. (abstract in English)
19. Makino T, et al. Committee for Medical Safety Report: example of minor incidents in the prescription of Kampo products in pharmacy. Kampo Med. 2020;71(4):394–401.
20. Chino A, Tsuji M, Yagi A, Terasawa K. Polipharmacy caused by Kampo prescriptions. Kampo Med. 2019;70(4):72–6.

General Theory of Kampo Medicine

2

Hideki Adachi, Shuji Yakubo, Takashi Ito, and Masamitsu Nakajima

1 Basic Theory of Kampo Medicine

Pathological conditions in Kampo medicine are described by the use of terminology and concepts different from those in Western medicine. These include deficiency-excess, cold-heat, and exterior-interior. Appropriate use of these terms and concepts leads to a correct understanding of Kampo medicine. The yin-yang is an overarching concept for these term groups.

1.1 Yin-Yang Theory

Hideki Adachi

The yin and yang theory is a philosophical concept that attempts to apprehend all phenomena from the two opposite but complementary aspects of nature, such as "yin and yang" and "male and female."

deficiency and excess		
deficiency	hollow and weak	pertains to yin
excess	full and strong	pertains to yang
cold and heat		
cold	being cold	pertains to yin
heat	being hot	pertains to yang
exterior and interior		
exterior	skin, muscles, joints, nerves, & tissues close to the body surface	pertains to yang
interior	internal organs, bones, & tissues deeper in the body	pertains to yin
Qi, blood[TM1], fluid[TM1]		
qi	circulating energy which is invisible	pertains to yang
blood[TM1] and fluid[TM1]	circulating substances that are visible	pertains to yin
The red substance is blood[TM1] and the white substance is fluid[TM1] or body fluids		

These terms compose pairs of two opposite but complementary qualities such as "yin and yang." The mutual relationships between these qualities are relative, because it is implied that there is a gradation (gradual change, tone gradient) between the complete shade (yin) and complete sunshine (yang). Otherwise, it can be said that shade and sunshine move toward each other via such a gradation. Terms that come under the concept of yin and yang possess such relativity and mutual transformation.

1.2 Five Phases

Shuji Yakubo

Dating back to ancient China, *gogyo*, the five phases theory, is based on the concept that all natural and anthropogenic phenomena can be divided into five categories by their properties. The character "gyo" (xing in Chinese) in *gogyo* means transforming qi under heaven, the character "go" (wu in Chinese) means the numeral five; the number originating from the five planets: Jupiter, Mars, Saturn, Venus, and Mercury.

These five categories correspond to Wood[TM1], Fire[TM1], Earth[TM1], Metal[TM1], and Water[TM1], respectively, as sym-

H. Adachi
Adachi Clinic, Tokyo, Japan

S. Yakubo
Department of Medicine, The Nippon Dental University School of Life Dentistry, Tokyo, Japan

T. Ito
Akashi Clinic Kanda, Tokyo, Japan

M. Nakajima (✉)
Division of Kampo Medicine and Pharmacognosy, Faculty of Pharmaceutical Sciences, Hiroshima International University, Higashihiroshima, Japan

Division of Kampo Medicine, National Hospital Organization Kure Medical Center, Higashihiroshima, Japan
e-mail: office@jsom.or.jp

Kampo Medical Literature Editorial Committee, The Japan Society for Oriental Medicine (ed.), *Complete Japanese Traditional (Kampo) Medicine*, https://doi.org/10.1007/978-981-96-7143-4_2

bolized by observations of natural phenomena and seasonal changes. The observations, properties, and seasons are summarized in Tables 2.1 and 2.2.

The five phases theory is also characterized by the generating and controlling relationships in which the individual elements influence each other (Fig. 2.1).

The generating relationship is one that promotes sequentially. Wood[TM1] generates Fire[TM1]: Wood generates fire when burning. Fire[TM1] generates Earth[TM1]: Fire changes to ash, which in turn becomes earth. Earth[TM1] generates Metal[TM1]: Metal is present on the earth. Metal[TM1] generates Water[TM1]: dew appears on metal surfaces, producing water. Water[TM1] generates Wood[TM1]: Wood is nourished by water to grow. Hence, generating initiates interactions in the sequence of Wood[TM1] →Fire[TM1] → Earth[TM1] → Metal[TM1] → Water[TM1] → Wood[TM1] to generate the next phase. In contrast, controlling is a relationship in which a phase restraining sequence. Wood[TM1] controls Earth[TM1]: Wood absorbs nutrients from the soil, so the soil becomes depleted. Earth[TM1] controls Water[TM1]: Earth dams up the overflowing water with an earthen embankment. Water[TM1] restrains Fire[TM1]: Water puts out fire: Fire[TM1] restrains Metal[TM1]: Fire vaporizes metal. Metal[TM1] restrains Wood[TM1]: a metal axe can cut down a tree. Hence, controlling inhibits interactions in the sequence of Wood[TM1] →Earth[TM1] →Water[TM1] →Fire[TM1] →Metal[TM1]→Wood[TM1] to restrains the subsequent phase.

These five phases influence each other in the two aspects of generating and controlling; all things change and recycle by their births and deaths and rises and falls. This is the philosophical basis of Oriental medicine.

1.3 Deficiency and Excess

Hideki Adachi and Takahi Ito

1.3.1 The Concept of Deficiency and Excess

Deficiency implies "hollow on the inside," whereas excess signifies "inside filled with something." Naturally, these are relative concepts that transform mutually. These apparently simple concepts have been associated with complex interpretations, thus leading to the explanation below.

Definition of Deficiency and Excess

There are several definitions of deficiency and excess, as listed below.

(a) A term describing the condition of the body's responses against pathogens: excess refers to remarkable resistance, while deficiency refers to weak responses.

(b) One of the guiding principles for analyzing the body's strength and constitution: excess refers to a strong constitution and deficiency refers to a weak constitution.

(a) and (b) are often used in Koho school, (a) and (c) are often used in Gosei school, while (c) is often used in traditional Chinese medicine.

Differentiation of Characteristics of Deficiency-Excess Theory in Japan and China

In Kampo medicine, a formula is determined on the basis of the clinical findings of a patient. Characteristically, discrimination of deficiency or excess is very likely to depend on the amount of abdominal strength (based on abdominal potential and the degrees of development and tension of abdominal muscles) as well as the amount of energy or qi, so-called being active or energetic. Unlike the view of deficiency-excess in Traditional Chinese Medicine, which deals with excess or deficiency of pathogenic qi and essential qi, Kampo medicine emphasizes the physical strength or resistance against a disease or diseases at that point in time. Between Japan and China, the same term "deficiency and excess" has different meanings.

1.3.2 Treatments Appropriate to Deficiency and Excess

Principles

Taking c) in 1 (1) above as an example, for deficiency, a c complement is tonified on the other hand, for excess, the draining formulas, etc., are used as a rule (see Chap. 3, Sects. 3.1.3, 3.1.4, 3.1.5, Chap. 4, Sect. 2.2.2). It is not simple, however, to determine the degree of deficiency or excess, and this determination-based therapeutic selection requires a certain level of experience and knowledge.

Examples

Examples are given for each of (a) to (c) in 1 (1) Definitions of Deficiency and Excess.

Extent of Resistance to Pathogens

If affected by influenza, the body will exhibit severe chilling and other strong resistances (responses) to the pathogen such as high fever and severe malaise. This state of intense disease-fighting responses (absence of sweating and strongly palpable floating pulses) is deemed an excess pattern, and *maoto*, *kakkonto*, etc. are prescribed.

On the other hand, in a case affected by common cold, the body experiences little chillness, showing weak resistance (responses) to the pathogen, such as mild fever and slight malaise. This state of weak disease-fighting responses (spon-

Table 2.1 Five-phase classification of vital activities

Five phases	Five zang organs	Five hollow viscera	Five tissues	Five sensory organs	Five flourishes	Five instincts	Five emotions	Five voices	Five exertions	Five colors	Five taste
Wood[TM1]	Liver[TM1]	Gallbladder[TM1]	Tendons	Eye	Nails	Soul	Anger	Shouting	Walking	Blue	Sour
Fire[TM1]	Heart[TM1]	Small intestine[TM1]	Blood vessels	Tongue	Facial complexion	Consciousness	Joy	Laughter	Use of eyes	Red,	Bitter,
Earth[TM1]	Spleen[TM1]	Stomach[TM1]	Fatty tissue	Mouth	Lips	Thoughts	Obsession	Singing	Sitting	Yellow,	Sweet,
Metal[TM1]	Lung[TM1]	Large intestine[TM1]	Skin and body hair	Nose	Body hair	Life energy	Anguish	Weeping	Lying down	White,	Pungent
Water[TM1]	Kidney[TM1]	Bladder[TM1]	Bones	Ears	Head hair	Willpower	Fright	Groaning	Standing	Black	Salty

Table 2.2 Five fundamental elements in nature and their properties

Wood[TM1]	Warming and extending, inflating, starting, generating wind, flourishing in spring, generating fire, controlling earth
Fire[TM1]	Causing fever, motivating, melting objects, rising, generating heat, flourishing in summer, generating earth and controlling metal
Earth[TM1]	Developing and nurturing, maintaining dynamic balance, generating moisture, flourishing in summer, generating metal and controlling water
Metal[TM1]	Cooling and solidifying, deflating, calming, generating dryness, flourishing in fall, generating water and controlling wood
Water[TM1]	Providing coldness and moisture, saving and preserving, sinking, generating chills, flourishing in winter, generating wood and controlling fire

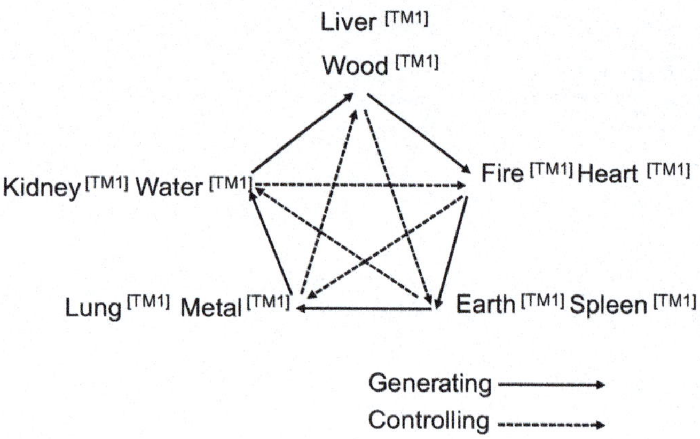

Fig. 2.1 Five elements theory

taneous sweating and weakly palpable floating pulses) is deemed a deficiency pattern, and keishito, etc. are prescribed.

The Patient's Physical Strength, Physique, and Constitution Are Assessed Comprehensively

People who are usually vigorous in physical strength, physique, and constitution are often symptom-free or suffer only minor symptoms, such as mild coughing and foreign sensation in the throat, even if affected by common cold. This state is deemed an excess pattern, which is a healthy condition not requiring Kampo treatments. People who are usually weak in physical strength, physique, and constitution are likely to catch a common cold, often suffering stubborn symptoms of a common cold with prolonged coughing etc. This state is deemed a deficiency pattern, and it is recommended that *hochuekkito,* etc., be taken daily.

Presence of Pathogen and Lack of Essential qi

Abdominal pain resulting from rapid ingestion of cold food or drink to cool the stomach (referred to as cold pathogen in Chinese medicine) is described as an excess pattern (excess cold pattern in this case). Abdominal pain from the lack of abdomen warming ability due to a lack of yang qi is described as a deficiency pattern (deficiency cold pattern in this case).

1.4 Cold and Heat

Hideki Adachi and Takashi Ito

1.4.1 The Concept of Cold and Heat

Needless to say, cold means being cold and heat means being hot. It is very important in Kampo medicine to determine whether a pathological condition is a "cold" or "heat" pattern, along with differentiation of deficiency and excess patterns. Differential diagnoses of cold and heat as well as deficiency and excess are the key factors in the therapeutic strategy.

Cold: A general term for subjective feelings of cold and objective findings of coldness.
Heat: A general term for subjective feelings of heat and objective findings of heat.

1.4.2 Treatment Appropriate for Cold and Heat

Principles

When the pathological condition is cold, heating medicines should be used to warm things up. When the pathological condition is heat, cooling medicines should be used to cool things down (see Chap. 3, Sects. 3.1.3, 3.1.4, 3.1.5, Chap. 4, Sect. 2.2.2). But there are some cases in which whether the condition is cold or heat cannot be determined easily.

Specific Examples

Heat

The pathological condition with subjective feelings of heat and objective findings of heat.

Of febrile diseases, pathological conditions are diagnosed and treated according to *Shanghanlun*, which describes the heat conditions as follows:

- aversion to cold and fever

In *Shanghanlun*, "fever" not only refers to elevation of body temperature, but also stands for heat on the exterior body surface, including feeling of aversion to cold or aversion to wind as well as sensation of heat, and conditions associated with body stiffness and pain. Generally, the pulse is floating. Aversion to cold is a feeling of being cold even under a comforter; aversion to wind is a feeling of being cold and desiring a comforter since it feels cold without it.

At the beginning of a disease, the presence of "fever" is indicative of early yang stage pattern, as described in

Shanghanlun, and heat pattern is diagnosed. Treatment in this case is to diffuse heat through sweating. Patients with floating and tight pulse and no sweating are finally diagnosed as early yang stage excess pattern. They are treated with *maoto* and the like. Patients with floating and relaxed pulse and spontaneous sweating are regarded as early yang stage deficiency pattern, with an indication of *keishito*. In contrast, the presence of aversion to cold with deep pulse and no feeling of heat are suggestive of the middle yin stage pattern, as described in *Shanghanlun*. These patients are generally regarded as having a cold pattern. In this case, *maobushi-saishinto* and the like are helpful.

- Alternating chills and fever

This is a comprehensive condition in which aversion to cold and fever occur alternately. Commonly, body temperature begins to rise in the afternoon, then after peaking, declines in the night. This type of heat, unlike "fever" that occurs in the very early stage of a disease, frequently develops several days after the onset; corresponding to the late yang stage pattern of disease transformation described in *Shanghanlun*. Such a patient is regarded as having heat pattern. The condition is frequently associated with fullness and discomfort in chest and hypochondrium, anorexia, string-like pulse, coating, tongue, and taste abnormality. Effective therapy is available with formulas with Bupleurum root such as *shosaikoto*.

- Whole body fever (*Shinnetsu*)

Whole body fever is systemic fever with deep pulse, not associated with sweating, as seen in late yang and middle yang stage pattern. This is a three-yang combined stage pattern described in *Shanghanlun*. Such a patient is regarded as having heat pattern. He or she also has burning sensation and aversion to heat (suffering from heat), usually not accompanied by aversion to cold or aversion to wind. However, aversion to wind is occasionally experienced in the late yang stage pattern. Also, aversion to cold on the back sometimes develops with three-yang combined pattern. *Shosaikoto* and the like are appropriate for the late yang stage pattern, while *byakkoto* is of choice for middle yang stage pattern and three-yang combined pattern (which is occasionally associated with sweating).

- Tidal fever

Body temperature rises at certain times in the day like a tide, associated with sweating in the whole body. There is no aversion to cold or wind, but aversion to heat (a condition in which the patient feels heat as pain) is evident. This medical condition corresponds to the middle yang stage pattern of disease transformation, as described in *Shanghanlun*, and is regarded as heat pattern.

Treatment with the formulas in jokito group including *daijokito* is effective.

- **Differentiation of heat pattern**

Even without a rise in the thermometer, pathological conditions may present with subjective feelings of heat such as sensitivity to heat, hot flashes, and feeling warmth when the body is touched. Objective findings of heat are not always present.

(a) Typical heat pattern

Patients are sensitive to heat even without elevation in body temperature, and experience heat.

sensation (*hoteri*) as revealed by palpation. The pulse tends to be tense and rapid. Urine is characterized by dark color and strong odor; stools also have a strong odor. Most patients experience thirst, and have thick and dark tongue coating.

(b) Fever-associated pathological conditions

A variety of fever-related pathological conditions are described in classics. Among these, the main conditions are as follows:

- Stagnated heat

This refers to the heat being retained with dampness in the body, and is associated with decreased urine volume. A diagnosis of heat pattern and excess pattern is considered. This condition is effectively treated with *inchinkoto* and the like.

- Deficiency heat

This is a condition where blood[TM1] and fluid[TM1] are lacking, and an excess of qi (normal or pathogenic) exists to cause heat. There was no term for deficiency heat in the classical Koho school; at present, the term "true cold with false heat" can be interpreted as being included in deficiency heat since it does not represent excess heat.

Rokumigan is indicated for a treatment to replenish fluid[TM1]. In addition, febrile symptoms can be caused by chronic fatigue and general weakness, and tonic formulas such as *kihito* are indicated.

- Heat with agitation

Heat with agitation is an uncomfortable sensation of heat and occurs in various pathological conditions. Formulas with

Gypsum, Coptis Rhizome, Rehmannia Root, and Rehmannia Root may be used.

- Vexing heat in the palms and soles (*Shusoku Hannetsu*)

This refers to a condition of uncomfortable heat sensation present in hands and feet and is described as a postpartum symptom in *"Kinkiyouryaku 金匱要略 (Synopsis of the Golden Chamber)"* and *sammotsuogonto* and *shosaikoto* are appropriate therapies.

- Vexing heat in the palms and soles (*Shusho Hannetsu*)

This refers to a condition of uncomfortable heat sensation present in palms and soles. *Unkeito* (温経湯) may be offered.

- True heat with false cold

A pattern presenting excess heat, but cold signs and symptoms appear due to excess heat.

Cold

The pathological condition with subjective feelings of cold and objective findings of reversal cold.

In the *Shanghanlun*, "cold" is included in the Yin stage patterns and early yin, middle yin, and late yin stage patterns of disease are described. The common feature is "cold," which should be treated by warming, using any of the following formulas: maobushisaishinto, shimbuto, shigyakuto, ninjinto, and keishikashakuyakuto. The pathological condition of subjective feelings of cold is primary, and objective findings of reversal cold are not present.

- Typical cold pattern

Even if the patient has elevated body temperature, he or she does not complain of feeling hot but does complain of coldness. This is the same as coldness being palpated on the body and limbs. The patient has deep and small pulse, which is likely to become slow (bradycardia). Urine is light colored and odorless, and stools have little odor. He or she may often have watery diarrhea, but usually does not experience thirst, and has thin and watery saliva with a uniformly smooth and glossy tongue and lesser tongue coating.

- Cold-associated pathological condition

A variety of cold-related pathological conditions are described in classics. Among these, the main conditions are as follows:

- Mixed cold and heat in hands and feet

The *Shanghanlun* discusses the medical condition in which a patient feels intense coldness in the limbs. This is called "mixed cold and heat in hands and feet" (which means qi can't reach the limbs and qi has to go around) or "cold sensation in limbs." Clinical findings include chilblains and pale limbs, suggesting poor peripheral circulation. In this case, tokishigyakuto and tokishigyaku-ka-goshuyushokyoto are used. Otsuka Keisetsu analyzed the cases in which these two Kampo formulas were effective and reported the conditions termed "abdominal colic syndrome A" (senki syndrome type A). This condition is characterized by coldness-induced aggravation of the chronic pain (low back pain, lower abdominal pain, headache, etc.) and other various complaints triggered by past coldness or surgery of the lower abdominal region. The pulse is deep and small or deep and thin, and is often too weak to be palpable.

- True cold with false heat (exterior heat and interior cold, interior cold and outer heat)

Despite the presence of possible febrile symptoms or signs on the body surface, the pathological condition is one of coldness in the depth of the body. In other words, there is an inconsistency between clinical findings and the pathological state. For example, the patient is sensitive to heat (if a heat pattern is considered, the urine should be reddish, very cloudy, and strong smelling, and the pulse should be tight), but presents with clear urine like water and a faint and weak pulse. Essentially this condition is a cold pattern, not a heat pattern. Treatment should focus on heat with formulas containing Processed Aconite Root, Ginseng, and Processed Ginger, such as shigyakuto.

1.5 Exterior and Interior

Hideki Adachi

1.5.1 A Concept of Exterior and Interior

Exterior and Interior and Exterior Pattern and Interior Pattern

In Kampo medicine, the terms exterior and interior are used to express the depth of the site where a disorder occurs. Exterior refers to the body surface, including the skin, mucous membrane, and throat. Interior stands for the depths of the body, which generally refers to the visceral organs, such as digestive organs. In addition, half-exterior half-interior pattern (area between exterior and interior) signifies a location between exterior and interior, which includes the bronchi, lungs, and liver.

Originally, the location indicated by exterior or interior is very rough and does not always represent specific viscera or tissue. Exterior pattern refers to signs and symptoms indicating that a disorder is located on the exterior; for example, "aversion to cold (with heat sensation)," "pains in the body and joints," "headache," and "sore throat."

Interior pattern refers to signs and symptoms indicating disorders located in the interior, for example, abdominal distention, abdominal pain, and diarrhea. Half-exterior half-interior pattern refers to signs and symptoms indicating disorders located in between, for example, alternating chills and fever, fullness and discomfort in chest and hypochondrium, and nausea and vomiting.

Inner and Outer (*Naigai*)

The *Shanghanlun* also uses the terms inner and outer, such as "half-ecterior half-interior (*Hangai Hanri*)." There is controversy regarding the interpretation of these terms. One group insists that exterior and outer have the same meaning, and interior and inner also have the same meaning. The other maintains that inner and outer are a relative concept: when the location of a disorder is fixed in a stage of disease transformation such as half-exterior and half-interior between exterior and interior at a given time, the part closer to the exterior is termed outer while the part closer to interior is called inner. The latter interpretation is often used when relatively distinctive locations are expressed in a wide range of half-exterior and half-interior.

1.5.2 Treatment Appropriate for Exterior and Interior

Treatment Appropriate for Each Stage of Disease Transformation

Concerning disease transformation, early yang stage pattern (heat pattern at exterior) is often treated with sweat inducing formulas such as keishito and maoto; late yang stage pattern (heat at half-exterior half-interior) is treated with harmonizing formulas such as shosaikoto; and middle yang stage pattern (heat pattern at interior) is treated with purgative formulas such as daijokito or formulas to clear heat such as byakkoto. For the treatment of Yin stage (early yin, middle yin, and late yin stage pattern) patterns, formulas for warming the interior are recommended such as keishikashakuyakuto, shimbuto, and shigyakuto.

1.6 Six Stage Patterns (Six Stage Patterns and Three-Yin and Three-Yang)

Hideki Adachi and Takashi Ito

1.6.1 A Concept of Six Stage Patterns

What are Six Stage Patterns? (Fig. 2.2 and Table 2.3)

The *Shanghanlun* classifies acute febrile diseases into six typical stage patterns.

Yang stage patterns of disease transformation are characterized mainly by heat. They consist of early yang stage pattern (heat at exterior), late yang stage pattern (heat at half-exterior half-interior), and middle yang stage pattern (heat at interior). Yin stages are characterized by cold. They consist of early yin stage pattern (cold at interior, in mild grade of disease), middle yin stage pattern (not only cold at interior but also occasionally cold at exterior and moderate), and late yin stage pattern (essentially cold at interior, but occasionally manifesting mixed conditions of upper heat and lower cold or true cold with false heat [exterior heat and interior cold], in severe stage of disease).

1.6.2 Transformation of Six Stage Patterns

When febrile disease occurs, it begins with early yang stage pattern, often followed a few days later by late yang stage pattern. Occasionally, however, the disease begins straightaway with middle yin stage pattern and does not feel like it begins at the early yang stage pattern. This is called direct strike into the middle yin stage pattern (without going through the early yang stage pattern). Otherwise, the early yang stage pattern can be followed by the middle yang stage pattern. In its various courses, the disease instead of resolving may become prolonged and reach the yin stage patterns, to finally end up in the late yin stage pattern.

Six Stage Patterns and Their Treatment

Yang Stage Pattern

- Early yang stage pattern

This is a stage of pattern transformation with pathogenic qi at exterior. The patient has a hot sensation accompanying aversion to cold or aversion to wind, headache, stiff neck and nape, and myalgia/ arthralgia, with floating pulse as a general rule. These signs and symptoms are collectively termed exterior pattern, meaning that the disorder manifests on the exterior.

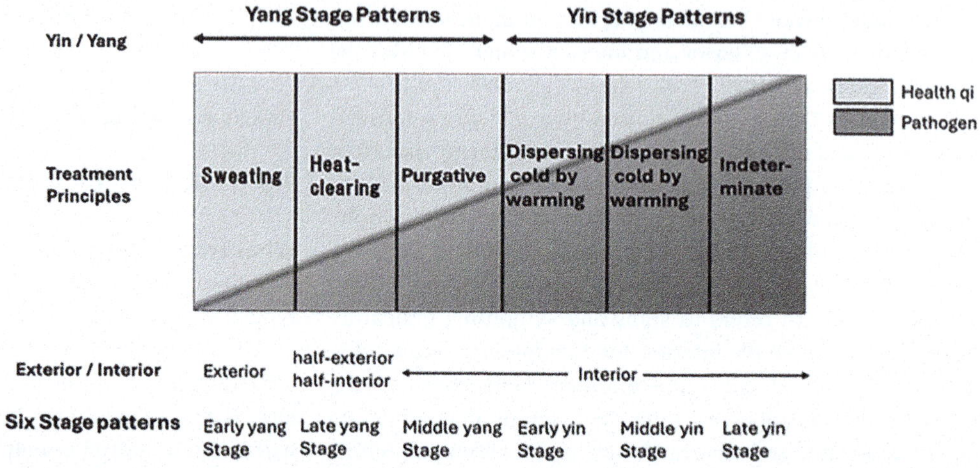

Fig. 2.2 Treatment principles of yin/yang, exterior/interior, and six stage patterns

Table 2.3 Summary of yang stage and yin stage

	Stage	Location of pathogens	Main symptoms	Severity	Deficiency and excess	Treatment principles
Yang pattern	Eary yang stage	Exterior	Floating pulse, headache, fever, aversion to cold, stiffness in the neck, arthralgia, muscle aches, no sweating, spontaneous sweating, normal tongue sign	No severe	Deficiency excess	Sweating
	Late yang stage	Half-exterior half-interior	Fullness and discomfort in chest and hypochondrium, alternating chills and fever, nausea and vomiting, discomfort in the mouth, dizziness, appetite loss, string-like pulse, dry white coating	↓	Deficiency excess	Heat clearing
	Middle yang stage	Interior	Persistent fever, abdominal distension, constipation, delirium, deep and tight pulse, slippery, surging and large pulse, thick dry white coating or yellow coating, hot-smelling sweat in the whole body	↓	Excess	Purgative
Yin pattern	Early yin stage	Interior	No fever, abdominal pain, diarrhea, flatulence, wet white coating	↓	Deficiency excess	Dispersing cold by warming
	Middle yin stage	Interior	Faint pulse, deep and fine pulse, anguish in the heart, watery diarrhea, reversal cold of the extremities, pale tongue, no coating, aversion to cold, declining energy, unconscious	↓	Deficiency	Dispersing cold by warming
	Late yin stage	Interior	Undigested food diarrhea, severe reversal cold of the extremities, cyanosis, aching heat in the chest, extreme weakness, deficiency heat, rarely sweating	Severe	Tangled deficiency and excess	Indeterminate

- Wind stroke and cold damage

In the *Shanghanlun*, febrile diseases are collectively termed cold damage. Nevertheless, mild and severe febrile diseases are named "wind stroke" and "cold damage," respectively. This is a somewhat complex terminological usage. In other words, the term cold damage has two meanings: (1) a generic term for febrile diseases and (2) a specific term for severe cases. This should be kept in mind.

Wind stroke is a condition of early yang stage pattern with mild symptoms such as aversion to cold, aversion to wind, and fever. It refers to the state in which the sensation of heat is accompanied by aversion to wind and is associated with spontaneous sweating, and floating and relaxed or floating and weak pulse. Such cases can be successfully treated with keishito and other formulas that act to cause sweating and vent called "releasing flesh" the wind stroke; this can harmonize/balance the exterior. The extent of this sweating action is like mild natural sweating (*Bijikan* in Japanese). Cold damage may be associated with intense aversion to cold from the beginning (reflecting the intensity of disease), and coexistence of exterior pattern (e.g., body pain, etc.) and interior pattern (e.g., gastrointestinal symptoms such as vomiting, etc.) as well as a floating and tight pulse. In such cases, appropriate treatment as a rule is formulas like maoto that strongly promote sweating, leading to a cure via mild sweating.

The use of this term varies in different texts whether the terms of wind stroke and cold damage are used only at early yang stage pattern (the initial stage of a febrile disease) or throughout the whole course of a febrile disease according to severity. Therefore, when reading the commentaries on the *Shanghanlun*, it is necessary to be careful about these terms.

- Malaria Like fever (alternating fever and chills disorder), and the status of strong heat sensation and mild cold sensation

The theory concerning disease subsequent to the early yang stage pattern, which is the late yang stage pattern, is as follows: If a disease that starts at early yang stage pattern (with pathogenic qi at exterior) does not cure even with induced sweating, in a few days it will often transform into late yang stage pattern (with heat at half-exterior half-interior). Sometimes, however, the disease may stay in early yang stage pattern, and present alternating fever and chills disorder like repeated rise and fall in body temperature as seen in malaria. In this case, the characteristic feature of early yang stage pattern, which is heat sensation associated with aversion to cold, remains.

This condition is described in the *Shanghanlun* as the state similar to alternating fever and chills disorder with great heat sensation and less cold sensation, as well as fever and aversion to cold. Keisetsu Otsuka interpreted this passage as follows: "the duration of fever is long whereas the duration of aversion to cold is short." From his own experiences, Ken Fujihira realized that while heat sensation is distributed throughout the whole body, aversion to cold is felt on the shoulders alone. Such a condition can be effectively treated with keishimaokakuhanto, keishinimaoichito, keishinieppiichito, and the like.

- Late yang stage pattern

This is the stage of disease transformation with pathogenic qi at half-exterior half-exterior. In late yang stage pattern, the disease transforms into a heat type of alternating aversion to cold and fever: body temperature rises with aversion to cold and the temperature rise subsides with appearance of heat sensation. Aversion to cold and heat sensation appear alternately. Actually, body temperature does not rise in the morning but rises gradually in the afternoon, reaches a peak in the evening, and subsides at midnight. Concurrently with alternating aversion to cold and fever, fullness and discomfort in the chest and hypochondrium in the hypochondrium also appear. This is a specific feature of this stage. The presence of discomfort in the chest and hypochondrium is the target for the use of formulas with Bupleurum root including shosaikoto. Such patients tend to have string-like pulse, white tongue coating, bitterness or taste changes in the mouth, and reduced appetite (sometimes associated with nausea). Symptoms of throat dryness, dizziness, and ear blocking also may occur.

Treatment is effective with formulas with Bupleurum root (such as shosaikoto), hangeshashinto group, shishikoto group, and others. These formulas each modulate and harmonize the whole, under a harmonizing principle. In this stage, in principle, strong cathartics or sweat inducing formulas are not used.

- Middle yang stage pattern of disease transformation

This is a stage of disease transformation with heat at interior.

- Tidal fever and formulas in jokito group

In middle yang stage pattern, the pattern of fever changes to tidal fever. Tidal fever means fever occurs at a certain time, concurrently there is spontaneous sweating enough to moisturize the whole body. The patient does not have the sensation of aversion to cold, but suffers heat sensation (aversion to heat). This is accompanied by abdominal distention, and constipation. Sometimes patients may talk deliriously when overwhelmed by fever. Pulse is deep and excess (strong). Basic treatment is purgation with formulas in jokito group such as daijokito and shojokito.

- Three-yang combined pattern and byakkoto

In addition to tidal fever that is treated with formulas in jokito group, middle yang stage pattern comprises another characteristic feature, three-yang combined pattern, for which byakkoto is appropriate. In three-yang combined pattern, the patient has burning sensation, with no aversion to cold as a rule (some patients feel slight aversion to cold on the back), but aversion to heat and with or without occasional spontaneous sweating. These manifestations are quite similar to those of a heat type whole body fever, as seen in late yang stage stage pattern of disease transformation. A patient also has much facial sebum, mouth irritation, and taste dysfunction. The patient may talk deliriously due to disturbed consciousness. Furthermore, the patient suffers severe thirst, not associated with decreased urine volume. The upper abdominal region is full and tense, along with pulse that is deep, smooth, and frequent, or large and surging. That is an excess pulse. A feeling of tension in the body similar to that of early yang stage pattern, mouth irritation similar to that of late yang stage pattern, abnormal taste, a fever-like body heat with a burning sensation, sweating similar to that of middle yang stage pattern, aversion to heat™, and abdominal distension all appear together. Hence, it is called the "combined disease of the three yang." However, the entity of the medical condition is heat at interior location and included in middle yang stage pattern. Some physicians claim that heat develops not only at exterior, but also interior and half-exterior half-interior pattern. Effective treatment is treat heat pattern (heat clearing therapy) with byakkoto, as a rule, rather than formulas in jokito group (the therapy for tidal fever).

Yin Stage Patterns

Among disease stages, early yin stage pattern, middle yin stage pattern, and late yin stage pattern are collectively referred to as Yin stage patterns. The essential nature of Yin stage patterns is cold at interior.

- Early yin stage pattern

This stage of disease transformation is characterized by cold at interior. The cold is mild but this pattern is associated with gastrointestinal symptoms such as abdominal distention and pain, vomiting, anorexia, and diarrhea. The pulse is also deep, and the abdominal strength often lack and this is occasionally accompanied by rectus abdominis muscle tension and epigastric stuffiness and resistance. Treatment with keishikashakuyakuto, ninjinto, or the like is effective.

- Middle yin stage pattern

This stage of disease transformation is characterized by cold at interior. This is sometimes accompanying cold at exterior. The cold is moderate and is represented by a pale face. Patients fatigue easily, want to lie down, and complains of dizziness, diarrhea, systemic pain, and occasional thirst (deficiency and thirst). Pulse is deep and faint, deep and thin, or deep and small. Some febrile diseases begin with middle yin stage pattern, which is termed "direct strike into middle yin stage pattern." Patients complain of sore throat and malaise, associated with chills rather than heat sensation, even in those with elevated body temperature. Appropriate formulas include maobushisaishinto, shimbuto, bushito, and shigyakuto.

- Late yin stage pattern

This is also a stage of disease transformation with cold at interior. but is likely to be associated with febrile symptoms. For example, the patient may present with mixed cold and heat: true cold with false heat, or upper heat and lower cold. This is a serious medical condition. Patients suffer coldness from the distal to the proximal limbs (coldness of limbs) but feels heat in the trunk, or cannot eat or may vomit even when hungry. Also, they have indigestion diarrhea associated with deep and slow pulse despite feeling heat on the body surface or in the upper body. These mixed symptoms are best treated by warming the interior with the formulas in shigyakuto group (including shigyakuto, bukuryoshigyakuto, and tsumyakushigyakuto).

Another Theory on the Six Stage Patterns

The six meridian patterns or disease stages are listed in the order of early yang stage pattern, middle yang stage pattern, late yang stage pattern, early yin stage pattern, middle yin stage pattern, and late yin stage pattern in all classics, including *"Shokanron 傷寒論 (Treatise on Cold Damage)"* and *"Koteidaikei 黄帝内経 (Yellow Emperor's Inner Classic)"*. Although it is difficult to understand from the modern perspective of three yin and three yang, it is clearly stated in the Heat Theory section of "*Somon 素問 (Basic Questions)*" that the sweating method is indicated for early yang stage pattern to late yang stage pattern. It is also stated that the purgative method is indicated for early yin stage pattern to late yin stage pattern. These were the correct method in ancient times.

The perception of pathological conditions, however, has changed greatly over time. In Japan, at the end of the Edo period, there was a tendency to regard *"Shokanron 傷寒論 (Treatise on Cold Damage)"* (actually *"Chukaishokanron 註解傷寒論 (Annotated Treatise on Cold Damage)"*) as absolute. A school emerged in this period that regarded the early yang stage pattern as exterior, middle yang stage pattern as inner, and late yang stage pattern as half-exterior half-interior, and late yang stage pattern as being the stage before middle yang stage pattern.

In addition, it should be noted that the understanding of the pathogenesis of the six meridian patterns changed drastically before and after the Northern Song Dynasty, although this will not be explained here.

Combination of Diseases

A pattern in the three yang-patterns that occurs primarily at one level, which also manifests on two or more levels, which can nevertheless be treated with one formula. (Refer to Chap. 3, Sect. 3.1.6)

Overlap

A disease caused by the overlapping of two diseases (patterns), treated with two formulas for each pattern. (Refer to Chap. 3, Sect. 3.1.6)

Destructive Stage

This is a destructive stage in which normally observed pathological features have changed due to inappropriate treatment. This includes not following the above-mentioned therapeutic principles based on combination and overlap as well as six stages of disease transformation (inducing sweating and releasing flesh for early yang pattern; harmonizing methods without sweating inducers for middle yang pattern; purgation or treating heat pattern for late yang pattern; interior-warming for yin stage patterns), and inappropriate dosage (excessive sweating, excessive purgation, etc). For successful treatment outcome, progress to the chaotic stage must be analyzed to find the mistake and the present pattern must be confirmed by physical examination. Chronic or intractable pathological conditions in the modern medical system are probably at such destructive stages. Careful review of the medical history and detailed physical examination will help in diagnosing the present pattern (six stage patterns, combination of diseases, or overlap of diseases) even for the destructive stage. This will lead to appropriate treatment, as mentioned above, and yield favorable outcomes. Even very complicated medical conditions can be resolved if the theory of overlap proposed by Ken Fujihira is applied. In this pattern, which is apt to be overlooked, medical conditions regarded as heat or excess patterns can be effectively treated by single or concurrent use of a formula for cold patterns. This approach takes into account theories by Shigenari Ogura, and others. Also, a breakthrough may be achieved by determination of cold or heat and deficiency or excess as well as examination of qi, blood[TM1], fluid[TM1], as described in the next section, instead of diagnosis based on six stage patterns.

1.7 Qi, Blood[TM1], and Fluid[TM1]

Hideki Adachi and Takashi Ito

These are physiological factors in the theory of Kampo medicine, and they are the three vital substances of the body to maintain homeostasis. Qi comprises inviable aspects and uniformly controls physical and mental activities. Blood[TM1] is a visible factor supporting material aspects. In one concept, the two elements of qi and blood[TM1] are the basis of all physiology.

1.7.1 Qi

The Concept of Qi

Qi refers to invisible action, function, or working that circulates throughout the body.

Qi Disturbance Pattern and Treatment

It is important that a certain amount of qi circulates throughout the body. Disruptions in qi circulation gives rise to various disorders.

Qi Deficiency

The activity of qi itself declines and gives rise to various dysfunctions. This 'inactive or low-spirited' condition is termed qi deficiency, which concurrently entails digestive dysfunction (deficiency of middle energizer). The patient complains of feeling tired and lethargic and presents with a weak pulse and soft abdomen (enough to be regarded as weak abdominal strength). Treatment involves the prescription of tonic formulas, such as hochuekkito, shikunshito, and rikkunshito, which contain ginseng and Astragalus Root. These formulas are also able to treat deficiencies in the upper abdominal region.

Qi Stagnation

This is the condition in which the circulation of qi is disturbed. Many patients complain of gas retention and associated feeling of fullness in the abdominal region. A depressive condition, stagnation of qi, can manifest as depression. This condition is really called qi depression. The following symptoms may occur as a result of qi stagnation:

- Obstructive discomfort in the throat (Inchu Sharen or Baikakuki)

This is an abnormal sensation in the laryngopharynx. The patient feels as if something like a piece of roasted beef or a plum kernel is caught in the throat, and cannot swallow it although wanting to swallow and cannot vomit although wanting to vomit. This abnormal sensation may be due to qi depression. Hangekobokuto is effective for this condition.

- Asthma

Occasionally qi stagnation may appear in a form of breathing difficulty like asthma and may be favorably treated with saibokuto, and hangekobokuto combined with makyokansekito, and the like.

- Ear blockage

Ear blockage may appear as a symptom of qi stagnation, although it may also develop in the middle yang pattern. Shisoin, shosaikoto combined with kososan, is used in some patients.

- Pain

Shigyakusan or kamishoyosan is sometimes applied for the treatment of stress-induced abdominal pain.

- Abdominal distension

As implied by the fact that the word qi also means gas, abdominal distention due to gas retention is also considered as qi stagnation.

Generally, formulas appropriate for qi stagnation and depression include kamishoyosan, hangekobokuto, and kososan. In addition, the formulas in jokito group, kumibinroto, shigyakusan, and daisaikoto are also effective for this condition. Furthermore, Magnolia Bark, Perilla Herb, Immature Orange, Rhubarb, and other crude drugs are useful for qi stagnation.

Qi Uprising pattern and Qi Counter Flow

This is a condition where the normal qi flow is disordered to produce a counterflow. This is due to a backflow of qi, which should normally flow from the center of the body (proximal) to the peripheries (distal), or from the upper half of the body to the lower half. Associated symptoms include palpitations, coughing, hot flash, vomiting, and feeling cold in the limbs.

- Palpitations

A condition where heart beats are perceptible, sometimes accompanied by discomfort. Ryokeijutsukanto, keishikaryukotsuboreito, and saikokaryukotsuboreito are used to treat this condition.

- Coughing

Coughing due to qi counter flow is often manifested as severe coughing. Bakumondoto and hangekobokuto are used to treat this condition.

- Vomiting

Vomiting due to qi counter flow is often manifested as a sudden heavy vomiting. Goshuyuto and hangekobokuto are used to treat this condition.

- Severe qi ascending counterflow (Honton)

This is a symptom described in the *"Kinkiyouryaku 金匱要略 (Synopsis of the Golden Chamber)."* The patient seems to suffer something like an attack toward the chest from the lower abdominal region in association with abdominal pain and fever, and falls into unconsciousness. At present, something like this attack is generally considered to be a hysterical attack. Hontonto from the *"Kinkiyouryaku 金匱要略 (Synopsis of the Golden Chamber)"*, ryokeikansoto, keishikakeito, and the like are effective.

- Counterflow of fire

The *Shanghanlun* describes a hypersensitive condition that occurs by heat treatment or burns. The main symptoms include palpitation, qi counter flow, and agitation and restlessness, which is similar to those of Honton. Keishikakeito, keishikanzoryukotsuboreito, and keishikyoshakuyaku-ka-shokushitsuboreiryukotsukyugyakuto are used. Many of the formulas used to treat qi counter flow contain Cinnamon Twig or Glycyrrhiza: for example, keishikyoshakuyakuto and shakanzoto.

1.7.2 Blood[TM1]

The Concept of Blood

Blood[TM1], circulating the body, is visible and red-colored. While qi represents action, function, and working, blood[TM1] is a visible component of the body, reflecting the nutritional and circulatory states.

Disorders of Blood[TM1] and Treatment

Blood[TM1] Deficiency

This is deficiency in blood[TM1], which not only appears as anemia, but also represents poor nutritional and circulatory conditions. The patient has dry skin, tendency toward atrophy, white and thin hair that is apt to fall out. Also, the limbs become lean enough to distinguish the tendons and joints.

Unlike qi deficiency characterized by fair skin, rather flabby body, soft and weak muscles as well as skin, and decreased activity, blood[TM1] deficiency is characterized by dark skin, lean body with a tendency to dehydrate. Also, the skin is firm along with the muscles and tendons and activity can be sustained .

Frequent formulas include shimotsuto, kyukikyogaito, renjuin, and unseiin, all of which contain shimotsuto (Japanese Angelica Root, Lindera Root, Cnidium Rhizome and Rehmannia Root). For dual deficiency of qi and blood[TM1], juzentaihoto, containing both shimotsuto and shikunshito, also effective for qi deficiency, is used.

However, the components Rehmannia Root and Cnidium Rhizome of shimotsuto may induce gastric symptoms in patients with decreased digestive function (deficiency of upper abdomen). In such cases, juzentaihoto may be preferable. Nevertheless, before prescribing juzentaihoto, shimotsuto, the deficiency of the upper abdomen should be thoroughly treated.

*Renjuin: ryokeijutsukanto and shimotsuto

Blood[TM1] Stasis

This means stagnant blood[TM1], specifically stagnation of the venous system and capillary vascular system can be imaged. Blood[TM1] stasis commonly occurs soon before, during, and after menstruation, and also in delivery, puerperium, and climacteric syndrome. Inflammation, bruising, hemorrhoids, and varix can also be included in blood[TM1] stasis. Confusion and bleeding are occur in febrile diseases associated with blood[TM1] stasis, and may result in significant modification of the pathological condition. The patient has resistance and tenderness in the lower abdominal region (*Shofuku Koman* [lower abdominal resistance and fullness], *Shofuku Kyuketsu* [lower abdominal cramp], etc.), along with sunken and rough pulse. In addition, the presence of blood[TM1] stasis is suggested by the following manifestations: (1) dry mouth (*Kokan*: the mouth is dried without thirst), (2) subjective feeling of abdominal distention (without objective distension), (3) feeling of heat with agitation, (4) purpura on the skin and mucosal membrane as well as capillary and venous distension, (5) dry and rough skin, (6) dark red or blue tongue, (7) purple spots on the lingual margin, (8) blue lips, (9) dark stools, (10) hemorrhagic tendency, (11) increased appetite, and (12) being impatient or irritable and tendency to blame others.

Blood[TM1] stasis resolving formulas, such as tokishakuyakusan, kamishoyosan, keishibukuryogan, nyoshinsan, tsudosan, and tokakujokito, are used in the treatment of blood[TM1] stasis based on the characteristics of each formula.

1.7.3 Fluids[TM1]

The Concept of Fluids[TM1]

Fluids[TM1] are visible and transparent, and circulate through the body. They can be visualized as humors.

Fluid[TM1] Disorders and Their Treatments

There is a wide range of pathological conditions related to fluids[TM1], including edema and inflammation which are involved in fluid[TM1] disorders. There are also many synonyms for the term fluids[TM1] (fluid[TM1], sputum, In [drink], dampness, etc.). In Japan, however, fluid[TM1]-related disorders (deviation from the normal) are often collectively called fluid[TM1] toxity (*Suidoku*) or fluid[TM1] retention (*Suitai*). Examples are as follows:

Dysregulation of Fluid[TM1] Metabolism

Manifest symptoms include edema, decreased urine volume, pollakiuria, vertigo or dizziness, orthostatic dizziness or syncope, dizziness or lightheadedness, headache, tinnitus, thirst, vomiting, and watery diarrhea. The pulse and abdominal pattern vary widely. Treatment depends on the condition of each patient, but formulas include goreisan, inchingoreisan, choreito, ryokeijutsukanto, shimbuto, tokishakuyakusan, and takushato. These formulas commonly contain crude drugs like Alisma Rhizome, Polyporus Sclerotium, rhizomes of *Atractylodes* spp., and Poria Sclerotium. These ingredients give formulas fluid[TM1] balance controlling or diuresis inducing properties.

Arthralgia, Arthritis, and Associated Edema

Formulas prescribed include keishikaryojutsubuto, eppikajutsuto, makyoyokukanto, and boiogito, which contain Ephedra, Rhizomes of *Atractylodes* spp., and Astragalus Root as components.

Fluid Retention in the Stomach

Splashing sounds are evident in the epigastric region. This condition is associated with belching, nausea, and/or vomiting. This condition is treated with shohangekabukuryoto, goreisan, ireito, bukuryoin, bukuryoingohangekobokuto, or bukuryotakushato. Fluid[TM1] retention in the stomach not only appears as a sign of fluid[TM1] disturbance, but can also develop as a result of reduced digestive function. In the latter case, ninjinto, shikunshito, rikkunshito, hangebyakujutsutemmato, and the like are effective.

Asthma and Rhinitis

Asthma and rhinitis are occasionally reflections of fluid[TM1] disturbance. In such cases, shoseiryuto or ryokankyomishingeninto is offered.

Fluid Deficiency

While the term fluid[TM1] retention comprehensively covers both water-rich and poor conditions, there is no established term to exclusively represent the latter alone. In this book, this state is denoted using the term fluid[TM1] deficiency. Typical symptoms include dry skin, thirst, and dehydration.

The term yin deficiency is not used here since it is similar to but distinct from fluid[TM1] deficiency. It has a different meaning of yin stage pattern and deficiency pattern and refers to a lack of yin fluid[TM1] with hot flash.

Many issues remain to be studied regarding "fluids (body fluids)" and "moisture."

1.8 *Gozo* (Five Zang Organs)

Shuji Yakubo

The five zang organs correspond to Wood[TM1], Fire[TM1], Earth[TM1], Metal[TM1], and Water[TM1] in the five elements theory. This concept represents the five functional units of the human body (Fig. 2.1). The *gozo* or five zang organs refer to the "solid organs"—liver[TM1], heart[TM1], spleen[TM1], lung[TM1], and kidney[TM1] in the human thoracic and abdominal cavities. In addition to five solid organs, there are five *fu* or empty organs in the human body—gallbladder[TM1], small intestine[TM1], stomach[TM1], large intestine[TM1], and bladder[TM1]. These five *fu* organs are positioned as complementary organs that assist in the functions of the five Zang organs. Another concept adds the triple-energizer[TM1] (this is believed to be the large veins) to five *fu* organs to comprise six *fu* organs. Modern medicine has no organ corresponding to the triple-energizer[TM1].

The functions of the five zang organs include both physical and mental functions. Disorders of these functions are considered to develop a wide variety of signs. Table 2.4 shows the functions of the five-zang *organs and signs suggestive of the* five zang organs abnormalities. Liver[TM1] corresponds to Wood[TM1], having hepatic functions as mentioned in modern Western medicine, such as nutrient metabolism and detoxication. Liver[TM1] is also associated with stabilization of the nervous system, mental stress, and the autonomic nerves. Heart[TM1] corresponds to Fire[TM1], having cardiac functions as mentioned in modern Western medicine, such as blood circulation. Heart[TM1] is also associated with mental activities such as consciousness and sleep. Spleen[TM1] corresponds to Earth[TM1], having gastrointestinal and digestive functions as mentioned in modern Western medicine, such as maintaining life through digestion and absorption. Spleen[TM1] is also associated with mental states such as depression. This concept is distinct from that of the spleen in modern Western medicine. This is attributable to the fact that Sugita Genpaku and others arbitrarily applied Kampo terms to translate a Dutch anatomy texts. Lung[TM1] corresponds to Metal[TM1], having respiratory functions as mentioned in modern Western medicine. Lung[TM1] also has a role with the skin, immunity, and water metabolism. It's also associated with mental states such as melancholy and grief. Kidney[TM1] corresponds to Water[TM1] and has renal functions and regulates water metabolism as mentioned in modern Western medicine. Kidney[TM1] is also associated with growth, development, and reproduction. It's associated with mental activities such as stabilizing thinking ability and judgment.

The fundamental principle for considering five zang organs is the five elements theory. For example, "Wood[TM1] generates Fire[TM1]," means that blood circulation in the heart[TM1] is accentuated by mental excitement of the liver[TM1]. In "Wood[TM1] restrains Earth[TM1]," the digestive and absorptive functions of spleen[TM1] are suppressed by the mental excitement of Liver[TM1]. In Kampo medicine, the five zang-organs concept involves the generating and restraining relationships based on the five elements theory, as described above. Therefore, there are only a few cases where any one of the five zang organs is disordered by itself. Thus, the five zang organs are not merely viewed from an anatomical viewpoint, but considered to be functional units associated with various metabolic and mental activities.

Table 2.4 Function of zang organs and symptoms of disorders in zang organs

Five zang organs	Function of zang organs	Symptoms of disorders in zang organs
Liver[TM1]	1. Mental stabilization 2. Metabolism and detoxification 3. Blood storage nutrition supply to the whole body 4. Maintenance of skeletal muscle tone Control of movement and balance	1. Irritability, irritation 2. Hives, jaundice 3. Menstrual abnormalities Anemia 4. Headache, shoulder stiffness, cramps, tension in the rectus abdominis 5. Swelling and pain in the hypochondrium area
Heart[TM1]	1. Maintenance of consciousness coordination of awareness activities 2. Sleep-wake rhythm regulation. 3. Blood circulation 4. Thermogenesis, secretion of sweat, thermoregulation	1. Impatience, agitation, poor concentration 2. Insomnia, lethargy, light sleep, excessive dream 3. Palpitation, bradycardia, arrhythmia, shortness of breath, chest compressions 4. Hot flush
Spleen[TM1]	1. Digestion and absorption, generating water and grain qi 2. Blood in a smooth, Preventing blood leaking 3. Myogenesis, maintenance of the muscles	1. Appetite loss, dyspepsia, nausea and vomiting, indigestion, abdominal pain, diarrhea, abdominal distension 2. Subcutaneous bleeding 3. Weakness, fatigue in the limbs, muscle atrophy. 4. Depression
Lung[TM1]	1. Intake of pectoral qi through respiration, supervision of qi flow 2. Generate of blood[TM1] and fluid[TM1] from water and grain qi 3. Control of skin function, maintenance of defense capabilities	1. Cough, expectoration, wheeze, nasal discharge, shortness of breath, difficulty breathing, chest congestion 2. Dry airway mucosa 3. Sweating disorders, itching, immunocompromise 4. Sorrow, distress
Kidney[TM1]	1. Growth, development, fertility control 2. Maintaining bone and tooth formation 3. Control of urinary function and water metabolism 4. Maintenance of respiratory capacity 5. Maintenance of thinking abilities, judgment and concentration	1. Diminished libido, infertility 2. Regressive change of bones, lumbago, deciduous tooth 3. Edema, nocturia, dry skin and eye 4. Dementia, impatience, fear, fright 5. Cataract, tinnitus

Diagnosis and Treatment

3

Katsutoshi Terasawa, Go Ito, Toshihiko Hanawa, Takao Namiki, Kazushi Uneda, Tadamichi Mitsuma, Mosaburo Kainuma, Hirozo Goto, Kazuo Mitani, and Masamitsu Nakajima

1 Patterns (General Concept)

Katsutoshi Terasawa

1.1 Basic Structure of Kampo Medicine

Kampo medicine is defined primarily by the two concepts "qi" and "yin and yang." Furthermore, "Kampo formulation" as a therapeutic agent is essential to the practice of this discipline. The present section describes the components of the diagnosis and treatment process in Kampo medicine.

1.1.1 Concept of Qi

Qi is the universal energy that pervades the environment of the earth. Kampo medicine considers all living organisms to be condensed forms of qi. Qi is invisible because it is energy. This idea of qi, which came from East Asian philosophy, is deeply rooted in daily life. For example, the term qi, used for natural phenomena, describes invisible energy. Similarly, there are terms with qi related to medicine (Table 3.1).

1.1.2 Theory of Qi, Blood[TM1], and Fluid[TM1]

The concept of qi plays a primary role in the assessment of clinical conditions in Kampo medicine, where physical disorders mean abnormal quantities or locations of qi (See Chap. 2, Sect. 1.7).

The International Classification of Diseases (ICD-11), Eleventh Edition, lists qi deficiency, qi counter flow and qi stagnation as qi disorders; blood[TM1] deficiency and static blood[TM1] as blood[TM1] disorders; and fluid[TM1] retention and lack of fluid[TM1] as fluid[TM1] disorders, along with their respective symptoms. The author has proposed diagnostic criteria (qi-body-fluid[TM1]score) for the Kampo physical conditions listed below (Tables 3.2, 3.3, 3.4, 3.5, 3.6, and 3.7).

1.1.3 Mind and Body Unity (These Two Are Inseparable)

As mentioned earlier, qi is the basic component that allows humans to exist as humans. It, therefore, supports all mental as well as physical functions and bodily structures. This is called "mind-body unity," and it is extremely important as a medical philosophy. This is because in modern natural sci-

K. Terasawa
Toyama University, Toyama, Japan

G. Ito
Oriental Medicine Therapy Center of Kitasato Institute Hospital, Kitasato University, Tokyo, Japan

T. Hanawa
Kitasato University Kitasato Institute Hospital, Tokyo, Japan

T. Namiki
International University of Health and Welfare Narita Hospital, Narita, Japan

K. Uneda
Department of Kampo Medicine, Aizu Medical Center, Fukushima Medical University, Aizuwakamatsu, Japan

T. Mitsuma
Department of Kampo Medicine, Aizu Medical Center Hospital, Fukushima Medical University, Aizuwakamatsu, Japan

M. Kainuma
Department of Japanese Oriental Medicine, Graduate School of Medicine and Pharmaceutical Sciences, Toyama University Hospital, Toyama, Japan

H. Goto
Hokusei Hospital, Toyama, Japan

K. Mitani
Nara Medical University/Mitani Family Clinic, Sakai, Japan

M. Nakajima (✉)
Division of Kampo Medicine and Pharmacognosy, Faculty of Pharmaceutical Sciences, Hiroshima International University/ Division of Kampo Medicine, National Hospital Organization Kure Medical Center, Higashi-hiroshima, Japan
e-mail: office@jsom.or.jp

Table 3.1 Concept of qi

Natural phenomenon	Ten-qi (weather), Ku-qi (air), Den-qi (electricity), Ji-qi (magnetism), Kei-qi (economy)
Medical terms	Gen-qi (vitality), Sei-qi (vitality), Byo-qi (illness), Kek-qi (vitality), Ei-qi (nutrition)

Table 3.2 Qi-blood[TM1]-fluid[TM1] score. Qi deficiency score

Body feels tired (now)	10
Lack of energy	10
Tires easily (tendency)	10
Sleepiness during the day	6
Loss of appetite	4
Easy to catch a cold	8
Easily surprised (easily startled)	4
Lack of power in eyes and voice	6
Tongue pale or swollen (sometimes teeth marked)	8
Weak pulse	8
Weak abdominal strength	8
Visceral atonic signs	10[a]
Weakness in the lower abdominal region	6[b]
Diarrhea tendency	4

When the sign is mild, 1/2 of the relevant score is given

A total score of 30 or more is considered qi deficiency

[a]Visceral atony signs include gastroptosis, renal ptosis, uterine prolapse, prolapse of the uterus, and anal prolapse

[b]Small abdominal distention refers to a decrease in abdominal wall tonus below the umbilicus

Table 3.3 Qi-blood[TM1]-fluid[TM1] score. Qi depression score

Depressive tendency	18[a]
Heaviness and headache	8
Stiffness in throat/throat tightness	12
Feeling of stuffiness in chest/feeling of tightness in the chest	8
Stiffness in hypochondrium/feeling of tightness in the costal region	8
Abdominal fullness	8
Symptoms change over time	8[b]
Difficulty getting up in the morning and not feeling well	8
Excessive gas	6
Frequent burping	4
Feeling of residual urine	4
Abdominal tympany	8

When the sign is mild, 1/2 of the relevant score is given

A total of 30 points or more is considered qi depression

[a]Depressive tendencies are determined based on symptoms such as depressed mood, lack of interest in things, and lack of appetite

[b]"Symptoms change over time" means that symptoms of the chief complaint change

Table 3.4 Qi-blood[TM1]-fluid[TM1] score. Qi counter flow score

Hot flash and cold feet	14[a]
Palpitations	8
Paroxysmal headache	8
Vomiting (minor nausea)	6
Coughing with anger	10
Attack of abdominal pain	6
Surprised easily	6
Sudden feeling of impatience/agitation	8
Facial flushing	10
Pulsations above the navel	14[b]
Cold lower limbs and extremities	4
Sweating in palms and feet/palmoplantar sweating	4

When the sign is mild, 1/2 of the relevant score is given

A total of 30 points or more is considered qi counter flow

[a]It is a feeling of heat in the upper body and a feeling of cold in the lower limbs at the same time. Certain signs are triggered when entering a room that is heated

[b]Supraumbilical palpitation refers to the pulsation of the abdominal aorta that can be felt when lightly touching the abdominal wall in the midline with the palm of the hand

Table 3.5 Qi-blood[TM1]-fluid[TM1] score. Static blood[TM1] score

	Male	Female
Pigmentation of the orbicularis oculi	10	10
Facial pigmentation	2	2
Skin hyperplasia[a]	2	5
Dark red lips	2	2
Dark red gums	10	5
Dark red-purple tongue	10	10
Detail[b]	5	5
Subcutaneous hemorrhage	2	10
Palmar erythema	2	5
Paraumbilical tenderness and resistance left	5	5
Paraumbilical tenderness and resistance, right	10	10
Paraumbilical tenderness and resistance midline	5	5
Ileocecal tenderness/resistance	5	2
Sigmoid tenderness/resistance	5	5
Hypochondriac tenderness/resistance	5	5
Hemorrhoids	10	5
Menstrual disorders	N/A	10

N/A Not Applicable

When the sign is mild, 1/2 of the relevant score is given

Total 20 points or less, non-blood[TM1] stasis; 21 points or more, blood[TM1] stasis; 40 points or more severe blood[TM1] stasis

[a]Roughness of skin and fissures on the skin

[b]Dilation of capillaries, spider hemangioma, etc.

ence, the mind and body are viewed as separate, and modern medicine, which is based on this dualism, tends to understand human existence with a bias toward the material aspects of the body. The philosophy of Kampo medicine, which considers the mind and body to be inseparable, is thought to become increasingly important in understanding human existence itself.

1.1.4 Yin-Yang Theory

The second aspect of understanding pathological conditions in Kampo medicine is the yin-yang theory. ICD-11 has adopted these terms along with their specific signs and findings. This theory gradually developed into a dualistic method of clinical practice wherein hypofunction and hyperfunction, exterior and interior, and heat and cold are the basic foundations (See Chap. 2 A-1).

Table 3.6 Qi-blood[TM1]-fluid[TM1] score. Blood[TM1] deficiency score

Decreased concentration	6
Insomnia, sleep disorders	6
Eye strain	12
Feeling dizzy	8
Cramps	10
Hypomenorrhea/Irregular menstruation	6
Poor complexion, dyspigmentation	10
Easy hair loss	8[a]
Dry and rough skin, redness of skin	14
Nail abnormalities	8[b]
Sensory disturbance	6[c]
Rectus abdominis muscle spasm	6

When the sign is mild, 1/2 of the relevant score is given
A total of 30 points or more is considered blood[TM1] deficiency
[a]Excessive dandruff on the head is also a sign of blood[TM1] deficiency
[b]Nails are brittle and cracked, and the nail beds are rough and cracked
[c]Numbness, such as tingling or numbness, sensation of being covered with skin, decreased sensation

Table 3.7 Qi-blood[TM1]-fluid[TM1] score. Fluid[TM1] retention score

Feeling of heaviness in the body	3
Pulsatile headache	4
Heaviness in head	3
Prone to car sickness	5
Dizziness/vertigo	5
Lightheadedness	5
Watery nasal discharge	3
Excessive saliva	3
Foamy sputum	4
Nausea/vomiting	3
Increased abdominal sounds	3
Morning stiffness	7
Edema tendency/splashing sounds of stomach	15
Pleural effusion, cardiac effusion, ascites	15
Pulsation in the supraumbilical region	5[a]
Watery diarrhea	5
Decreased urine output	7
Polyuria	5

When the sign is mild, 1/2 of the relevant score is given
Fluid[TM1] retention is defined as a total of 13 points or more
[a]Pulsation in the supraumbilical region: increased pulsation of the abdominal aorta palpable in the umbilical region

1.1.5 Variable Clinical Conditions

The basic structure of Kampo medicine has been mentioned above. However, another important characteristic is that clinical conditions are viewed not as fixed entities but as changeable over time.

Let us consider a case of influenza. The initial symptoms may be chills or discomfort in the nasal cavity. This is followed by fever, headache, arthralgia, and myalgia. Symptoms of the upper and lower respiratory tracts follow. Usually, treatment is given at this point, and the fever resolves, and the patient is cured. However, patients with low vitality may develop pneumonia, go into shock, and die. In other cases, the patient may have a persistent fever, cough, anorexia, and diarrhea even after the fever has broken. In Kampo medicine, the early stage of the illness is generally referred to as the "first stage of yang pattern" and is called the early yang stage. The third stage of the yin pattern is called the late yin stage and is similar to the state of shock, with hypotension, peripheral circulatory failure, and decreased metabolic rate. The period of prolonged fever, cough, and anorexia after the resolution of fever is called the "second stage of yang pattern," or the late yang stage of the disease.

Even in chronic diseases, the rate of transition may be slow, but it is still considered to be in transition from a yin pattern to a yang pattern, or from a yang pattern to a yin pattern. Although this concept differs from modern medicine, which determines the name of a disease based on histopathological findings or various diagnostic criteria and develops treatment strategies in a somewhat fixed manner, we believe that this recognition of the changeable nature of the disease in Kampo medicine will be an important factor in the future development of therapeutics.

This classification of stages of infectious disease (six-stage patterns) is also listed in ICD-11.

1.2 Characteristics of Kampo Formulas

Kampo medical formulas generally contain several crude drugs mixed in fixed amounts. Each formula is indicated for the treatment of various clinical conditions, which are called the characteristics of the formulas.

Each crude drug has various medicinal properties, and it is unique in that it applies yin-yang theory to its medicinal properties. For example, aconite, dry ginger rhizome, return, and medicinal evodia have the property of increasing the production of heat in the body and are called medicines with properties and actions of warming. On the other hand, *Gypsum*, *Rheum*, *Bupleurum*, *Coptis japonica*, and *Scutellaria baicalensis* have the property of suppressing heat production in the body and are called heat-clearing formulas. In general, the rule is to use cooling medicines for positive conditions and warming medicines for negative conditions in order to normalize the condition.

There are approximately 300 types of Kampo extract formulations in common use, but only 147 are currently covered by medical insurance. These formulas are not a random mixture of herbs but rather a combination of herbs designed to restore the yin-yang of biological reactions or the imbalance of the qi, blood[TM1], and fluid[TM1] systems.

In other words, each Kampo extract formulation has its own specific indications for a particular condition, which is called the character of Kampo formulas.

For example, kakkonto consists of Ephedra herb (麻黄), Cinnamon Bark (桂皮), Pueraria Root (Common Kudzu Root) (葛根), Peony Root (芍薬), Jujube Fruit (大棗), fresh ginger rhizome (生姜), and Glycyrrhiza root (liquorice root) (甘草). Ephedra herb and cinnamon bark produce heat to enhance the flow of qi and blood[TM1]; pueraria root, peony root, and Glycyrrhiza root relax muscles in the neck and back. Jujube fruit, ginger rhizome, and Glycyrrhiza root buffer the gastric mucosa and thereby protect the stomach from the actions of Ephedra herb and cinnamon bark. Kakkonto is used when the body exhibits hyperfunction (excess pattern) with concomitant stiffness in the neck and back, headache, and cold in the early stages of infectious disease. This formulation may not be beneficial in patients with yin conditions or yang conditions with hypofunction (deficiency pattern). Each formula, in other words, has its own therapeutic window or spectrum.

1.3 What is a Pattern?

In Kampo medicine, a pattern is a diagnosis. This perspective, however, is very different from diagnosing chronic hepatitis or diabetes in Western medicine. In order to determine the pattern, the original parameters of Kampo medicine are used. The parameters are yin-yang, deficiency or excess of qi, blood[TM1], and fluid[TM1]. Thus, a pattern is "a diagnosis obtained by applying the pathognomonic method of Kampo medicine."

Furthermore, the characteristic feature of this "pattern" is that it results in "a probable indication for the formula(s)."

Therefore, the academic definition of pattern is as follows: "Pattern refers to the symptoms a patient is exhibiting at the moment, based on basic concepts such as qi, blood[TM1], fluid[TM1], yin and yang, deficiency and excess, cold and heat, exterior and interior, five organs, and six-stage patterns. It is a diagnosis that is obtained by comprehensively recognizing symptoms that indicate the specificity of the condition and provides instructions for treatment." The specificity of the condition here refers to abdominal signs and findings from the radial artery.

As mentioned above, the patient's clinical condition is considered to change over time. The phrase "at the moment" is thus necessary because Kampo diagnosis changes along with the patient's clinical progress. First, patients are categorized based on the theory of qi, blood[TM1], fluid[TM1], and yin-yang theory. Subjective symptoms such as sensitivity to cold and heat and dull feelings are essential information for this process; Kampo medicine is known as the "medical system with mind-body unity" due to this characteristic.

Symptoms that indicate "the specificity of the condition" are those that are important in selecting the most appropriate Kampo formula among the categories narrowed down by yin-yang, excess deficiency, etc. Specifically, abdominal symptoms such as fullness and discomfort in the chest and hypochondrium, epigastric stuffiness and resistance, and paraumbilical tenderness and resistance, as well as the degree of tension and size of the radial artery.

Let us give an example of this process. In the early stages of infection, when fever, excess pulse, and no spontaneous sweating are found, the Kampo diagnosis is early stage and excess pattern. In this pattern, formulas for the treatment are indicated, such as daisaikoto, maoto, and kakkonto. The three formulas are differentiated by the specific symptoms of mental restlessness in daisaikoto, wheezing and joint pain in maoto, and the presence of muscle tension in the back of the trunk in kakkonto. If the patient shows stiffness in the back of the trunk, kakkonto is the treatment of choice. In this case, the symptom is described as "a condition of the early yang stage, for which kakkonto is the first choice." The customary term used to describe this is "kakkonto pattern."

Signs presenting the specific properties of the clinical condition are important signifiers that assist the Kampo physician in selecting the most appropriate treatment. That is, the categories for treatment are narrowed down based on yin-yang or hypofunction/hyperfunction concepts.

1.3.1 Formulation Corresponding to the Pattern

The above explanation of pattern implies that first, the Kampo physicians must acquire knowledge of categorizations as well as skills in diagnosis. Second, it is necessary for them to learn about the categories into which each formulation resides and the specific signs helpful in identifying which formulation to give to the patient.

Diagnosis in Kampo medicine is made by a combination of assessing clinical conditions and selecting formulas to prescribe as therapeutic agents. The relationship between these steps is like the one between lock and key. Since ancient times, the term "formulation corresponding to pattern" has been used because of the close correspondence between a formula and a pattern.

2 Diagnostics of Kampo Medicine

For examination, the office should be well-illuminated by natural light, and the room temperature should be maintained appropriately so that unclothed patients do not feel cold. Examinations of Kampo medicine are also part of the diagnostic and treatment processes.

2.1 Four Diagnostic Examinations

Go Ito and Toshihiko Hanawa

In Kampo, "four diagnostic examinations" are performed. These examinations are inspection, listening, inquiry, and palpation. A Chinese character for listening means hearing and smelling. So the two meanings of auscultation and olfaction are included in the listening examination. In addition, the Chinese character for palpation means not only cutting but also touching (palpation includes pulse examination, abdominal examination, and back examination). Tongue diagnosis is included in the inspection. These examination methods employ the physician's four senses of vision, hearing, olfaction, and touch to determine the patient's pattern and thus follow concrete procedures for processing prescriptions.

2.2 Visual Inspection

Go Ito and Toshihiko Hanawa

Inspection of Kampo medicine is almost the same as that of modern medicine. It includes observation of the patient's movement, gait, and abnormal movement when they enter the office. General observations include the patient's nutritional status, body shape, size, posture, muscle tone, skeletal deformities, edema, skin color/tone, skin dryness/dampness, and sweating. This is followed by specific observations, including the complexion, light in the eyes, facial expression, ocular and conjunctival conditions, hair and nail conditions, intraoral and tongue conditions (tongue diagnosis), and oral mucosal and gingival conditions. Among the inspectional assessments, tongue diagnosis has a special role and is explained in detail later in this chapter.

2.2.1 Overall Observation

Movement and Gait

To detect a deficiency or excess of qi and blood[TM1], it is important to know whether the patient moves or walks fast or awkwardly. If physical movement and walking manner are speedy and normal, the patient's ability to fight the disease may be considered substantial. If movement is slow or clumsy, it implies a state of enfeeblement or the presence of illness involving qi, blood[TM], fluid[TM1], or the five zang organs.

Physique

The doctor first observes the strength of the patient's reaction to the disease by assessing his or her physique and musculature. During the visual examination, physique and complexion are inspected to determine whether the patient has the appearance of strength to recover from disease (so-called excess pattern) or whether he or she is emaciated and weak (so-called deficiency pattern). Obese individuals do not necessarily have excess patterns, but their body size indicates that their muscles and bones are firm. On the other hand, people with a delicate physique or those who are obese due to lack of exercise or obesity from water retention often have a deficiency pattern even if they are fat at first glance. A person like this, with weak bones, who is obese and tends to sweat as soon as getting tired, doesn't settle down even when sleeping, and frequently catches a mild cold and gets blood[TM1] impediment is called a "respectable delicate person" in "*Jinguitaolue*."

Skin

Skin conditions indicate the general nutritional status and blood circulation and, therefore, should be observed carefully. Dry appearance is frequently linked to blood[TM1] deficiency.

Considerable differences may be observed in the skin according to the patient's age and sex, but generally, skin of good color and moderate moisture and shine is normal. Hyperhidrosis of the face and above the neck tends to be induced by qi counter flow. Dry skin, poor nourishment state, and cracks on the skin with atrophy and keratotic abnormality are symptoms of lack of blood[TM1] deficiency. In such cases, formulas based on shimotsuto (四物湯) may be used. Pigmentation, bloodshot appearance with marble pattern, capillary dilatation, or subcutaneous hemorrhage of skin suggests static blood [TM1] is considered. Skin symptoms due to phlebeurysm or arteriosclerosis obliterans, frostbite, Raynaud phenomenon by collagen diseases, or scleroderma may also imply static blood[TM1]. If there are those static blood[TM1] findings, the prescription is often selected from a blood[TM1] stasis-resolving formula (駆瘀血剤).

Perspiration

Naturally sweating is called "spontaneous sweating (*jikan*)," cold sweat is "deficiency sweat (*kyokan*: 虚汗)," and no sweat when to sweat is "absence of sweating (*mukan*)." Patients who tend to spontaneously sweat may have exterior [TM] deficiency and fluid [TM] retention, which may be treated with formulas containing Astragalus root (黄耆). Most patients who perspire with less sticky and low-viscosity sweat under conditions that do not normally cause sweating have exterior [TM] deficiency, such as "deficiency sweat," and may be treated with formulas such as keishito (桂枝湯) and keishikaogito (桂枝加黄耆湯). In some cases, the heat on the exterior of the body is taken away, and the sweat gets cold and complains of cold sweat. On the other hand, sweat with high viscosity is mainly caused by interior heat (*rinetsu*), which is seen in the indication of the drug in the late yang stage pattern or the middle yang stage pattern. (See "Abnormal sweating.")

2.2.2 Sectional Observation

Eyes

The brightness and emptiness of the eyes, when the patient enters the office, are important determinants of the degree of deficiency or excess of qi and blood [TM1]. Powerful eyes are suggestive of either fullness or normal qi. Empty, faint eyes are suggestive of qi deficiency (*kikyo*) and qi depression (*kiutsu*). Consider prescribing hochuekkito (補中益気湯) for those with qi deficiency, nyoshinsan (女神散) for qi stagnation (*kitai*) or qi counter flow (*kigyaku*) with both qi and blood[TM1] deficiency, kyukichoketsuin (芎帰調血飲) for qi stagnation with static blood[TM1], and tsudosan (通導散) for those with excess pattern. On the other hand, the feeling that the eyes protrude or are irritated suggests abnormalities in the liver[TM1] as well as a sympathetic tone. Redness of the eyes suggests reluctance and bleeding (blood[TM1] fever) associated with fever. On the other hand, slanted eyes or being in an impatient or irritable state is suggestive of liver[TM1] abnormality, or high tension in the sympathetic nervous system, while red eyes are suggestive of qi counter flow and blood[TM1] heat (*ketsunetsu*). When there is qi counter flow and blood[TM1] heat, consider kamisyoyosan (加味逍遙散).

Complexion

Complexion is an important determinant of the degree of deficiency or excess of qi and blood[TM1]. Flushing of the skin may be suggestive of conditions such as blood heat, qi counter flow, and static blood[TM1]. A dark red color tends to be symptomatic of static blood[TM1].

Pallor may be suggestive of conditions such as qi deficiency, blood[TM1] deficiency, and fluid[TM1] retention. Puffy eyes may be suggestive of fluid[TM1] retention and darkish eye circles may be suggestive of kidney[TM1] deficiency and static blood[TM1]. A yellowish complexion suggests spleen[TM1] deficiency, blood [TM1] deficiency, or jaundice. Tokishakuyakusan (当帰芍薬散) or keisibukuryogan (桂枝茯苓丸) is considered for facial telangiectasia; pigmentation and dark circles under the eyes are signs of static blood[TM1].

Scalp Hair

Thin hair, lusterless hair, and excessive hair loss may be suggestive of blood[TM1 deficiency. Circular alopecia is often related to depression. For example, consider keisikaryukotsuboreito (桂枝加竜骨牡蛎湯) in cases of significant hair loss due to deficiency pattern, juzendaihoto (十全大補湯) for a wide range of hair loss with both qi and blood[TM1] deficiency, and daisaikoto (大柴胡湯) or saikokaryukotsuboreito (柴胡加竜骨牡蛎湯) for alopecia areata with qi stagnation or liver[TM1] qi stagnation.

Nails

Fragile nails with vertical ridges or cracks around the nails and the nail bed skin may be suggestive of blood[TM1] deficiency. Juzentaihoto (十全大補湯) is used for both qi and blood[TM1] deficiency, and blood[TM1] stasis-resolving formulas are used for dark red nails suggestive of static blood[TM1].

Lips of Mouth and Gingivae

Dry lips and angular stomatitis are linked to spleen[TM1] deficiency, blood[TM1] deficiency, and fluid[TM1] deficiency. Weak children with dry lips and spleen[TM1] deficiency are likely to present with a shokenchuto-pattern (小建中湯証) pattern. Dark-purple-colored lips and gingivae may be suggestive of static blood[TM1], and pale-colored lips suggest blood[TM1] deficiency. When the lips are dry from static blood[TM1], unkeito (温経湯) may be used. When there is a fluid deficiency with blood[TM1] deficiency, ninjin'yoeito (人参養栄湯) may be used. Angular stomatitis reflects digestive organ (spleen[TM1] and stomach[TM1]) disorders, and aphtha in the mouth reflects excessive heat of five zang organs, especially heat in the heart[TM1]. Orento (黄連湯) is used for the angular stomatitis in the stage from early yang stage to late yang stage pattern, hangeshashinto (半夏瀉心湯) is used for that in the late yang stage, and inchinkōto (茵陳蒿湯) is used for that in the middle yang stage.

2.3 Tongue Diagnosis

Go Ito

Originally, the origin of the tongue examination method was in ancient China. An oracle bone script was excavated from sites of the Shang Dynasty in ancient China 3000 years ago. It has a fortune-telling of tongue disease, which is now considered to be the oldest tongue disease notation. In ancient Chinese medicine, the tongue was a mirror that reflected the condition of the body. Diseases in the viscera and states of mind were thought to appear as changes in the tongue.

2.3.1 History of Tongue Diagnosis

In ***Huangdi Neijing***, which is a medical text of ancient China, there are already notations of morphological changes such as tongue curl, tongue rigidity, tongue wilt, and short tongue. In the 32nd chapter of ***Suwen*** (part of the *Huangdi Neijing*), it is stated that "yellow moss" appears on the tongue when there is a fever due to pneumonia. In ***Shanghanlun,*** written after the common era, there is also a description of "white moss" and descriptions such as using shishishito (梔子豉湯) for those with tongue coating during the early illness stage and byakkokaninjinto (白虎加人参湯) for those with dry tongue. In addition, some tongue findings, such as "yellow moss" and "blue tongue," are cited in ***Jinguitaolue***. Subsequent texts also contained tongue findings or were systematized as a tongue examination method after the ***Records***

of Golden Mirror was written in the Yuan Dynasty in the twelfth century. The ***Records of Golden Mirror*** is considered to be the oldest specialized text on tongue coating in China, but it is now lost. In 1341, ***Mr. Ao's Records of Golden Mirror*** was compiled by Du Ben. Originally 12 types of tongue coatings were described, and later 24 types were added to make a total of 36 types. Subsequently, with the rise of the warm illness school in the sixteenth century, the method of diagnosing tongue coating developed dramatically. In 1668 (Qing Dynasty), in the ***Tongue Model on Cold Damage*** written by *Cho To*, 9 types of tongue moss were described. The tongue was classified into white, yellow, black, ashen, crimson, purple, slightly cherry-colored, indigo-colored, and cold pregnancy damage, and there were 120 tongue coatings.

In Japan, due to the influence of those classical Chinese texts on tongue diagnosis, *Takayuki Tsuchida* published the ***Zettaizusetsu*** in the Edo period (1835). This text divides tongue coating into four classifications on the basis of color (white, yellow, black, and red) and 35 subclassifications. *Mosai* emphasized the benefits of the tongue inspection, stating that "Signs of differences between yin and yang, exterior and interior, deficiency and excess, and cold and heat are always seen on the tongue, unlike pulse diagnosis, which is difficult to perform." *Mosai* stated that "The objective is to develop standards for diagnosing diseases by not only observing the color, luster, thickness, and lesions of tongue coating, but also giving attention to the movement and tremors of the tongue." This deserves special consideration.

In 1813, *Kuronaga Nojo* published the ***Kokujifukuzetsuzukai***, which presents abdominal examination and tongue examination findings and the corresponding treatments (Kampo formulas). *Gencho* published volume one of the ***Kokujifukuzetsuzukai*** for his disciples as a textbook of his lectures on abdominal and tongue examinations. He suggested that tongue coating is the priority in diagnosing the signs and symptoms of cold damage, and yellow coating and black coating should always be linked to fever. White coating is also commonly linked to fever, and a thin, whitish-red coating is commonly linked to a cold. Diagnosis requires careful evaluation. 91 Kampo formulas are suggested in the ***Kokujifukuzetsuzukai***, mainly from the ***Shanghanlun***, linked to 91 tongue findings and 91 abdominal findings. The big difference between Japanese texts and older *Chinese* texts is that *tongue illustrations are printed in color.*

In Western medicine, on the other hand, it is recorded in 1828 that the tongue was observed for knowing the stage of health [1]. In 1918, Faber wrote the phrase "tongue is the mirror of stomach," which became the norm today, so that changes in the tongue are associated with stomach issues. In contemporary Japanese Kampo of the Koho school, as well as in acupuncture and moxibustion, comprehensive patterns are not determined solely by examination of the tongue.

2.3.2 Key Points of Tongue Examination

The tongue can be used to obtain long-term physical information such as constitution as well as acute systemic metabolic states such as fever and dehydration or chronic changes in gastrointestinal function such as constipation and gastritis.

The upper and lower surfaces of the tongue are also known as the dorsal and ventral surfaces of the tongue, respectively. The back of the tongue is called the root of the tongue, the center is called the middle of the tongue, and the tip is called the apex of the tongue. The dorsal surface is covered with several types of papillae, including filiform, fungiform, circumvallate, foliate, and conical papillae. The tongue inspection focuses on filiform papillae, which are distributed evenly over the entire dorsal surface of the tongue, and fungiform papillae, which occur sporadically on the same surface.

Only the surface of the epithelium (stratified squamous epithelium) of the filiform papillae (not the other papillae) is keratinized. Tongue coating (*zettai*) is produced by weak exfoliation of the epithelium of filiform papillae and increases bacterial propagation. The growth of tongue coating, incidentally, is associated with factors such as sleep, drinking, smoking, constipation, fever, and hypermetabolism. The formation of tongue coating is associated with the pH and the secretory volume of saliva, the condition of the oral flora or filiform papillae. Tongue capillaries are at the center of each papilla, but the color tone in the blood vessels cannot be seen through papillae except for fungiform papillae because they are not keratinized. Therefore, it may be recognized through fungiform papillae as red spots in heat patterns and as stasis spots in static blood[TM1] patterns. (see Red spots/Stasis spots)

Observing the tongue always requires a certain amount of light, but the color of the tongue differs depending on the light source, such as a light bulb, fluorescent light, LED, penlight, and natural light. Generally, it must be taken into account that fluorescent light is bluish and the natural light of the morning sun or sunset or in the light bulb may be reddish. At the time of examination, it is necessary to have the tongue stuck out as far as possible to observe the root of the tongue. But if the tongue is moved in and out many times or placed in the supine position, the color tone of the tongue may change because the blood flow may change. When the tongue coating has an unnatural color, such as green or purple, it is necessary to make sure that patients have not taken anything that colors the tongue, such as candy or beverages, just before.

Tongue findings are called tongue signs (*zetsusyo* or *zetsuko*). There are two major tongue inspection procedures: inspection of the tongue texture (*zetsushitsu*: tongue itself) and inspection of the tongue coating (*zettai*: tongue coating). In the inspection of the tongue texture, ①tongue color, ②tongue shape, and ③tongue motion are assessed. In the inspection of tongue coating, ①coating texture and ②coating color are assessed.

2.3.3 Types of Tongue Examination Findings

There are the following types of tongue examination findings currently used (Table 3.8).

(The numbers in parentheses in this section correspond to the explanation in Fig. 3.1.)

2.3.4 Tongue Color (Fig. 3.1)

The color of the tongue body itself, excluding the tongue coating, is evaluated.

Pale

Pale tongue (*tanpakuzetsu*) (tongue color ①) is less red than normal light red tongue and indicates the presence of circulatory disturbances and erythroid depletion such as ischemia and anemia, edema, or hypoproteinemia. In other words, the pathology of either the qi deficiency or the blood[TM1] deficiency, or both, is possible. Formulas such as shikunshito (四君子湯) or hochuekkito (補中益気湯) that include ginseng (人参), Astragalus root (黄耆), atractylodes rhizome (白朮), and poria sclerotium (茯苓) are used for qi deficiency, and formulas such as shimotsuto (四物湯) that include Japanese Angelica root (当帰), Rehmannia root (地黄), atractylodes rhizome (白朮), and ass glue (阿膠) are used for blood[TM1] deficiency.

In the case of the yang deficiency, with a pale white-colored tongue, this is often accompanied by enlargement (*handai*) and teeth marks (*shikon*) from edema of the tongue. In this case, formulas such as bushirichuto (附子理中湯) that include processed aconite tuber (附子) and Processed Ginger (乾姜) are used.

Table 3.8 Differentiation of tongue examination findings

Tongue findings	**Tongue body**	**Color**	Pale, (pale red), light red, red (crimson red), dark red (crimson), light purple, purple, red-purple, bluish-purple, blue
		Shape	Enlargement, thin teeth marks, fissures, red spots, stasis spots, stasis macules, prickles, varicose vein
		Condition	Shortness, atrophy, protruding, licking, wryness, tremor
	Tongue coating	**Texture**	None, thin, little, thick, greasy, putrid, lateralized, exfoliative (geographic), dry, moist
		Color	White, yellowish-white, yellow, gray, black, hairy black

The color tone of tongues between pale and light red is called *pale red tongue* (*hentanzetsu*) (tongue color ②) in Chinese medicine and indicates a mild condition of pathology of pale tongue, but the treatment is almost the same as that for the pale tongue.

Light Red

Light red tongue (*tankōzetsu*: 淡紅舌) (tongue color ③) is the normal tongue color. This color was also called slight red (*bikō*) in the Edo period of Japan.

Red

Red tongue (*kōzetsu*) (tongue color ④) is darker than the normal pale red tongue. This color is also called pure red (*junko*) or vermilion (*shu*) in the classic texts of the Edo period of Japan.

This color indicates fever, dehydration, and static blood[TM1], and is often linked to heat patterns, including both excess heat and deficiency heat. The common causes of red tongue due to fever are telangiectasia or hyperemia and congestion, or hemoconcentration due to dehydration in the interstitium of the tongue. Red tongues like the mirror tongue (*kyomenzetsu*) may also be attributed to the atrophy of the lingual papillae or tongue mucosa.

Formulas such as kamishoyosan (加味逍遙散), that include Mentha herb (薄荷), Japanese Angelica root (当帰), Moutan Bark (牡丹皮), gardenia fruit (山梔子), etc., are used for red tongues caused by heat patterns or static blood[TM1]. Formulas such as byakkokaninjinto (白虎加人参湯), which contain gypsum (石膏) and Anemarrhena rhizome (知母), are used for those caused by interior heat or dehydration in the middle yang stage pattern.

In addition, the color of the tongue is bright red, and the color tone between red and crimson is called "*crimson red tongue* (*ko-kozetsu:* 紅絳舌) (tongue color ⑤)" in Chinese medicine, and it is regarded as a mild stage of crimson tongue, and the treatment is similar to a red tongue or a crimson tongue according to another pattern.

Dark Red and Crimson

Dark red (*ankō*) color is darker than red, and another name for this is *anseki* (暗赤). It was called *sinko* (深紅) in the Edo period of Japan and crimson (*ko*)" in traditional Chinese medicine.

Dark red tongues (*ankōzetsu*) (tongue color ⑥) have been attributed to the middle yang stage syndrome of acute febrile illnesses or fluid[TM1] deficiency. This is yin deficiency in Chinese medicine, but it is also observed in heat patterns or static blood[TM1] (瘀血) with dehydration. It may be caused by the concentration and stagnation of blood flow at the capillary level, which leads to oxygen desaturation of the blood and produces a dark red color.

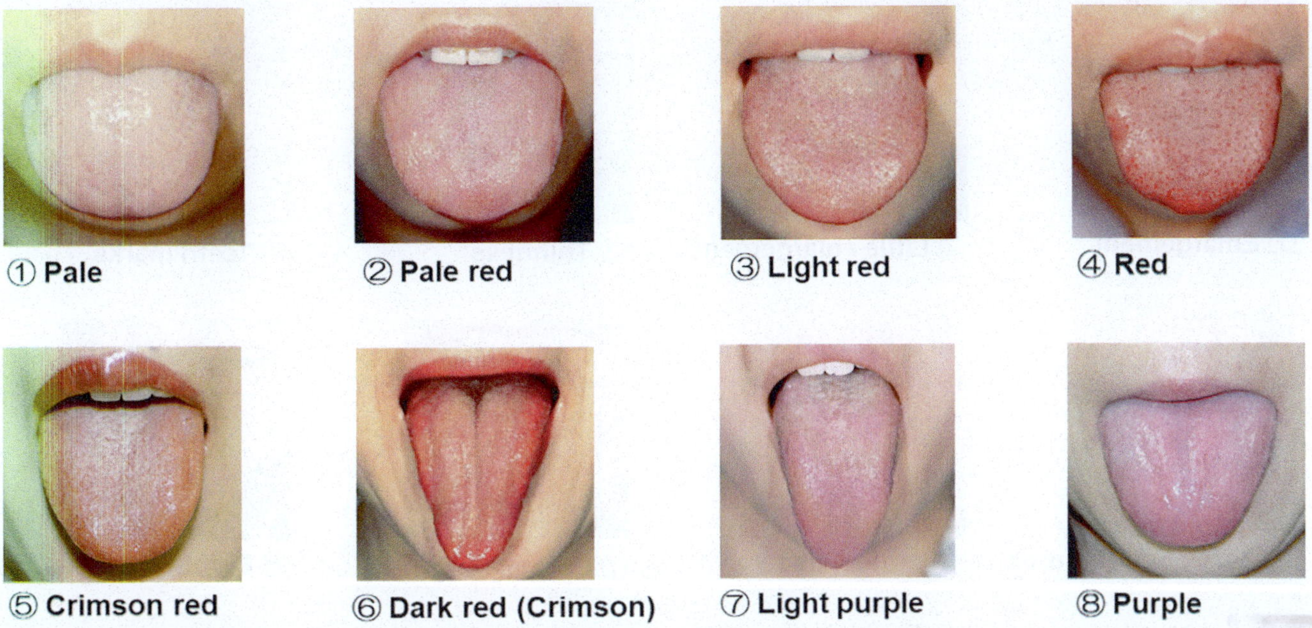

Fig. 3.1 Tongue color. ① Pale: pale, enlarged tongue with light teeth marks and thin white coating. ② Pale red: pale red enlarged tongue with thin white coating. ③ Light red: light red tongue with thin white coating. ④ Red: red slightly enlarged tongue with teeth marks, red spots, and a thin white coating. ⑤ Crimson red: crimson red and slightly enlarged tongue with a white greasy coating. ⑥ Dark red (crimson): dark red tongue with a small yellow coating. ⑦ Light purple: light purple tongue with a small white coating on the root. ⑧ Purple: purple enlarged tongue with thin white coating

When static blood[TM1] is strong, blood[TM1] stasis-resolving formulas (駆於血剤) are considered. If it is accompanied by severe fluid[TM1] deficiency or atrophy of the papillae and the mucous membrane of the tongue, formulas to nourish yin, which contain Rehmannia root (地黄), Ophiopogon Tuber (麦門冬), and Adenophora root (沙参), such as rokumigan (六味丸), bakumondoto (麦門冬湯), or jiinkōkato (滋陰降火湯), are considered.

Purple and Blue

Light purple tongue (*tanshizetsu*) (tongue color ⑦) in which the whole tongue color is bluish, was called slight blue and pale blue in the Edo period. It is often seen in people who suffer from cold or cold syndrome (hieshō) and is probably caused by poor circulation in the tongue due to blood[TM1] deficiency and sympathicotonia. Formulas for resolving blood[TM1] stasis such as tokishigyakukagoshuyushokyoto (当帰四逆加呉茱萸生姜湯), that contain Japanese Angelica root (当帰), Peony Root (芍薬), Cnidium Rhizome (川芎), and Rehmannia root (地黄) are considered.

Purple tongue (*shizetsu*) (tongue color ⑧) is a finding of poor blood circulation or static blood[TM1]. The purple and bluish-purple-colored tongue is frequently attributed not only to an increase of venous blood flow, such as venous dilatation or congestion, but also to anoxia, such as cyanosis in the tongue. Of the purple tongues, *the red-purple and dry tongue* is static blood[TM1] when it comes from heat patterns, and *the bluish-purple and moist tongue* is static blood[TM1] caused by yang deficiency or cold patterns. Formulas for resolving blood[TM1] stasis such as keishibukuryogan (桂枝茯苓丸) or tokakujokito (桃核承気湯) are considered [2].

Blue tongue (*seizetsu*) is even more bluish than the bluish-purple tongue and is considered to be a condition in which the cold is strong and static blood[TM1] progresses. Treatment is similar to bluish tongue, and formulas for resolving blood[TM1] stasis are considered.

2.3.5 Tongue Shape (Fig. 3.2)

The tongue consists of muscles that allow for food intake. In general, a thick and large tongue has well-developed muscles and indicates a good appetite and strong digestion, whereas a thin and small tongue has small muscles and indicates a poor appetite and weak digestion.

Enlargement

Enlarged tongue (handaizetsu) (tongue shape ①) is a thick and corpulent tongue that is large enough to force the mouth open with margins that protrude beyond the lips.

This is known as macroglossia in Western medicine and is also seen in patients with acromegaly, hypothyroidism, and Down's syndrome. It is attributed to hypertrophy of a group of muscles in the tongue and edema of the tongue body.

In Kampo medicine, an enlarged tongue usually bears teeth marks as dental indentations; when it reflects condi-

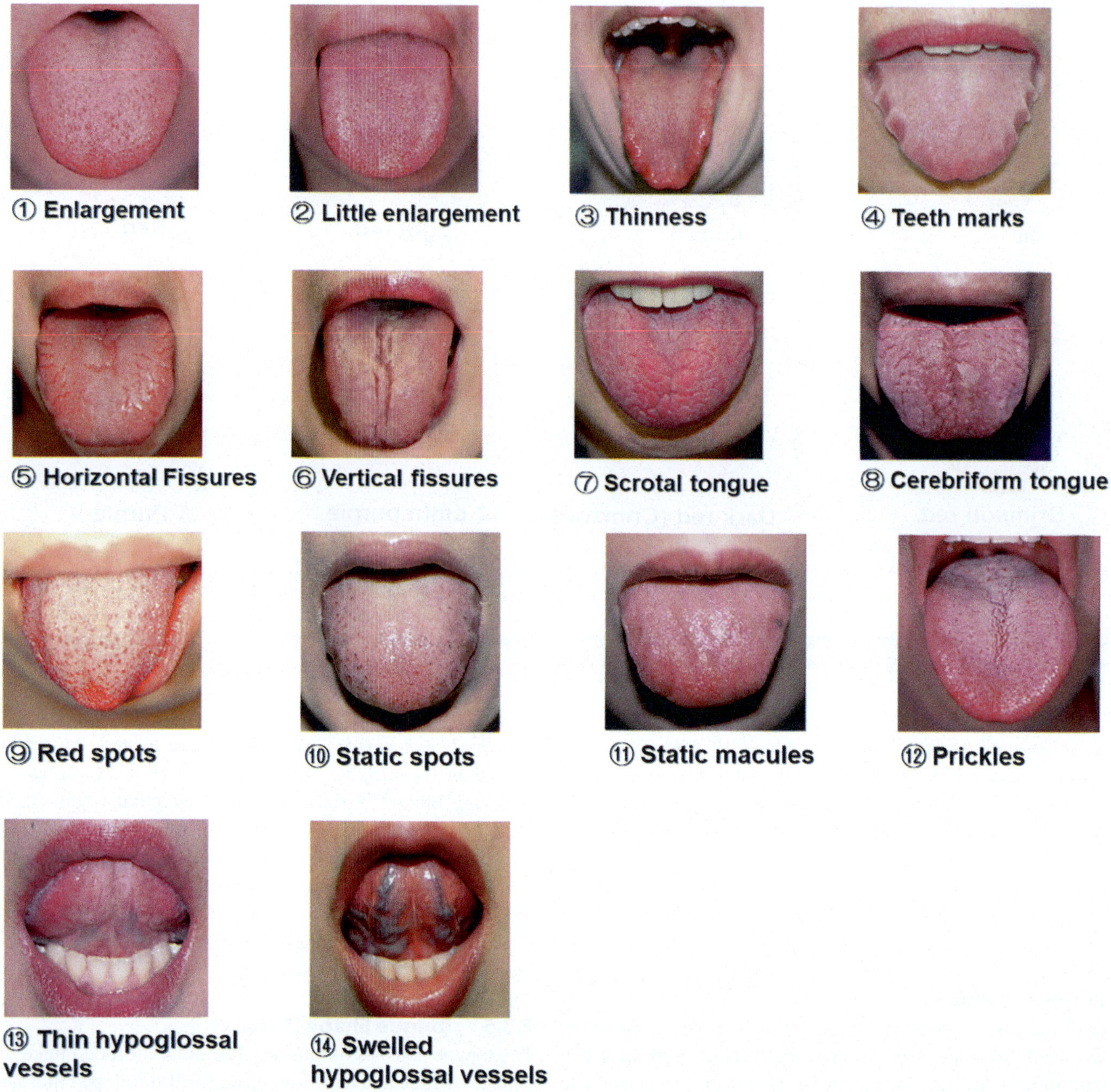

Fig. 3.2 Tongue shape. ① Enlargement: light red enlarged tongue with red spots and a small white coating. ② Little enlargement: light red little enlarged tongue with red spots and a thin white coating. ③ Thinness: crimson red thin tongue with teeth marks and small yellow greasy coating. ④ Teeth marks: pale red enlarged tongue with vivid teeth marks and thin white coating. ⑤ Horizontal Fissures: crimson red enlarged tongue with horizontal fissures on the edge and small white coating. ⑥ Vertical fissures: light red tongue with vertical fissures in the middle and a small yellow coating. ⑦ Scrotal tongue: red-purple enlarged tongue with scrotum-like fissures and a thin, dry, white coating. ⑧ Cerebriform tongue: blue-purple enlarged tongue with cerebriform fissures and thin white coating. ⑨ Red spots: light red tongue with red spots on the tip and thick white coating. Static spots: slightly enlarged purple tongue with teeth marks, static spots on the edge, and white greasy coating. Static macules: light red enlarged tongue with static macules on the edge and thin white coating. Prickles: light red enlarged tongue with white prickles in the center and white coating. Thin hypoglossal vessels: light red normal tongue with thin deep lingual veins on the ventral tongue.Swelled hypoglossal vessels: red tongue with dark-blue distended deep lingual veins on the ventral tongue

tions of qi deficiency and fluid[TM1] retention, formulas treating qi disorders and fluid[TM1] -regulating formulas are used, and when a bluish enlarged tongue with dental indentations is diagnosed as yang deficiency, yang-tonifying formulas such as shimbuto (真武湯) are used.

For reference, a slightly larger tongue in which tongue margins fill the corners of the mouth is called "a little enlarged tongue" (tongue shape ②) in traditional Chinese medicine and is often seen in normal people with a big appetite.

Thin

Thin tongue (*sōhakuzetsu*) (tongue shape ③) is a relatively small and thin tongue, also called *souhetsu*. It is often caused by underdevelopment or atrophy of the intralingual muscles, which reflects qi deficiency, blood[TM1] deficiency, or fluid[TM1] deficiency. It usually results from poorly developed muscles in the tongue and tongue muscle hypotrophy. It may be diagnosed as indigestion due to constitutional weakness, eating disorders, and loss of appetite, but it may also be congenital.

Teeth-Marks Fissured

Teeth-marked tongue (*shikonzetsu*) (tongue shape ④) are dental indentations of the tongue along the maxillary or mandibular dental arch and are observed in patients with qi deficiency, spleen[TM1] deficiency, fluid[TM1] retention, etc., and also in yang deficiency with enlargement of the tongue.

For the treatment of teeth-marked tongue, consider formulas containing ginseng (人参) and Astragalus root (黄耆) for qi deficiency or spleen[TM1] deficiency, yang-tonifying formulas like shimbuto (真武湯) for yang deficiency, and fluid[TM]-regulating formulas for fluid[TM1] retention.

The teeth-marked tongue can also be caused by pressing the tongue forward against the anterior dentition in anxious patients. In this case, the cause is not fluid[TM1] retention, so the size of the tongue is normal.

Fissures

A fissured tongue (*sūretsuzetsu*) (tongue shape ⑤) is a tongue with a crack or wrinkle that develops on its surface, and this is also called "*retsumonzetsu.*" There are vertical types, horizontal types, and mixed types of fissures. In the Edo period, a kind of vertical type (tongue shape ⑥) was called *jinretsu*, *jinjiretsu*, and *jinjimon,* the shape of a Chinese character for a man (人). In Western medicine, this is called *lingua plicata* (*sūjōzetsu*), *scrotal tongue* (*innōzetsu*) (tongue shape ⑦), and *cerebriform tongue* (*nōkaijozetsu*) (tongue shape ⑧) by the appearance of the fissures.

Fissured tongue may be congenital or familial, increasing from adolescence, especially in women in their 30s. In addition, it is seen as a partial symptom of Melkersson-Rosenthal syndrome, and it is said to occur in 80% of Down syndrome and 27% of psoriasis vulgaris.

A fissured tongue normally does not need to be treated because it is not a disease. Treatment is needed, however, if inflammation is observed with redness or pain in the tongue. In Kampo, it is associated with a deficiency of blood[TM1] and fluid[TM1]. When the tongue is pale in color, it indicates blood[TM1] deficiency or deficiency of both qi and blood[TM1], and when red in color, it indicates fluid[TM1] deficiency; formulas like seinetsuhokito (清熱補気湯)* or bushirichuto (附子理中湯)* (ninjinto + processed aconite root) may be used.

Red Spots

Red spots (*kōten*) (tongue shape ⑨) are scattered red spots on the dorsal surface of the tongue, especially at the tip of the tongue. The spots are called *kōsei* in the classic literature of the Edo period. Because fungiform papillae are not keratinized, their blood vessels are visible. If capillary vessels in the fungiform papillae become hyperemic or dilated, the papillae become redder and appear as red spots with increased red blood cells.

Red spots are commonly observed in patients presenting with heat pattern or static blood[TM1], and formulas such as kamishoyosan (加味逍遙散) that contain Moutan Cortex (牡丹皮) and gardenia fruit (山梔子) are used to treat this.

Stasis Spots

Stasis spots (*often*) in the tongue (tongue shape) are scattered dark brown to purplish-black spots on the dorsal surface of the tongue, which corresponds to *kokuten* in the classic literature of the Edo period. Stasis spots visible from the outside are presumed to be capillary vessels that become rusty in color due to stagnation of blood in the fungiform papillae, which has destroyed red blood cells with oxidized hemoglobin. This indicates static blood[TM1] in Kampo, and formulas for resolving blood[TM1] stasis are used.

Static Macules

Static macules (*ohan*) (tongue shape) are flat and bluish-purple to purplish-black macules on the dorsal tongue surface. It may also be caused by dilation of veins near the surface of the tongue.

This indicates static blood[TM1] in Kampo, and formulas for resolving blood[TM1] stasis are used.

Prickles

Prickles (*bōshi*)" (tongue shape) are lingual papillae visible as pampas grass-like prickles on the surface of the tongue, especially along the central groove of the tongue. Black protrusions are called black thorns (*kokushi*). It can be observed at the febrile stage of infectious disease. The protrusions are caused by the proliferation and keratinization of filiform papillae.

In Kampo, prickles with a yellow coating on the red tongue are indicative of exuberant heat of the gastrointestinal tract, and daisaikoto (大柴胡湯), etc., are considered.

Varicose Vein

Varicotic veins (*jōmyakudochō*) (tongue shape) are engorged veins, tortuous veins, or small spots by veinlet stasis that appear on the ventral surfaces of the tongue. These are caused by congestion of venules and are signs of static blood[TM1]. It is the same as venous engorgement of hypoglossal vessels in Chinese medicine. It indicates static blood[TM1], and formulas for resolving blood[TM1] stasis are used.

The term "sublingual vein" has been used in tongue examinations of Kampo, but the official anatomical name for the veins that are normally visible under ventral surfaces of the tongue is deep lingual vein (tongue shape). The sublingual vein is not visible because it is the vein through the inside of the tongue from the sublingual glands. In Chinese medicine, veins on the ventral surface of the tongue are sometimes referred to as "hypoglossal vessels," but it should be noted that some texts refer to it idiomatically as "sublingual vein."

2.3.6 Tongue Condition (Fig. 3.3)

Abnormal movement and conditions of the tongue are examined.

Shortness

A tongue condition in which it does not stretch and appears to be contracted is called short tongue (*tanshukuzetsu*) (tongue condition ①). The term (*tanzetsu*) was used for this in the Edo period of Japan. The short tongue is diagnosed in ankyloglossia, etc., but congenital ones are considered normal.

Atrophy

The condition in which the tongue is flaccid and weak and does not move well is called atrophied tongue (*inanzetsu*) (tongue condition ②).

The atrophied and pale tongue indicates a deficiency of both qi and blood[TM1], and juzentaihoto (十全大補湯), etc., is considered. The dark red and dry tongue with atrophy indicates a lack of fluid[TM1], or deficiency heat associated with fluid[TM1] deficiency (in Chinese medicine, yin deficiency with effulgent fire). Formulas that have a tonifying effect of fluid[TM1] and humor (yin-tonifying effect), such as rokumigan (六味丸), bakumondoto (麦門冬湯), and jiinkokato (滋陰降火湯), are considered.

Protruding and Licking

A tongue condition in which the tip of a tongue is characterized by stretching out of the mouth but being unable to retract back into the mouth is called the protruding tongue (*tozetsu*), and another condition in which the tip of a tongue is repeatedly thrust and retracted back into the mouth or licked is called licking tongue (*rozetsu*); this term was also used in the Edo period of Japan.

Licking the tongue is more likely to occur in feverish conditions such as stomach heat and stomach fever and in those who often lick their lips to relieve dryness of their oral cavity and lips. Byakkokaninjinto (白虎加人参湯) is considered for this condition.

Wryness

The tongue is characterized by deviating to one side (right or left) while protruding out of the mouth and is called a wry tongue (*waisyazetsu*) (tongue condition ③). The wry tongue is often associated with cranial neuropathy, such as hemiplegia due to stroke.

Tremor

A tongue condition with uncontrollable trembling is called the tremor (*sen*) or the tremor tongue (*zetsusen*), and the term *senzetsu,* with the same meaning, was used in the Edo period of Japan. Tremor tongue is associated with cranial nerve disorders such as Parkinson's disease.

A pale red-colored tongue with tremor indicates qi and blood[TM1] deficiency or qi deficiency, and Kampo formulas such as juzentaihoto (十全大補湯) and hochuekkito (補中益気湯) are considered.

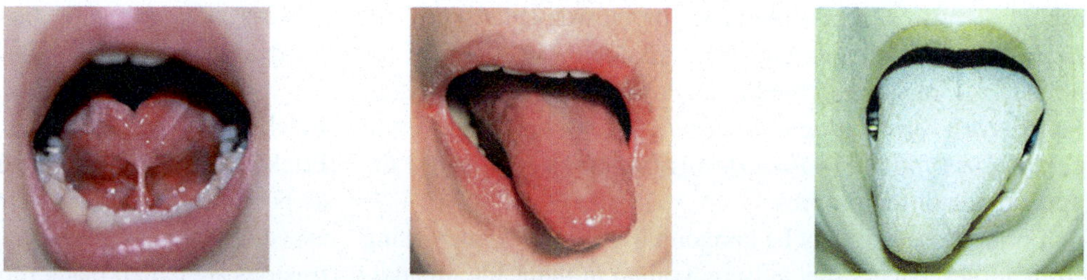

① Shortness ② Atrophy ③ Wryness

Fig. 3.3 Tongue condition. ① Shortness: light red shortened tongue. ② Atrophy: dark red atrophied wry tongue with a small smooth coating. ③ Wryness: purple wry tongue with a thick, dry, white coating

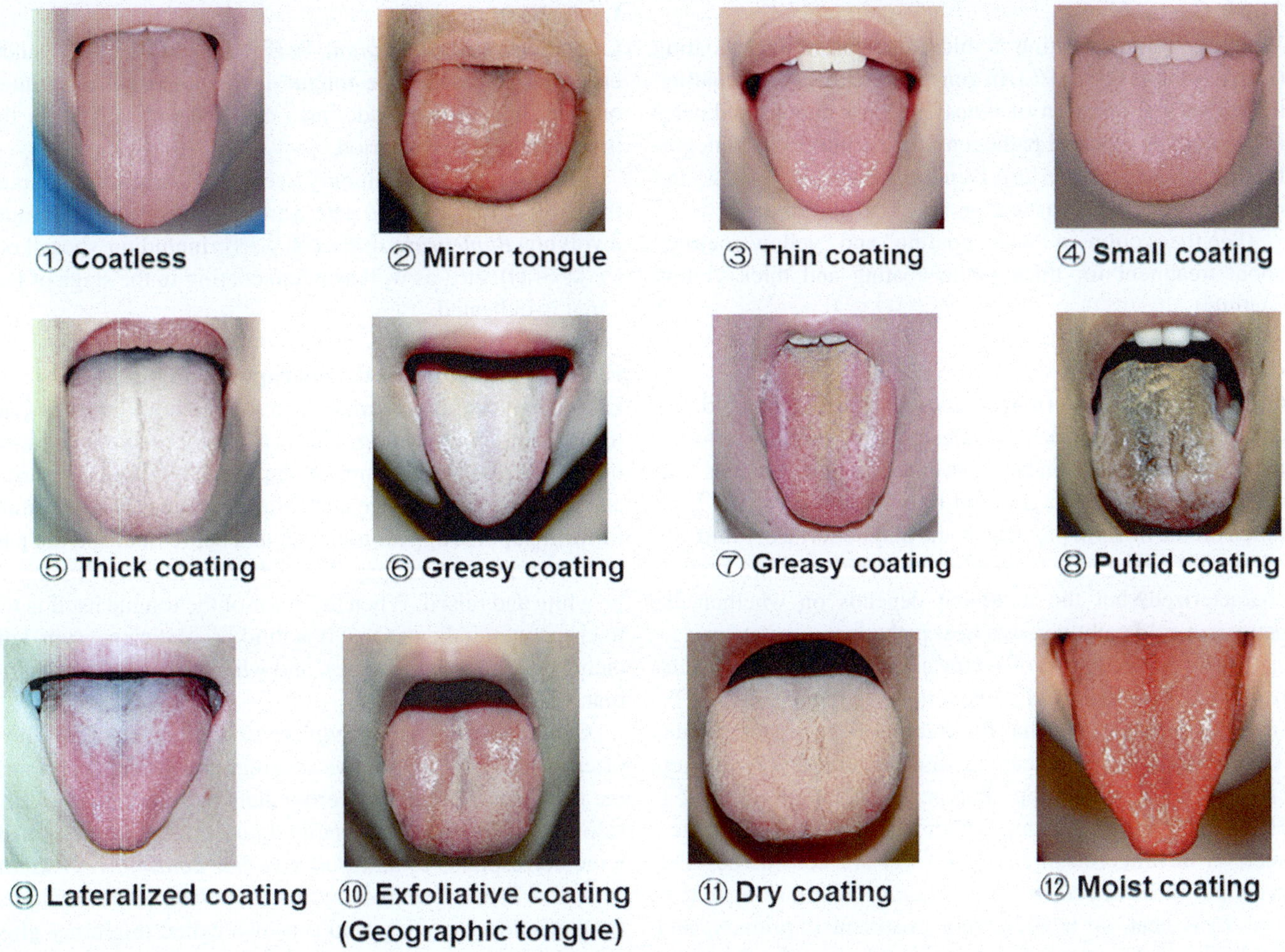

Fig. 3.4 Coating texture. ① Coatless: light purple dry tongue with no coating. ② Mirror tongue: crimson red and enlarged dry wry tongue with a smooth coating like a mirror. ③ Thin coating: light red tongue with thin white coating. ④ Small coating: light red and slightly enlarged tongue with a small white coating. ⑤ Thick coating: purple tongue with static spots and thick white coating. ⑥ Greasy coating: light red tongue with white and double yellow greasy coating. ⑦ Greasy coating: red tongue with red spots and burnt yellow greasy coating in the center. ⑧ Putrid coating: blue tongue with black putrid coating. ⑨ Lateralized coating: red-purple tongue with a lateralized thick white coating on the root. Exfoliative coating (geographic tongue): light red enlarged tongue with white exfoliative coating. Dry coating: light red enlarged tongue with yellowish-white dry coating. Moist coating: crimson red tongue with a moist, smooth coating

2.3.7 The Texture of Tongue Coating (Fig. 3.4)

Coating thickness and shedding of the coating are examined.

No Coating

The tongue with no coating (*mutai*) (tongue texture ①) allows the color of the tongue body itself to be clearly visible since there is no coating due to atrophy, disappearance, or immatureness of filiform papillae.

The crimson and dark crimson "mirror tongue " (tongue texture ②) that is often seen in the elderly appears in cases of extreme heat pattern or fluid[TM1] deficiency. Formulas like rokumigan (六味丸) with yin-tonifying effects are considered for the latter case. When a light red or pale tongue is present in the cases of deficiency of both qi and blood[TM1], juzentaihoto (十全大補湯) or kihito (帰脾湯) is considered.

Thin Coating and Little Coating

When the tongue coating is thin, this is called thin coating (*hakutai*) (tongue texture ③). When the tongue coating is mild and the extent is partial or small, it may be called little coating (*bitai*) (tongue texture ④). A thin tongue coating with little exfoliation of cells from keratinized filiform papillae indicates the condition of a patient with normal or mild lesions.

(See the section on "white coating/whitish-yellow coating" about treatment for thin white coating or yellowish coating.)

Thick Coating

When the tongue coating is thick, it is called thick coating (*kōtai*) (tongue texture ⑤). In general, the thicker the coating, the longer the duration of illness. A thick coating indicates invasion of an external pathogen into the interior or phlegm-fluid[TM1] retention (*tan'in*). Dentures, difficulty eating, and reduced strength in mastication may also contribute.

(See the section on "white coating" and "yellow coating" about treatment for thick white coating and thick yellow coating.)

Greasy Coating

Greasy coating (*jitai*) (tongue texture ⑥⑦) is sticky and viscous like oil; the surface granules are fine and adhere to the tongue surface. Its condition is attached to the mucus and rotten food residue, in addition to epithelial cells that have fallen off the filiform papillae on the tongue surface. Fluid[TM1] retention (*suitai*) and food retention (*shokutai*) are mainly characterized, but the treatment depends on whether the cause is a cold pathogen or a heat pathogen.

The principal cause of *white greasy coating* (*hakujitai*) (tongue texture ⑥) is cold, and treatment to regulate fluids[TM1] (*risui*) is primary, and that for clearing heat is subordinate. The formulas for both heat clearing and fluid[TM1] regulation (清熱利水剤), including Polyporus Sclerotium (猪苓), Hoelen (茯苓), and Artemisia Capillari Spica (茵蔯蒿), etc., such as inchingoreisan (茵陳五苓散) are considered. The principal cause of *yellow greasy coating* (*ōjitai*) (tongue texture ⑦) is heat, so heat-clearing treatment is primary, and fluid[TM1] regulating treatment is subordinate. The formulas for clearing heat [TM1], which include Coptis rhizome (黄連), Phellodendron bark (黄柏), and Scutellaria root (黄芩), etc., such as orengedokuto (黄連解毒湯) and orento (黄連湯), are taken into consideration.

If food[TM] retention (*shokutai*) is severe, formulas such as nichinto or rikkunshito, including Pinellia Tuber (半夏), Magnolia Bark (厚朴), and Citrus Unshiu Peel (陳皮), are used.

Putrid Coating

Putrid coating (*futai*) (tongue texture ⑧) is characterized by the accumulated coating with coarse granules and dirty color on the tongue surface, and the greasy coating is hard to peel off, whereas the putrid coating is easy to peel off.

The long tongue coating may be accompanied by bacterial or fungal infections (such as Candida). The putrid coating basically shows a heat pattern and is caused by food retention and fluid[TM1] retention. This is also seen, however, in the late stage of deficiency heat, which in Chinese medicine is called yin deficiency with internal heat and is caused by chronic wasting disease and dehydration. In this case, jiinshihoto (滋陰至宝湯), etc., which have yin-enriching effects, are considered.

Lateralized Coating

Lateralized coating (*hentai*: 偏苔) (tongue texture ⑨) indicates the coating of the tongue inclines toward the center, outside, left, or right side; also called *hentai* (邊苔) in the literature of the Edo period.

This coating is commonly seen in the transitional stage from the early yang to late yang stage, and the formula involving *Bupleurum radix* (柴胡剤), including shosaikoto (小柴胡湯), etc., as well as white coating in the stage of late yang, is indicated.

Exfoliative Coating and Geographic Tongue

Exfoliative coating (*hakutai*) is a tongue with irregular partial exfoliation of coating. This is a disorder of keratinization of the mucosal epithelium of the tongue caused by partial atrophy or disappearance of filiform papillae. The immature filiform papillae appear to be red and depressed, and the part of the mature filiform papillae with keratinization appears to be white and raised. When the color of the tongue itself is red to crimson, it indicates that it is fluid[TM1] deficiency(yin deficiency in Chinese medicine), and when it is pale, it indicates that it is qi deficiency.

Geographic tongue (*chizujozetsu*) (tongue texture) is most often seen in the exfoliative coating, and it was mentioned the marks looked like the vermiculate pattern 'chusai' in the Edo period. Tongue examination in traditional Chinese medicine corresponds to an *exfoliative-like coating* (*ruihakutai*) or *flower-like exfoliative coating* (*kahakutai*) with scattered small shedding coating, and it is also called migratory glossitis in Western medicine.

The tongue is commonly seen in patients with psychosomatic, immune, and allergic disorders, and it is also considered that it is associated with pustular psoriasis or atopic tongue change because it has been reported that it is associated with 80% of pustular psoriasis and 45% of atopic disease. Asymptomatic ones do not require Kampo treatment, but if they become inflamed or hurt, consider yin-tonifying formulas (補陰剤) or qi-tonifying formulas (補気剤).

Dry Coating and Moist Coating

Dry coating is called *kantai* (乾苔) (tongue texture), and for a *moist coating*, the term *sitsu* (湿) (tongue texture) is used. Dry tongue was also used the term *kan* (乾) or *kanso* (乾燥), and a *damp tongue coating* was used the term *jun* (潤), and *slippery tongue* coating by excessive fluid was used the term *katsu* (滑) in the Edo period.

The degree of wetness of the tongue depends on the amount of saliva secretion, viscosity, swallowing amount, evaporation amount, etc., and is very useful for knowing the signs of water retention in the whole body and the degree of water metabolism. In emergencies and emergency medicine of modern medicine, dry tongue is also a finding that helps to determine the patient's immediate condition of dehydration.

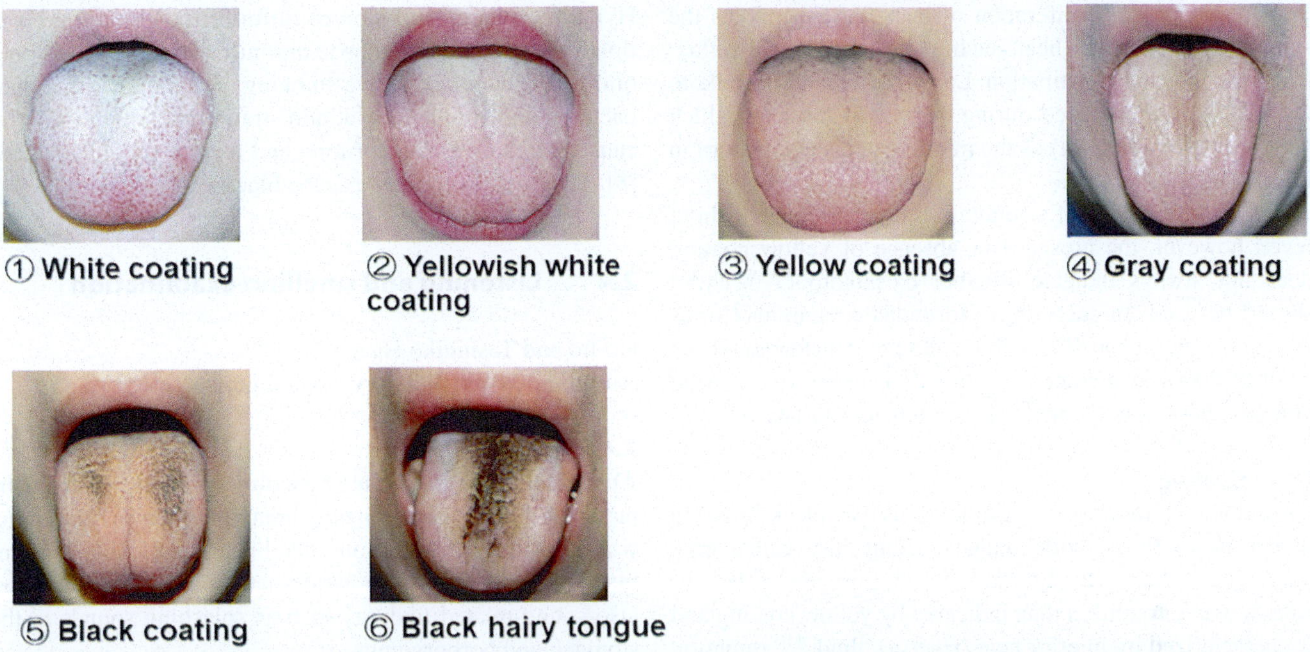

Fig. 3.5 Coating color. ① White coating : pale red enlarged tongue with teeth marks, red spots, and thick white coating. ② Yellowish-white coating : light red and slightly enlarged tongue with static spots. and yellowish-white greasy coating on the root. ③ Yellow coating : light red and slightly enlarged tongue with yellow greasy coating. ④ Gray coating : light red and slightly enlarged tongue with gray greasy coating and burnt yellow coating in the center. ⑤ Black coating : slightly red and slightly enlarged tongue with a thin white coating and a double black dry coating. ⑥ Black hairy tongue : light red tongue with white coating and black hairy coating in the center

In the case of dry coating (*kantai*) with yang pattern, byakkokaninjinto (白虎加人参湯) is considered for patients with yang pattern and fluid[TM1] deficiency, and blood[TM1] stasis-resolving formula (駆於血剤) is also considered for patients with yang pattern and static blood[TM1]. On the other hand, *slippery coating* (*katsutai*) that makes the tongue surface wet with excessive saliva is also called "*kida*" and is a sign of a yin pattern for which ninjinto (人参湯) is indicated.

2.3.8 Color of the Tongue Coating (Fig. 3.5)

White Coating

White coating (*hakutai*) (coating color ①) is a coating covered with epithelial cells of filiform papillae that are degraded by keratinization but remain on the tips of the papillae.

A thin white coating (*hakuhakutai*) or part of a *little white coating* (*bihakutai*) is a normal tongue finding usually seen in healthy subjects and indicates an exterior pattern with a small number of epithelial vesicles of the papillae that have fallen off due to keratinization attached to the filiform papillae.

It indicates conditions such as the late yang stage pattern and spleen[TM1] and qi deficiency, such as stagnation or impairment of digestive function. Bupleurum root (柴胡)-containing formulas, including shosaikoto (小柴胡湯), and formulas containing Pinellia Tuber (半夏), Atractylodes Japonica, A. Ovata (朮), and Poria Sclerotium (茯苓) are considered for white coating and thick white coating. For the treatment of common chronic diseases without fever, however, the presence or absence of white coating does not always indicate whether shosaikoto (小柴胡湯) should be used or not. In other words, shosaikoto (小柴胡湯) can be used under the condition without white coating. As a rule, cathartics are not used when the white coating is present on the tongue.

In addition, for white-thick coating (*kōhakutai*) and *white greasy coating* (*hakujitai*) that are seen in pathological conditions such as stagnation or impairment of digestive function (the deficiency of spleen[TM1] and qi), consider supplements such as rikkunshito (六君子湯).

Moreover, yellowish-white coating (or light-yellow coating) (*ouhakutai*) (coating color ②), a mixture of white coating and small amounts of yellow coating, corresponds to '*little yellow coating* (*bioutai*: 微黄苔)' in the classic literature of the Edo period and shows the process of transition from exterior pattern to interior pattern. It indicates impairment of the digestion caused by the middle yang stage pattern or febrile disease, for which the formula involving Bupleurum radix (柴胡剤) and the formula involving Rhubarb (大黄剤) are considered.

Yellow Coating

Yellow coating (*ōtai*)(coating color ③) is a yellowing of tongue coating caused by further degeneration of cells of filiform papillae and proliferation of bacteria and reflects the symptoms of stomach heat, such as heartburn, acid reflux, stomachache, and constipation. Laxatives such as daisaikoto (大柴胡湯) may be used during periods of fever and thick yellow coating (*kouōtai*) as the middle yang stage pattern in infectious diseases.

For the treatment of common chronic diseases without fever, however, the presence or absence of yellow coating does not always indicate whether daisaikoto (大柴胡湯) should be used. In such cases, formulas containing Coptis Rhizome (黄連) and Rhubarb (大黄) are considered. If the color of the coating changes from yellow to brown (or burnt yellow), daisaikoto (大柴胡湯) is often appropriate.

Gray Coating

Gray coating (*kaitai*) (coating color ④) is pale black (gray) to dark brown colored with tongue coating, also called gray tongue (*kaizetsu*) in the literature of the Edo period. It indicates a worse condition than indicated by yellow coating and is characterized by interior heat (*rinetsu*), fluid[TM1] retention (*tannin*), and cold dampness. If the gray coating becomes worse, it will turn into a black coating and show an interior pattern, and the treatment is similar to that for a black coating.

Black Coating and Hairy Black Tongue

Black coating (*kokutai*) (coating color ⑤) colored black with tongue coating, is seen at the peak of fever and in serious stages of disease, in the middle yang stage or late yin stage mainly, and indicates an interior pattern. Black coating tongue is also called black tongue (*kokuzetsu*) in the literature of the Edo period. Black coating is commonly seen in patients receiving long-term antibiotic therapy [6], post-elimination therapy of *Helicobacter pylori*, and terminally ill cancer patients recently. Bacteria producing black or brown water-soluble pigment or bacteria producing hydrogen sulfide (H_2S), which, by binding to iron and calcium, stains tongue coating, may contribute to the formation of black coating. Candida infection as a secondary infection may also be a cause.

In Kampo medicine, patients exhibit two fever patterns: An excess heat pattern that requires purgation using rhubarb-containing formulas (大黄剤) such as daijokito (大承気湯) and a deficiency and cold pattern due to yin deficiency or yang deficiency that must be treated with [interior cold pattern]-treating formulas such as processed aconite root-containing formulas (附子剤), including shimbuto (真武湯).

The hairy black tongue (*kokumōzetsu*: 黒毛舌) (coating color ⑥) is characterized by prominent extension of the filiform papillae and fluffing compared to the black coating tongue [7], and is often diagnosed with a more serious disease than the black coating tongue. The black hairy tongue is accompanied by hyperkeratosis of hair-type keratin. Hypertrophy and extension of filiform papillae and prevention of decidual keratin due to chronic irritation such as poor oral hygiene and excessive smoking, and the growth of fast bacteria and mold after administration of antibiotics [6], cause the change of color tone and texture into hairy black [8]. Treatment is the same as the black coating.

2.4 Listening and smelling examination

Go Ito and Toshihiko Hanawa

Auscultation and olfactory examination are performed.

2.4.1 Auscultation

Auscultation in Kampo medicine directly diagnoses from the patient's voice characteristics, breathing sounds, coughing, wheezing, dyspnea, delirious talk, hiccups, belching, abdominal rumbling, etc. In the abdominal examination, there are also sound-related findings such as splashing sounds in the stomach and borborygmus.

Speech and Voice

Powerful and brisk speech indicates fullness of healthy qi, and good coordination of qi blood[TM1], fluid[TM1]. A clear, vigorous voice often indicates an excess pattern; a high-pitched voice and incessant talking often indicate a heat pattern or excess pattern; a low-pitched voice and few words often indicate a cold pattern or deficiency pattern; and a faint, low-pitched voice often indicates a deficiency pattern. Speech in a hoarse or feeble voice may be a sign of qi deficiency. A low-pitched and feeble voice is one of the traditional keys for prescribing hochūekkitō as a formula for qi deficiency.

Coughing and Breathing Sounds

Coughing and wheezing can be easily heard during the listening examination. Moistening formulas such as bakumondōtō are selected to treat dry coughs, while formulas to treat fluid disturbance such as shoseiryūtō are used to treat productive coughs. Also, depending on the nature of breathing sounds, shortness of breath and shallow breath are judged.

Borborygmus

Peristaltic sound that is heard even when the stomach is not empty is linked to gastrointestinal disorders and coldness of spleen[TM1] and stomach[TM1].

If a loud rumbling sound in the bowel (so-called thunder in the abdomen) is heard, formulas such as hangeshashintō for yang pattern or bushikōbeitō for yin pattern are appropriate. Daikenchūtō should be considered when the stomach and intestines move erratically.

2.4.2 Olfactory Examination

Diagnosis of abnormalities in the body may be made by sniffing scents such as body odor, halitosis (sputum, gastric acid, alcohol, acetone, etc.), pus odor, discharge odor, stool odor, and urine odor.

In the Edo period, *Shuan Kagawa* confirmed that listening examinations included both olfactory examinations and hearing examinations. Also, *Chin-an Goto* advocated the importance of olfactory examinations such as hot odor, pus odor, axillary odor, bad breath, genital odor, and discharge odor.

Body odors are noted in olfactory examinations in modern medicine. Diabetes is suspected if there is a ketone odor, and kidney disease or hepatic encephalopathy is suspected if there is an ammonia odor. Sinusitis or periodontal disease is suspected if the breath has a rotten odor. An acidic odor on the breath indicates gastric hyperacidity or gastroduodenal ulcer. When the breath smells of stools, intestinal obstruction is suspected. Likewise, breath smelling like old beer is possibly gout, and smelling like sweet sputum is a sign of bronchiectasis.

In Kampo medicine, when the scent of excretion, such as body odor, pus odor, or leukorrhea, is strong, it is diagnosed as a yang pattern or excess pattern. When such odors are weak or absent, it is diagnosed as normal, yin pattern, or deficiency pattern. When the odor of halitosis, stools, or urine is strong, it is often diagnosed as a yang pattern, heat pattern, or excess pattern. When the odor is weak or absent, it is often diagnosed as a yin pattern, cold pattern, or deficiency pattern.

2.5 Inquiry

Go Ito and Toshihiko Hanawa

"Inquiry" refers to finding out about the patient's complaints and their background factors by talking with patients or their families. Therefore, in Kampo medicine interviews, special emphasis is placed on the patient's minor complaints and symptoms, in addition to general medical histories such as occupational history, family history (family structure and medical history, marriage history, etc.), preferences and habits (smoking, drinking, sleeping, eating), medical history (surgical history, blood transfusion history, medication history, etc.), and current medical history. Inquiry is characterized by searching for a solution together with the patient from a holistic standpoint in combination with the medical findings. This is nothing but the "medical interview" of modern medicine. In addition to the patient's complaints, the therapist must actively ask whether there are symptoms, so the symptom questionnaire items are inevitably detailed and diverse. In addition, in Japanese Kampo, the treatment is determined based on the pattern (*zuishochiryo*). Therefore, the final prescription must be judged comprehensively by combining the results of the other examinations in addition to the inquiry.

2.5.1 Key Points of the Interview in Kampo

The primary goal of Kampo medicine is to help patients perform activities of daily living more comfortably by improving their subjective symptoms. Kampo practitioners should help patients describe in their own words their conditions and enter the words as heard into the medical record. It is not uncommon that signs which seem to be insignificant in modern medicine are important and diagnostic in Kampo medicine. Such signs include a bitter taste in the mouth, dry mouth with no desire to drink, sensation of a lump in the throat, growling sounds in the stomach even when it is not empty, difficulty in speaking due to excessive salivation, cold feet even in the midsummer with several socks on, insomnia due to hot feet, weather-sensitive pain, severe sweating on the neck and face, and so on.

In order to narrow down the formula, Kampo practitioners consciously ask about the nature/conditions/distribution of the patient's complaint, concomitant symptoms, work stress, and lifestyle, as well as exacerbation and improvement factors of the complaints. For example, if the exacerbating factor of a headache is menstruation, a formula for resolving blood[TM1] stasis is indicated, and if the pain is from the posterior neck to the back of the head, a formula containing Pueraria Root is a strong candidate.

The following items are important information for Kampo diagnosis and treatment, so one must note these carefully at the time of the interview.

- Elapsed time: In acute diseases, it is useful to estimate the stage of the disease and the time of recovery based on the number of days elapsed since the onset of the disease. In chronic diseases, the elapsed time from onset and the duration of the disease help to estimate the stage of the disease and the time for recovery.
- Medical history: Practitioners will ask how past events relate to current distress from the perspective of etiology and sequelae.
- Treatment history: Information on the effectiveness of Kampo medicines used so far may be an important hint for understanding the patient's pathology and deciding on a formula.
- Exacerbating and alleviating factors: Exacerbation due to cold or heat (cold pattern, heat pattern), improvement or deterioration when warming up in a bath (cold pattern, heat pattern), worsening due to rainy weather or the approach of low pressure (fluid[TM1] retention), exacerbation from afternoon to night (qi deficiency), exacerbation from evening to night (static blood[TM1]), pain when moving (static blood[TM1]), pain when moving (static

blood[TM1]), pain when standing still or moving the site of pain (qi counter flow, qi stagnation), etc.

- Stool characteristics: For patients with loose stools and a tendency to diarrhea and for those with constipation who have abdominal pain and diarrhea when using laxatives, attention should be paid not only to laxatives such as rhubarb, glauconium, and hemp fruit, but also to Kampo prescriptions containing herbal medicines such as moutan bark, peach seed, and gardenia fruit.
- Menstruation and menopause: Although limited to women, it is important not only for gynecological symptoms such as irregular menstruation, menstrual pain, infertility, and climacteric disturbance but also for understanding the relationship with other symptoms such as mental state and defecation status.
- Allergies: If patients have allergies to cinnamon (cinnamon bark), wheat, yam (Dioscorea Rhizome), seri, or mitsuba (Japanese Angelica root, Cnidium Rhizome), avoid prescribing formulas that contain these or other ingredients that belong to the same family.

2.5.2 Symptom Questionnaire Items

It is important for Kampo practitioners to ask the following questions about the main complaints and symptoms. It should be noted that even if the symptoms are similar, the formulas are different for different patterns, and the final prescription is determined by integrating the patterns obtained from examinations such as inspection examination (*boshin*) with tongue examination (*zetsushin*), listening examination (聞診), inquiry (問診), pulse examination (*myakushin*), abdominal examination (*fukushin*), and back examination (*haishin*).

Fever and Sensation of Heat

In times past, when there were no thermometers, fever was diagnosed by local or general heat, burning sensation, etc. Fever is usually viewed as a yang pattern, but there are two different types of heat, “excess heat (*jitsunetsu*),” and “deficiency heat (*kyonetsu*),” and fever also occurs in yin pattern. The heat that appears on the surface of the body is "exterior heat [TM1] (*hyonetsu*)," the heat felt objectively by touching the surface of the skin is "high fever (*dainetsu*)," and the heat inside the body is "interior heat (*rinetsu*)." In treatment, exterior heat is basically removed by promoting sweating with a releasing exterior formula, and interior heat is removed by promoting defecation with a laxative. Aside from this, whole-body fever refers to an elevation of body temperature without sweating and the external pattern of the middle yang stage pattern. “Aversion to heat (*onetsu*)” refers to a condition in which the patient suffers from an unbearable fever, which is an excess internal pattern of the middle yang stage. “Alternating chills and fever (*oraikannetsu*)” refers to a condition in which fever and chills alternate and is fever in the late yang stage. In addition, a condition in which the patient suffers from heaviness in the chest due to fever is called “heat with agitation (*hannetsu*).” A condition in which there is a periodicity in raised body temperature just as the tide rises and falls is called “tidal fever (*chonetsu*).” A condition in which heat retention causes dysfunction in the organs is called “bind heat (*ketsunetsu*).” In addition to this, there is "true cold with false fever (*shinkankanetsu*)" that is actually a cold pattern, but this is easy to mistake for a heat pattern. Also, there is "true heat with false cold" that is actually a heat pattern, but this is easy to mistake for a cold pattern, but these discriminations are important (See Chap. 3, Sect. 3.1.3).

Burning Sensation and Hot Flashes

"Burning sensation" is a common word for "frenzy with fever" in Japan, and “hot flashes” are redness in the face or part of the body, both of which are symptoms of so-called, qi counter flow, blood[TM1] deficiency (血虚), and blood[TM1] heat (*ketsunetsu*: fever associated with bleeding and anemia). The formulas considered for hot flashes due to qi counter flow with coldness in the lower limbs (*hienobose*) are nyoshinsan or kamishōyōsan. Unkeitō is considered for hot flashes due to blood [TM] deficiency. In addition, blood[TM1] heat (*ketsunetsu*) is both a deficiency and an excess pathology. When the face is flushed and the mouth and throat are dry, this is excess heat (*jitsunetsu*), for which sammotsuōgontō is indicated.

When the foot is hot and one is unable to sleep, this is deficiency heat [TM1] (*kyonetsu*). Since this is a deficiency of blood[TM1] and fluid[TM1], consider formulas such as jiinkokato, jiinshihoto, and bakumondoto, which contain ingredients that supplement fluids such as ophiopogon tuber, asparagus tuber, and Anemarrhena rhizome. Otherwise, sammotsuōgontō, a yin-tonifying and heat-clearing formula containing Rehmannia root, is indicated. When there are burning sensations with cold at the end of the limbs, tokishigyakukagosyuyusyokyoto should be considered.

Aversion to Cold and Aversion to Wind

Aversion to cold (*okan*) refers to a feeling of chill with shivering, which is usually an exterior pattern, such as in the early stages of a common cold. Occasionally it indicates an interior pattern such as interior cold (*rikan*) and signs of yang and yin patterns in some cases.

Dislike of wind because of cold sensations when exposed to the wind is called “aversion to wind (*ofu*).” Consider the formulas keishito, kakkontō, and maōtō for aversion to cold and wind with exterior pattern, and shinbuto (真武湯) for aversion to cold (See Chap. 2, Sect. 1.6).

Coldness and Intolerance of Cold

According to *Shanghanlun,* subjective coldness is "*kan*" and objective coldness is "*rei*." Reversal cold of extremities is called "reversal of qi (*ketsu*)." Though coldness may be limited to the hands and feet in mild cases, it is explained by two patterns of yin and yang. A yin pattern with a cool sensation in the extremities and watery diarrhea due to coldness in the body (internal cold) is called cold syncope (*kanketsu*), and the therapeutic rule is warming. A yang pattern with inflammation in the interior (internal organs) and heat trapped in the body with cold sensation of extremities is called heat syncope (*nekketsu*), and the therapeutic rule is cooling.

In medical examination, an objective condition in which coldness spreads from the tips of the extremities in a retrograde manner, causing severe cold, is called "reversal (objective) cold of the extremities (*shusoku-ketsurei*)." A subjective sense of coldness from the tips of extremities caused by hypersensitivity to external cold stress is called "reversal (subjective) cold of the extremities (*shusoku-ketsukan*)." In addition, feeling chills in one's hands and feet is called "cold in the extremities (*shusoku-kan*)," and the state that is neither hot nor cold is called "warm in the extremities (*shusoku-on*)."

The basic distribution pattern of cold and heat in the body is classified into the next four types. ① "reversal cold of the extremities (*shusoku-ketsukan*)," which is cold from the tips of extremities, ② "upper heat and lower cold (*jonetsu-gekan*)," in which cold of the lower extremity (lower cold) is accompanied by heat signs in the upper part of the body (upper heat), ③ "external hot and internal cold (*hyonetsu-rikan*)," which is warm or hot on the surface of the body but cold inside the body, and ④ "cold in both external and internal (*hyori-gukan*)," in which there is cold on both the exterior and interior. Each of these types corresponds to four basic types of cold and types of patients with cold: (1) distal limb type, (2) lower limb type, (3) internal type, and (4) systemic type.

For treatment consider ōrentō for upper heat and lower cold of the abdomen, hachimijiōgan for lower body cold (lower cold) such as upper heat and lower cold (*jōnetsu-gekan*) or inferior limb type cold, and tōkishigyakukagoshuyushōkyōtō for reversal cold of the extremities (*shusokuketsukan*).

In addition, if cold is accompanied by external heat and internal cold (*hyonetsu-rikan*), if it is internal type and interior cold is strong, consider formulas containing aconite root, such as tsūmyakusigyakutō*. Otherwise, consider unkeitō if heat with agitation (*hannetsu*) or exterior heat (*hyonetsu*) is strong.

Consider formulas containing aconite root for "cold in the extremities (*shusokukan*)" in which one feels a chill; tōkishigyakukagoshuyushōkyōtō for prolonged reversal cold of the extremities (*shusokuketsukan*), chilblains, or extremity chills, and distal limb type cold; and for reversal (objective) cold of the extremities (*shusokuketsurei*). For cold in both external and internal (*hyori-gukan*) or systemic type cold, consider formulas containing aconite root, such as shigyakutō* or tsūmyakusigyakutō*or goshuyutō. Otherwise, when coldness is caused by spontaneous sweating from exterior [TM] deficiency, consider keishitō.

(* dry ginger + processed aconite root + glycyrrhiza)

Dyshidrosis (Hyperhidrosis, Sweating from the Hands and Feet, Night Sweats, etc.)

Hyperhidrosis is called "profuse sweating (*takan*)." Boiogito (防已黄耆湯) is considered for hyperhidrosis in flabby and sweaty people, and kamishoyosan (加味逍遙散) is considered for sweating caused by qi counter flow, such as excessive sweating from the face during menopause.

Excessive sweating only from the head is called "*zukan*," and formulas like saikokeishikankyoto (柴胡桂枝乾姜湯) are considered. Sweating only from the neck upwards is cited in the ***Shanghanlun***, and inchinkoto (茵陳蒿湯) is considered if patients are in the middle yang stage pattern. Excessive sweating on the palms and soles, regardless of heat, is called "sweating in the hands and feet (*syusokukan*)" and is often psychogenic sweating due to tension. Sigyakusan (四逆散) or hangekobokuto (半夏厚朴湯) is considered for such qi stagnation or qi counter flow rooted in sympathetic nerve overstrain.

Night sweating is called "stolen sweats (*tōkan*)," and is commonly caused by a tendency toward lack of body fluid combined with feverishness and mental excitement. This is also seen in people with the tendency of fluid[TM1] retention, frailty, and those in a state of chronic exhaustion.

Consider saikokeishikankyotoō (柴胡桂枝乾姜湯) for night sweats with a lack of body fluid due to yin deficiency or deficiency pattern in the late yang stage pattern, hochuekkito (補中益気湯) and ogikenchuto (黄耆建中湯) for night sweats of qi deficiency, and formulas containing Astragalus root such as juzentaihoto (十全大補湯) for both qi and blood[TM1] deficiency.

Eating Disorder (Hyperorexia and Anorexia)

Illness does not always reduce appetite but also can increase appetite. When static blood[TM1] is prominent, for example, appetite may be excessive with increased food intake and recurrence of hunger sensation shortly after eating. This hyperorexia was described as "swift digestion with rapid hungering" in classical texts such as ***Huangdineijing***. Formulas like teitoto (抵当湯) are considered for these hunger sensations caused by static blood[TM1]. Moreover, premenstrual syndrome (PMS) may cause excessive appetite before menstruation, and patients with constipation may complain of increased appetite.

Anorexia has numerous causes, such as gastrointestinal disorders, psychosomatic disorders, and febrile diseases. Also, people who prefer sweets are often spleen[TM1] deficient. As a general principle of Kampo treatment, for example, when spleen[TM1]-stomach[TM1] deficiency and kidney[TM1] deficiency occur together, treatment should begin by tonifying spleen[TM1]-stomach[TM] deficiency. For appetite loss due to spleen[TM1] deficiency, formulas to enhance gastric mucosal defense or to promote gastric emptying, such as shikunshito (四君子湯), hochuekkito (補中益気湯), and rikkunshito (六君子湯), are considered. Even if Rehmannia root is indicated, such as in hachimijiogan (八味地黄丸) or formulas containing Ephedra herb, such as kakkonto (葛根湯), Rehmannia root and Ephedra herb should be used with caution because these may aggravate gastrointestinal symptoms for patients with appetite loss or weak digestion.

Sleep Disturbance (Insomnia and Hypersomnia)

Neurotic insomnia and depressive insomnia are the major types of insomnia. Coptidis Rhizoma, Poria, Polygalae Radix, and Zizyphi Semen are commonly added to formulas for the treatment of insomnia. The major cause of neurotic insomnia is often "vexation of deficiency type (*kyohan*)," which is a consumptive disease such as weakness and fatigue (*kyorō*). If patients with this type of insomnia complain of fatigue, difficulty in falling asleep, restlessness, and excessive night sweats (*tōkan*), formulas such as saikokeisikankyoto (柴胡桂枝乾姜湯) or sansoninto (酸棗仁湯) may be indicated for treatment. San'oshashinto (三黄瀉心湯) or oōrengedokuto (黄連解毒湯) may be considered for insomnia patients with red complexion, irritability, and hypertension. Yokukansan (抑肝散) and yokukansankachimpihange (抑肝散加陳皮半夏) may also be considered for insomnia patients with anger about anything, along with restlessness.

In depressive insomnia, consider formulas such as kihito (帰脾湯), kamikihito (加味帰脾湯), or kanbakutaisoto (甘麦大棗湯) for patients with deficiency patterns and daisaikoto (大柴胡湯) or saikokaryukotsuboreito (柴胡加竜骨牡蛎湯) for robust patients with fullness and discomfort in the chest and hypochondrium (*kyōkyō-kuman*).

In addition, chikujountanto (竹茹温胆湯) is also indicated for difficulty with sleep due to severe coughing. Kakkonto (葛根湯) may be effective when the main cause of insomnia is extreme stiffness in the shoulders and back in intense patients. It should be used with care, however, because it also has a stimulating effect. Sleep disorders include not only insomnia but also hypersomnia (lethargy), in which patients do not feel rested, no matter how much sleep they get, and drowsiness continues. Sansoninto (酸棗仁湯), which is used for insomnia, may also be effective for hypersomnia.

Urination Disorder (Pollakiuria, Dysuria, Incontinence, Enuresis, and Miction Pain)

In Kampo medicine, issues with excretion of fluid are called "fluid[TM1] retention." Easy discharge or increase in urine volume is called "spontaneous urination (*shobenjiri*)," and oliguria or dysuria is called "inhibited urination (*nyofuri*)." Difficulty in urination or anuria is called "difficult urination (*shōbennan*)," and urinary incontinence is called "enuresis (*inyo*)." When the color of urine is clear white, it indicates a yin and cold pattern. When the color of urine is yellow or reddish, it indicates a yang and heat pattern.

As for decreased urine volume, consider it in relation to other symptoms, goreisan (五苓散) for conditions with thirst, or choreito (猪苓湯) for conditions with thirst and no sweating.

As for polyuria and frequent urination caused by prostatic hypertrophy, consider hachimijiogan (八味地黄丸) for conditions with thirst and weakness or paresthesia of the lower abdomen (*shofukufujin*). For pollakiuria caused by aseptic cystitis or hyperactive bladder, consider choreitogoshimotsuto (猪苓湯合四物湯) or seishinrenshiin (清心蓮子飲).

Hochuekkito (補中益気湯) has been used to treat urinary incontinence, but hachimijiogan (八味地黄丸) is preferred for patients with urinary incontinence accompanied by weakness or paresthesia of lower abdomen (*shofukufujin*). For enuresis in children, keishikaryukotsuboreito (桂枝加竜骨牡蛎湯) should be considered. As for miction pain, consider formulas such as choreito (猪苓湯) and gorinsan (五淋散) for urination pain, and choreitogoshimotsuto (猪苓湯合四物湯) for urination pain with hematuria.

Defecation Disorder (Constipation, Soft Stools, and Diarrhea)

Most constipation with hardened stools indicates a yang excess pattern, while most diarrhea and loose stools indicate a yin deficiency pattern. However, heat dysentery (*netsuri*), which is acute diarrhea with melena (*rishitsu*) caused by fever, and lower body heaviness (*geju*), which is a sense of incomplete defecation and an urge to defecate without the ability to defecate, are signs of a yang excess pattern. Tenesmus (*rikyu-koju*) is a spasmodic condition with difficulty in defecation and abdominal pain despite frequent and urgent desire to defecate.

Rhei Rhizoma (大黄) is the preferred treatment for constipation, but it is often inappropriate for patients with weak gastrointestinal function, which is known as spleen[TM1] and stomach[TM1] deficiency.

In such cases, gardenia fruit (山梔子), Hemp Fruit (麻子仁), and Zanthoxylum Fruit (山椒) should be used appropriately. Alternating constipation (also called spastic constipation) that alternates between diarrhea and constipation, is basically considered to be constipation. In this case, consider kamishoyosan (加味逍遙散) or goshakusan (五積散), with additional ingredients for liver[TM1] and spleen[TM1] harmonization.

As for diarrhea, chronic functional diarrhea is called *sessha*, and acute infectious diarrhea is called *rishitsu*. Rhubarb (大黄) is used for a short period of time for bacterial diarrhea (as *rishitsu*), and then a formula for regulating of spleen[TM1] and stomach[TM1] (that is, gastrointestinal function) is prescribed.

Since sennoside, the main component of rhubarb, has a laxative effect only after being changed to rheinanthrone by intestinal bacteria, it should be noted that antibiotics may reduce the laxative activity of rhubarb due to changes in intestinal flora. If there are symptoms such as dry mouth, decreased urine output, or edema, as in conditions like acute enteritis, goreisan (五苓散) or saireito (柴苓湯) is considered.

Chronic constitutional diarrhea (*sessha*) is related to spleen[TM1] and stomach[TM1] deficiency or kidney[TM1] deficiency. Ninzinto (人参湯) is good for gastric symptoms, and shimbuto (真武湯) is good for diarrhea due to cold. As for lienteric diarrhea, shokentyuto (小建中湯), ogikentyuto (黄耆建中湯), or keihito (啓脾湯) is considered.

In the case of irritable bowel syndrome accompanied by diarrhea or constipation with urgent abdominal pain, keishikashakuyakuto (桂枝加芍薬湯) should be considered for diarrhea type and mixed type, and keishikashakuyakudaioto (桂枝加芍薬大黄湯) should be considered for constipation type.

Lassitude and Easy Fatigability

Lassitude, such as easy fatigability and sluggishness, is the most common symptom among all complaints. Common causes are generally qi deficiency or deficiency of both qi and blood[TM1], but there are also various other pathologies such as mental stress (qi stagnation), depression (liver[TM1] qi stagnation), and decreased energy metabolism (kidney[TM1] deficiency or yang deficiency).

For those caused by qi deficiency, formulas such as sikunshito (四君子湯) or hochuekkito (補中益気湯) are considered among the qi-tonifying formulas (補気剤). For those caused by deficiency of both qi and blood, juzentaihoto (十全大補湯) and ninjin'yoeito (人参養栄湯) are considered.

For those caused by qi stagnation and liver[TM1] qi stagnation, shigyakusan (四逆散) is considered. For those caused by kidney deficiency or yang deficiency, hachimijiogan (八味地黄丸) and bushirichuto (附子理中湯) are considered.

Heaviness of the Body

Symptoms that make the body feel heavy may be present in fluid[TM1] retention (*suitai*), as well as in the late yang stage pattern, the middle yang stage pattern, and the middle yin stage pattern. For cases of fluid[TM1] retention, ryokyojutsukanto (苓姜朮甘湯) is considered when the waist (low back) feels cold and heavy; otherwise, boiogito (防已黄耆湯) is considered when the body is heavy and sweaty and the wind causes discomfort.

For those in the late yang stage pattern, when the whole body is heavy and it is impossible to turn over, saikokaryukotsuboreito (柴胡加竜骨牡蛎湯) should be considered. For those in the middle yang stage pattern, when the body is heavy and has malaise due to constipation, daijokito (大承気湯) should be considered. For those in the middle yin stage pattern, when the body is heavy and there is diarrhea or a cold and a strong desire to lie down, shimbuto (真武湯) should be considered.

Forgetfulness

Forgetfulness is called *kibō* in traditional Kampo, and it means often forgetting. It is regarded as one of the symptoms of kidney[TM1] deficiency and static blood[TM1]. For age-related forgetfulness, kamikihito (加味帰脾湯) and ninjin'yoeito (人参養栄湯), which include Polygala Root (遠志), should be considered. For forgetfulness related to cerebrovascular disease, formulas such as orengedokuto (黄連解毒湯), hachimijiogan (八味地黄丸), and chotosan (釣藤散) are considered. For Alzheimer-type dementia, toōkishakuyakusan (当帰芍薬散), kihito (帰脾湯), or kamiuntanto (加味温胆湯) is considered.

Irritability

In general, irritability is regarded as qi counter flow or a symptom of liver[TM1] abnormality, and in Chinese medicine, it is considered to be a pathological condition of liver[TM1] fire blazing upward or effulgent liver[TM1] fire. Formulas containing Bupleurum root (柴胡), such as kamishoyosan (加味逍遙散), may be used for qi counter flow. Frowning while speaking, irascibility, haste, and insomnia may be treated with yokukansan (抑肝散) or yokukansankachimpihange (抑肝散加陳皮半夏). When irritability is accompanied by tendencies of nervousness or depression, kambakutaisoto (甘麦大棗湯) is considered for deficiency pattern, and saikokaryukotsuboreito (柴胡加竜骨牡蛎湯) is considered for excess pattern.

Headache and Heaviness of Head

The formula for headaches and heaviness of the head is determined in relation to signs of coldness, gastrointestinal symptoms, stiff shoulders, static blood[TM1], etc. For migraines, goshuyuto (呉茱萸湯) and senkyuchachosan (川芎茶調散) should be considered. For tension headaches associated with stiff shoulders, kakkonto (葛根湯), keishikakakkonto (桂枝加葛根湯), and chotosan (釣藤散) should be considered. In addition, goshakusan (五積散) is used for headaches caused by coldness; hangebyakujutsutemmato (半夏白朮天麻湯) and hochuekkito (補中益気湯) are used for headaches caused by spleen[TM1] deficiency with weakness in the gastrointestinal tract; kamishoyosan (加味逍遙散) is used for female static blood[TM1], and hachimijiogan (八味地黄丸) is used for those caused by kidney[TM1] deficiency and aging. In addition, for headaches associated with fluid[TM1] retention, which tend to occur when the weather changes, especially a decrease in air pressure, formulas like goreisan (五苓散) are considered.

Tinnitus and Hearing Loss

Formulas for tinnitus or hearing loss are determined in relation to their causes, such as genetics, aging, trauma, and stress. For transient tinnitus and hearing loss caused by diseases like Ménière's, consider formulas that tonify the kidney[TM1] such as hachimijiogan (八味地黄丸). For those associated with aging, formulas containing Bupleurum radix (柴胡剤), such as kamikihito (加味帰脾湯) and sigyakusan (四逆散), are considered. For stress-related hearing issues, qi-regulating formulas such as hangekobokuto (半夏厚朴湯) are considered. In many cases of tinnitus due to aging, the therapeutic goal is more to reduce symptoms than a complete cure. When tension in the neck and shoulder muscles is strong, the symptoms will worsen, so attention should also be paid to shoulder stiffness and posture.

Vertigo and Dizziness on Standing Up

Vertigo, which is characterized by rotation, is caused by disorders in the periphery of the vestibular nerve nucleus, such as the semicircular canals, vestibular nerves, and otoliths, while dizziness, which is characterized by non-rotation, is said to be caused by abnormalities in the brainstem or cerebellum or left-right differences in cerebral blood flow. Dizziness on standing up and orthostatic hypotension are thought to be caused by abnormal autonomic nervous system balance or anemia involved in maintaining cerebral blood pressure during standing.

In Kampo medicine, dizziness and vertigo are associated with many things, including fluid[TM1] retention, qi counter flow, qi deficiency, and blood[TM1] deficiency. For rotational vertigo, which is called *gen'un*, goreisan (五苓散) is considered, and for vertigo due to fluid[TM1] retention or qi counter flow, kamishoyosan (加味逍遙散) is considered. For floating dizziness, which is called *zugen*, hangebyakujutsutenmato (半夏白朮天麻湯) is considered. For dizziness upon standing (orthostatic hypotension), considered to be due to qi deficiency, and for dizziness due to blood[TM1] deficiency and anemia, tokishakuyakusan (当帰芍薬散) is used. For dizziness experienced by elderly people with a sense of being about to fall, shimbuto (真武湯) is used according to the pattern.

Decreased Visual Acuity, Eye Strain, and Dry Eyes

Among the five zang organs, the liver[TM1] is not only involved in the regulation of blood storage and circulation, skeletal muscles and movement, nutrition and metabolism, menstruation, the autonomic nervous system, and mental activity, but it also has functions related to the eyes. Eye disorders are therefore often regarded as symptoms of blood[TM1] deficiency and liver[TM1] insufficiency (decreased liver function). Shimotsuto (四物湯) or formulas containing shimotsutō should be considered for symptoms such as eye strain, blurred vision, intolerance of glare, and dry eyes.

In addition, formulas like kakkonto (葛根湯) or keisikakakkonto (桂枝加葛根湯) may be effective for symptoms such as photosensitivity, glare, and dry eyes caused by decreased light reflex of the pupils and suppression of lacrimal gland secretion. This is due to sympathetic nerve tension in the eyes mediated by the superior cervical ganglion associated with stiff neck and shoulders caused by lifestyle, such as heavy use of personal computers. Also, symptoms such as decreased visual acuity and blurred vision are caused by decreased blood flow in the visual area of the brain due to decreased blood flow in the vertebral artery.

Sensation of a Lump in the Throat

The feelings of choking and blockage and discomfort in the throat are known not only as obstructive discomfort in the throat (*inchūsyaren:* sensation of a lump in the throat) but also as plum-stone qi (*baikakuki*). Hangekobokuto (半夏厚朴湯) is famous as a remedy for globus hystericus, which is due to qi stagnation.

If this symptom is regarded as hypersensitivity in the mucous membranes of the throat, treatment options will expand. Because "qi rising and thrusting against the chest" is one of the therapeutic targets of ryokeijutsukanto (苓桂朮甘湯) and "disturbance in the throat" is one of the therapeutic targets of bakumondoto (麦門冬湯), and both are associated with qi counter flow, these formulas can be prescribed for these symptoms.

When symptoms such as abdominal fullness are also present, bukuryoin (茯苓飲) or bukuryoin-go-hangekobokuto (茯苓飲合半夏厚朴湯) may be indicated.

Thirst, Dry Mouth, and Dry Lips

In Kampo medicine, thirst (*kōkatsu*), a feeling of dryness in the mouth with a desire to drink, is distinguished from dry mouth (*kōkan*), a lack of fluid in the mouth without a desire to drink.

The formulas to be considered for thirst and decreasing urine volume are goreisan (五苓散); for thirst and fever symptoms, byakkokaninjinto (白虎加人参湯); for dry mouth, jiinkokato (滋陰降火湯). Dry lips are symptoms of pathologies such as spleen[TM1] deficiency, lack of fluid (yin deficiency), blood[TM1] deficiency, and static blood[TM1].

Shokentyuto (小建中湯) should be considered for spleen[TM1] deficiency, rokumigan (六味丸) for lack of fluid (yin deficiency), and unkeito (温経湯) for blood[TM1] deficiency accompanied by static blood[TM1]. Otherwise, for other static blood[TM1] conditions, formulas for resolving blood[TM1] stasis should be prescribed according to the condition.

Respiratory Disorder(Cough, Dyspnea, and Shortness of Breath)

Consider formulas such as bakumondoto (麦門冬湯) for nonproductive coughs in the upper respiratory tract from inflammation caused by a common cold or colds; otherwise, consider seihaito (清肺湯) or chikujountanto (竹茹温胆湯) for coughs accompanied by phlegm. Coughs indicated for bakumondoto (麦門冬湯) are violent and paroxysmal coughs. Coughs indicated for seihaito (清肺湯) are coughing and phlegm associated with bronchiectasis. Chikujountanto (竹茹温胆湯) is indicated for cases where cough and phlegm are prolonged and there is insomnia. In addition, jiinkokato (滋陰降火湯) is considered for coughs in elderly patients who have dry tongue and dehydration (yin deficiency). For dry cough and dyspnea due to bronchial asthma, consider formulas according to the occurrence, such as gokoto (五虎湯), makyokansekito (麻杏甘石湯), and shimpito (神秘湯) at the time of coughing attack, and saibokuto (柴朴湯) for prevention.

In Kampo, shortness of breath is called "short air (*tannki*)," and shortness of breath is also called "little air (*shoki*)." Shakanzoto (炙甘草湯) is considered when shortness of breath is accompanied by tachycardia or arrhythmia, and ryokeijutsukanto (苓桂朮甘湯) is considered when it's accompanied by dizziness or palpitations.

Dysgeusia

There are various causes of dysgeusia (taste abnormalities), such as idiopathic, psychogenic, drug-induced, zinc deficiency, iron deficiency, and post-respiratory infection. According to the *Shanghanlun*, "the late yang stage pattern (少陽病期) is characterized by a bitter taste in the mouth, thirst, and dizziness." In Kampo medicine, bitter taste in the mouth is an indication for formulas containing Bupleurum radix (柴胡剤). Care must be taken in using such formulas, however, as dysgeusia can also be caused by aging, tooth decay, gingivitis, dental prostheses, or other drugs.

On the other hand, "neutral in mouth (*kōtyuwa*)" indicates a harmonious state in which there are no abnormalities such as dry mouth, bitter mouth, and insensitivity to taste (*kōfujin*).

When there are symptoms of chills in the back, the middle yang stage pattern (陽明病) shows severe thirst (thirst with agitation), while the middle yin stage pattern (少陰病期) is characterized by neutrality in the mouth. Incidentally, a change in normal taste is called a deficiency of taste (*kotyufujin*). For the loss of taste (no taste) due to qi deficiency brought about by exhaustion, hochuekkito (補中益気湯) should be considered. Otherwise, for conditions like blood[TM1], deficiency, lack of fluid[TM1] (yin deficiency), dry mouth, and fluid[TM1] retention, formulas that take into account the cause of each taste abnormality should be prescribed.

Salivation

In general, raw spit is caused by excessive secretion of saliva due to stimuli from the senses of sight, taste, and hearing when seeing, eating, or hearing about sour foods such as lemons or pickled plums.

Overflow of saliva (*kida*), in which saliva overflows in the mouth and drips from the tongue when the mouth is opened, indicates that the stomach may be cold. This symptom is the target for ninjinto (人参湯). In addition, overflow of saliva is not only caused by excessive secretion of saliva but may also be caused by a decrease in the ability to swallow saliva due to excessive tension or age-related dysphagia (See Chap. 3, Sect. 2.3.7).

Belching

Belching is a symptom of reverse flow of gases in the stomach back to the esophagus, such as fast eating, aerophagia, or decreased stomach peristalsis. Belching is commonly called *aiki* in Kampo medicine. Formulas such as hangekobokuto (半夏厚朴湯) for epigastric stuffiness with resistance (*shinkahiko*) on abdominal examination and hangeshashinto (半夏瀉心湯) for aerophagia are considered.

Heartburn and Epigastric Discomfort

Heartburn is a symptom of discord of stomach qi (*ikifuwa*). This is called fluid and gas retention in the stomach in Chinese medicine. Heartburn is caused by chlorhydria (gastric hyperacidity) and gastric acid reflux (*ryuin*) into the esophagus. The symptom of gastric acid reflux into the oral cavity is called *donsan*. Formulas like hangeshashinto (半夏瀉心湯) for heartburn with nausea and choijokito (調胃承気湯) for heartburn with constipation are considered.

Epigastric discomfort is caused by decreased gastric motility and decreased gastric acid secretion, or food [TM1] retention and indigestion due to gastric ptosis. Formulas like hangeshashinto (半夏瀉心湯) for epigastric discomfort with epigastric stuffiness and resistance and rikkunshito (六君子湯) for epigastric discomfort from spleen[TM1] deficiency or fluid[TM1] retention in the stomach are considered.

Nausea and Vomiting

Symptoms of nausea and vomiting are caused by stimulation of the vomiting center in the stomach and brain. In Kampo medicine, these are thought to be symptoms caused by discord of stomach qi, which is gastrointestinal dysfunction; otherwise, stomach heat (inflammation and hyperemia of the upper gastrointestinal tract), fluid[TM1] retention, and qi counter flow.

For those symptoms caused by gastrointestinal dysfunction, goshuyuto (呉茱萸湯) or hangeshashinto (半夏瀉心湯), which contain Pinellia Tuber (半夏), Citrus Unshiu Peel (陳皮), Euodia Fruit (呉茱萸), and Ginger (生姜), are prescribed. In addition, choijokito (調胃承気湯) should be considered for inflammation or hyperemia of the upper gastrointestinal tract. Otherwise, goreisan (五苓散), shohangekabukuryoto (小半夏加茯苓湯), or bukuryoin (茯苓飲) should be considered for vomiting due to fluid[TM] retention from decreased gastric motility and gastric juice retention. Hangekobokuto (半夏厚朴湯) should be considered for vomiting due to qi counter flow caused by such things as mental excitation, and shosaikoto (小柴胡湯) for vomiting caused by cold with abdominal finding of fullness and discomfort in chest and hypochondrium (*kyokyokuman*).

Abdominal Distention, Stomach Growling, and Excessive Gas

Abdominal distention indicates a deficiency and excess pattern. Formulas such as keisikashakuyakuto (桂枝加芍薬湯) or daikentyuto (大建中湯) may be used for deficiency patterns with soft, swollen abdominal fullness, and jokitō-group formulas (承気湯類) such as choijokito (調胃承気湯) or tokakuzyoōkito (桃核承気湯) may be used for excess patterns of abdominal fullness with firm distention. Stomach growling is a good indication for hangeshashinto (半夏瀉心湯). And passing of much gas is an indication for hangekobokuto (半夏厚朴湯) or jokito-group formulas (承気湯類).

Abdominal Pain

Abdominal pain is a common symptom. For spasmodic pain of the intestinal tract, formulas based on the combination of peony root (芍薬) and glycyrrhiza (甘草), such as shakuyakukanzoto (芍薬甘草湯) and keishikashakuyakuto (桂枝加芍薬湯), are commonly used. In addition, anchusan (安中散), containing the analgesic Corydalis tuber (延胡索), and formulas for resolving blood [TM1] stasis such as keishibukuryogan (桂枝茯苓丸) or tokakuzyokito (桃核承気湯), are indicated for menstruation-related abdominal pain. Otherwise, gosyakusan (五積散) is considered for abdominal pain caused by cold, and tōkishigyakukagosyuyusyokyoto (当帰四逆加呉茱萸生姜湯) or tsudosan (通導散) is considered for lower abdominal pain caused by cold, such as colic.

Since there are many types of abdominal pain, and the Kampo formulas used for them are also highly diverse, consider the formula according to each pattern.

Muscle Pain, Joint Pain, and Nerve Pain

The sites of pain caused by static blood[TM1] do not move and tend to become worse at night, probably because peripheral circulation is worse at night. Pain from qi deficiency tends to worsen during the day and subside during the night, pain from qi stagnation may frequently move, and pain from wind-dampness often responds to changes in weather.

Symptoms of rheumatoid arthritis and migraine may worsen in response to reduced atmospheric pressure, and this is attributed to the state of 'dual attack of wind-dampness' in Kampo medicine.

Basically, for pain caused by static blood[TM1] (e.g., ischemic pain), formulas for resolving blood[TM1] stasis such as sokeikakketsuto (疎経活血湯), keishibukuryogan (桂枝茯苓丸), or tokakuzyokito (桃核承気湯), should be considered.

For nerve and musculoskeletal pain, select formulas containing ephedra (麻黄剤) such as kakkonto (葛根湯), yokuininto (薏苡仁湯), and makyokansekito (麻杏甘石湯), as well as formulas containing processed aconite root-containing (附子剤) such as keisikajutubuto (桂枝加朮附湯), daibofuto (大防風湯), and goshajinkigan (牛車腎気丸). Jidabokuippoō (治打撲一方) is for bruising, while shakuyakukanzoto (芍薬甘草湯), which contains peony root, is good for pain and muscle spasms such as cramps and acute lower back pain. Choose Kampo formulas according to the symptoms and pattern.

Stiff Neck, Stiff Shoulders, and Stiff Back

Stiffness as an indication for keisito (桂枝湯) is characterized as "stiff in the head and neck (*zukōkyō*)" with strong muscle tension from the occiput to the nape of the neck, or "stiff from the occiput down to the back (*kohaikyo*)" with strong muscle tension from the occiput down to the back, and is sometimes accompanied by headaches (Fig. 3.6).

Stiffness as an indication for kakkonto (葛根湯) is greater than "stiff from the occiput down to the back," the indication

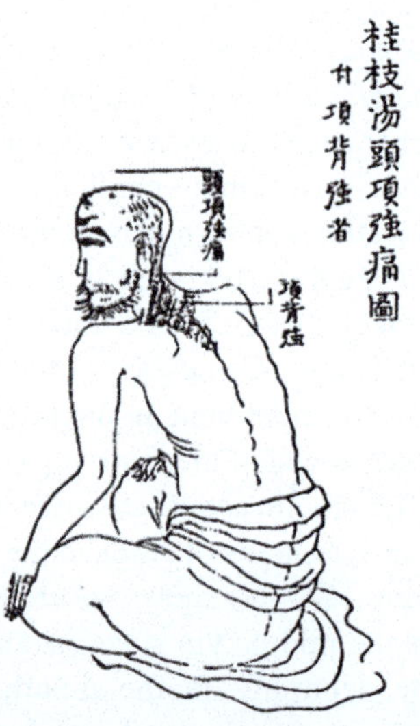

Fig. 3.6 The picture of the abdominal diagnostic pattern of keisito(桂枝湯証図)stiffness in head and neck(頭項強) and stiffness from neck down back (項背強) "Fukusyokiran-yoku (腹証奇覧翼)" by Yoshitora Wakuda. (Collection of Kyoto University Library)

for keisito (桂枝湯), and is often felt as stiffness from the occiput straight down the Bladder meridian line to the back and waist (Fig. 3.7).

If the patients have a weak gastrointestinal function and cannot use formulas containing Ephedra (麻黄剤), consider keisikakakkonto (桂枝加葛根湯), which adds only Pueraria root (葛根) to keisito (桂枝湯). In addition, "stiffness in the occiput and neck (*keikōkyō*)," in which primarily the neck is stiff, is also an indication for shosaikoto (小柴胡湯) along with fullness and discomfort in the chest and hypochondrium (*kyōkyō-kuman*) and stuffiness and resistance below the hypochondrium (*kyōka-hikō*) (see Fig. 3.8). In general, it is said that the stiffness that formulas containing Bupleurum root (柴胡剤) are effective for is broad stiffness in the longitudinal direction from the shoulders along the trapezius muscle.

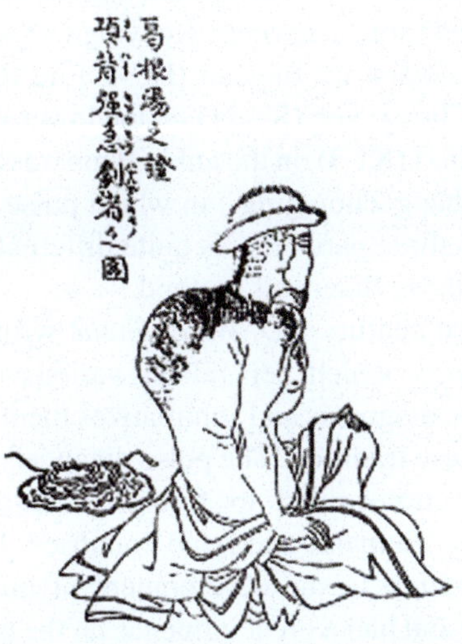

Fig. 3.7 The picture of the abdominal diagnostic pattern of kakkonto (葛根湯証図)(項背強急)"Fukusyokiran (腹証奇覧)" by Bunrei Inaba. (Collection of Kyoto University Library)

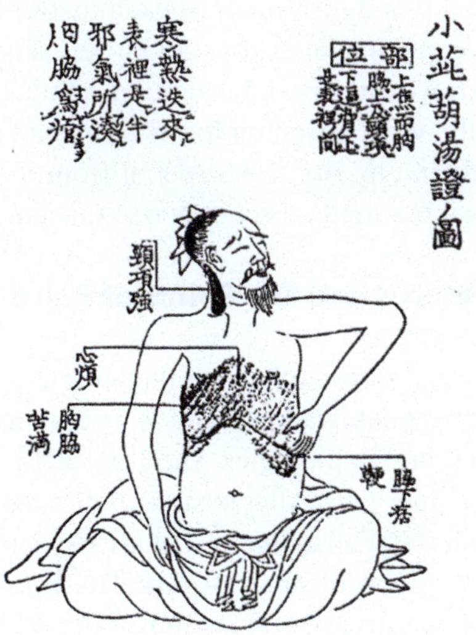

Fig. 3.8 The picture of the abdominal diagnostic pattern of shosaikoto (小柴胡湯証図)"Fukusyokiran-yoku (腹証奇覧翼)"by Yoshitora Wakuda. (Collection of Kyoto University Library)

This is said from the relationship between the Foot Taiyang Bladder meridian and kakkonto (葛根湯), used during the early yang stage, and that between the Foot Shaoyang Gallbladder meridian and formulas containing Bupleurum root formulas (柴胡剤), used during the late yang stage. Also, if there is "excessive muscle tension extending from the shoulder down the back (*kenpaikokyu*)" due to stress or other reasons, the indication of "muscle tension from the shoulder down the back" should be considered (See Chap. 3, Sect. 2.9.1).

Brittle Nails, Hair Loss, and Dry Skin

These symptoms are generally regarded as signs of blood[TM1] deficiency. The basic treatment is shimotsuto (四物湯). If Rehmannia root (地黄) causes indigestion, treatment should begin by prescribing a formula for the spleen[TM1] deficiency such as shikunshito (四君子湯) or rikkunshito (六君子湯). After this, formulas for both qi and blood[TM1] deficiency such as jyuzentaihoto (十全大補湯), are considered. Formulas to treat qi deficiency, such as ogikentyuto (黄耆建中湯), may also be effective.

Skin Itching

The patient's skin should be palpated to determine whether it is hot or not and dry or moist. If there is exterior heat due to atopic dermatitis or eczema, prescribe orengedokuto (黄連解毒湯) with its clearing effect. If the skin is wet with heat or sweating, shofusan (消風散) or jumihaidokuto (十味敗毒湯) are considered. When associated with yin deficiency or dry skin without heat, such as senile pruritus, tokiinshi (当帰飲子) is considered. In addition, for urticaria, which is dry but has heat and becomes moist when it becomes inflamed, kakkonto (葛根湯), saikokeishito (柴胡桂枝湯), and inchingoreisan (茵陳五苓散) are considered.

Chilblains

Chilblains are caused by poor peripheral circulation. If chronic exposure to cold stress is the cause, tokishigyakukagoshuyushokyoto (当帰四逆加呉茱萸生姜湯) may be used.

Decreased Libido

Decreased libido is a sign of kidney[TM1] deficiency. Disorders of organs, both spleen[TM1] and stomach[TM1] (digestive disorder) and liver[TM1] abnormality, or qi deficiency may cause decreased libido in both men and women from adolescence to middle age. Consider formulas such as hachimijiogan (八味地黄丸) for kidney[TM1] deficiency, saikokaryukotsuboreito (柴胡加竜骨牡蛎湯) for excess pattern with abnormalities of liver[TM1] caused by stress, etc., keishikaryukotsuboreito (桂枝加竜骨牡蠣湯) for deficiency pattern due to stress, etc., and hochuekkito (補中益気湯) for spleen[TM1] and stomach[TM1] disorders and qi deficiency.

2.6 Palpation

Go Ito and Toshihiko Hanawa

The Chinese character (*kanji*) for cut (切) also means touch, and palpation (*sesshin*), which includes this character, means that a doctor precisely touches the patient's body to perform a medical examination. Pulse examination and abdominal examination are vital parts of palpation. The ancient people said that diagnosis of external invasions (acute febrile illness) should be mainly based on pulse examination, and diagnosis of internal damage (chronic constitutional illness) should be based mainly on abdominal examination. Thus, pulse examination is considered important for the diagnosis of acute illness, and abdominal examination is essential for the diagnosis of chronic illness.

The palpation includes "back examination," in which the back is examined, but back examination is seldom performed today even though there are various descriptions in the texts of the Edo period, and *Kagawa Shuan* explained the importance of back examination, "*shihai,*" along with abdominal palpation, "*anpuku* (按腹)," in his book *Ippondogyoyoigen*. In the treatments of acupuncture and moxibustion, however, back examination is often performed to determine the selection of acupuncture points (See Chap. 3, Sect. 2.9.1).

In addition, practitioners should always palpate the hands and feet to determine, for example, whether a sense of coldness is objective or both objective and subjective. At the same time, the coldness of fingers, toes, abdomen, and back should also be palpated. If there is objective cold, the pathophysiology is considered from the distribution pattern of cold and heat (See Chap. 3, Sect. 2.5.2). At the same time, findings such as heat and heat sensation in the extremities are also important for capturing the pathophysiology of cold and fever [TM1] (See Chap. 3, Sect. 2.5.2).

2.7 Pulse Diagnosis

Go Ito and Toshihiko Hanawa

2.7.1 History of Pulse Diagnosis

Pulse diagnosis has been emphasized since ancient times in Chinese diagnostic technology, and it was widely used for diagnosing disease around the second century BC. In the Han Dynasty, two pulse-taking sites, the elbow and the shin, were used for a pulse diagnosis method called the "phase pulse method." Around the second century AD, the body was divided into three parts—the upper part (head), the middle part (hands), and the lower part (feet)—and each part was further divided into three parts—heaven, person, and earth—for a total of nine sites (3 × 3). After the end of the Han Dynasty, the pulse diagnosis method to be used in Chinese medicine was completed as "the three positions and nine indicators method." This system is found in the *Huangdineijing*, an ancient medical text. After that, the pulse diagnosis on the radial artery of the wrist from the *Huangdineijing* was expanded as in the pulse diagnosis of *Nanjing*. This is a classical text on acupuncture, and the method of single palpation at the radial artery of the wrist (*sunkou*) was established as the "single wrist pulse-taking method."

On the other hand, *Zhang Zhongjing* presented 27 diagnostic methods in the *Shanghanlun*, and his method of pulse diagnosis used three acupoints: Renying (ST-9) on the upper part (neck), *sunkou* or Taiyuan (LU-9) on the middle part (hand), and Chongyang (ST-41) on the lower part (foot), and alternately Taixi (KI-3) on the ankle. This was the "three-part method of Zhang Zhongjing," in which pulse palpation was performed in three parts; this is quite different from the current Kampo pulse diagnosis method.

In the third century AD, *Wang Shuhe* wrote the *Maijing (Pulse Classic)*, which generalizes various theories about Chinese pulse diagnosis and summarizes them into 24 symptoms of Chinese tradition. The pulse diagnosis method of the *Maijing* was transmitted to foreign countries, including Korea, Japan, Vietnam, and Arab countries. It thus made a great contribution to the development of pulse science in each country and had a great influence on the pulse diagnosis method of Western medicine.

In Japan, pulse diagnosis by the pulse-taking method on the wrist (six-position pulse diagnosis/pulse diagnosis of difference in six pulse positions) (Fig. 3.9) based on the *Nanjing* has been used mainly for medical examinations of acupuncture and Kampo medicine by the Gosei School since the Azuchi-Momoyama period. In addition, another pulse-taking method on the wrist based on the *Maijing* came into use for Kampo medicine by the Koho school from the Edo period. Both pulse-taking methods continue to this day.

2.7.2 Features and Key Points of Pulse Diagnosis

Since the pulse is constantly changing, it is excellent for capturing instantaneous changes and is useful for diagnosing rapidly changing pathologies such as acute diseases. In Kampo medicine, pulse diagnosis is performed not only to check the pulse and arrhythmias but also to gain information for determining treatment strategies. The Kampo physician measures the wrist pulse of the radial artery. The index finger goes on the point *sunko* (cūn kǒu), and the ring finger goes on the point *shakuchu* (chí zhōng), and both these fingers are in contact with the middle finger on the point *kanjo* (guān shàng), which is the pulsation slightly to the inside of the styloid process of the radius. Generally, these three points on the wrist for pulse diagnosis are usually referred to together as "*sun-kan-shaku*" (Fig. 3.9).

In the Koho school, the state of the pulse at *sun-kan-shaku* is generally diagnosed together (Fig. 3.10). In acupuncture and the Gosei School, these pulse diagnosis points are assessed individually to diagnose by comparison of each of the three pulses, which is known as "six-position pulse diagnosis" (Fig. 3.9).

The pulse is taken by lightly pressing the sites of measurement and then gradually increasing the pressure. During pulse examination, the condition of not only the radial artery but also supporting tissues is examined. In modern Kampo medicine, pulse examinations often do not emphasize the difference between the left and right pulses and the differences between *sun-kan-shaku*. In cases of pulseless disease (aortitis syndrome), however, the difference may be of great diagnostic significance. If there is a clear difference in pulse between the left and right wrists, the condition of the wrist with the weaker pulse may be useful for the diagnosis of chronic illness. In rare cases of "recurrent pulse," however, with an abnormality in the position of the radial artery passing over the upper side of the styloid process, it should be noted that the pulse may not be palpated in the fixed position.

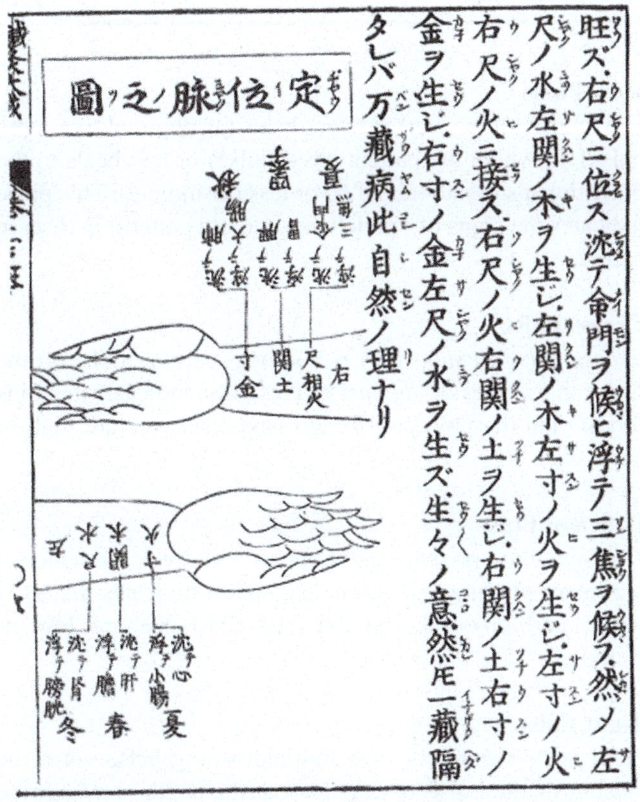

Fig. 3.9 Six position pulse diagnosis "Sinkyubassuitaisei" Ippo Okamoto. (Keio University, media center)

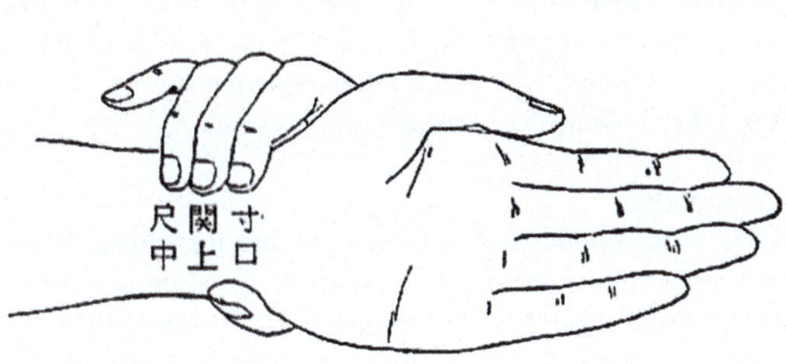

Fig. 3.10 Pulse examination "Toyoigaku Gaisetsu" Yoshio Nagahama

2.7.3 Pulse Types

There are about 28 types of pulse qualities in traditional chinese medicine, including floating (浮), sunken (沈), rapid (数), slow (遅), deficient (虚), excess (実), tight (緊), relaxed (緩), surging/large (洪•大), fine/small (細•小), slippery (滑), rough/stagnant (渋•濇), wiry (弦), hollow (芤), soggy/soft (濡•軟), hidden (伏), weak (弱), faint (微), skipping (促), bound (結), intermittent (代), long (長), short (短), drumskin (革), firm (牢), dissipated (散), stirred (動), and racing (疾).

Pulse diagnosis findings that provide clues to Kampo medicine are called pulse patterns (*myakusho*) or pulse signs (*myakukō*). *Typical pulse diagnosis findings used for Kampo medicine today* are the pulses (1–7) shown in Table 3.9. Among these, the most important pulse qualities are "the six pulses," as shown below: (1) depth (floating and sunken), (2) speed (rapid and slow), and (3) strength (excess and deficient).

The major pulse characteristics to be determined by pulse palpation are ①Depth (surface—deep),

In modern Japanese Kampo medicine, the six pulse characteristics of ①depth—floating and sunken, ②strength—excess and deficient, and ③ speed—rapid and slow—are important for basic pulse examination.

A schematic diagram of the criteria for pulse diagnosis is shown below (Fig. 3.11).

Table 3.9 Typical pulse diagnosis findings used for Kampo medicine today

	Characteristics	Pulse diagnosis
1.	**Depth**	**Floating and sunken**
2	**Speed**	**Rapid and slow**
3.	**Strength**	**Excess and deficient**
4.	Tension	Tight, relaxed, and wiry
5.	Width	Large and small
6.	Smoothness	Slippery and rough
7	Irregularity	Bound and intermittent

Bold text indicates important qualities

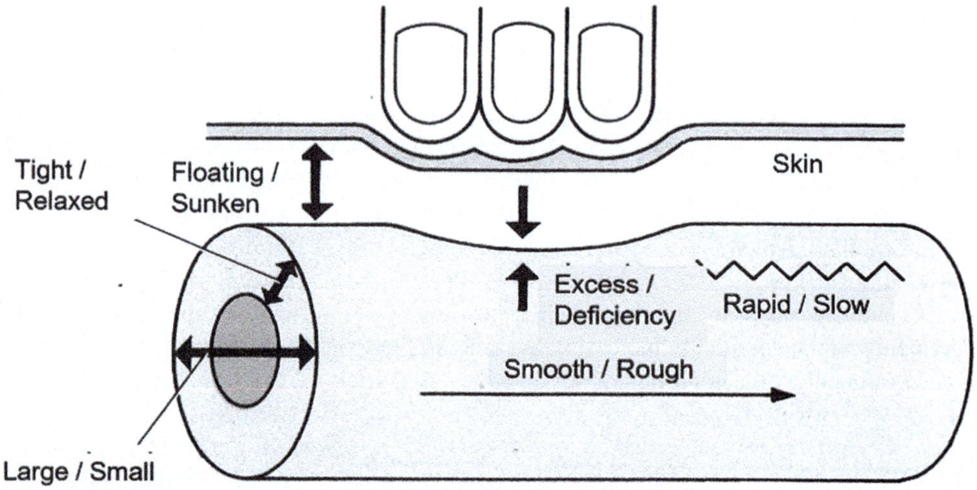

Fig. 3.11 Schematic diagram of pulse qualities used for diagnosis. (Source: Katsutoshi Terasawa: case studies in Japanese oriental [Kampo] medicine)

2.7.4 Main Pulse Findings and Clinical Findings

Normal Pulse

The pulse of a healthy person shows the middle in (1) depth, (2) speed, (3) strength, (4) tension, (5) width, and (6) smoothness, with (7) no irregularities. This pulse is called the *normal pulse* (*heimyaku*).

Floating Pulse

A floating pulse (*fumyaku*) feels like the artery floats just under the skin and is clearly felt by a light touch of the finger. The pulse is taken with light pressure on the site of measurement and then gradually increasing the pressure. In general, the floating pulse indicates that the site of the disease reaction is "exterior [TM1]." A floating pulse found in the early stages of acute febrile disease is suggestive of an exterior pattern because the blood flow rate in the vessel is increased and the vessel wall is pushed up from the inside. A floating pulse detected in patients with chronic non-febrile diseases suggests a deficiency pattern.

Sunken Pulse

A sunken pulse (*chinmyaku*) is a pulse that cannot be detected with a light touch but can be felt by deep and strong pressure. In general, the sunken pulse indicates that the site of the disease reaction is interior. This means that the disease is moving inward (interior pattern) and may also suggest edema or water retention.

Rapid Pulse

Rapid pulse (*sakumyaku*) is a fast pulse, and the patient's pulse is 6 or more beats to the practitioner's breath (about 90 or more per minute). There are two different types of heat states: excess heat and deficient heat. The rapid pulse indicates a fever sign (heat pattern) in disease states.

Slow Pulse

Slow pulse (*chimyaku*) is fewer beats (as opposed to a rapid pulse), in which the patient has 4 pulses or less beats to the practitioner's breath (about 60 or less per minute). This pulse indicates the signs of yin deficiency (cold pattern) in disease nature.

Excess Pulse

Excess pulse (*jitsumyaku*) is a strong resistant pulse to the finger that is pressed against it. This pulse indicates that qi is robust, and the physical strength and resistance are high or excessive.

Deficient Pulse

Deficient pulse (*kyomyaku*) is a pulse with weak resistance to the finger pressing against it. This pulse indicates that qi is weak, and physical strength and resistance are low or lacking.

Tight Pulse

Tight pulse (*kinmyaku*) is a thin and strong pulse when the tension of the pulse is examined at the depth at which the pulse is most clearly felt. This pulse indicates conditions such as excess, pain, cold, and the strength of the disease response.

Relaxed Pulse

Relaxed pulse (*kanmyaku*) is a slow pulse rate of about 65 beats per minute, which is not slower than a slow pulse, and this pulse indicates a weak disease response.

Wiry Pulse

Wiry pulse (*genmyaku*) is a straight and taut pulse, like a musical string to the touch. In general, it is slightly less taut than a tight pulse. Some references describe the differences in characteristics as "a wiry pulse does not shake left and right, while a tight pulse shakes left and right." A wiry pulse is often detected in the late yang stage pattern.

Rough Pulse

Rough pulse (*jūmyaku* or *shokumyaku*) is sluggish and irregular with delayed propagation of the pulse felt in the three fingers and is associated with sluggish circulation (*ukketsu*), fluid[TM1] retention (*tannin*), and static blood[TM1]. This pulse is thought to be caused by hypovolemia, decreased cardiac output, and increased blood viscosity.

Slippery Pulse

Slippery pulse (*katsumyaku*) is a pulse that spreads quickly and smoothly, is felt in the three fingers, and feels like a ball rolling. It shows the heat pattern, excess pattern, and yang pattern and is also seen in pregnant women. In the old days, it was considered one of the signs of pregnancy.

Bound Pulse

Bound pulse (*ketsumyaku*) is characterized by slow beats (less than 60 beats/min) that pause transiently or at irregular intervals. It corresponds to bradyarrhythmia, usually seen in patients with various blocks, certain extrasystoles, sinus bradycardia with auxiliary contractions, and atrial fibrillation, extrasystoles, and sinus bradycardia with escape rhythms.

Intermittent Pulse

Intermittent pulse (*daimyaku*) is described as a pulse that pauses at regular intervals, and the duration of each pause may be exceptionally long. In modern medicine, it is seen in second-degree atrioventricular block, premature ventricular contraction (including staged pulse), etc.

2.7.5 Other Pulse Findings and Clinical Diagnosis

Surging Pulse and Large Pulse

A wide pulse is called a *surging pulse* (*kōmyaku*) or *large pulse* (*daimyaku*). When the pulse is strong, it indicates yang, or heat, and when it is weak, it indicates deficiency. The large pulse is only wide, not undulating.

Fine Pulse and Small Pulse

A narrow pulse is called a *fine pulse* (*saimyaku*) or *small pulse* (*shōmyaku*) and indicates yin or cold.

Faint Pulse

A faint pulse (*bimyaku*) is a slight and hard-to-feel pulse and harder to palpate than a fine pulse. It indicates a collapse of spirit and a decrease in blood volume in peripheral circulation due to bleeding or dehydration, shock, or a decrease in blood pressure.

Soggy Pulse and Soft Pulse

Soggy pulse (*jumyaku* or *nanmyaku*) is a pulse that is floating but thin and weak and which disappears when more pressure is applied. It indicates a deficiency pattern and decreased cardiac function and is thought to be caused by constriction of blood vessels due to decreased intravascular pressure.

Weak Pulse

A weak pulse (*jakumyaku*) is a pulse that is sunken, thin, and weak. It is a pulse that is palpated only with strong pressure, but it disappears when pressed more strongly. This pulse indicates a lack of qi and blood[TM1].

Hidden Pulse

Hidden pulse (*fukumyaku*) is an extremely sunken pulse that is felt only when the pressure is strong enough to reach the bone. The pulse itself is a powerful and kind of excess pulse and appears in severe pain, sudden consciousness disturbance, or shock.

Hollow Pulse

Hollow pulse (*kōmyaku*) indicates an empty blood vessel that is clearly felt when pressed lightly, but it collapses when pressed a little stronger. It is a pulse that feels like it is hollow, like pressing the stalk of a long green onion. This is a serious pulse that indicates vascular collapse due to bleeding.

Skipping Pulse

Skipping pulse (*sokumyaku*) is a pulse that seems to stumble for a moment and resumes a fast beat and indicates yang.

2.7.6 Combined Pulse Examinations

Clinically, the pulse quality is often a combination of multiple pathological pulses (combined pulse qualities) rather than one. The features and clinical indications of combined pulse qualities (*kenmyaku*) are described below.

Combined Pulse Often Seen in Acute Diseases

- **Floating-rapid-weak pulse**
  A floating-rapid-weak pulse is a pulse that instantly feels weak and without tension when touched lightly and disappears when strongly pressed. This pulse indicates an exterior heat pattern. This pulse can be treated with formulas such as keishito (桂枝湯).
- **Floating-rapid-tight pulse**
  A floating-rapid-tight pulse is a pulse that feels strong and tense when lightly touched and indicates an exterior heat pattern and increased metabolism in the upper body. This

pulse can be treated with formulas containing ephedra, such as maoto (麻黄湯) and kakkonto (葛根湯).

- **Sunken-excess pulse**
  Sunken-excess pulse is a pulse that is strong on heavy pressure and indicates the need for purgation with formulas containing rhubarb (大黄剤).
- **Sunken-slippery pulse**
  Sunken-slippery pulse is a pulse indicating the presence of interior heat, and treatment with gypsum-containing formulas (石膏剤) is indicated.
- **Sunken-weak pulse**
  Sunken-weak pulse is a pulse that is not felt with light pressure and is barely felt with heavy pressure. A *sunken-moderate-weak pulse* indicates an interior cold pattern. This pulse indicates impaired metabolism, for which formulas containing processed aconite root (附子剤) are indicated.

Common Pulse Qualities in Chronic Diseases

- **Floating-weak pulse**
  Floating-weak pulse is a pulse indicating interior deficiency, in which the yang qi escapes. *Paradoxical large and no strength pulse* (散大無力) is an indication for hochuekkito (補中益気湯); *floating-large-faint* pulse is an indication for formulas containing processed aconite root (附子剤); *floating-weak-slow pulse* is an indication for shōkenchuto (小建中湯).
- **Floating and excess pulse**
  Floating and excess pulse is a pulse indicating multiple simultaneous pathogens, for which formulas such as sweat-inducing formulas (発汗剤), fluid[TM1] regulating formulas (利水剤), and purgative formulas (瀉下剤) may be indicated. Diseases associated with chronic pain may be treated by sweat-inducing formulas such as yokuininto (薏苡仁湯).
- **String-like-fine pulse**
  String-like-fine pulse is a pulse indicating the late yang stage pattern, fluid disturbance, or a prolonged but not significantly deficient condition. Shosaikoto (小柴胡湯) may be used, but sweat-inducing formulas, purgative formulas (瀉下剤), or emetic formulas (吐剤) must not be used.
- **Sunken-slow-excess pulse**
  Sunken-slow-excess is a pulse suggestive of an interior excess pattern (e.g., constipation), for which purgative formulas such as choijokito (調胃承気湯), shoijokito (小承気湯), and daisaikoto (大柴胡湯) are indicated.
- **Sunken-tight pulse**
  Sunken-tight pulse indicates respiratory distress, palpitations, decreased urine output, and edema due to water stagnation. Formulas such as mokuboito (木防已湯) and ryokeijutsukanto (苓桂朮甘) are indicated by this pulse.
- **Sunken-rough pulse**
  Sunken-rough pulse is a pulse that indicates static blood[TM1] and pain/numbness pattern. Sunken-excess-rough pulse is suggestive of static blood[TM1], for which formulas to treat blood[TM1] stasis such as tokakujokito (桃核承気湯) and keishibukuryogan (桂枝茯苓丸), are indicated. A sunken-weak-rough pulse may also indicate the complication of blood[TM1] deficiency.
- **Fine-slow pulse**
  A fine-slow pulse is a pulse indicating the presence of coldness in the extremities. If the subjective feeling of reversal cold in the extremities is present, formulas such as tokishigyakuto (当帰四逆湯) and tōkishigyakukagosyuyusyokyoto (当帰四逆加呉茱萸生姜湯) may be indicated. If the objective finding of reversal cold at the extremities is present, formulas such as goshuyuto (呉茱萸湯), shimbuto (真武湯), and bushiorityuto (附子理中湯) may be considered.
- **Large-weak pulse**
  A large-weak pulse is a pulse indicating severe fatigue and loss of stamina, for which formulas such as juzentaihoto (十全大補湯) and hochuekkito (補中益気湯) may be indicated.

2.8 Abdominal Diagnosis

Go Ito and Toshihiko Hanawa

2.8.1 History of Abdominal Diagnosis

In the abdominal diagnosis of the *Nanjing*, which was the first such system in ancient Chinese medicine, disease was judged based on the position and nature of the moving qi (pulsation). The pattern (証) and the treatment plan were determined, and the prognosis was discussed.

The pulsation palpated in the umbilical region was called the interrenal palpitations (*jinkan-no-dō*) (Fig. 3.12), and this

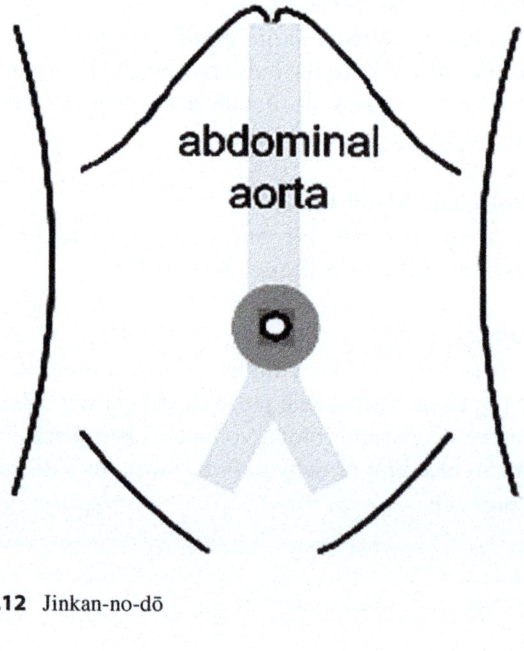

Fig. 3.12 Jinkan-no-dō

pulsation below the navel was considered to be the source of vitality and the most important finding.

Areas on the abdomen are allotted to the "five zang organs" in the Nanjing system. The liver[TM1] area is on the left side of the navel, the heart[TM1] area is above the navel, the spleen[TM1] area is on the navel, the lung[TM1] area is on the right side of the navel, and these were where pulsations were palpated.

The difference in the system of abdominal diagnosis between the Shanghanlun and the *Nanjing* is that abdominal diagnosis directly serves as an instruction for treatment. Even though the prescription is determined, the prognosis is not mentioned at all. There are a few observations about abdominal diagnosis in the *Shanghanlun* and *Jinguiyaolue*, but the details of findings are often unknown. Therefore, it is no exaggeration to say that most of the abdominal diagnosis findings currently used were created in Japan (Fig. 3.13).

The development of abdominal diagnosis is unique to Japan, and it is given particular importance in the practice of Kampo medicine. As to the reason for the development of abdominal diagnosis in Japan, *Osuka Keisetsu* (大塚敬節) speculated that the treatment similar to the techniques of abdominal palpation (abdominal massage) by Zen priests in the Muromachi period (1392–1575) influenced the abdominal examinations in later generations. These techniques were summarized by *Zen priest Taga Hōin* and documented in the book *Fukushinnohō* (Methodology of abdominal diagnosis) preserved at the Taga Yakushi temple.

It is believed that *Mubunsai* (夢分斎), who was a Zen priest during the Azuchi-Momoyama period, was taught abdominal diagnosis at the same time as the acupuncture techniques from this *Taga Hōin*. These techniques were then transmitted from *Mubunsai* to *Misono Isai* (1557–1616). *Misono* developed a method of acupuncture, striking the head of the needle with a small hammer (*dashin*), and had great success in the use of this style of acupuncture and his Mubun-style abdominal diagnosis. The text, *Mubun-style dividend diagram of zang-fu organs* (Fig. 3.14), is the definitive record of the *Mubun*-style abdominal diagnosis, and this system is still used by some acupuncturists today.

These early techniques of abdominal diagnosis were based on the *Nanjing* system and mainly proposed by acupuncturists, and it is worth mentioning that Zen priests and acupuncturists played important roles in the genesis of the abdominal diagnosis.

The techniques of abdominal diagnosis by the *Nanjing* system also influenced the abdominal diagnosis of the Gosei School of Kampo, which compiled and published the text "*Shinbyō kigai*" by *Taki Motokata* (Fig. 3.15). This text was later translated into Chinese by *Matsui Misao* in the Meiji period (1888), and this was the first text of Japanese Kampo medicine published in China.

While the techniques of abdominal diagnosis based on the *Nanjing* system had a great impact on the Gosei School

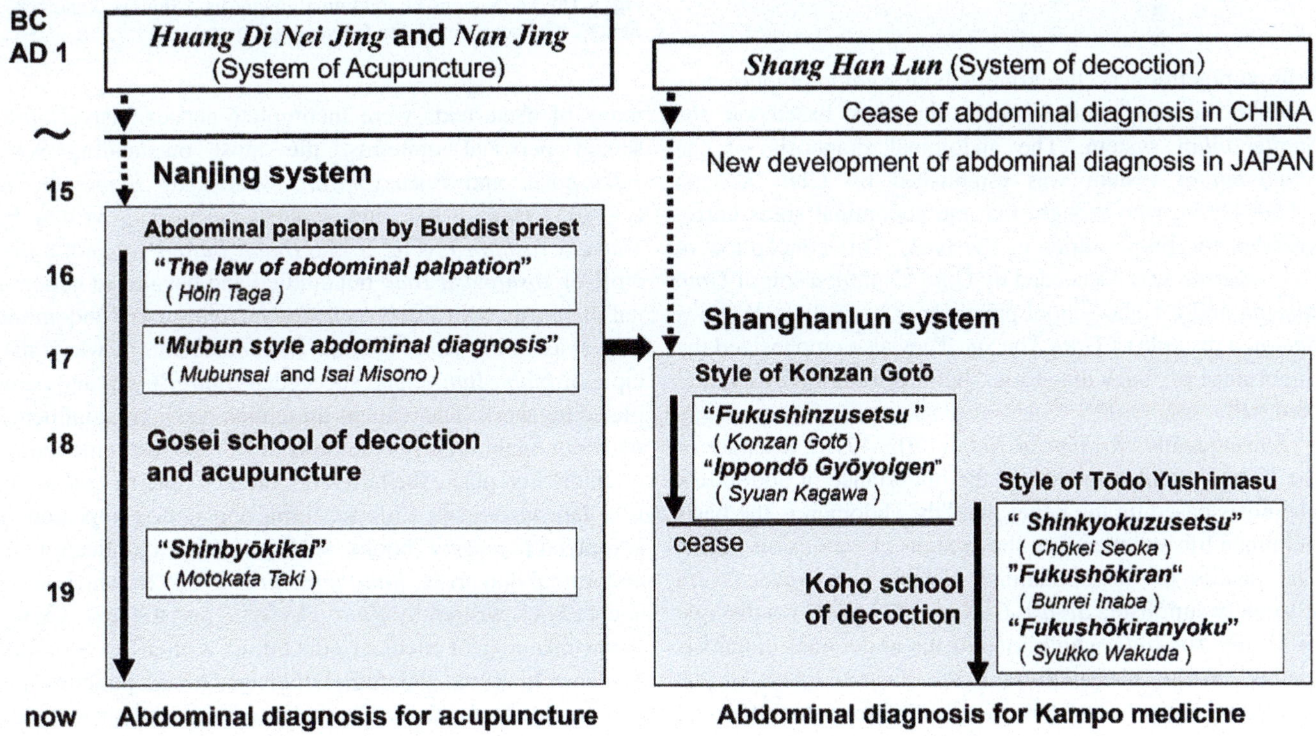

Fig. 3.13 History of abdominal diagnosis

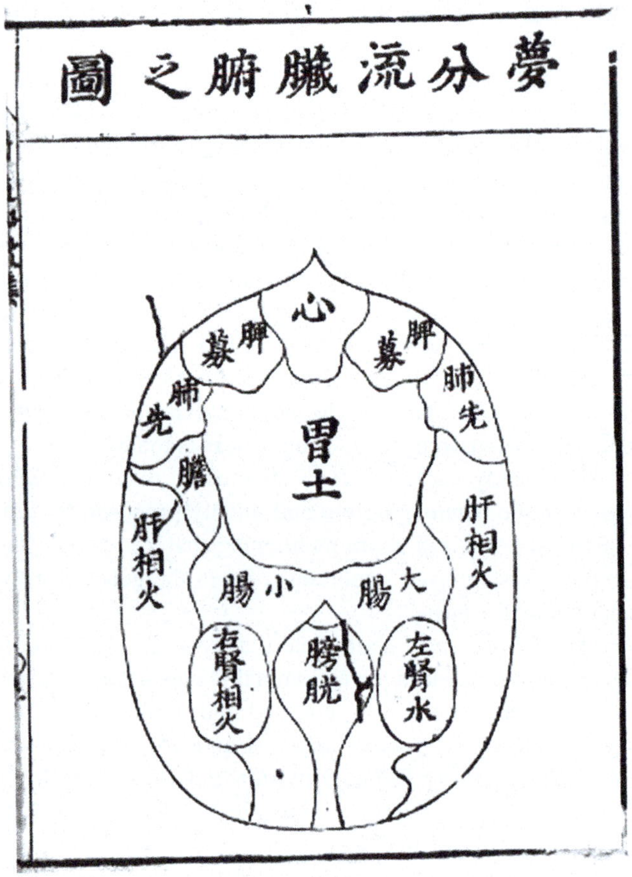

Fig. 3.14 The Mubun-style diagram of zang-fu organs. "Shindō hiketusyu (鍼道秘訣集)". (Collection of Kyoto University Library)

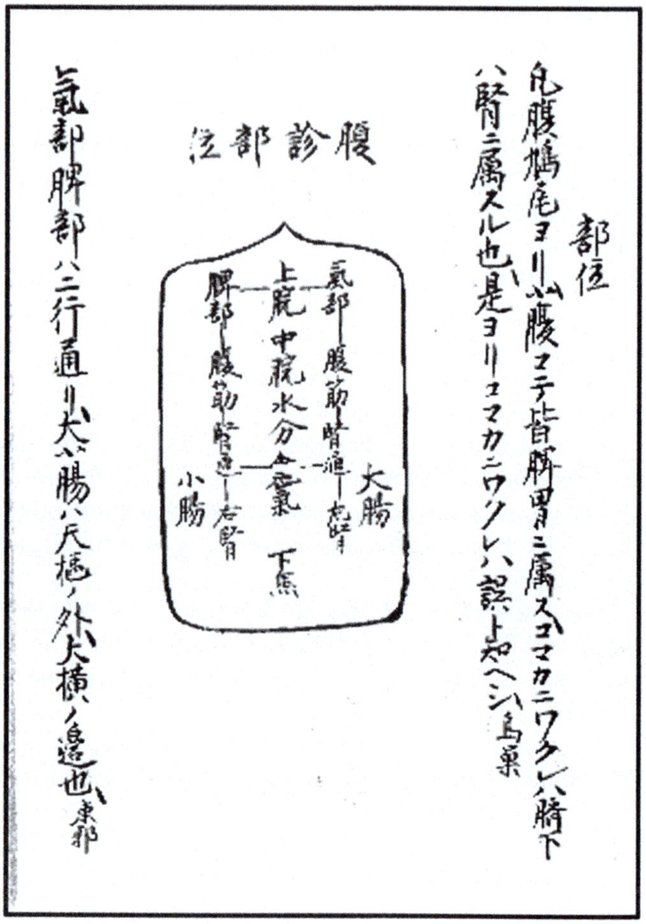

Fig. 3.15 The regions of abdominal diagnosis. "Shinbyo kigai (診病奇侅)". (Collection of Kyoto University Library)

Kampo practitioners, the Koho School Kampo practitioners used techniques of abdominal diagnosis based on the *Shanghanlun* system. The abdominal diagnosis of the *Shanghanlun* system was established by *Goto Konzan* (1659–1733), who thought that the abdominal signs corresponded to abnormalities of the back. This conception of *Goto Konzan* was succeeded by *Goto Chinan,* a son of *Gotō Konzan* and a Koho school practitioner, as well as *Kagawa Shuan*, a disciple of *Goto Konzan*. They also emphasized the importance of "back diagnosis," but this tradition eventually died out.

Subsequently, *Yoshimasu Todo* (1702–1773), a leader of the Koho School, emphasized the importance of abdominal diagnosis based on the belief that "the abdomen is the basis of human life and therefore shows signs of various diseases." The details of his abdominal diagnosis, however, were extremely simplistic. *Se-oka Chokei* (1733–1781), a disciple of *Yoshimasu Todo* who mastered the abdominal diagnosis method, wrote *Sinkyokuzusetu*, an illustrated text of the abdominal diagnosis. Thus, *Se-oka* influenced abdominal diagnosis methods of later generations, such as in texts like *Kohōbinran,* written by *Rokkaku Shigeto* (六角重任). While many of these texts were incomplete and exclusively presented personal opinions, the most outstanding were *Fukushōzui* and *Fukusyōkiran,* written by *Inaba Bunrei* (?~1805) (Fig. 3.16), and *Fukushokiranyoku,* written by *Wakuda Yoshitora.* (Fig. 3.17). *Inaba Bunrei* was not a disciple of *Yoshimasu Todo* but studied and developed abdominal diagnosis with *Tsuruya Yasuhide*, a master of abdominal diagnosis in the Koho school. *Wakuda Yoshitora* was a disciple of *Inaba Bunrei* and succeeded *Bunrei's* will and completed his work. The texts of these men had a great influence on abdominal diagnosis methods in Kampo medicine today.

In the first place, the term abdominal diagnosis (*fukushin*) is a Japanese-made Chinese term, and it first appeared in seventeenth-century books such as Kuno's collection of abdominal diagnosis, *Kunoharashinsyu* (1652), which is the source book written by *Kuno Gen'etsu*, and the text *Ikyoseii* (right meaning of medical education) written by *Kusakari San'etsu*. In effect, abdominal diagnosis for acupuncture and abdominal diagnosis for herbal medicine influenced each other to create various abdominal examination texts in the Edo period.

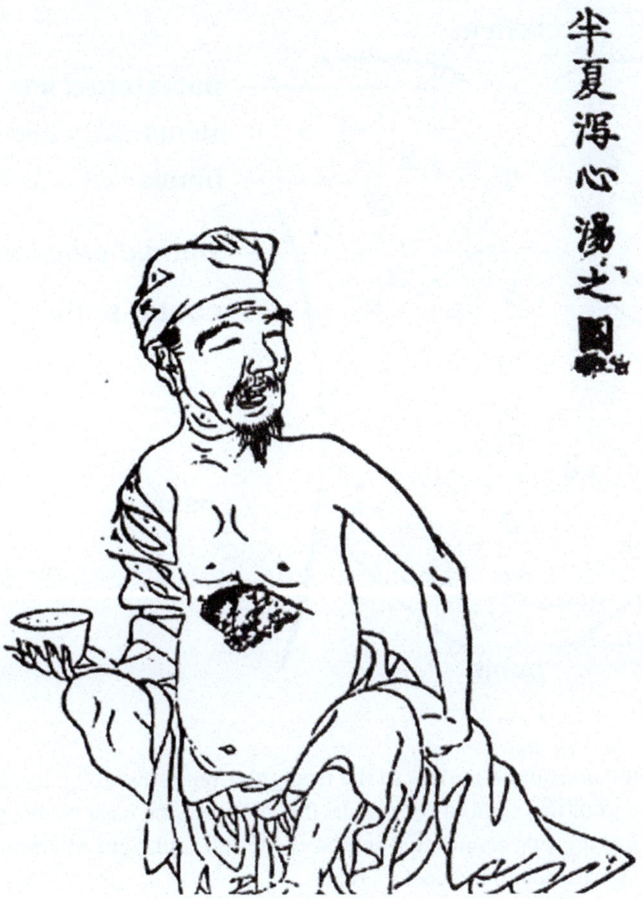

Fig. 3.16 Illustration of abdominal diagnostic pattern of hangeshashintō. "Fukusyokiran" by *Inaba Bunrei.* (Collection of Kyoto University Library)

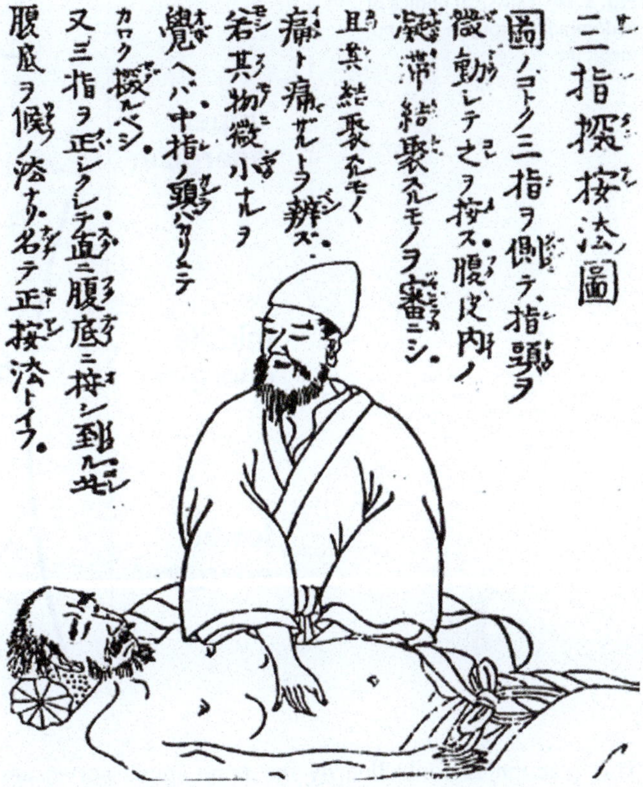

Fig. 3.17 Illustration of abdominal examination. "Fukusyōkiran-yoku" by *Wakuda Yoshitora.* (Collection of Kyoto University Library)

Otsuka Keisetsu listed a total of 106 publications on abdominal diagnosis (36 publications on *Nanjing*-based methods, 37 on *Shanghanlun*-based methods, 5 on combinations of both, and 28 which he did not read) in his book, "Classification of Literature on Abdominal Diagnosis."

2.8.2 Characteristics and Key Points of Abdominal Examination

While findings of pulse diagnosis capture changes in minute detail, findings of abdominal examination are often continuous findings, which last from hours to days, so they can reflect not only acute diseases but also chronic pathologies.

As a rule, abdominal examination in Kampo medicine is traditionally performed with the examiner sitting on the left side of the patient (Fig. 3.17). Generally it is performed with the patient relaxed, with the legs extended in the supine position. This is in contrast to the position for abdominal examination in Western medicine, which is performed from the right side of the patient with the patient's knees bent. This is because, in Western medicine, mainly loosening the abdominal wall is required, and the abdominal wall needs to be relaxed to examine the condition of abdominal organs. In Kampo medicine, on the other hand, the abdomen is examined to investigate how abnormalities of abdominal organs as well as the body overall appear on the abdomen based on the condition of the abdominal wall, such as tension and tenderness. Abdominal examination should be done by softly touching the abdomen using one or both hands. It should be noted that pressing the abdomen too hard will cause pain and tension in the abdominal wall and prevent correct findings.

In general, abdominal examination should be done slowly for frail persons by stroking the abdomen with warm hands. For robust, middle-aged men, the tender points should be checked by quickly pressing with the fingers. In abdominal examination, it is important not only to detect tender points and resistance but also to feel for warmth, coldness, moistness, and dryness with the palm of the hand. If typical findings are obtained by this examination, question the patient again about symptoms associated with the findings.

Tender points are areas in which pressing on the skin causes pain or discomfort and indicates the existence of lesions under the skin or deeper in the body cavity. When there is inflammation, nerve injury, or reduced blood flow in internal organs, the peritoneum, or the mesentery, visceral pain, somatic pain, or visceral motor reflex may cause involuntary contraction of abdominal skeletal muscles (tetany).

Fig. 3.18 Classical names of abdominal regions in Kampo medicine

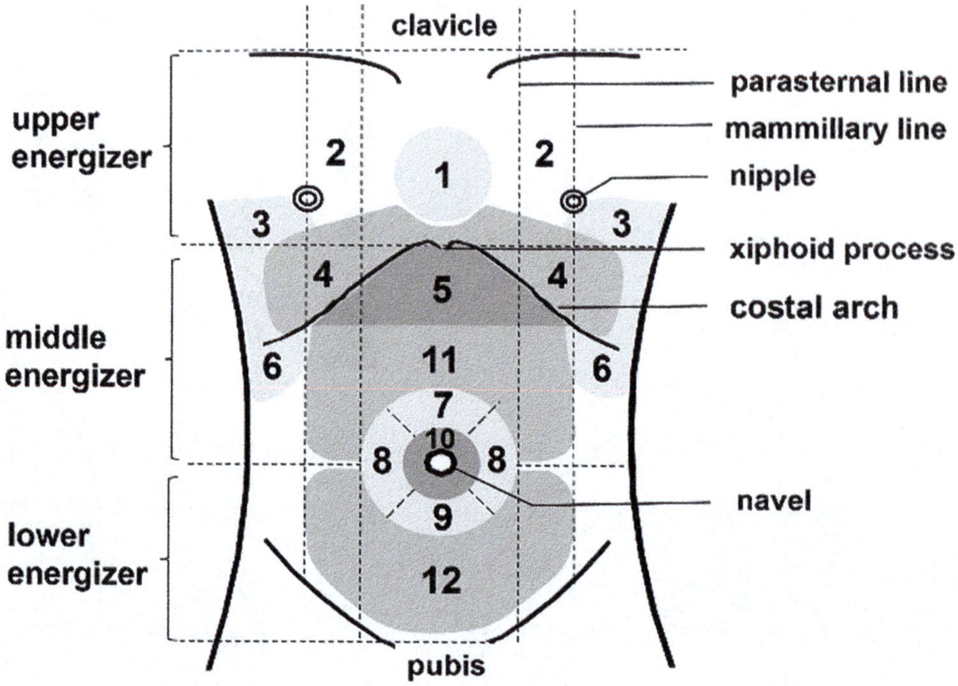

This reaction is controlled by the same spinal nerve, and there is increased sensitivity (hyperalgesia) in the domain of the same spinal nerve. As a result, this may cause tenderness in local regions (skin and muscles) controlled by that spinal nerve. Therefore, from the presence or absence of tenderness, the abdominal examination can diagnose changes resulting from changes in blood flow to the tissue, such as static blood[TM1] and blood[TM1] deficiency.

2.8.3 Nomenclature of Abdominal Regions in Kampo Medicine

In naming the abdominal regions in traditional Kampo medicine (Fig. 3.18), the trunk is divided into three sections. The cardiothorax above the diaphragm is the *upper energizer*, the area from above the navel to the diaphragm is the *middle energizer*, and the lower abdomen from below the navel to the pubic bone is the *lower energizer*. These are respectively called *jōshō, chūshō,* and *geshō* in Kampo medicine. Furthermore, in the thorax above the costal arch, the area between the left and right mammillary lines and under the clavicle is known as *mune* (chest) or *kyō,* and the area lateral to the mammillary line is known as *waki* (side) or *kyō.*

In addition, the entirety of the area above the costal arch from the chest to the side is called *kyokyō* (chest and sides), the ribs of the costal arch are called *kyōroku* (sides and ribs), and the area below the costal arch is called *kyōka* (hypochondrium). Furthermore, the area of the xiphoid process is called *kaku* (diaphragm); above it is *shin* (heart)," below *shin* is *shinka* or *shinge* (epigastrium or below the heart). Moreover, the area *shinka* refers to the triangular region with the lower end of the xiphoid process as the apex and the base connecting the two points that intersect the left and right mammillary lines and the costal arches.

In the abdomen, the area above the navel (upper abdomen) is called *daifuku,* and the area below the navel (lower abdomen) is called *shōfuku.* When the term *fuku* is used in Japanese classic texts, it generally refers to the upper abdomen, and in this case, *shōfuku* is used to refer to the lower abdomen. Either side of the umbilicus is called *seibō* or *saibō* (paraumbilicus), the area above the umbilicus is called *seijō* or *saijō* (supraumbilicus), and the area below the umbilicus is called *seika* or *saika* (infraumbilicus), while just below the umbilicus is called *seitei* or *saitei* (umbilical bottom) (Fig. 3.18). The range of the supraumbilical, subumbilical, and left and right umbilical areas is approximately within a circle centered on the navel and with its margins on the parasternal line. The mammillary line and parasternal line in modern medicine almost coincide with the course of the stomach meridian of acupuncture on the chest and abdomen.

2.8.4 Types of Abdominal Examination Findings

The types of abdominal examination findings that provide clues for Kampo diagnosis are *abdominal patterns* or *abdominal signs*; these are called *fukusyō* (腹証) or *fukukō* (腹候), respectively. The types of abdominal findings are comprehensively determined by not only palpation but also visual inspection and auscultation, as shown in Table 3.10.

Table 3.10 Types of abdominal diagnostic findings of Kampo medicine

Type classification	Diagnostic findings	Kampo names	Japanese letter
Confirm by palpation	Epigastric stuffiness and rigidity Abdominal urgency Weakness or paresthesia of lower abdomen Lower abdominal contracture Lower abdominal taut Cord in abdominal midline Resistance and distention in the lower abdomen Epigastric pulsation below the xiphoid process Supraumbilical pulsation Infraumbilical pulsation	*sinka-hiken* *rikyū* *shōfuku-fuzin* *shōfuku-kōkyū* *syōfuku-genkyū* *seichūshin* *shōfuku-kōman* *shinka-ki* *seizyō-ki* *seika-ki*	心下痞鞕 裏急 小腹不仁 小腹拘急 小腹弦急 正中芯 小腹鞕満 心下悸 臍上悸 臍下悸
Palpation with inspection	Strong protruding abdominal wall or obtuse costal arch Weak and caved in abdominal wall or acute costal arch Excessive tension in rectus abdominis muscle Abdominal fullness with firm distention of excess type Abdominal fullness with soft swelling of deficiency type Visible peristaltic discord	*jisshō* *kyoshō* *fukuchokukin-renkyū* *jituman* *kyoman* *zendō-fuon*	実証 虚証 腹直筋攣急 実満 虚満 蠕動不穏
Palpation with auscultation	Fluid[TM1] retention in stomach Splashing sound Fullness and distention of the whole abdomen	*inai-teisui* *shinsuion* *fukman*	胃内停水 振水音 腹満

(continued)

Table 3.10 (continued)

Type classification	Diagnostic findings	Kampo names	Japanese letter
Palpation with tenderness	Epigastric stuffiness and resistance Stuffiness and resistance below hypochondrium Fullness and discomfort in chest and hypochondrium Severe tenderness in epigastric region Epigastric tightness and stuck feeling Abdominal wall contracture Tenderness in the ileocecal region Tenderness in the sigmoid colon region Tenderness in the iliac fossa Resistance and severe tenderness in the left iliac region Tenderness in the paraumbilical region Umbilical pain	*shinka-hikō* *kyōka-hikō* *kyōkyō-kuman* *kekkyō* *shinka-shiketsu* *fukuhi-kōkyū* *kaimōbu-attsū* *esuzyōbu-attsū* *chōkotsukabu-attsū* *shōfuku-kyūketsu* *seibō-attsū* *seitsū*	心下痞鞕 脇下痞鞕 胸脇苦満 結胸 心下支結 腹皮拘急 回盲部圧痛 S状部圧痛 腸骨窩部圧痛 小腹急結 臍傍圧痛 臍痛

2.8.5 Main Abdominal Findings and Clinical Diagnosis

Strong and Protruding Abdominal Wall and Weak and Caved in Abdominal Wall

Obtuse costal arch and acute costal arch

The elasticity and tone of the abdomen are assessed. Abdominal strength is usually divided into five stages: excessive, slightly excessive, moderate, slightly deficient, and deficient. The degree of the disease response is determined by examining *the deficiency and excess based on the unevenness and strength of the abdominal wall.*

In general, when viewed from the side, the *abdominal wall that is firm and protruding* above the ribcage (over the horizontal line of the sternum), which is called a paunchy abdomen, is diagnosed as excess pattern (*jisshō*). Conversely, *the abdominal wall that is weak and caved in* from the ribcage (under the horizontal line of the sternum) is diagnosed as a deficiency pattern (*kyoshō*) (Fig. 3.19).

However, the soft and bloated abdomen that protrudes from the ribcage may also be caused by qi deficiency (*kikyo*), so the assessment of whether it is deficient or excessive should be made by palpation.

Persons with an *obtuse* costal arch in the epigastric region are often diagnosed as excess pattern (*jisshō*). Those with *acute costal arch* are often diagnosed as deficiency pattern (*kyoshō*) (Fig. 3.20). Clinically, abdominal strength is judged on whether it is strong or not, because those with weak abdominal strength and poor muscle tone tend to have an insufficient disease response, and the use of purgative formulas (containing Ephedra herb, rhubarb, and gypsum) is not advisable. In such cases, tonic formulas (containing ginseng, Astragalus root, and processed aconite root) are commonly used.

Epigastric Stuffiness, Epigastric Stuffiness and Resistance

Epigastric severe tenderness

Epigastric stuffiness that is only a subjective full sensation in the epigastric region is called *sinka-hi* (Fig. 3.21), and

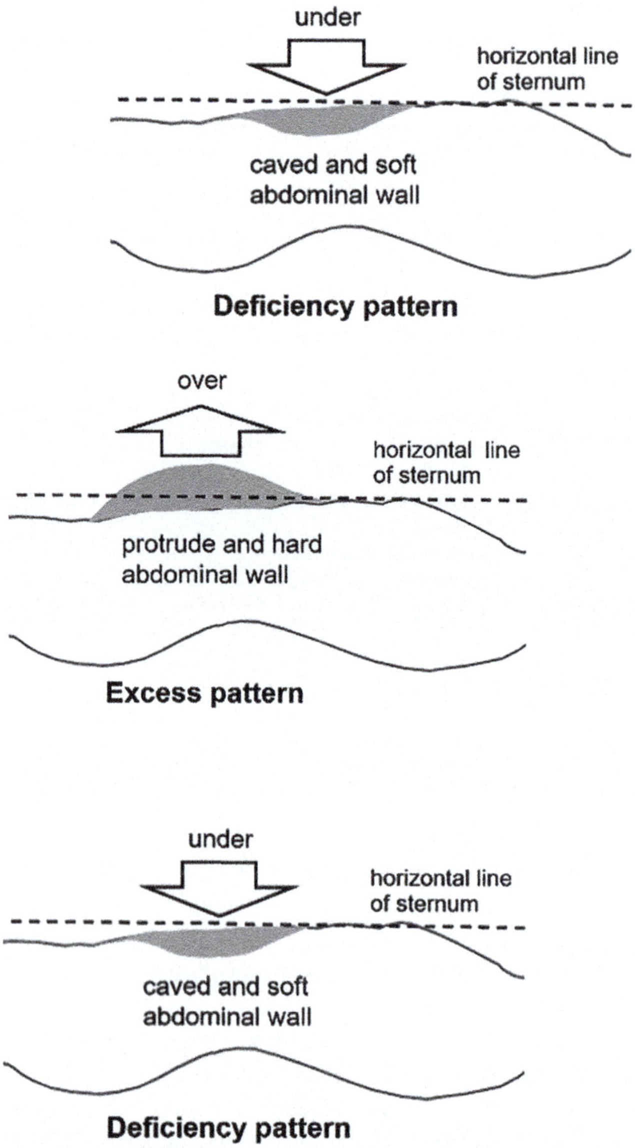

Fig. 3.19 Deficiency and excess patterns diagnosed by unevenness of abdominal wall

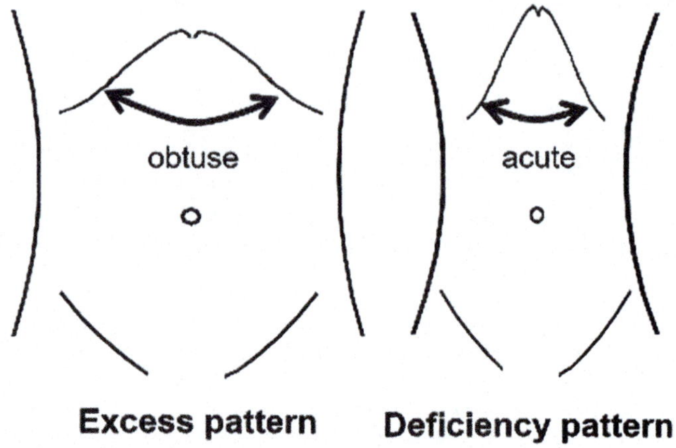

Fig. 3.20 Excess and deficiency patterns diagnosed by angle of costal arch

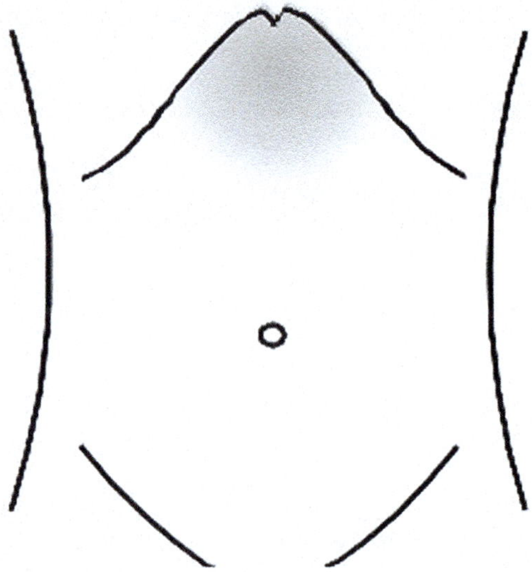

Fig. 3.21 Shinka-hi

epigastric stuffiness with resistance that is a subjective full sensation with objective resistance in the epigastric region is called *sinka-hikō* or *shinge-hiko* (Fig. 3.22). In practice, tenderness is commonly noted in patients with *shinka-hikō*, and *more severe tenderness in* the *epigastric region than shinka-hikō* may be called *kekkyō* (Fig. 3.22).

Treatment should be performed according to the pattern, keeping in mind that this epigastric region is a reaction zone of the stomach, duodenum, pancreas, and gallbladder, and is also the area where viscera-related pain refers [9].

For *shinka-hikō* with signs of water stagnation in the background, formulas containing Coptis rhizome, Ginseng, Bupleurum root, and Pinellia tuber, such as hangeshashinto (半夏瀉心湯) or ninjinto (人参湯), may be considered. If there are no signs of water stagnation and *kyōkyōkuman* (fullness and discomfort in the chest and hypochondrium) is present at the same time, formulas containing Bupleurum root *(Saikozai)* such as shosaikoto (小柴胡湯), and daisaikoto (大柴胡湯), are often indicated. For *kekkyo* (結胸), saikanto (shosaikoto + shokankyoto) is considered.

Epigastric Stuffiness and Rigidity

Epigastric stuffiness and rigidity without elasticity, like thin plywood, is called *shinka-hiken* (Fig. 3.23). The resistance is wider and stronger than that of the *shinka-hikō*.

One of the causes may be signs such as hepatomegaly due to right heart failure, suggesting the possibility of heart, liver, or kidney disease. In this case, consider mokuboito (木防已湯).

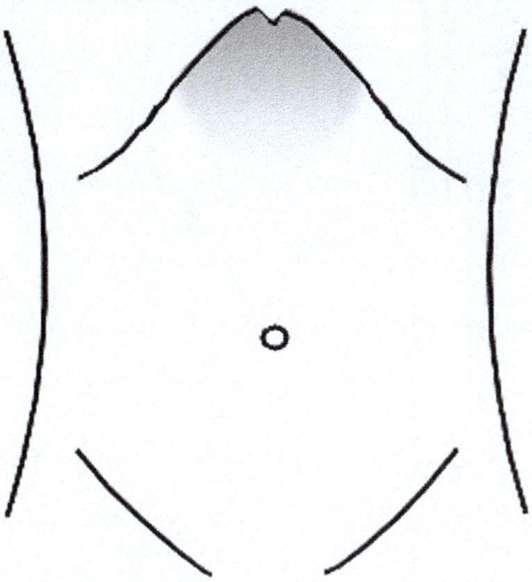

Fig. 3.22 Shinka-hikō and Kekkyō

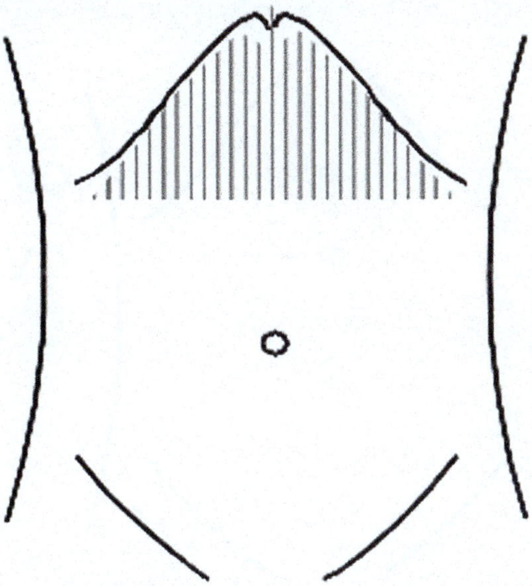

Fig. 3.23 Shinka-hiken

Fullness and Discomfort in the Chest and Hypochondrium

Stuffiness and resistance in lower hypochondrium

Fullness and discomfort in the chest and hypochondrium are called *kyōkyō-kuman* (Fig. 3.24). The term *kyōkyō-kuman* described in the classic literature originally refers to the subjective symptoms of discomfort in the area from the chest to the side, *kyōkyō*. In modern Kampo medicine, the main findings of *kyōkyō-kuman* have been *fullness with the rigidity and tenderness of hypochondrium*, but *stuffiness and resistance with tenderness in the lower hypochondrium* is a finding corresponding to the classic *kyōka-hikō* (Fig. 3.25) and is often present at the same time as *kyōkyō-kuman* (Fig. 3.24).

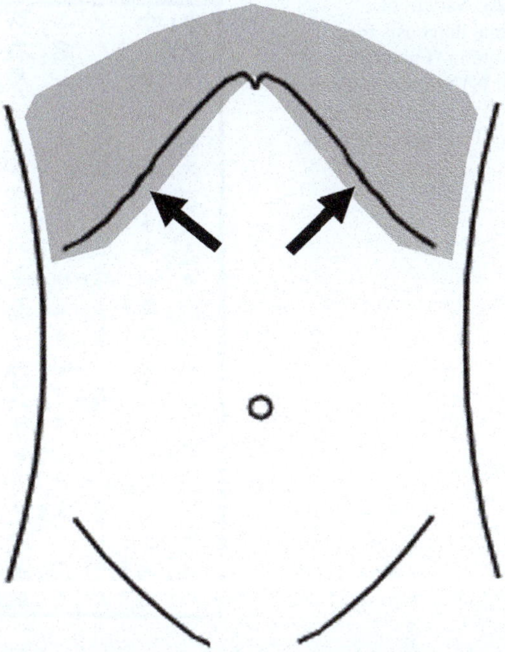

Fig. 3.24 Kyōkyō-kuman

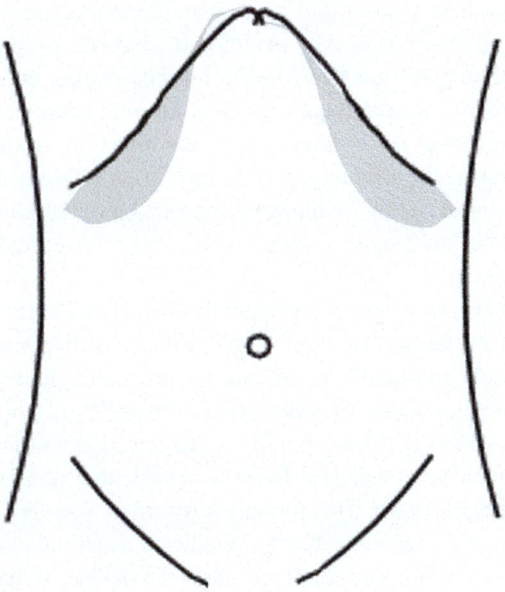

Fig. 3.25 Kyōka-hikō

According to the *Fukusyōkiran*, since resistance and discomfort are difficult to detect on the surface, it is necessary to press the fingers from the costal margin into the subcostal region of the hypochondriac region, that is, toward the side of the chest, and see if there is a reaction (Fig. 3.26 ⇓).

Ōtsuka Keisetsu also wrote, "*kyōkyō-kuman* refers to the patient's own feeling of fullness in the chest and sides, but to examine this objectively, the doctor should push the thumb into the chest cavity from the hypochondrium. If there is

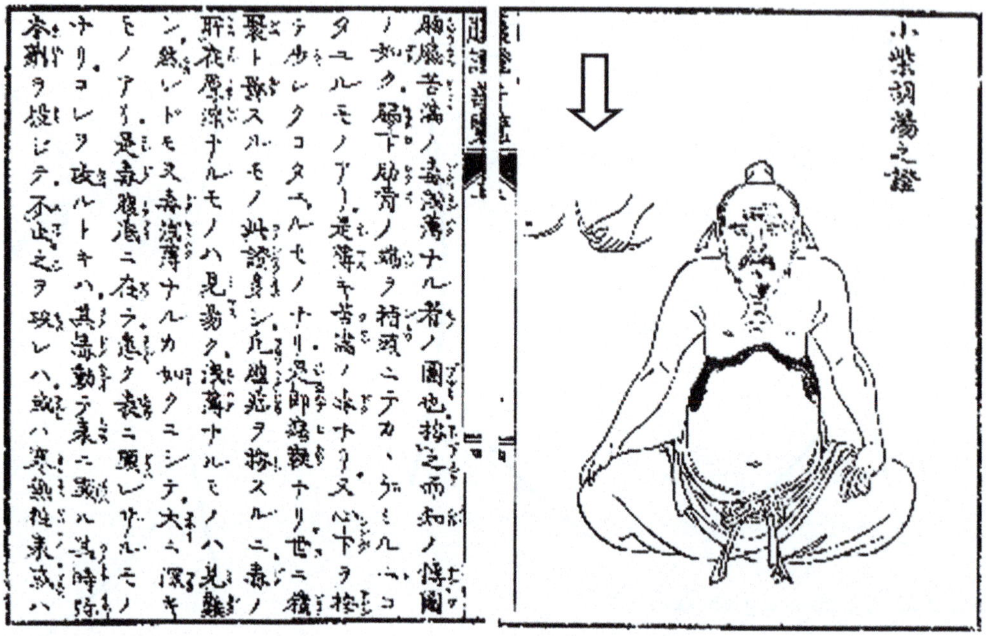

Fig. 3.26 Pattern of abdominal diagnosis for shosaikotō in "Fukusyokiran (腹証奇覧)"written by Bunrei Inaba (稲葉文礼). (Collection of Kyoto University Library)

kyōkyō-kuman, resistance will be felt at the fingertip, and the patient will feel suffocated and complain of pain.'

It is also believed that rigidity and tenderness in the side of the chest are caused by irritation of visceral afferent fibers by pathological reactions in the internal organs around the diaphragm, causing hyperalgesia of afferent neurons such as the intercostal nerve mediated by the reflex arc in the same segment of the thoracic spinal cord. Then efferent neurons cause resistance by involuntary contraction of the muscles in the subcostal region, such as the transverse abdominis muscles.

Kyōkyō-kuman may appear on both the left and right sides or just on the left or right in the margins of hypochondria. Relatively frequently it appears on just the right side. The condition of *kyōkyō-kuman* reflects liver[TM1] qi stagnation (*kanki-ukketsu*), which is a more advanced state of *qi deficiency* and is considered to be a typical finding of the late yang stage pattern. This finding is regarded as a very important target in Japanese Kampo medicine as an indication for formulas containing Bupleuri radix (柴胡剤). It has been pointed out that *kyōkyō-kuman* is associated with diseases of organs that are located above and below the diaphragm, such as chronic hepatitis, splenomegaly, hepatomegaly, and pneumonitis, or just mental stress. As for treatment, both *kyōkyō-kuman and kyōka-hikō* have indications for formulas containing Bupleuri radix (柴胡剤) such as shosaikoto (小柴胡湯), daisaikoto (大柴胡湯), shigyakusan (四逆散), and saikokaryukotsuboreito (柴胡加竜骨牡蛎湯).

Epigastric Tightness and Stuck Feeling

Shinka-shiketsu (Fig. 3.27) was regarded as the abdominal pattern or indication for saikokeishito (柴胡桂枝湯) in the *Shanghanlun*. *Otsuka*'s interpretation that "*shinka-shiketsu* is a state with stuck feeling in hypocardia (*shinka*) along with *tense rectus abdominal muscles in the hypochondrium*" is generally accepted today. *Terasawa Katsutoshi,* however, added the finding of "tenderness at the acupoint CV12.

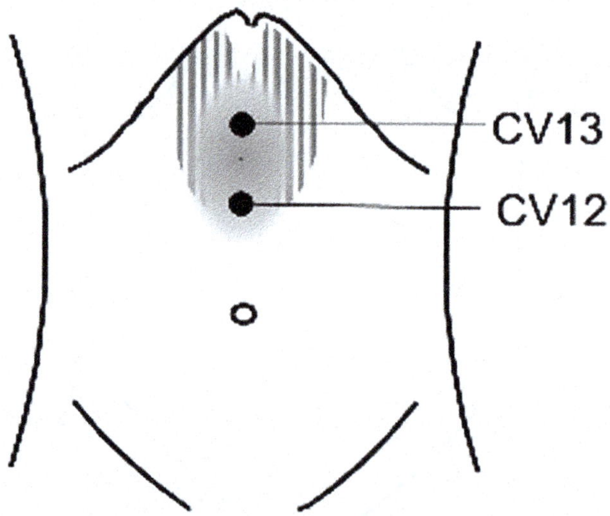

Fig. 3.27 Shinka-shiketsu

According to the *Fukushokiranyoku*, since saikokeishito (柴胡桂枝湯) is the formula prescribed during the transition period from early yang stage pattern to late yang stage pattern, the abdominal pattern is characterized by *shinka-shiketsu* rather than *kyōkyō-kuman* in the late yang stage pattern. In addition, *shi-ketsu* means the tightness and clogged feeling around CV12 and CV13 in the epigastric region, with "substance in the stomach." CV12 and CV13 are acupoints on the Conception Vessel, and "substance" here refers to inflammatory lesions in the stomach (Fig. 3.33). In other words, *shinka-shiketsu* is the finding of *epigastric tightness and a stuck feeling* that appears around the acupoints CV12 to CV13, as in cases of gastritis.

Splashing Sounds and Fluid[TM1] Retention in Stomach

The splashing sounds heard over the abdomen when pressing and releasing repeatedly with a wrist action are called *shinsui-on. The splashing sounds heard over the epigastric region* especially are called *shinkabu-sinsuion* or *fluid retention in the stomach* (*inai-teisui*) (Fig. 3.28). *Water*[TM1] *qi signs under the epigastric region* (*sinka-suiki*) have almost the same meaning.

The epigastric splashing sound on abdominal examination is thought to be a sign of fluid[TM1] retention (*suitai*). It is produced when the gastric wall is relaxed and there are a certain amount of gastric juices and air in the stomach. It is considered such sounds are likely to occur when, instead of being excreted, gastric juices and air are retained in the stomach. The state of the stomach is weakened, such that its smooth muscles are relaxed and the peristalsis is decreased, as in cases of gastroptosis.

It should be noted that in patients with gastroptosis, the stomach moves below to the lower umbilical region, and splash sounds can occasionally be detected on the lower abdomen, as shown by the broken line (Fig. 3.29).

This is suggestive of vagus nerve dysfunction, which is often accompanied by other signs of autonomic nerve dysfunction. The sound may also be caused by fluid[TM1] retention in the third portion of the duodenum or jejunum. This is called *shinsui-on* (splashing sound). Formulas for treating fluid disturbance which contain Poria Sclerotium (茯苓), Atractylodes Rhizome (白朮), and Pinellia Tuber (半夏), such as rikkunshito (六君子湯), may be used.

Excessive Tension in the Rectus Abdominis Muscle
Abdominal wall contracture

Excessive tension of the rectus abdominis muscle is called *fukuchokukin-renkyū* (Fig. 3.30). In classical Kampo terms, it was called *nihonbō,* which means "two sticks," and also *nidaichiku,* which means "two big bamboos." This finding is usually bilateral but may also be unilateral (tighter on one

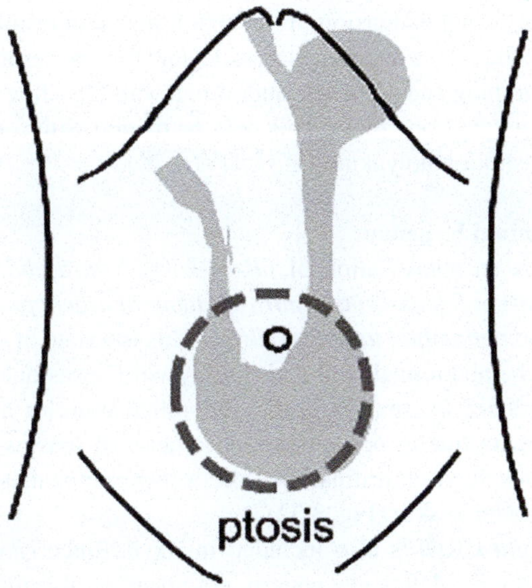

Fig. 3.29 The case of shinsuion (splash sound due to gastric ptosis)

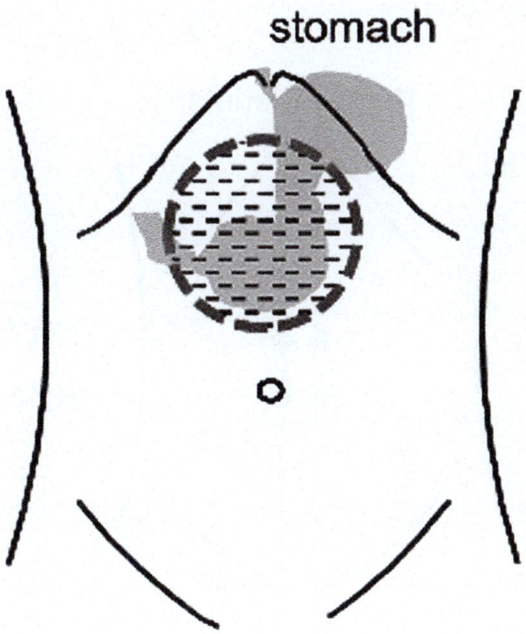

Fig. 3.28 Shinkabu-shinsuion

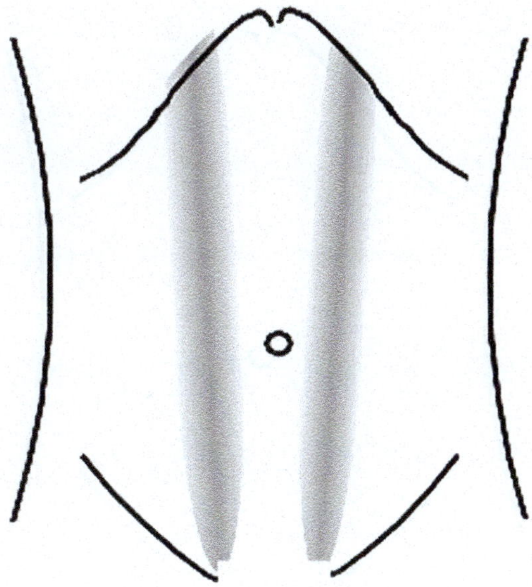

Fig. 3.30 Fukutchokukin-renkyū

side) or appear only on the upper abdomen. Tension in the muscle usually develops symmetrically, but it may only be on one side or the upper abdomen. The tension in the upper rectus abdominis muscle is attributed to the middle thoracic cord, and the lower rectus abdominis muscle to the lower thoracic cord. The tension may not be due to muscle contraction caused by visceral motor reflexes but to compensatory excessive tension from hypotonicity in abdominal muscle groups other than the rectus abdominis muscle or from decreased abdominal pressure.

Shigyakusan (四逆散) may be used for patients with an excess pattern, and shokenchuto (小建中湯) may be used for patients with a deficiency pattern.

Fukuhi-kōkyū (Fig. 3.31) refers to *abdominal wall contracture*, which is tension in the abdominal skin or muscles, such as the rectus abdominis muscle, and this causes abdominal cramping and pain. The abdominal wall feels like touching a thin plywood plate. This may be treated with formulas like keishikashakuyakuto (桂枝加芍薬湯).

Abdominal Urgency

Rikyū is an abbreviation of *fukuri-kokyū* (*intra-abdominal restraint*) or *fukuri-kyūtsū* (*intra-abdominal urgent pain)* and refers to *abdominal urgency* (*rikyu*). This is a state of cramping in the abdominal wall and rigidity with occasional pain. It is induced by spasms in the abdominal muscles and the peritoneum due to peritonitis, and otherwise spasms in the intestines due to intestinal dilation or hyperperistalsis under the abdominal skin (Fig. 3.32).

Fukuhi-kōkyū is also included in *rikyū*. Since *rikyū* is a symptom of a deficiency pattern, not laxatives, formulas like shokenchuto (小建中湯) and daikenchuto (大建中湯) should be considered for the purpose of relieving distension. In addition, *abdominal urgency after defecation and acute pain in the abdominal area* are called *rikyū-kōjū.*

Umbilical Pain

Umbilical pain, which is a tenderness that is developed when pressed directly on the upper side of the umbilical ring, is called *seitsū* or *saitsū* (Fig. 3.33); a cord-like object may be palpated at the same points of tenderness. It is also called "Otsuka's umbilical pain" because it is one of the indications for using kakkonto (葛根湯) devised by Otsuka Keisetsu.

Seitsū tends to appear between the acupuncture points KI16 and KI17 on the kidney meridian and develops any-

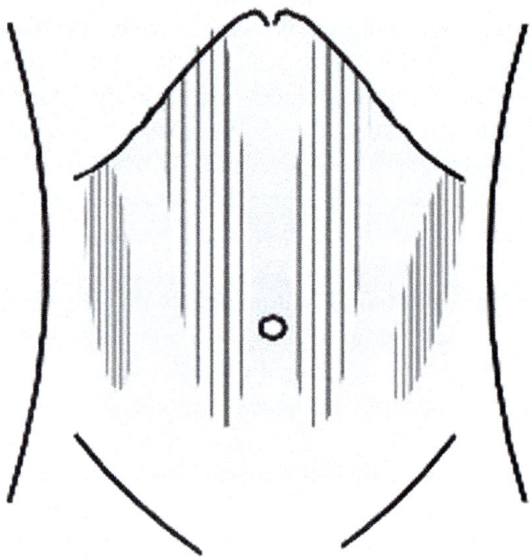

Fig. 3.32 Rikyū

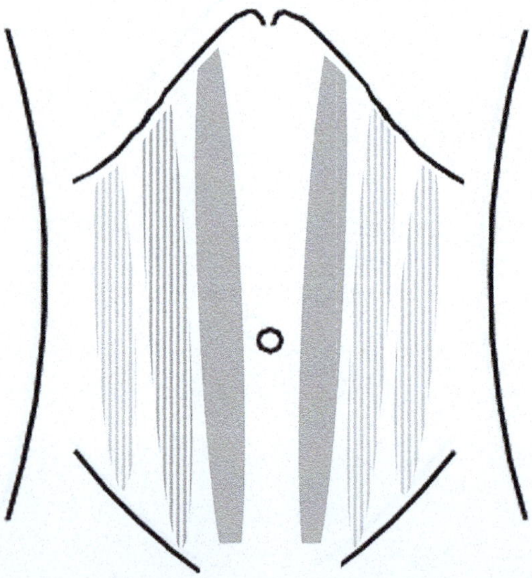

Fig. 3.31 Fukuhi-kokyu Fukutchokukin

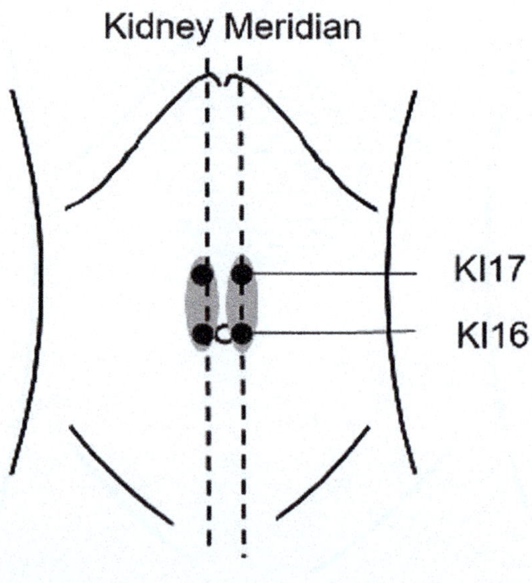

Fig. 3.33 Seitsu

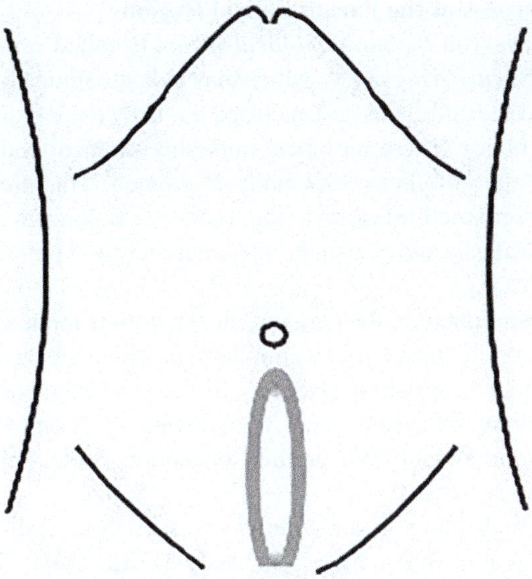

Fig. 3.34 Shōfuku-fujin

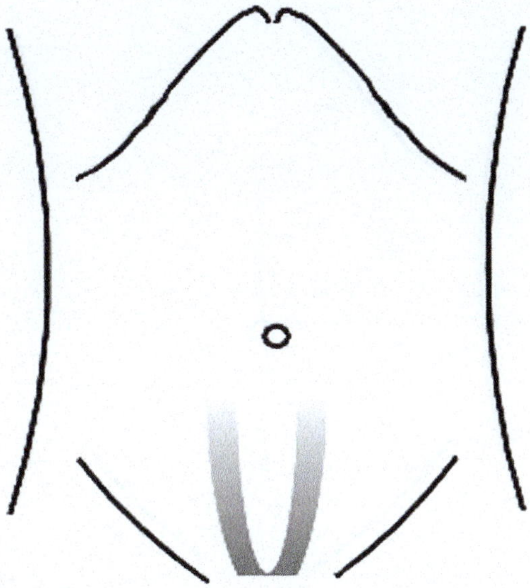

Fig. 3.35 Shōfuku-kōkyū

where on the upper umbilical ring, obliquely or to either side.

Weakness or Paresthesia of the Lower Abdomen

Lower abdominal contracture and lower abdominal taut

Weakness or paresthesia of the lower abdomen is called *shōfuku-fujin* (Fig. 3.34), and *seika-fujin*. These two are almost synonymous, although there is a slight difference between the lower abdominal region and the area under the umbilicus. Originally, *fujin* referred to paresthesia such as dullness, numbness, and sometimes hypersensitivity, but diagnoses of abdominal patterns now include degraded states in which the tone of the abdominal wall is reduced.

Lower abdominal contracture, that is cramping of lower abdominal muscles, such as the rectus abdominis muscle, is called *shōfuku-kōkyū* (Fig. 3.35). *Lower abdominal tautness so that cramping of lower abdominal muscles extends to the upper abdomen* is called *shōfuku-genkyū* (Fig. 3.36).

The linea alba is composed of the fusion of abdominal muscle aponeuroses, such as the sarcolemmas of rectus abdominis muscles, which separates the left and right rectus abdominis muscles at the midline. As the linea alba is thinner in the infraumbilical region than in the supraumbilical region, a decrease in the tone of the linea alba caused by aging or physical weakness may result in numbness or "*fujin*" in the infraumbilical region.

The above abdominal findings are diagnosed as kidney deficiency and indicate formulas containing Rehmannia root and processed aconite root, such as hachimijiogan (八味地黄丸) or shimbuto (真武湯).

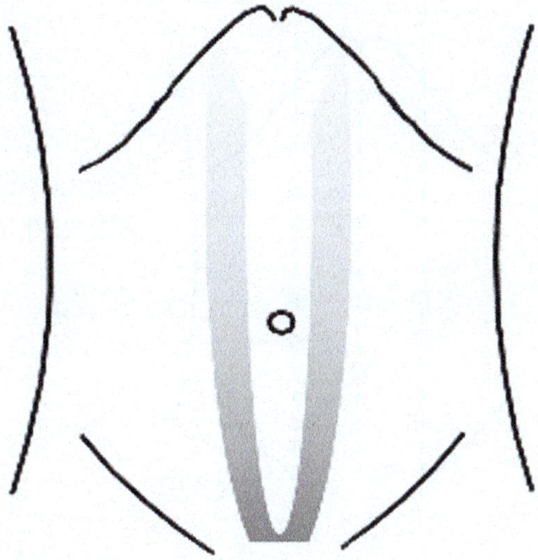

Fig. 3.36 Shōfuku-genkyū

Cord in the Abdominal Midline

The cord in the abdominal midline that is a palpable funicle under the linea alba in the infraumbilical region and supra-umbilical region is called *seichūshin* (Fig. 3.37). It tends to appear in aged, skinny, or frail individuals. The term *seichūshin* was coined by Keisetsu *Otsuka* (大塚敬節), but there were descriptions of "sinewy tension along the midline on the Conception Vessel" in texts on abdominal diagnosis of the Edo period.

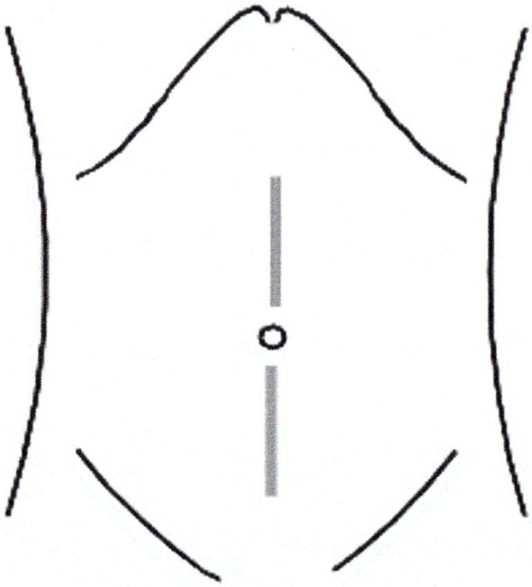

Fig. 3.37 Seichūshin

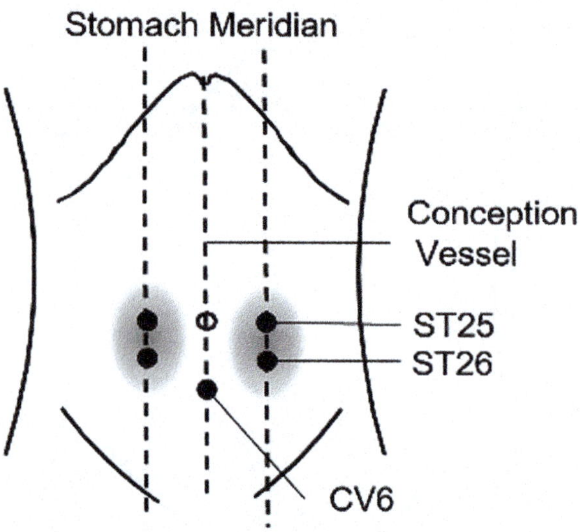

Fig. 3.38 Seibō-attsū

Anatomically, the *seichūshin* that appears in the supraumbilical region is the falciform ligament of the liver, including the round ligament, which is the persistent umbilical vein and artery. Otherwise, the *seichūshin* that appears in the infraumbilical region is the median umbilical fold, including the median umbilical ligament. The cord may become palpable from the outside when the linea alba becomes loose and the surrounding connective and fat tissues decrease due to aging, etc.

Seichūshin in the supraumbilical region is an indication for formulas such as ninjinto (人参湯), and that in the infraumbilical region is an indication for formulas containing processed aconite root such as hachimijiogan (八味地黄丸).

Tenderness of the Paraumbilical Region

Tenderness in the paraumbilical region is called *seibō-attsū* or *saibō-attsū* (Fig. 3.38), which may indicate static blood[TM1] around the umbilicus and enclosed tissue by the left and right coxal bones. There may be a horseshoe-shaped tender area below the umbilicus, especially in women. This area from the lower small intestine to the transverse colon is a zone of hyperesthesia and is also the site where referred pain appears [10].

In acupuncture, the paraumbilical region is related to acupoints on the upper to lower abdomen, which are associated with microcirculation disorders of the gastrointestinal tract and urogenital system, such as ST25 and ST26 on the stomach meridian and CV6 on the Conception Vessel below the umbilicus.

Formulas to treat static blood[TM1], such as keishibukuryogan (桂枝茯苓丸) and tokishakuyakusan (当帰芍薬散), may be used.

Tenderness in the Ileocecal Region
Tenderness in the right iliac fossa

Tenderness in the ileocecal region is called *kaimōbu-attsū* (Fig. 3.39), and *tenderness in the right iliac fossa* is also called (*migi-chōkotsu-kabu-attsū* (右腸骨窩部圧痛) (Fig. 3.40).

Tenderness in the ileocecal region, also known as a sign of appendicitis, is the site where hyperesthesia and related pain appear due to abnormalities in the ovaries, fallopian tubes, cecum, and ileocecal region [10, 11].

This finding may be one of the symptoms of static blood[TM] caused by congestion or ischemia in the intestinal tract of the ileocecal region, adnexa, or venous plexus around the fallopian tubes may also play a role. Formulas to treat

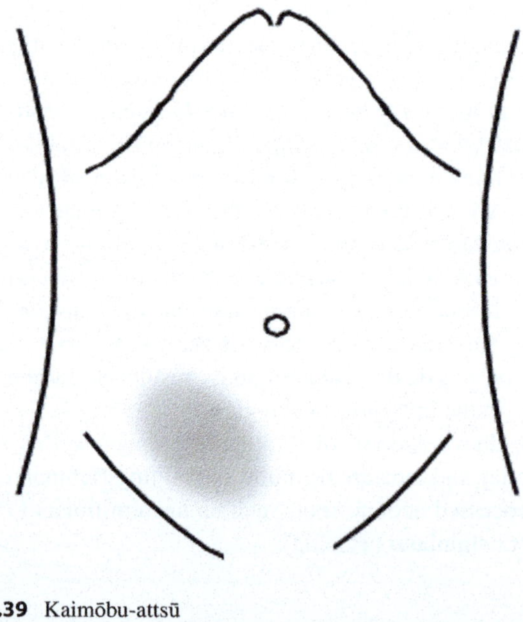

Fig. 3.39 Kaimōbu-attsū

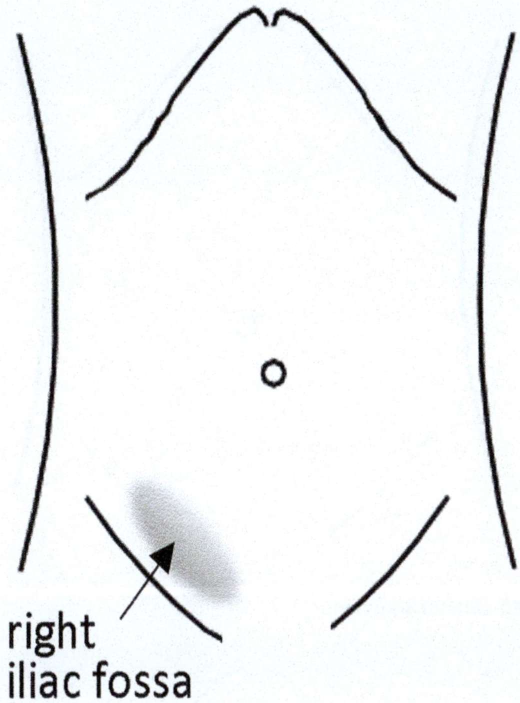

Fig. 3.40 Migi-chōkotsu-kabu-attsū

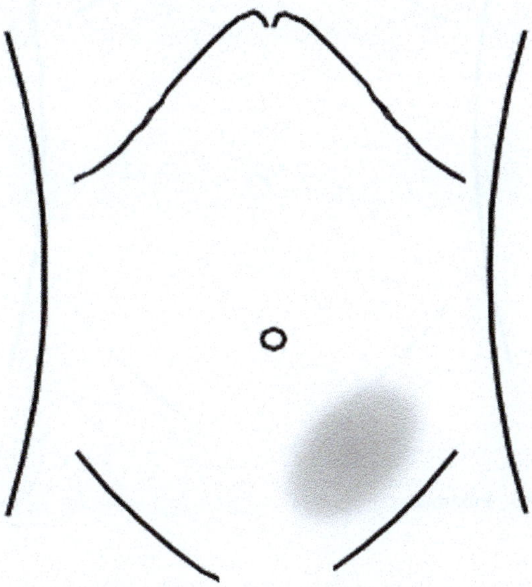

Fig. 3.41 Esuzyōkettchōbu-attsū Esuzyōkettyōbu-attsū

static blood[TM1], such as daiobotampito (大黄牡丹皮湯), may be used.

Tenderness in the Sigmoid Colon Region and Tenderness in the Left Iliac Fossa

Resistance and severe tenderness in the left iliac region

Tenderness of the sigmoid colon region is called *esujōketchōbu-attsū* or *esujōbu-attsū* for short (Fig. 3.41),

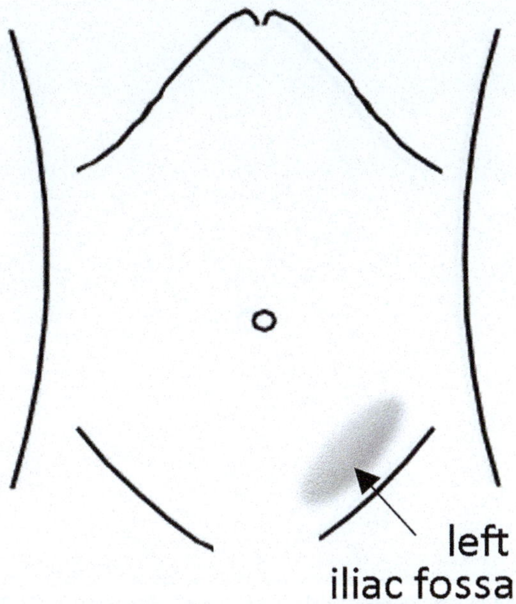

Fig. 3.42 Left Tyōkotsukabu-attsū

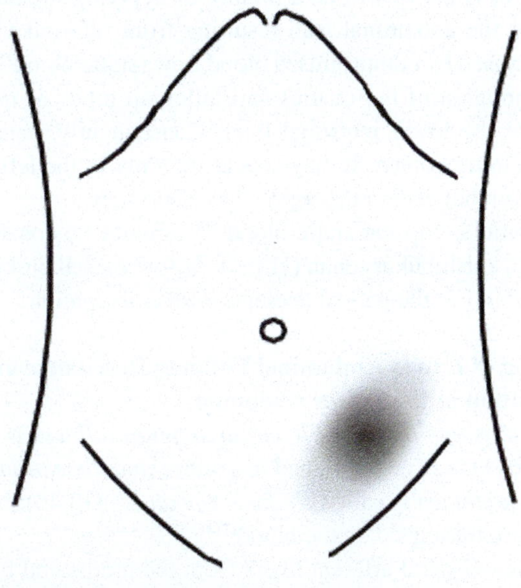

Fig. 3.43 Shōfuku-kyūketsu

and *tenderness in the region of the left iliac fossa* is also called left *chōkotsu-kabu-attsū* (Fig. 3.42). Tenderness of both the sigmoid colon region and the left iliac fossa is thought to be evidence of static blood[TM1] of the sigmoid colon, descending colon, or adnexa uteri. *Resistance and severe tenderness in the left iliac region* that is easily induced by scraping is called *shōfuku-kyūketsu* (Fig. 3.43).

This region is the equivalent site for the area of hyperesthesia and referred pain generated by issues of the ovaries and fallopian tubes that are sensory controlled by T12-S4 spinal nerves and issues of the sigmoid colon and the descending colon that are sensory controlled by T12-S2 and

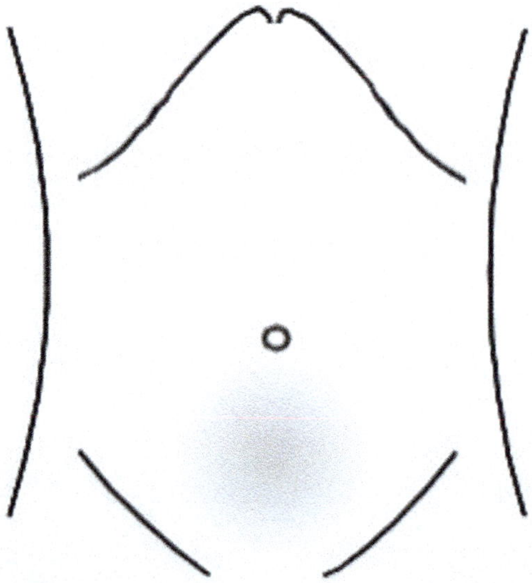

Fig. 3.44 Shōfuku-man

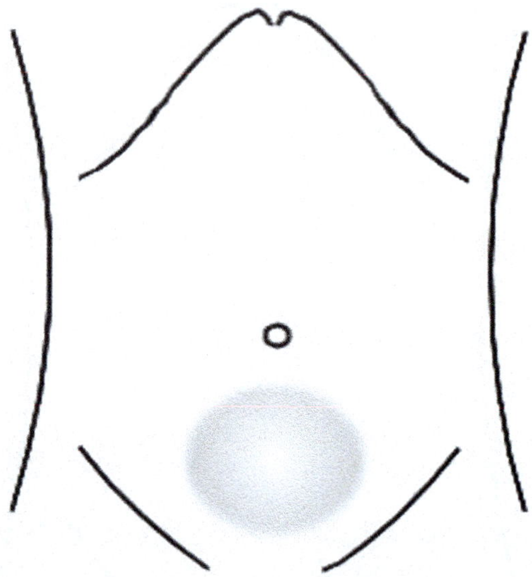

Fig. 3.45 Shōfuku-kōman

S1-S3 spinal nerves, respectively. Therefore, *shōfuku-kyūketsu* is thought to be a finding of hyperalgesia and tension in the abdominal wall resulting from referred visceral pain caused by compromised blood flow (static blood[TM1]) or inflammation of the ovaries and fallopian tubes or referred pain of the lower intestinal tract. Consequently, it is more common in women. It may appear not only in the left lower abdomen but also in the right lower abdomen.

Formulas to treat static blood[TM1] should be considered, such as keishibukuryogan (桂枝茯苓丸) or tokakujokito (桃核承気湯), if the patient presents with constipation.

Feeling of Lower Abdominal Fullness/Resistance and Distention in the Lower Abdomen

The subjective feeling of lower abdominal fullness is called *shōfuku-man* (Fig. 3.44), and *resistance and distention in the lower abdomen* is called *shōfuku-kōman* (Fig. 3.45); both of them are findings of static blood[TM1].

Since visceral afferent fibers from the uterus and bladder enter T10-L2 of spinal nerves and correspond to the dermatomes from the lower abdomen to the inguinal region, the lower abdomen is also the site of visceral pain and hyperesthesia. This is sometimes accompanied by tenderness due to abnormalities in these organs.

This may be an indication for formulas to treat static blood[TM1] such as unkeito (温経湯) or keishibukuryogan (桂枝茯苓丸) for *shōfuku-man*, and keishibukuryogan (桂枝茯苓丸) or daiobotanpito (大黄牡丹皮湯) for *shōfuku-kōman*.

Fullness and Distention of the Whole Abdomen
Abdominal fullness with firm distention of excess type
Abdominal fullness with soft swelling of deficiency type

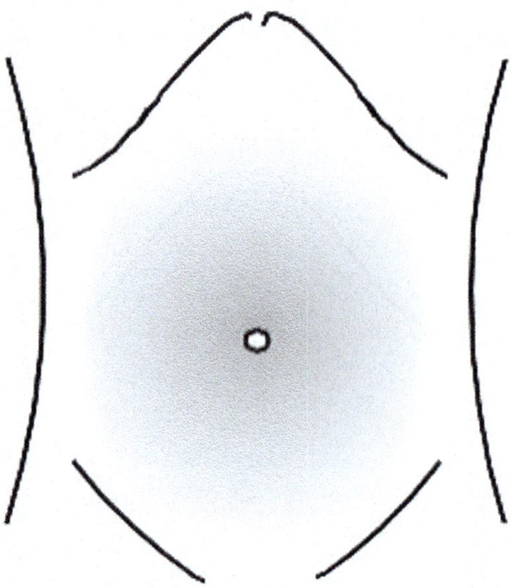

Fig. 3.46 Fukuman

Fullness and distension of the whole abdomen are called *fukuman* (Fig. 3.46), and this is sometimes accompanied by *tympanitic resonance with tapping* caused by gas in the intestines. *Fukuman* is caused by retention of stool or gas in the intestinal tract or ascites.

It is classified into two types: one type refers to *abdominal fullness with firm distention of excess type*, or *jitsuman*, and the other type is *abdominal fullness with soft swelling of deficiency type*, or *kyoman*. Both types are caused by qi stagnation. *Jitsuman* is caused by severe constipation, and *kyoman* is caused by retention of bowel gas and ascites due to intestinal relaxation and hypoperistalsis.

Jitsuman may be treated with formulas in the jokito-group such as (承気湯類), bofutsuseisan (防風通聖散), daisaikoto (大柴胡湯), and intinkoto (茵陳蒿湯). *Kyoman* may be treated with keishikashakuyakuto (桂枝加芍薬湯) or shokentyuto (小建中湯). For *kyōman* due to ascites, water may be regulated by goreisan (五苓散) or by treatment according to the cause.

Visible Peristaltic Discord

Visible peristaltic discord of the intestines, which is visible through weak abdominal walls and is often accompanied by abdominal pain, is called *zendō-fuon* (Fig. 3.47). In the *Fukushō Kiran*, the classical text of abdominal diagnosis from the Edo period, visible abnormal peristalsis was perceived as movement of a snake or eel. In the case of gastrointestinal dysfunction due to cold or paralytic ileus, it is caused by distended intestines when gas or fluid moves in the intestinal tract due to stagnation or peristalsis.

This movement occurs sporadically and usually does not affect the passage of intestinal contents. It may be usually treated with daikenchuto (大建中湯) etc., but not for mechanical ileus brought about by obstruction or strangulation. In mild cases, ninjinto (人参湯) or shokentyuto (小建中湯) may be indicated.

Abdominal Pulsation

Epigastric pulsation below the xiphoid process, supraumbilical pulsation, and infraumbilical pulsation

Abdominal pulsation, which is strongly palpable at the abdominal aorta, is called *fukubu-dōki*. For *epigastric pulsation below the xiphoid process*, especially, the term *shinka-ki* is used. Likewise, *seijō-ki* is used for *supraumbilical pulsation*, and *seika-ki* for *infraumbilical pulsation* of the abdominal aorta (Fig. 3.48).

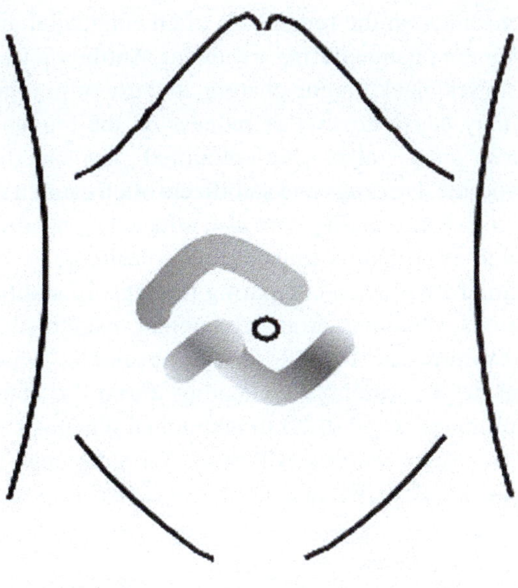

Fig. 3.47 Zendō-fuon

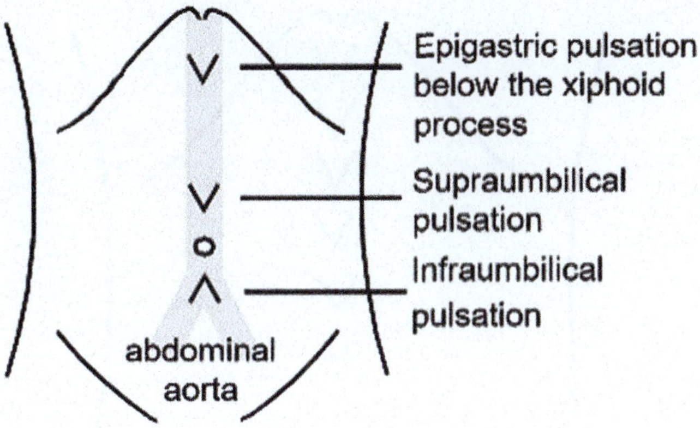

Fig. 3.48 Fukubudoki (shinkaki, *seijōki, seikaki*)

This is caused by transmission of pulsation from the abdominal aorta to the abdominal wall and depends on the balance between the tension in the abdominal muscles and abdominal wall, tone of the sympathetic nerves, hardening of the arterial walls, and thinning of the abdominal wall.

Pulsation of the abdominal aorta is felt by light pressure on the abdominal wall or can be seen on the abdominal surface in patients with deficiency patterns, who have thin and relaxed abdominal walls. In the elderly, the aortic bifurcation may be pulled downward due to spinal deformity and arteriosclerosis, which may cause a strong pulse to be felt in the infraumbilical region (*seika-ki*).

Pulsation of the abdominal aorta may be strong and readily transmitted to the abdominal wall in patients with an excess pattern characterized by high sympathetic tone (*shinka-ki* or *seijō-ki*).

Shinka-ki may be treated with ryokeijutsukanto (苓桂朮甘湯). *Seijō-ki* may be treated with saikokaryukotsuboreito (柴胡加竜骨牡蛎湯) for those with an excess pattern and keishikaryukotsuboreito (桂枝加竜骨牡蛎湯) or shakanzoto (炙甘草湯) for those with a deficiency pattern. Yokukansan (抑肝散) or yokukansankachimpihange (抑肝散加陳皮半夏) may be used for the cases with strong and straight pulsation from the umbilicus up to the xiphoid process (Fig. 3.49).

2.9 Other Palpations

Go Ito

2.9.1 Back Diagnosis

Back diagnosis (*haisin*) may reveal abnormalities even when no abnormalities are found in the abdominal diagnosis. In general, there are characteristic back patterns such as stiffness from the nape to back (*kohaikyō*), stiffness from the sides of the neck to occiput (*keikōkyō*), stiffness of the occiput (*zukōkyō*), and the finding of excessive muscle strain extending from the shoulder to the back (*kenpaikōkyū*).

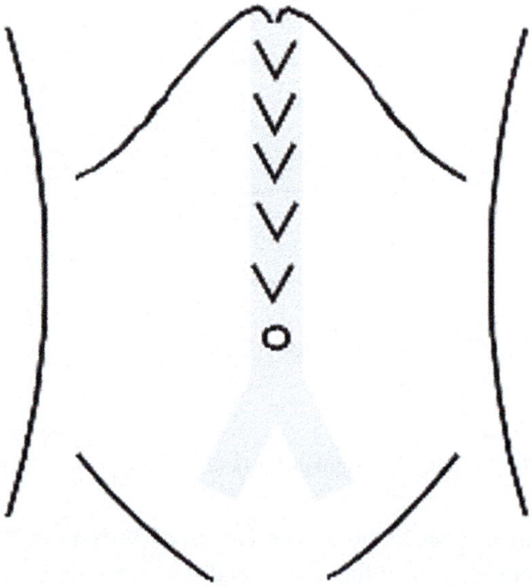

Fig. 3.49 Fukubudoki. (shinkaki, *seijōki, seikaki*)

Typically the findings of stiffness of the occiput and stiffness from the nape to the back are indications for keishito (桂枝湯) (Fig. 3.13). Acute stiffness from the nape down to the back (*kohaikyōkyū*) is famous as the indication for kakkonto (葛根湯) (Fig. 3.14).

In addition to these, it is also important to perform a back examination to detect abnormalities such as indurations and tenderness at bladder meridian points that run in two rows along both sides of the spine (known as back Shu or transport points). In particular, acupuncture points, such as BL13 (Feishu, *hai-yu*), BL15 (Xinshu, *shin-yu*), BL18 (Ganshu, *kan-yu*), BL19 (Danshu, *tan-yu*), BL20 (Pishu, *hi-yu*) & BL21 (Weishu, *i-yu*), BL23 (Shnshu, *jin-yu*), BL25 (Dachangshu, *daichō-yu*), BL27 (Xiaochashu, *shōtyō-yu*), and BL28 (Pangguangshu, *bōkō-yu*) are closely related to the visceral distribution of sympathetic nerves to the lungs, bronchi, heart, liver, gallbladder, stomach, kidney, large intestine, small intestine, and bladder. So, these points are indispensable for the diagnosis and treatment of visceral diseases.

Persons with weak abdominal strength may have thin and contracted back muscles. Stiffness in the scapulae and back of the neck should also be palpated. Reactive points associated with internal organs may appear on the back.It is also important to observe the left-right differences in the dorsal muscle groups (erector spinae, rhomboid muscles, multifidus, etc.) and the torsions and distortions in the spine.

2.9.2 Palpation of Meridians

According to Nagahama Yoshio, "The method to detect abnormalities by directly palpating meridian and collateral is called *meridian palpation* (*sekkei*); this is an indispensable examination method in the Gosei School and especially in acupuncture practice." That is to say, *sekkei* was not only a diagnostic method performed for acupuncture and moxibustion but was also used by the Gosei School of Kampo medicine.

In Yanagiya Sorei's text, *Gateway to the Art of Acupuncture and Moxibustion* (*Shinkyu Ijyutsu no Mon*), he writes that "excess" in meridian palpation is "a tactile sensation such as a linear induration, lump, sticky substance (static blood[TM1]), an aggregation of small masses, a rodlike substance, a platelike substance, a bonelike mass, presence of tenderness, etc.," while "deficiency" in meridian palpation refers to changes such as concavity, depression, pruritus induced by palpation, local softness or weakness, and pleasurable feeling when pressed." Localized cold and heat sensation and skin abnormalities (e.g., moles, papules, pigmentation) are also abnormal meridian palpation findings.

Since the 12 meridians are located bilaterally on both sides of the body, it is important to gently press each acupoint and carefully compare each pair of points to detect tenderness or paresthesia and then to examine for other abnormalities by palpation of the meridian. It should also be noted that these abnormal acupoints are also treatment points in acupuncture practice.

2.10 Summary of the Practice of Kampo Medicine

2.10.1 Precautions for the Four Examinations

The examiner should be mindful of how the findings relate to the current illness and whether they are significant or not. Findings that change as treatment progresses are significant. However, findings that are subject to change, findings that are difficult to change, and changes due to natural causes need to be reconsidered. For example, fissures and static macules on the tongue are often congenital and usually may not change during treatment. Antibiotic treatment often causes black tongue coating, and use of psychotropic drugs may cause erosion or redness on the tongue. Pulse qualities may also be modified by medication. Antihypertensive drugs and stabilizers often cause a sunken, slow pulse. Since findings are also affected by meals, drinking water, examination time, etc., it is desirable to examine at a similar time when comparing findings. In addition, the indications obtained from abdominal examination and pulse examination may differ. For example, what were thought to be findings indicating formulas containing Bupleurum radix (柴胡剤) in abdominal diagnosis may be found to require starting with tonic formulas such as shokenchuto (小建中湯) due to the presence of a deficient pulse.

2.10.2 Significance of Kampo Diagnosis

Needless to say, modern Kampo medicine, as a diagnostic modality, needs to be supplemented by diagnostic techniques of modern medicine. For example, early cancers cannot be detectable by Kampo diagnostic methodology alone. Kampo medical examination that relies on the five senses has its limitations compared to modern medical examinations with advanced science and technology. Tongue, pulse, and abdominal pattern are not diagnostic results of "local" findings but are assessments for imbalances in the whole body and disease-fighting action of the body that is trying to return to normal. It can also be interpreted as empirical knowledge of visceral-somatic reflex or as an image in which various disease reactions of the living body are projected on the abdominal wall like images on a screen. It is expected that the diagnostic technology of Kampo will be further elucidated and utilized with scientific knowledge with the progress of science and medicine in the future.

3 Therapeutics Overview

3.1 Treatment Processes

3.1.1 Introduction

Takao Namiki

The essence of Kampo treatment resides in treatment by pattern identification. The treatment by pattern identification refers to an ideal state where the pattern of Kampo medicine (pattern of formula) is completely consistent with the diagnostic pattern (pattern of illness) obtained by the "four examinations" in Kampo. Treatment by pattern identification can be executed by matching a pattern of Kampo medicine to the pattern of illness. Specifically, a formula suitable to the patient's pattern is determined by adjusting the choice and dose of the crude drug written in the formula codex. In Japan, however, extract preparations in use in many clinical settings are available as ready-made pharmaceuticals. Therefore, not all patterns, including chief complaints (or treatment targets), can be covered comprehensively.

There are two methods of choosing a Kampo medicine according to its effect on the target disease.

Orthodox treatment or *seichi*: A therapeutic method of normalizing a pathologic condition by administering a formula countering the effect of the properties of the disease (e.g., medicines with properties and action of heat for cold patterns, medicines with properties and action of cold for heat patterns).

Unusual opposite treatment or *hanchi* (*jyuchi*): A therapeutic method of prescribing formulas with the same action as the disorders. In practice, this treatment promotes a cure just as with orthodox treatment. This method is used in cases of true cold with false heat, true heat with false cold, and the like (e.g., for an early yang stage pattern, the fever-promoting crude drug *mao* is used).

3.1.2 Treatment Sequences

Takao Namiki

"Kampo Medicine in Practice" (in Japanese), a comprehensive commentary on Kampo treatments published in Japan early in the Showa period, describes treatment sequences in terms of general rules for Kampo treatment applicable to actual clinical settings. This general rule is applicable to modern Kampo treatments (steps 1 and 2 are described in separate sections).

1. When deficiency and excess patterns coexist, first tonify the deficiency, and then attack the excess—tonifying first, draining second.
2. First tonify the deficiency in the exterior, then attack the excess in the interior —exterior first, interior second.
3. Treat simultaneously both diseases in the exterior and interior—some exceptional cases exist, e.g., an exterior pattern develops because the excess has turned to deficiency.
4. When it is difficult to diagnose a pattern of deficiency and excess, first consider the condition as a deficiency pattern.
5. If an acute disease occurs as a complication in the course of treating chronic disease, the acute disease should be treated first.

3.1.3 Therapeutic Methods

Takao Namiki

As shown in Table 3.11, there are general rules and their exceptions, as well as coexisting conditions.

- **Deficiency and excess**

Tonifying methods and draining methods used to treat deficiencies and excesses, respectively, are described in separate sections.

- **Acute disease (general principles of treatment advocated in the "*Shanghanlun*")**

(a) **Exterior-first, interior-second, acute-first, and chronic-second**

Refer to the "Overlap of Diseases" section.

"Exterior-first, interior-second" is the general rule (known as "Exterior-first, interior-second is the rule").

In exceptional cases, the above rule is broken to first manage any condition requiring emergency treatment, followed by treatment of any relatively mild condition (known as "acute-first, chronic-second is an emergency order").

For details, see Chap. 3, Sect. 3.1.6.

(b) **Overlap of diseases and combination of diseases**

Table 3.11 Therapeutics

		Method	Exceptions, overlaps, and combinations of diseases
(I)	Deficiencies and excesses		
	Excess pattern	Draining	Tonify first, drain second
	medium (excess, deficiency) pattern	Pattern-dependent	
	Deficiency pattern	Tonifying	Tonifying and draining methods performed concurrently
(II)	General rules of treatment advocated in the ancient Chinese medical text "*Shanghanlun*" (the six-stage patterns)		
(a)	Exterior and interior patterns (treatment sequences in acute diseases)	Exterior first, interior second	Acute-first, chronic-second Concurrent treatment of two patterns (mixture of medications): conditions at close locations of disease may be treated concurrently
(b)	(Acute diseases) overlaps of diseases	Exterior first, interior second Concurrent treatment of two patterns (mixtures of medications)	
	(Acute diseases) combinations of diseases	To be treated primarily with a single formula	
(III)	Cold and heat		
	Heat patterns	Heat-clearing formulas	(Exception) warming and tonifying formulas
	Cold patterns	Warming and tonifying formulas	(Exception) heat-clearing formulas
	Cold-heat medium patterns	Pattern-dependent	
	Mixed cold and heat	Pattern-dependent	
(IV)	(Subacute to chronic stage, sudden deterioration of condition) treatment of qi, blood[TM1], fluid[TM1]		
	Qi counter flow	Qi-descending formulas	
	Qi stagnation	Qi-regulating formulas	
	Blood[TM1] deficiencies	Qi-tonifying formulas	
	Static blood[TM1]	Blood[TM1] stasis-resolving formulas	
	Fluid retention (due to fluid[TM1] excess)	Fluid-regulating formulas	
	Yin deficiencies (due to fluid[TM1] deficiency immeasurable)	Yin nourishing formulas	(For any deficiency heat) mixture of heat-clearing formulas
	Qi deficiencies	Qi-tonifying formulas	

These concepts are not discussed here but are described in detail in another section.

Cold and Heat

The general rule is to prescribe a formula with properties and action of heat for cold patterns and a formula with properties and action of cold for heat patterns (*seichi*). In the case of upper heat and lower cold (mixed cold and heat), however, both true cold with false heat and true heat with false cold are likely, so a treatment in accordance with the pattern will be performed.

Example) True heat with false cold: In the pathology of early yang stage patterns in cold damage, chills apparently like a cold pattern can develop despite the condition essentially being a heat pattern. This condition is managed mainly using a formula with crude drugs having the action of heat, such as Ephedra (*mao*).

Example) True cold with false heat: In conditions to be treated with *tokishigyakukagoshuyushokyoto* (early yin stage pattern), the essential pattern is cold sometimes with cold feet and a false hot upper half of the body.

Qi, Blood[TM1], Fluid[TM1]

The general rule of treatment is as follows: Tonify deficient factors of qi, blood[TM1], and fluid[TM1], and drain any excess. In actual clinical settings, some factors can be concurrently in excess or deficient. In such cases, treatments for respective signs are used in combination. Qi, blood[TM1], fluid[TM1] treatments are described in detail under the Qi, Blood[TM1], Fluid[TM1] see Chap. 2, Sect. 1.7.

3.1.4 Symptomatic Approach and Fundamental Approach (Treatment in View of the Pathologic Cause)

Takao Namiki

The term "symptomatic approach" refers to "treating the condition according to its disease pattern," whereas the term fundamental approach is defined as "treating the condition targeting the root of the disease" [12].

Differences between symptomatic and fundamental approaches are described in Table 3.12. Make the right judgment considering which needs to be given priority, symptomatic approach or fundamental approach. A symptomatic approach is not always inferior to a fundamental approach. It

Table 3.12 Differences between fundamental and symptomatic approaches

	Fundamental approach	Symptomatic approach
Pathologic condition targeted for treatment	The root cause of the condition	Manifested set of symptoms (including symptoms unrelated to the cause)
Viewing the pathologic condition targeted in treatment in terms of old versus new	The root cause is often an old condition The radical root and manifested condition often develop concurrently	Although the condition develops as symptoms from the root cause in some cases, new symptoms develop later in other cases
Form of cure	Many signs, including associated signs, are ameliorated without sequelae by a fundamental approach alone	No root treatment is expected with a symptomatic approach alone. On the contrary, a fundamental approach often ameliorates symptoms targeted by a symptomatic approach
Treatment causality	Kampo-based causal treatment	So-called symptomatic treatment

is a general rule to make a fundamental approach for radical treatment. However, if any condition, such as time required, hampers a causal treatment, a symptomatic approach may be taken first to achieve a quick amelioration of symptoms, even though it will not completely cure the disease. In addition, a fundamental approach and a symptomatic approach may be used concurrently.

Details on Treatments Using a Fundamental Approach and/or a Symptomatic Approach

(a) **Cases with priority given to symptomatic treatment**

This may be viewed as a symptomatic treatment. If the condition worsens and any severe or intolerable symptom develops, their signs may be managed preferentially (Fig. 3.1). In the ***Shanghanlun***, an ancient Chinese medical text describing acute febrile diseases, the "acute-first, chronic-second" concept (acute disease is treated first, and relatively slow conditions are treated later) is described as an exceptional therapeutic approach (refer to Chap. 3, Sect. 3.1.6). This approach corresponds to cases with priority given to a symptomatic approach.

Example 1: Cases with Priority Given to a Symptomatic Approach

- Sprains

  Treatment of pain (symptom) (poultices, medications)

  → Mild cases will be cured.

  (severe conditions requiring a fundamental approach: blood stasis-resolving medications, plaster casts, surgery, etc.)
- During the course of lumbago treatment with *hachimijiogan*, pain intensified; *shakuyakukanzoto* was added to the regimen.
- → After the condition stabilized, lumbago treatment with *hachimijiogan* alone was resumed, and this led to a cure.

  Fundamental approach: *hachimijiogan*

  Symptomatic approach: *shakuyakukanzoto*

(b) **Priority given to etiological treatment (fundamental approach)**

When the condition is relatively stable (gradual remission period, etc.), or when the condition is changing slowly, priority is given to a fundamental approach (Example 2). This approach is expected to strengthen or improve the constitution to prevent exacerbations and recurrences.

Example 2: A Successful Case of Treatment with Priority Given to a Fundamental Approach

Cough variant asthma

The chief complaint of coughing was eased at first with *makyokansekito*. When the medication was discontinued, however, coughing recurred repeatedly in the pollen season. For this reason, the pattern was re-examined. Qi stagnation with a sensation of obstruction in throat was found, and abdominal examination revealed fullness and discomfort in the chest and hypochondrium. Thus, *saibokuto* was used for a while as a prophylaxis to prevent recurrence of asthma. As a result, there were no longer recurrences in the pollen season; *saibokuto* alone was used for several years, and the medication was terminated.

Symptomatic approach: *makyokansekito*

Fundamental approach: *saibokuto*

(c) **Concurrent use of a fundamental approach and a symptomatic approach**

In cases where exacerbations and gradual remissions occur repeatedly in relatively short cycles, and neither one can be resolved faster, and in cases where the signs targeted by a fundamental approach and a symptomatic approach cannot be distinguished, a fundamental approach and a symptomatic approach are performed concurrently (Example 3).

Example 3

A patient with chronic cystitis: Repeatedly recurring symptoms of cystitis were treated with *hachimijiogan*.

→ During the course of treatment, hematuria developed, with symptoms of acute cystitis; *choreito* was used to treat this condition.

(Commentary) The patient was being treated for chronic cystitis that required a fundamental approach (*hachimijiogan*).

A formula for acute cystitis symptoms that require a symptomatic approach (choreito) was used in combination.

3.1.5 Tonifying Methods and Draining Methods

Takao Namiki

This is an introduction to tonifying and draining methods and a description of their clinical applications. The properties and actions (whether a formula for tonifying or for draining) of various extract formulas and the medicinal properties of crude drugs are described in a separate section (See Chap. 4, Sect. 2.2.2, and Chap. 9).

In modern Kampo, a tonifying method is defined as "a therapy to help overcome physical and mental weakness and impaired functions." The draining method is defined as "a therapy to attack the pathogen" [13]. Chapter 69 of the ***Nanjing***, an ancient Chinese medical text, states, "Tonify conditions with deficiencies, and drain conditions with excesses." For various pathologic deficiency patterns in illness, various tonifying methods with respective designations are used (Table 1.1).

For the qi, blood[TM1] and fluids[TM1], tonifying methods such as qi-tonifying, blood[TM1]-tonifying, and yin-enriching methods are available. In addition, there are some cases where warming and tonifying are performed for cold and heat, and exterior patterns are tonified in exterior deficiency patterns (Case 1).

It is a general rule to use a draining method for the treatment of excess patterns (Table 1.2).

In all cases, the appropriate treatment is performed to remove the source of illness, including releasing the exterior of any pathogen, heat clearing for any feverishness, and purgation for any food stagnation (Case 2).

Coping with Complex Conditions

In actual clinical settings, complex conditions can occur, which require the use of both a tonifying method and a draining method. Appropriate prescriptions are formulated with the pattern in mind. If a tonifying formula and a draining formula are combined carelessly, crude drugs having mutually contradictory medicinal properties will be used concurrently. Therefore, it is necessary to consider other methods of administration, such as taking different prescriptions at different times. In addition, some patients have both a deficiency and an excess, and some formulas consist essentially of a tonic formula and a purgative formula to ensure long and safe use by striking a balance between deficiency and excess (*unseiin*, etc.).

For some conditions, the sequence of the draining method and tonifying method should be taken into account. For example, if the patient's healthy qi has been affected, it is necessary to first restore healthy qi before starting a draining method (tonifying first, draining second). Otherwise, if the physician is unable to determine which to start first (draining method or tonifying method), treatment should be started for deficiency to ensure safe care. In such cases, qi is first supplemented using a tonifying method, and then the condition is treated using a draining method (Case 3).

However, use of a tonifying method can contrarily have an adverse effect, and a draining method can be performed to an extent that does not consume healthy qi. Therefore, the patient should be carefully examined before determining the therapeutic policy and modifications.

For classification of formulas by indication, refer to Chap. 4, Sect. 2.2.2.

Case 1: A 55-Year-Old Woman

Chief complaint: General malaise

History of past illness: Breast cancer treated at 48 years of age

History of present illness: The patient had recently been busy working and anxious about many things, including personal troubles in her department. Since her fatigue did not resolve even after a rest on a holiday, she visited a nearby clinic.

Vital signs: Height 157 cm, weight 52 kg, blood pressure 123/83 mmHg, pulse rate 72 beats/min

Pulse examination: Slightly deep, weak. Tongue examination: A swollen, wet, pale white tongue.

Abdominal examination: Slightly weak abdominal strength, extreme skin dryness.

Diagnosis: Both qi and blood[TM1] deficiency are present. When *juzentaihoto* was prescribed, the severity of the chief complaint was reduced by half in about 3 months.

(Commentary) The patient was considered to have depleted healthy qi because of business and stress; *juzentaihoto* was prescribed to supplement both qi and blood[TM1].

Case 2: A 13-Year-Old Boy

Chief complaint: Fever

History of present illness: An essentially healthy boy.

A high fever of 39 degrees developed on the day before the first visit. He had pharyngeal pain and arthralgia. He had little thirst. He tested positive for influenza at his family doctor.

Vital signs: Reddening is present in the throat. No sweat on the body.

Auscultation: No abnormality in respiratory sound.

Pulse examination: The pulse was floating and tense. Tongue examination: Dry red tongue.

An excess pattern in the early yang stage was suspected; *maoto* was prescribed thrice daily with the patient's age in mind.

(Course) When *Maoto* was taken twice, sweating started, and the fever began to decline. At the same time, the arthralgia and pharyngeal pain decreased. Normal temperature was restored in 2 days, and the arthralgia was ameliorated.

(Commentary) The pathogen (influenza) was removed by inducing sweating with *maoto* (releasing the exterior).

Case 3: A 48-Year-Old Woman (Housewife)

Chief complaint: Sensation of fatigue, hot flash, lower limb coldness

History of past illness: She contracted uterine cancer 2 years before.

History of present illness: The above symptoms developed 6 months before. When the condition was not treated with the expectation for spontaneous amelioration, recent sensations of fatigue and hot flashes became frequent. She is unable to have a sound sleep because of the night sweats. She was unable to undergo hormone replacement therapy for hot flashes because of her history of past illness, so she visited a clinic for Kampo treatment.

Present status: 155 cm, 60 kg, blood pressure 140/88 mmHg

Pulse examination: Deep, slightly weak, slightly stringy. Tongue examination: Dark red with pale white coating.

Abdominal examination: Slightly weak abdominal strength, mild fullness and discomfort in chest and hypochondrium, and there were also paraumbilical points with tenderness and resistance.

Diagnosis: Qi deficiency and static blood[TM1]. *Hochuekkito* (tonifying therapy first) was started to treat marked qi deficiency. The fatigue and night sweats decreased after 1 month of oral medication. Thus, the qi deficiency was considered to have mostly resolved. When *keishibukuryogan* (draining therapy second) was used concurrently, the hot flashes and stiff shoulders began to resolve. After oral medication for 3 more months, these symptoms, as well as lower limb coldness, were ameliorated.

(Commentary) Although both qi deficiency (tonic formula) and static blood[TM1] (draining formula) needed to be addressed, the concurrent use of tonic and draining formulas was considered difficult because of the marked qi deficiency. Therefore, *hochuekkito* (tonifying first) was administered, followed by *keishibukuryogan* (draining second). If the deficiency pattern is not considered severe, the two formulas may be taken concurrently.

3.1.6 Combinations of Diseases and Overlaps of Diseases

Kazushi Uneda and Tadamichi Mitsuma

Combinations of diseases and overlaps of diseases are conditions involving more than one of the six-stage patterns, and they are treated with different therapeutic policies.

What is a Combination of Diseases?

A pattern in the three yang patterns (early yang stage pattern, late yang stage pattern, and middle yang stage pattern) that occurs primarily at one stage, which also manifests in two or more stages where the condition is treated with only one formula for the primary pattern. This phenomenon occurs mainly in acute diseases.

(a) **Combination of diseases in early yang stage pattern and middle yang stage pattern (Case 1)**

Although an early yang stage pattern (formula 1: exterior pattern) is accompanied by diarrhea (formula 2: interior pattern), a formula for the treatment of early yang stage patterns (typically *kakkonto*) is also effective against diarrhea. If the chief complaint is vomiting without diarrhea, *kakkonkahangeto* is indicated.

(b) **Combination of diseases in early and late yang stage patterns (Case 2)**

Although symptoms in late yang stage patterns, such as vomiting, diarrhea, and abdominal pain, are associated with an early yang stage pattern (formula 3: exterior pattern), *ogonto*, a therapeutic formula for late yang stage patterns (formula 4: half exterior and half interior pattern), is indicated. *Ogonkahangeshogato* may also be used for severe nausea.

(c) **Combination of diseases in the three yang stage patterns (Case 3)**

While involving an early yang stage pattern formula (formula 5: exterior pattern), a late yang stage pattern (formula 6: half exterior and half interior pattern), and a middle yang stage pattern (formula 7: interior pattern), this condition is treated with *byakkoto* or *byakkoto*-similar formulas in view of its major location of disease as an interior pattern.

Commentary: Although formula 5, or *kakkonto,* may be indicated for the early yang stage pattern without spontaneous sweating, formula 6 is used because the late yang stage pattern for which a Bupleurum root (*saiko*) formula is most likely indicated. Formula 7 is used in the middle yang stage pattern for which *byakkokaninjinto* may be indicated.

In this case, the formulas 5 and 6 could not be used alone or mixed together (mixture of *saiko* formula and *kakkonto*) to achieve a cure.

(d) **Combination of diseases in middle yang stage pattern and late yang stage pattern**

Daijokito (or a *jokito* group formula) is indicated for the excess heat in an interior pattern with diarrhea. Some authors, however, do not recognize this condition as a combination of diseases.

Case 1: 30-year-old woman: She experienced chills 2 days before, then a mild hot sensation and stiffness in the nape of her neck (signs of formula 1). Slight tenesmus and odorous watery feces (signs of formula 2). No spontaneous sweating, floating pulses, and a medium (between excess and deficiency) pattern (formula 1). *Kakkonto*, an indication for middle yang stage patterns, was prescribed, and the various symptoms, including an interior sign (diarrhea), disappeared in about 12 h. The condition was diagnosed as diarrhea due to a combination of early yang stage pattern and middle yang stage pattern. (Partially modified from Ref. [4].)

Case 2: Woman in her 30s: *Headache developed in the morning of the day before her visit, with a hot sensation* (exterior pattern: formula 3). *Starting in the morning of the day of her visit, she frequently experienced diarrhea with abdominal pain, borborygmus, tenesmus, and strong fecal odor, along with nausea* (half exterior and half interior pattern: formula 4). *Pulses were slightly floating and slightly tight (*pattern of formula 3). *Tongue coating was thin and white* (pattern of formula 4). Abdominal strength was moderate with bilateral full-length tension in the rectus abdominis. *Ogonto*, a formula indicated for late yang stage patterns, was prescribed. Her headache was mitigated 1 hour later. The hot sensation and diarrhea disappeared after three doses in total. Although some findings seemed to be in early yang stage pattern (exterior patterns), the condition was considered to be a combination of diseases based on late yang stage patterns.

Case 3: Man about 40 years of age. He caught a common cold, for which he took *kakkonto* ineffectively. Several days later, he experienced chills in the afternoon *and then much sweating and intensifying* stiffness in the nape of his neck (signs of formula 5). *A bitter taste in the mouth, a dry white coat on the tongue, and severe fullness and discomfort in the chest and hypochondrium* (signs of formula 6). *Thirst but no diuretic abnormality. Hot flush in the face, hot sensation on the entire surfaces of the chest and abdomen, but cold sensation on the back* (signs of formula 7). This condition was considered to be a combination of diseases in the three yang stage patterns; *byakkokaninjinto* was taken by itself, and the various symptoms were mitigated in 20 min. (Partially modified from Ref. [5].)

Overlap of Diseases

A state in which multiple patterns coexist concurrently that can be treated with multiple (usually two) formulas for respective patterns. On the other hand, many chronic conditions, in particular, often involve different patterns that are not always mutually related, and these conditions are deemed an overlap of diseases in its broader sense.

An overlap of diseases can occur among the six-stage patterns, sometimes within the same stage (Fig. 3.50). Overlap of diseases for *shosaikoto* and *saikokaboshoto**, which are both indicated for late yang stage patterns. The *shosaikoto* pattern, which is relatively close to the body surface (early yang stage), is treated first.

**Saikokaboshoto*: A formula prepared by adding sodium sulfate (Glauber salt) to *shosaikoto* or *daisaiko*.

Next, some methods are available to treat overlaps with multiple formulas indicated for the coexisting patterns.

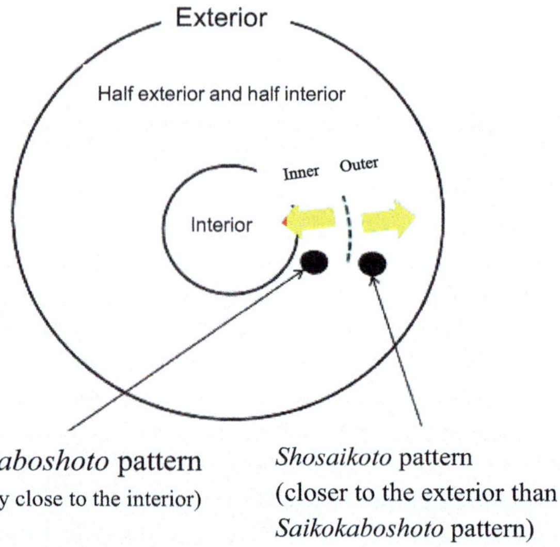

Fig. 3.50 Overlap of diseases at the same level (late yang stage pattern)

(a) **Treatments in systematic sequence**

- **Treating the exterior before the interior (exterior pattern first, interior pattern second)**

Following the general rule for the treatment of overlaps in diseases, exterior patterns are treated first, and interior patterns are treated second. Any exterior pattern (early yang stage pattern), such as chills or fever, should be treated first. After the exterior pattern has disappeared, *daijokito* (laxative) and other formulas that act on interior patterns (middle yang stage patterns) are used.

Following the "exterior pattern first, interior pattern second" rule, exterior patterns (relatively close to the surface) should be treated first, and interior patterns (relatively close to the inside) should be treated second. For example, in an overlap of diseases in a late yang stage pattern (half exterior/half interior pattern), *shosaikoto* patterns that are relatively close to the surface are treated first, and *saikokaboshoto* is administered second for patterns that are relatively close to the inside (See the figure).

- **Treating the acute before the chronic (acute disease first, chronic disease second) (Case 4)**

This is a therapeutic approach to meet the situation. Even in the presence of an exterior pattern, any concurrent interior pattern is preferentially treated if the interior pattern is in an emergency. For example, if the patient with an overlap of diseases in an early yang stage pattern (exterior pattern) and a middle yang stage pattern (interior pattern) has considerable agony due to constipation, the middle yang stage pattern (interior pattern) is treated first. However, because of a violation of the exterior first, interior second rule, the pattern can change in quality (this phenomenon is known as collapse pattern). In chronic diseases, deficiency patterns or cold patterns are often treated preferentially. This approach may be considered to be a kind of the "acute pattern first, chronic pattern second" rule, also known as the "tonifying first, draining second" rule.

Case 4: An Acute Disease First, Chronic-Second, or Tonifying First, Draining Second Case

Male in his 60s.

Chief complaints: Heavy sensation of epigastric stuffiness, vertigo, headache, shoulder stiffness

History of current illness: The patient developed symptoms on the day after the Great Earthquake that occurred several months before. Epigastric discomfort appeared several days every week.

History of illness and comorbidity: Coronary bypass surgery and implanted defibrillator for myocardial infarction

Family history: The patient's mother died at 92 years of age after the earthquake.

Pulse examination: Deep and slightly excessive

Tongue examination: Dark red, thick, dry, white coating

Abdominal examination: Swollen, high abdominal strength. Epigastric stuffiness and resistance, bilateral fullness and discomfort in the chest and hypochondrium, and bilateral abdominal muscle tension mainly in the upper abdomen, all intense.

Course of treatment: To treat the condition suspected to be in a yang pattern and excess pattern, *daisaiko*to was prescribed but was ineffective. Because his epigastric area was cold during the exacerbation of his epigastric symptoms, and this lessened upon warming with a pocket warmer, *a yin pattern was suspected. So his formula was switched to Ninjinto (taken before meals.) The epigastric discomfort lessened, and the general condition improved* (acute-first pattern). His *shoulder stiffness and headache*, however, were not mitigated, so *daisaikoto* was again prescribed, in combination with *ninjinto* (after meals), and this treatment was effective.

(Commentary) *Daisaikoto*, which had been previously ineffective, was effective after treatment of the painful yin pattern.

(b) **Concurrent treatments**

- **Mixture of formulas (Case 5)**

For concurrent patterns of close locations of disease, formulas indicated respectively may be used in a mixture (for any overlapping crude drugs, the one of higher content alone should be used). For example, in the presence of both an early yang stage pattern (exterior pattern) and a late yang stage pattern (half exterior and half interior pattern) in a transition (transfer) from the former stage to the latter, *saikokeishito*, a mixture of *keishito* (indicated for exterior patterns) and *shosaikoto* (half exterior and half interior pattern), may be indicated.

Case 5: A Case of Mixing Formulas

50-year-old female. Her skin rash, which developed more than 1 year previously, was diagnosed as toxicoderma and treated but remained to be ameliorated. Punctate to macular reddening and pigmentation in the whole body.

History of illness: Total hysterectomy and total ovariectomy for hysteromyoma.

Height 148 cm, weight 50 kg, reddish face

Pulse examination : Deep and excess

Tongue examination: Dark red, moderate dry white coating

Abdominal examination: Slightly swollen abdomen with high abdominal strength, severe epigastric stuffiness and resistance, and severe fullness and discomfort in chest and hypochondrium. Severe abdominal muscle tension at the center of the upper abdomen. A hypogastric pattern was noted with intense resistance and severe tender pain beside the umbilicus.

Course of treatment: Both signs and symptoms indicating late yang stage excess patterns, daisaikoto and tokakujokito, a blood stasis-resolving formula, were mixed. One week later, the skin rash was ameliorated, and the itching disappeared 3 weeks later.

(partially modified from Reference [7])

- **Combination (Case 4)**

Two formulas or more, not mixed together, are separately taken at time intervals. A combination is often used for conditions at different disease levels, such as the simultaneous presence of a yang pattern and a yin pattern.

The formulas in the combination are usually taken at intervals of at least 30 min, such as in the morning and afternoon or before and after meals within the same day. They may be taken alternatively every 2 days. In such cases, it is a general rule that a warming and tonic formula indicated for yin deficiency patterns is taken first, and a heat-clearing purgative formula indicated for yang excess patterns is taken second (tonifying first, draining second).

Concomitant medication (Case 4): The condition was a coexistence of a pattern indicated for *ninjinto* and another for *daisaikoto*, and the two formulas were used in combination without being mixed together.

3.1.7 Kampo Medicine Efficacy Determination

Mosaburo Kainuma

Introduction

Kampo practitioners often get inquiries from their patients: "When do you determine the effect of your Kampo treatment after administration?" "Are Kampo medicines quickly effective?" and "How long is Kampo medicine to be taken?" It is recommended that the efficacy of Kampo treatment, including the occurrence of adverse drug reactions, be determined in distinct ways for acute diseases and chronic diseases. In this section, we describe specific times for efficacy determination and other aspects in their respective cases.

Efficacy Determination in Acute Diseases (See Case)

In the early stages of acute diseases such as the common cold and influenza, clinical symptoms are ameliorated to some extent in about 10 min after taking a dose. If the treatment is ineffective 30 min later, treatment errors (choice of formula, method of taking medicine, health maintenance) should be suspected. One oral dose taken by way of trial may also be useful for choosing a formula. The same principle applies to other acute diseases. An effect is obtained within 30 min for conditions including painful muscle cramps, menstrual pain, allergic rhinitis, and nasal discharge. If the symptoms are not ameliorated, assume that the Kampo diagnosis was incorrect, and consider switching the formula to another. In acute diseases, treatment may be completed if the condition has been ameliorated completely.

Case: A 22-year-Old Male

Chief complaints: Chills, fever, systemic arthralgia

History of present illness: He is essentially a healthy person. While driving a car accompanying his mother, the patient experienced severe chills. Upon outpatient clinic arrival, he had chills and a fever. He tested positive for influenza.

Physical findings: Height 170 cm, weight 75 kg, pulse rate 108 beats/min, body temperature 39.6 °C, hot flush in the face, no sweating on body surfaces.

Pulse examination: Floating, excess, and rapid

Diagnosis: An excess pattern in the early yang stage with thirst was noted. The condition was diagnosed as indicated for *daiseiryuto*.

(Course) 2.5 g of *maoto* and 2.5 g of *eppikajutsuto*, which are substitutes for *daiseiryuto*, were dissolved together in hot water, and this mixture was administered for trial purposes. The patient's body temperature decreased to 37.5 °C, and he returned home.

The mixture was taken three times more at 3-h intervals, and his body temperature fell under 37 °C on the day after his return home.

(Comments) Trial use of a mixture of *maoto* and *eppikajutsuto* was useful in the early diagnosis and treatment.

- **Efficacy determination in chronic diseases** (Table 3.13)

In chronic diseases, the first priority should be given to ameliorating the main symptoms. Generally, an effect of Kampo medicine becomes perceivable in several days to about 2 weeks. This, however, is not always the case for the most troublesome symptom. Other symptoms such as poor appetite, sleep, and excretion are often improved rather than the main symptom. In addition, objective findings may improve in advance of the symptoms. The effect of Kampo medicine is determined as follows in chronic diseases: When the Kampo medicine has been taken for 1–2 months, the effect should be judged as to whether "the main symptom of the patient" has resolved. If no amelioration is observed in subjective symptoms or objective findings, the patient should be managed with formula changes and other measures. At the same time, instructions are provided to help decrease stress, dietary and other lifestyle irregularities, lack of exercise, and other likely causes of physical imbalance. These efforts are made concurrently and continued to the end of the treatment. In chronic diseases, treatment may be continued in some cases until normalization of Kampo medicine findings, in addition to symptom amelioration. Treatment may be continued for about 1–2 years after remission, in view of seasonal changes.

Table 3.13 Efficacy determination in chronic diseases

	Key points	Policy	
After 1–2 weeks	Did the patient's appetite, sleep, excretion, and other health signs improve?	The same formula is continued.	
	Were the subjective symptoms ameliorated?		
After 1–2 months	How about amelioration of the main symptom?		
	Amelioration of subjective symptoms and objective findings	Yes	The same formula is continued. Life guidance→Towards the end of treatment [a]
		No	Formula switch

[a]Treatment may be continued until normalization of Kampo clinical findings in some cases, and may be continued for about 1–2 years after remission, in view of seasonal changes

- **Adverse drug reaction onset times, symptoms, and measures taken after treatment discontinuation (Table 3.14)**

Pseudoaldosteronism as induced by glycyrrhiza is the most common adverse drug reaction. Symptoms such as hypokalemia, edema, and hypertension develop. Although there is no particular trend for the association between duration of use and onset, cases of onset within 3 months reportedly accounted for approximately 40% of the study population. The first priority should be given to treatment termination doses of Kampo medicines for ethical use. In the case of decoction doses, the glycyrrhiza content may be reduced, or glycyrrhiza may be removed from the formula.

Interstitial pneumonia is a less common but serious adverse drug reaction. The most common onset time is around 2 months after treatment initiation. Interstitial pneumonia, however, can develop in a few cases as early as 1 week of treatment, possibly because of previous sensitization. It is often caused by a crude drug contained in the formula, with *Scutellaria* root (Scutellariae Radix) considered to be one such crude drug, and a supporting report is available. Therefore, the following precautions should be exercised in prescribing Kampo medicine, especially a formula

Table 3.14 Adverse drug reaction onset times, symptoms, and measures taken after treatment discontinuation

Crude drug	Adverse drug reaction	Major symptoms	Post-dose common onset time	Measures
Glycyrrhiza discontinuation	Pseudoaldosteronism	Hypertension, edema, weakness, etc.	Within 3 months for approximately 40% of patients [3]	Extract granules
				→ reduction or discontinuation
				Decoctions
				→ Only Glycyrrhiza dose reduction or discontinuation of Glycyrrhiza
Scutellaria root	Interstitial pneumonia	Fever, coughing, short breath	Within 2 months [4]	Discontinuation with oxygen and steroid administration
	Liver disorders	Absence of subjective symptoms (common), jaundice	Within 3 months [3]	Discontinuation
Gardenia fruit	Mesenteric phlebosclerosis	Abdominal pain - diarrhea, nausea - vomiting	5 or more years [6]	Oral dosing discontinuation Intestinal resection in serious cases

containing *scutellaria.* Oxygen saturation (SpO_2) should be measured when fever, coughing, dyspnea, lung sound abnormality (crepitus), and the like develop after taking the Kampo medicine. When a decreased SpO_2 level is found, treatment with the Kampo medicine should be discontinued. Chest radiography and other examinations should be performed immediately, and appropriate measures such as administration of adrenocortical hormones must be taken.

Formulas containing *Scutellaria* can cause liver disorders. In 80% of cases, liver disorder develops within 3 months after starting the medication, and blood sampling reportedly should take place within 3 months. More recently, it was reported that mesenteric phlebosclerosis can develop with long-term administration (often 5 years or more) of a formula containing gardenia fruit (*sanshishi*). Kampo medicine for ethical use containing gardenia fruit should not be prescribed carelessly. If there is any sign or test finding suggestive of mesenteric phlebosclerosis, the medication should be discontinued, and appropriate countermeasures should be taken (refer to Chap. 4, Sect. 3.3.3).

- **Changes in subjective symptoms and objective findings and efficacy determination**

In the manifestation of therapeutic effects, subjective symptoms and objective findings are often ameliorated in advance of test data improvements. Therefore, it is recommended that first attention be paid to symptoms and general clinical findings when determining the efficacy. On the other hand, an approach with priority given to therapeutic effect, despite some undesirable actions and the extremely unpleasant taste of the Kampo medicine, is often inappropriate for Kampo treatment, including compliance with oral medication dosage. It should be noted, however, that a special phenomenon known as paradoxical healing response can occur infrequently (paradoxical healing responses are described in the next section) (Table 3.14).

- **Special transient responses in Kampo medicine——paradoxical healing responses**

Paradoxical healing responses are various symptoms that are suspected to be adverse drug reactions that develop temporarily after taking a Kampo medicine, and these symptoms disappear later as the medicine is used continuously. As far as reports go, paradoxical healing responses often develop within 3–4 days after the start of medication, and this is followed by a dramatic amelioration of the condition. However, the patient often discontinues their treatment soon after experiencing symptom aggravation after taking a Kampo medicine. They consider the aggravation as an adverse drug reaction, but it is difficult to determine whether the aggravation is a transient paradoxical healing response or an adverse drug reaction.

Responding to inquiries: Patients sometimes inquire about the acceptability of taking the Kampo medicine despite symptom aggravation. In such cases, it is safer to determine how to deal with the situation only after discontinuing the medication and examining the patient. However, another instruction in view of paradoxical healing responses is feasible: "Continue the oral medication for 2–3 more days, and discontinue if your symptoms get worse. If your symptoms no longer get worse, continue the oral medication, since the symptoms are likely transient responses." Of course, it is preferable for the patient to achieve transient responses to symptoms without a paradoxical healing response. It is very difficult, however, to determine whether various responsive symptoms that develop temporarily after taking Kampo medicines are paradoxical healing responses. Adequate caution should be exercised when providing the latter advice.

Fig. 3.51 Outline of mutual transitions of the six-stage patterns

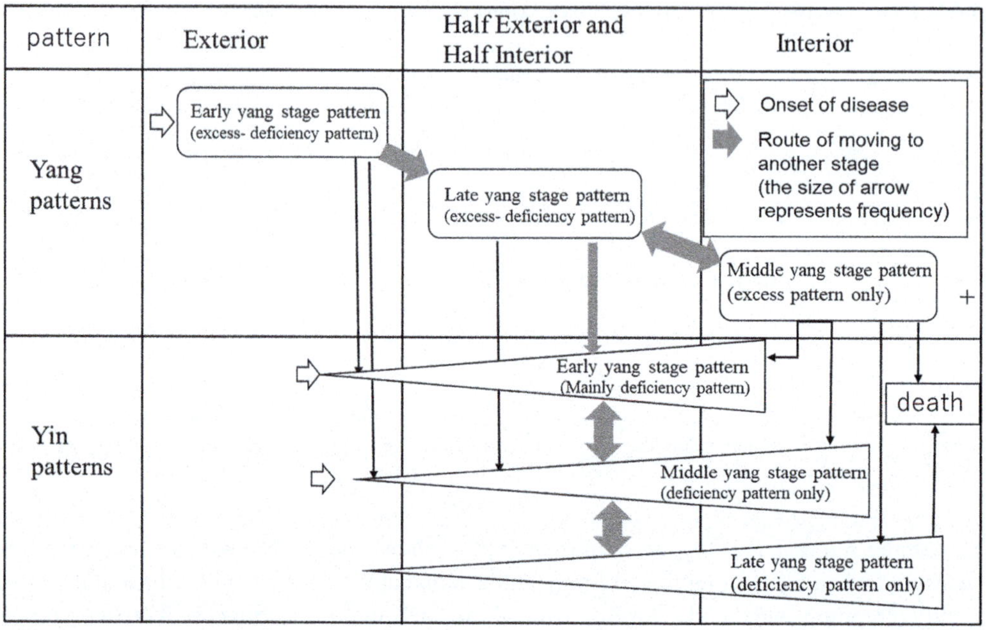

3.1.8 Pathological Changes During Treatment

Hiromi Gotoh

Introduction

"Patterns," as stated in Kampo medicine, change over time. It is important that the formula be modified (formula change) according to any change in pattern (pathological change). Assessments are made according to the pathological changes based on the concepts of the six-stage patterns, qi, blood[TM1], fluid[TM1], and the five zang organs.

The Six-Stage Patterns and Pathological Changes (see Fig. 3.51)

The concept of the six-stage patterns is often used to manage pathological changes in the acute stage (for details of the six-stage patterns, refer to another section). The figure shows such pathological changes. The initial onset site of the pathologic condition occurs in the early yang stage pattern, early yin stage pattern, and middle yin stage pattern. If the treatment is ineffective in any pattern, the target is shifted to another site in another pattern as indicated by the arrows in the figure. Usual courses of the six-stage patterns are described below. An early yang stage corresponds to the initial onset of disease. A cure can be achieved with appropriate treatment. However, this stage often shifts to a late yang stage in cases with decreased physical strength or potent action of any complicating factor. A middle yang stage is a state characterized by the presence of powerful external pathogens and fully mobilized physical strength. This does not occur in all cases. An early yin stage is found when complete remission has not been attained from an early yang stage pattern or late yang stage pattern or after a middle yang stage has been ameliorated and physical strength remains. A middle yin stage is a progressed condition with weakened physical strength. A late yin stage corresponds to shock.

The following points are important for the differential diagnosis of the six-stage patterns.

(I) Initial onset of disease corresponds not only to an early yang stage pattern, as in the common cold developing with a fever, but also to an early yin stage pattern, as in acute gastroenteritis in the elderly, or a middle yin stage pattern, as in the common cold with a sensation of coldness. (II) The course is not consistent; we often encounter transitions from the early yang stage pattern to the middle yang stage pattern, to the early yin stage pattern, and to the middle yin stage pattern, and from the late yang stage pattern to the middle yin stage pattern. (III) In yang patterns, it is easy to distinguish early, late, and middle yang stage patterns because the primary locus of the disease in the body is the exterior, half exterior and half interior, and interior, respectively. In yin patterns, on the other hand, it is sometimes difficult to distinguish early, middle, and late yin stages because the primary locus of the disease in the body is the interior.

In respiratory disease, for example, a fever due to upper airway inflammation is treated with *maoto* and the like prescribed for an excess pattern suspected from pulse examination and other findings in an early yang stage pattern. When a cure occurs, no further treatment will be required. In the event of new symptoms, such as persistent slight fevers, bad taste in the mouth, and prolonged coughing that develops in the afternoon with no amelioration of the existing symptoms, a transition to a late yang stage will be diagnosed. Then the formula will be changed to *saikokeishito* and the like. If symptoms aggravate, with persistent high fevers or intensifying thirst, in special cases, the condition will be identified as a middle yang stage pattern, and the formula will be changed to *byakkokaninjinto* and the like. In general, if a disease persists in a late yang stage, a transition to an early yin stage will be diagnosed, and the formula will often be changed to a formula like *ninjinto*, taking into account loss of physical strength. If general malaise becomes severe, a formula for the middle yin stage, such as *shinbuto*, will be used. If the treatment is ineffective and the condition further worsens with aggravated malaise, indigestion, diarrhea, and other symptoms, a transition to a late yin stage will be diagnosed, and a formula for the late yin stage, such as *bukuryoshigyakuto*, will be administered.

In addition, the concept of the six-stage patterns involves therapeutic methods for complex conditions known as combinations of diseases, overlaps of diseases, and simply comorbid diseases. For details, refer to another section (Chap. 3, Sect. 3.1.6).

Qi, Blood[TM1], Fluid[TM1], and Pathological Changes

The concept of qi, blood[TM1], and fluids[TM1] and their pathological changes is that formulas are chosen based on changes in the main symptoms associated with qi, blood[TM1], and fluids[TM1]. Examples are given below.

1. [Change from blood[TM1] stasis to fluid[TM1] retention] The patient had menstrual irregularity and cold sensitivity and was taking oral doses of *tokishakuyakusan*, a prescription for blood[TM1] stasis. In winter, she experienced aggravation of the cold and stiffness in her hands and feet, and her formula was changed to *shinbuto*, a prescription for fluid[TM1] retention. According to the concept of the six-stage patterns, this case can be described as a change from the early yin stage pattern to the middle yin stage pattern.
2. [Change from qi stagnation to blood[TM1] stasis] The patient, somewhat depressive with a sensation of a foreign object in the throat, was taking oral doses of *hangekobokuto*, a prescription for qi stagnation. After hot flashes and other climacteric symptoms developed, her formula was changed to *kami-shoyosan*, a prescription for blood[TM1] stasis.
3. [Switch from treatment for qi deficiency to treatment for both qi deficiency and blood[TM1] deficiency] The patient had epigastric stuffiness and was taking oral doses of *rikkunshito*, a prescription for qi deficiency. After appetite improved but the patient developed anemia and rough skin, the formula was changed to *juzentaihoto*, a prescription for both qi deficiency and blood[TM1] deficiency.

The Five Zang Organs and Pathological Changes

The concept of the five zang organs and their pathological changes is that formulas are chosen based on changes in main symptoms associated with the five zang organs. Examples are given below.

1. [Switch from treatment for the heart to treatment for the kidney[TM1]] The patient experienced numbness and cold in lower limbs while taking oral doses of *shaku-kanzoto*, a prescription for cardiac abnormalities, to treat palpitations. Since weakness of the lower abdominal region was found in the Kampo abdominal examination, the formula was changed to *goshajinkigan*, a prescription for renal abnormalities.
2. [Switch from treatment for the liver[TM1] to treatment for the lung[TM1]] The patient was taking oral doses of *yokukansan*, a prescription for hepatic abnormalities, to treat irritability. For patients with aggravating nasal discharge due to pollenosis in winter, the formula is changed to *shoseiryuto*, a prescription for pulmonary abnormalities.
3. [Switch from treatment for the kidney[TM1] to treatment for the spleen[TM1]] The patient had lumbago and was taking oral doses of *hachimijiogan*, a prescription for renal abnormalities. Although the lumbago was ameliorated slightly, epigastric stuffiness developed, so *ninjinto*, a prescription for the spleen[TM1], and *hachimijiogan* were mixed together. This mixture was taken orally.

Quick Change of Prescription and Continuation of Prescription (Table 3.15)

There are two contradictory concepts of quick change of prescriptions and continuation of prescriptions to treat pathological changes in the course of treatment. In principle, both are based on the principle of choosing a formula corresponding to pattern identification. Hence, it is necessary to quickly change the formula for changes in the disease pattern in some cases, and in other cases it is better to continue treatment with the same formula without any changes. To ensure the appropriate judgment, it is important that the timing of changing the formula be determined based on careful examination of the patient's condition.

In the case reported below, the change to the prescription of *kanzoshashinto* corresponds to a **quick change of prescription** (a). Although various formulas were prescribed and administered, the symptoms were not ameliorated at all, so the formula was quickly changed to *kanzoshashinto*. Soon after the formulation change, the symptoms were generally ameliorated, so the formula was continued despite transient abdominal pain in the morning and afternoon, and the symptoms were eventually ameliorated. **Continuation of prescription** (b) was effective in this case.

Table 3.15 Quick change of prescription and continuation of prescription

	Quick change of prescription	Continuation of prescription
Definition	To change a formula to another occasionally according to disease pattern change	To continue the same formula without changing to another when there is no pattern change
Clinical measures	**(I) Cases where formula A ineffective** When formula A is ineffective (a pattern change), change the formula to another quickly **(II) Cases where formula A is ineffective** When formula A does not produce an amelioration (a wrong pattern), change the formula to another	**(I) Cases where formula B is used for chronic disease** We are sometimes unable to know whether formula B is suitable to the patient's disease pattern because its short-term use is not effective or is unlikely to be effective. If formula B ameliorates symptoms other than the chief complaints or makes the patient feel better with treatment, formula B will be continued

(Note) *Kanzoshashinto* is usually not used for abdominal pain.

A case report about a quick change of prescription and continuation of prescription by Keisetsu Otsuka. The patient was a 27-year-old unmarried woman. She had been suffering from diarrhea for about 10 years. (omitted) *Jinreibyakujutsusan was* prescribed for 2 weeks, but no change occurred. Hence, **the formula was changed to *shinbuto*** (a). It was taken for 2 weeks, but no change occurred. Hence, the formula was changed to ***ifusan*** (a). This formula also failed, and the patient experienced diarrhea four times in a day and complained of physical dullness. Therefore, **the formula was changed back to *jinreibyakujutsusan*** (a). The next morning, the patient became very sick in the stomach and experienced severe gastric pain. In addition, epigastric stuffiness developed, and also her appetite decreased.

I noticed my wrong choice of formulas and determined the new pattern, ***kanzoshashinto*** (a). Though diarrhea continued four times on Sunday morning, the new formula was started in the evening of the day. It was highly effective. She had no bowel movement Monday through Friday, except once with soft stools on Friday, with no bowel movement on Saturday. On Sunday, spontaneous defecation of favorably hard stools occurred once. In addition, the epigastric stuffiness disappeared with good comfort, and appetite increased. However, the patient complained of abdominal pain after breakfast and dinner. Therefore, *the same formula (**kanzoshashinto**) was administered for 1 week. Then spontaneous defecation occurred every day or every 2 days, and the abdominal pain lessened in severity. The same formula continued to be administered* (b). *Thereafter, the patient became generally able to have normal defecation, with no more malaise in the early morning, although she did experience diarrhea infrequently.*

Points to Note on Pathological Changes During Treatment

The patients' stages are diagnosed from the perspective of six-stage patterns. Based on this diagnosis, and in view of the concepts of qi, blood[TM1], and fluids[TM1] and the five zang organs, the formula is changed to an appropriate one. Furthermore, it should be taken into account that the condition can sometimes change in special ways, such as combinations of diseases, overlaps of diseases, and comorbid diseases (refer to Chap. 3, Sect. 3.1.6). With regard to changing formulas, it is desirable that both quick change of prescription and continuation of prescription always be kept in mind.

3.2 Disease Before Onset *(Mibyo)*

Kazuo Mitani

3.2.1 Introduction

In the *Shikichoshintairon* (theory of seasonal health conditioning) chapter of *Huangdi Neijing, Suwen* (Basic Questions), it is said, "A good physician does not begin treatment after a disease develops but begins the treatment before the onset. Treat disease before its onset or prepare for the situation before the war starts." Hence, it is important that practitioners instruct patients to live their daily lives in accordance with the principles of yin and yang while he or she is not yet ill but somehow unwell. The classics place importance not only on medications but also on diets and exercises in the treatment of disease.

3.2.2 What is Disease Before Its Onset?

In Kampo medicine, the term health condition before its onset (*mibyo)* is defined as "a disease that has not developed or the physical condition before its onset" [14]. In Kampo medicine, causes of disease are explored in two categories: internal causes (internal injury) and external causes (external contractions). Specifically, a health condition before its onset is induced by incipient "invasion of pathogenic qi" or external contractions (affected by external pathogens) [14], resulting in internal injury (some of the five zang and six fu organs are injured) [14]. Hence, a health condition before its onset is a state where pathogenic qi has invaded the body but has not yet damaged the five zang organs. It can also be viewed as a condition where no disease has developed, even after the invasion of pathogenic qi, because nutrient qi and defensive qi in the body work sufficiently. Nutrient qi and defensive qi represent the activities of physiological functions involved in all aspects of human life, and this means the body's defense reactions, including immune response. Kampo medicine is comprised of purgative formulas, which are based on the body's biological response to pathogens (sweating, emetics, draining), and tonic formulas, which act to increase the body's resistance. Thus, importance is placed on adjusting the body's defense systems.

3.2.3 Clinical Practice Based on the Concept of Treating Health Condition Before Its Onset: The Way of Modern Kampo Medicine

This concept is the major feature of Kampo medicine practices. Japan's modern medical practices are based on Western medicine. Kampo medicine is practiced in an environment where patients enjoy the world's most advanced treatments, including university hospitals. Therefore, Kampo medicine is never in conflict with Western medicine. Instead, Kampo medicine is made available while patients make the best use of Western medical approaches. The patient presents with a wide variety of subjective symptoms (deconditioning) and first wishes to receive allopathic drug therapy. When there is no pathological finding, however, Kampo medicine, including doses of Kampo formulas, as well as acupuncture, moxibustion, and dietetic guidance, is offered.

"Doctor, Kampo treatment is received simply by taking Kampo medicines, isn't that so?" This is true in some respects, but health is not achieved by "simply taking medicines." What are the wide variety of phenomena occurring in the patient's body without being perceived by the patient? This is explored by Kampo practitioners together with their patients. A therapeutic plan suitable for the patient is made by carefully checking his or her nutrient qi and defensive qi, which vary even if the attacking force (external contraction) is the same. This is the treatment of health condition before its onset.

Patients ask, "No abnormal findings were found in my examination. Then, why do I feel so ill now?" Now, let's begin here. We Kampo practitioners always want to follow our patients' experiences. Nutrient qi and defensive qi cannot be observed without collaboration between the practitioner and the patient. We cannot enjoy the desired efficacy of any Kampo treatment without understanding the essentials of the patient's complaints and identifying the health condition before its onset.

3.2.4 Looking at Lifestyle-Related Diseases (Internal Damage) as an Example

In recent years, a wide variety of examinations have become available not only in outpatient clinics but also in health checkups, and abnormal test values are often reported without subjective symptoms. In such situations, we can proceed with the concept of health condition before their onset in mind. We start treatment to prevent disease from developing even when no symptom is manifested despite signs of internal damage or the condition worsening. This concept will be increasingly important in the future. Lifestyle-related diseases, such as hyperlipidemia, diabetes, and hypertension, may be viewed as diseases to which the concept of health condition before its onset is applicable. In the fields of rheumatoid arthritis and psychosomatic medicine, good results can be obtained by thinking about "What is the health condition before its onset in this patient?" (see Table 3.16). Conditions like "no energy" and "unable to sleep" should be managed with health condition before its onset in mind, rather than focusing on treating the present illness (refer to Chap. 3, Sect. 3.1.4).

Table 3.16 Examples of treatments based on health condition before its onset concept

Hyperlipidemia	Kampo medicines, diet therapy (medicinal cooking)
Diabetes	Kampo medicines, diet therapy (medicinal cooking)
Hypertension	Kampo medicines, acupuncture and moxibustion, diet therapy (medicinal cooking)
Rheumatoid arthritis	Kampo medicines, acupuncture and moxibustion, Daoyin and *anma* massage, diet therapy (medicinal cooking)
Psychosomatic medicine	Kampo medicines, acupuncture and moxibustion, Daoyin and *anma* massage, diet therapy (medicinal cooking)

3.2.5 Conclusion

While symptoms may be described as physical responses (prophylaxis), we are usually conscious of unpleasant symptoms as incipient disease and want to treat them without delay. However, symptoms have many benefits to the body. For example, meal-induced diarrhea (diarrhea due to food poisoning) is attributable to our body's "healing power" to eliminate pathogens. Fevers conquer pathogens to mitigate the condition by sweating. As such, the treatment in view of the health condition before its onset may be considered to be quite a proactive therapeutic approach to allow the body to restore health based on its spontaneous healing power.

3.3 Healthcare and Diets

Kazuo Mitani

3.3.1 Overview

As it has long been said, "Prioritize health maintenance over medicine." It is important to think about "health maintenance" in our daily lives. They say, "Disease often recurs because of inadequate health maintenance due to negligence, when the disease could have been cured completely." Medicines are

Table 3.17 Lessons from *Yojo-kun*

General rules	Reduce anger and anxiety and remain mentally calm
	Avoid overeating and do adequate exercise suitable to oneself
	Follow your own rules in daily activities and avoid doing physically harmful things
	Make efforts to prevent disease from developing, rather than starting treatment after the onset
	Do everything in moderation, and live a harmonized life
	Regardless of the amount of money you have, find pleasure in your own life
	Breathe slowly and sometimes take a deep in breath
	Avoid staying up late at night and take care to have good sanitation
Diets	Eat foods while warm (at appropriate temperature)
	Eat foods adjusted to the physical condition during gastrointestinal disorders or other troubles (do not eat foods that take time to digest, such as meats, spicy foods, and viscous foods)
	Take lightly seasoned foods, and avoid overeating strongly seasoned foods and fatty foods
	Avoid taking (too much of) cold food, raw food (equal to cold food), and hard food (food taking time to digest)
	Eat foods of a wide variety in a good balance
	Take less food at dinner than at breakfast
	Avoid eating indigestible foods, such as big fish and poultry or fish skins
	Avoid overdrinking
	Have meals of low salt content
Sex life	The sexual desire is the strongest of human desires, and we must restrain ourselves when young and thereafter
Housing	Stay in an adequately bright room, avoiding a long stay in a dark room with yin qi
Sleep	Sleep on your side at bedtime. Sleeping in a supine position causes sickness and an anxious feeling. Sleeping with the hands on the chest produces a nightmare
Excretion	Do not suppress defecation or urination, and eliminate it early
Medicines	There is no medicine for perpetual longevity. Live out your allotted span of life
	Use cold water when taking a medicine for food poisoning. Hot water activates toxicity
Aging	Enjoy everyday life quietly and control anger and selfish desires
	Avoid overdoing

( ) is extra explanation by the Japanese supervisor of this publication

unwanted, but health maintenance is necessary for a disease to be cured. In Kaibara Ekiken's *Yojo-kun* (Health Cultivation Instructions), food is described as being very important. When the disease is treated using medicines and foods in combination, healthy qi should not be affected. Having what's called spontaneous healing power, our body works spontaneously to get healthy. Avoid violating natural principles. This is the essence of health maintenance. While the indication of a particular food item is often emphasized, it is important that the food taken be in harmony with the season and the patient's age and constitution. Taking a particular food item in excess reduces harmony, which in turn can affect healthy qi.

The key points for healthcare described by Kaibara Ekiken in *Yojo-kun* are shown in Table 3.17.

3.3.2 Conclusion

Anxiety about health largely involves not only the disease as it is but also issues of daily living in a diseased state. Medicine cannot be effective without a good supply of food, clothing, and shelter. Recovery from disease depends on how the patient realizes his or her potential for spontaneous healing. Specifically, resistance to infections and balanced organic functioning are essential. This chapter emphasizes how dietary and other lifestyle factors are important issues for health maintenance and allow medical care to work well. On the other hand, worries about delayed disease recovery can work the other way, as stated in the proverb, "Struggling with health maintenance emaciates you." Although choosing the appropriate formula is key to successful treatment, in Kampo practice, it is no exaggeration to say that successful treatment depends on how instructions are provided to ensure reasonable health maintenance that suits each person's lifestyle. (See the table above.)

References

1. Edwards M. Put out your tongue! The role of clinical insight in the study of the history of medicine. Med Hist. 2011;55:301–6.
2. Faber A. Zschr klin Med 85:319–334. Berlin: Verlag von August Hirschwald; 1917
3. Beavens DW, Brooks SE. A colour atras of the tongue in clinical diagnosis. Wolfe Medical; 1988.
4. Dawson TAJ. Tongue lesions in generalized pustular psoriasis. Br J Dermatol. 1974;91(4):419–24.
5. Marks R, Czarny D. Geographic tongue: sensitivity to the environment. Oral Surg Oral Med Oral Pathol. 1984;58:156.
6. Ren J, Zheng Y, Du H, et al. Antibiotic-induced black hairy tongue: two case reports and a review of the literature. J Int Med Res. 2020;48(10)
7. Manabe M, Lim HW, Winzer M, Loomis CA. Arch Dermatol. 1999;135(2):177–81.
8. Schlager E, St. Claire C, Ashack K, et al. Am J Clin Dermatol. 2017;18:563–9.
9. Haubrich B. Gastrointestinal symptoms: clinical interpretation. Philadelphia: BC Decker; 1991. p. 23–58.
10. Jones CM, et al. Digestive tract pain: diagnosis and treatment, experimental observation. New York: Macmillan; 1938. p. 7–42.
11. Bockus HL. Symptomatology; abdominal pain and discomfort. In: Bockus HL, editor. Gastroenterology, vol. 1. Philadelphia: W. B. Saunders; 1974. p. 64–5.
12. The Editing Committee for Dictionary of Kampo Medicine, the Japan Society for Oriental Medicine, edt. The dictionary of Kampo medicine (basic terms). Kyoto: Medical Yukon; 2020. p. 35.
13. The Editing Committee for Dictionary of Kampo Medicine, the Japan Society for Oriental Medicine, edt. The dictionary of Kampo medicine (basic terms). Kyoto: Medical Yukon; 2020. p. 32–3.
14. Japan Society for Oriental Medicine. Mibyo, external contractions, internal damages in the Dictionary of Kampo Medicine, 2020.

Crude Drugs and Formulas

4

Toshiaki Makino, Tatsuhiko Suzuki, Yoshiharu Tobina,
Kazuyoshi Kawazoe, and Tatsuya Nogami

1 General Remarks on Pharmacognosy

Toshiaki MakinoTatsuhiko Suzuki, Yoshiharu Tobina and Kazuyoshi Kawazoe

Terms Referring to the Medicinal Substances Used in Traditional Medicine

In modern European and American culture, the medicinal substances derived from natural sources used in traditional medicine are commonly called as "herbs," "herbal medicines," or "botanical medicines." In the old European and American culture, such substances had been called as "crude drugs," and they had used the medicines derived from not only plants (herbs) but also animal tissues and minerals. However, after the active chemical ingredients had been isolated from these medicines, the custom using medicines derived from animals and minerals had been disappeared, and they are using only the medicines derived from plants in traditional or alternative medicine.

However, East-Asian traditional medicine including Kampo medicine has still been using the medicinal substances derived from animals and minerals. For example, Gypsum is commonly prescribed in the formula of Kampo medicine, but since Gypsum is not derived from plants but from minerals, it cannot be called as "herbal medicine." In China, such substances are called as "Chinese medicines"; however, in Japan, "Kampo medicines" refers not to the medicines composed of a single substance derived from natural sources but to the mixture of such medicinal substances (formula).

Therefore, in this book, the medicines composed of a single substance derived from natural sources prescribed in Kampo medicines are expressed as "crude drugs," since this term is scientifically right and is officially used in Japanese Pharmacopoeia.

Crude drugs is the term that refers to a naturally derived material used as a pharmaceutical agent after simple processing such as drying and cutting. Japanese Pharmacopoeia supervised by the Ministry of Health, Labor and Welfare, Japan, defines crude drugs as the medicinal parts of animals and plants, cell contents, secretions, extracts or minerals, etc. Until about 200 years ago, before chemistry was fully developed, all pharmaceutical products were derived from crude drugs. In Western medicine, with the subsequent development of chemistry, the active chemical ingredients (compounds or pure substances) contained in crude drugs were isolated one after another, and then, these pure substances have been used as the pharmaceutical agents. Therefore, the occasions to use crude drugs as the source of pharmaceutical products have decreased. In Kampo medicine, on the other hand, crude drugs are still used for pharmaceutical products as the raw materials of Kampo prescriptions or formulas.

T. Makino (✉)
Department of Pharmacognosy, Graduate School of Pharmaceutical Sciences, Nagoya City University, Nagoya, Japan
e-mail: office@jsom.or.jp

T. Suzuki
Faculty of Pharmaceutical Sciences, Teikyo Heisei University, Tokyo, Japan

Y. Tobina
Onchido Yakazu Clinic, Tokyo, Japan

K. Kawazoe
Division of Natural Medicine and Therapeutics, Department of Clinical Pharmacy, School of Pharmacy, Showa Medical University, Tokyo, Japan

T. Nogami
Department of Kampo Medicine, Tokai University School of Medicine, Isehara, Japan

Kampo Medical Literature Editorial Committee, The Japan Society for Oriental Medicine (ed.), *Complete Japanese Traditional (Kampo) Medicine*, https://doi.org/10.1007/978-981-96-7143-4_4

Most of the sources of crude drugs are medicinal plants. Since prehistoric times, human beings have used specific parts of specific plants for the treatment of various diseases, and have empirically developed the methods for using medicinal plants. For example, in Japan, the aerial part of *Swertia japonica* and *Geranium thunbergii* has been used empirically for digestive diseases. However, when medicinal plants are collected as wild products, they are not called crude drugs but are simply called "medicinal plants" or "medicinal herbs."

1.1 The Borderline Between Pharmaceuticals and Non-pharmaceuticals

Keywords: Functional foods, Raw materials exclusively used as pharmaceuticals.

In our lives, foods are the first commercial products derived from natural materials. The primary purpose of purchasing foods is to satisfy hunger and to maintain our vital activity. However, for the purpose of further improving our health, functional foods (so-called healthy foods) derived from natural materials are commercially distributing in markets. On the other hand, the purpose of using crude drugs is to prevent or treat diseases. Since crude drugs may have side effects, they are distributed as the pharmaceutical products.

When distributing the products that are made from naturally derived materials and are intended to be taken orally in Japanese market, we have to follow "the list of raw materials exclusively used as pharmaceuticals" (so-called the borderline of pharmaceuticals to non-pharmaceuticals), which is a notification on February 25, 2022, from the Director of the Pharmaceutical and Living Hygiene Bureau, the Ministry of Health, Labor and Welfare (Table 4.1). This document determines the essential ingredients (raw materials) used exclusively as pharmaceuticals. In this list, 232 plant-derived materials and 21 animal-derived materials are listed as "exclusively pharmaceuticals," and the products made from them can only be distributed as pharmaceutical products. In other words, the products made from naturally derived ingredients that are not "exclusively pharmaceuticals" on this list can be distributed as functional foods.

Table 4.1 The part of the list of raw materials exclusively used as pharmaceuticals (so-called the borderline of pharmaceuticals to non-pharmaceuticals) revised on February 25, 2022

Names	Alias names	Medicinal parts	Others
Khat		Leaves	
Arnica		Root bark, Whole herb	
Ogon	Baikal skullcap	Roots	Its stems and leaves are non-pharmaceuticals.
Obaku	Amur cork tree	Barks	Its leaves and froots are non-pharmaceuticals
Kuzu	Kudzu	Roots	Its seeds, leaves, flowers, and starch from this plant are non-pharmaceuticals

In this list, the names of animals, plants, and minerals as well as their medicinal parts are specified, and even if the materials are derived from plants of the same species, they can be classified as pharmaceutical raw materials or food (non-pharmaceutical) raw materials depending on their parts. For example, *kuzu*, which is one of the components of Kakkonto, is the dried root of *Pueraria lobata* from which periderm has been removed, and it is classified as "exclusively pharmaceuticals." However, the seed, leaf, flower of *Pueraria lobata,* and the starch prepared from the root of *Pueraria lobata* are classified as non-pharmaceuticals. Since the root of *Pueraria lobata* itself classified as "exclusively pharmaceuticals," it can only be sold by pharmacists or registered sales clerks in pharmacy. However, since the starch extracted from it is non-pharmaceuticals, everyone can sell the products such as *kuzumochi* and *kuzuyu* (cake and gruel made from starch collected from the root of *Pueraria lobata*, respectively) as food products. When non-pharmaceuticals are distributed as food products, there is no strict quality regulation as for the pharmaceuticals; therefore, inferior products can also be distributed, and general consumers have to select and consider their quality good or bad when purchasing. In addition, since it is not permitted for foods to indicate the efficacy of a specific disease name (health claims), the ambiguous expressions such as "for those who are concerned about some symptoms" are displayed as the functionality.

1.2 Folk Medicines and Kampo Medicines

Keywords: Folk medicines, Kampo medicines, *Kan*-medicines, Japanese traditional pharmaceutical products, *Wakan*-medicines, Crude drug products, Manufacturing Kampo products.

As mentioned above, human beings have used medicinal plants in ethnic groups all over the world, and we have accumulated the experiences such that even ordinary people can judge how to use the specific part of the specific medicinal plant for specific diseases. For example, in Japan, there are customs to use the aerial part of *Geranium thunbergii* as an antidiarrheal, and that of *Swertia japonica* as a stomachic. In European countries, the leaves of *Digitalis purpurea* are used as a cardiotonic medicine, and the seeds of *Colchicum autumnale* as an analgesic for gout. Such crude drugs have been used by the experiences within ethnic groups, and these kinds of crude drugs are called **folk medicines**. The unique folk medicines have been handed down from ancient times to the present day within ethnic groups around the world. Such folk medicines are also used as raw materials for developing new chemical medicines, and new medicines such as digitoxin from *Digitalis* leaves and colchicine from *Colchicum* seeds have been developed and used as modern medicines.

Based on the experiences of using folk medicine, the medical theory (see Chap. 1, Sect. 1.1) including the contents corresponding to physiology, pathology, and pharmaceutical therapeutics in modern medicine has been developed. Then, crude drugs have been used under the medical theory. Folk medicines are the herbal medicines that are simply used for the symptoms without medical theory of pharmaceutical therapeutics, and since there are no theories to make the prescriptions using herbal medicines, crude drugs belonging to folk medicines are often used as a single material without making formula.

Kampo medicines refer to the medicines used under the theory of Kampo medicine explained so far. In most cases, multiple herbal materials are combined according to the theory of pharmaceutical therapeutics described later (exceptions are Kanzoto, only *kanzo*, and Dokujinto, only *ninjin*). Most of the crude drugs used as the raw materials of Kampo medicines are those used in ancient Chinese medicine, which is the origin of Kampo medicine (they are sometimes called as ***Kan*-medicines**, i.e., *Kan* is the Japanese pronunciation of the ancient Han dynasty in mainland China. *Kan*-medicines can be said to be folk medicines in ancient China). In the subsequent development of history, crude drugs unique to Japan had been added into Kampo medicines. Such unique crude drugs in Japan have been sometimes called as the same names of crude drugs as those in China, that is, the different pharmaceutical substances have been called as the same names in Japan and mainland China.

On the other hand, in Japan, there are medicinal products called **Japanese traditional pharmaceutical products**, which had been called as the patent medicinal products in the old days. The famous ones are *Daranisuke*, *Hyakuso*, *Yomeishu*, and *Rokushingan*. Among these, *Daranisuke* and *Hyakuso* belong to the folk medicines because they use *obaku* alone, but *Yomeishu* and *Rokushingan* are different from the typical folk medicines since they are composed of multiple crude drugs. In addition, when combining these multiple crude drugs, the original prescription derived from ancient China had been changed by adding folk medicines unique in Japan to the prescription, or to modify the herbal components according to detailed symptoms. Some of these Japanese traditional medicinal products can be said to be Kampo medicines because they were based on Japanese unique Kampo medical theory, which was the standard medicine of the past. However, these traditional Japanese medicinal products are classified as the conventional crude drug products (non-Kampo crude drug products) under the Pharmaceutical Affairs System in Japan.

In European countries, crude drugs, which were originally folk medicines, have come to be used under the medical theory of Western medicine, and some of them have been used in Japan with the introduction of Dutch medicine in the latter half of the Edo period. These crude drugs are sometimes called as **Western crude drugs**. Some of them, such as senna, the dried leaves of *Senna alexandrina*, are still used alone even now. However, other Western crude drugs are sometimes used as the components in the prescription (formula), and the multiple crude drugs are combined based on the theory of Western medicine. In Japan, Western crude drugs are prescribed in the pharmaceutical products to improve colds or gastrointestinal function, or as nourishing tonics, etc., that are used as over-the-counter (OTC) products.

In contrast to *Kan*-medicines, Japanese folk medicines are sometimes called ***Wa*-medicines** (*Wa* refers to ancient Japan). However, since some *Kan*-drugs had been introduced from ancient China to Japan and become established as Japanese folk medicines, and *Wa*- and *Kan*-medicines are often duplicated. Therefore, the classification of them is sometimes combined, and the term ***Wakan*-medicines** is commonly used. By combining *Wakan*-medicines and Western crude drugs, it is possible to cover all medicinal products derived from crude drugs in Japan.

In Japan, crude drugs themselves are also distributed as the pharmaceutical products, of which 176 items are listed in the National Health Insurance Drug Price Standard, and most of them are used for preparing Kampo products by formulating them based on Kampo medical theory (the term *XX-to* as Kampo formula institutionally refers not to the pharmaceutical products (extract granules, decoctions, tablets, etc.) derived from crude drugs but the mixture of crude drugs that cannot be taken directly under the Pharmaceutical Affairs System in Japan). In addition, other pharmaceutical products are manufactured by processing and preparing the single crude drug or the mixture of them as raw materials, and by processing (formulating) them into easy-to-drink dosage forms such as tablets or granules in pharmaceutical industries. In Japan, pharmaceutical products derived from crude drugs are roughly divided into **Kampo products** and **crude drug products** (non-Kampo crude drug products). The former is derived from typical Kampo formulations, and the latter is derived from Japanese folk medicines, Japanese traditional medicines, and Western crude drugs. The latter sometimes composes the combination of multiple crude drugs, but some crude drugs are approved as the crude drug products even if they consist of a single crude drug. Most of the crude drug products are distributed as OTC drugs, but a small number of them such as the laxative made from *Sennna* leaves, the therapeutic agent for edema from the aerial part of *Melilotus officinalis* (melilot), and for urinary lithiasis from the bark of *Quercus salicina* have been approved and

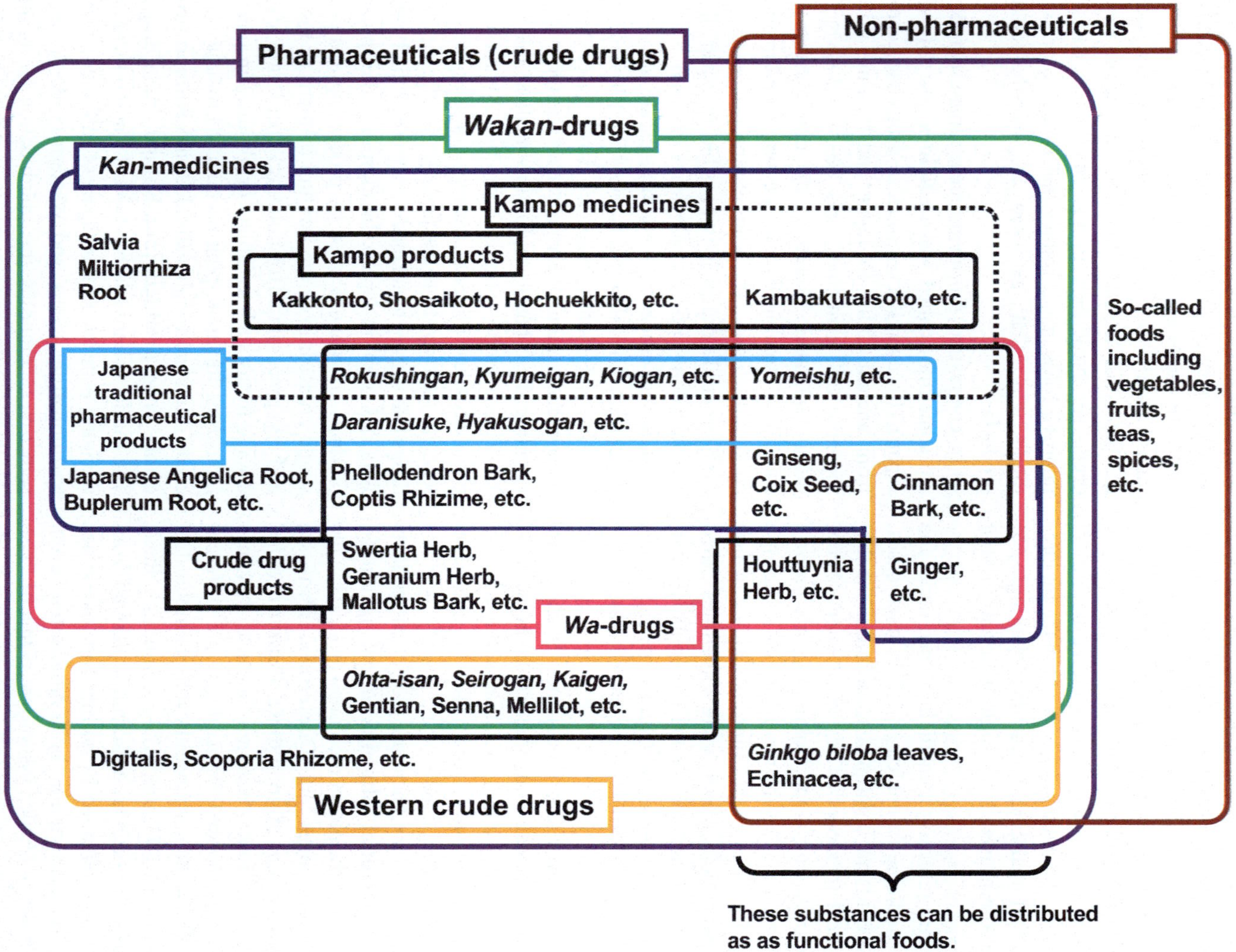

Fig. 4.1 Classification of the products that are taken orally using natural substances in Japan. Although folk medicines are not shown in this figure, those used with single crude drug generally correspond to folk medicines

Table 4.2 Drug classification of ethical, pharmacy, and over-the-counter (OTC) drugs in Japan

Ethical Drugs						
Pharmacy drugs				Over-the-counter (OTC) drugs		
Prescription drugs	Ethical drugs other than prescription drugs	Pharmacy-made pharmaceuticals	Pharmaceuticals requiring guidance	1st category	2nd category	3rd category
Pharmacist can sell them by the prescriptions issued by physicians.	In principle, pharmacist can sell them by the prescriptions issued by physicians. But if necessary, pharmacist can sell without prescription.	Pharmacist can sell them without prescription. Pharmacist also can sell them online if permitted by government.	Pharmacist can sell them without prescription. Pharmacist cannot sell them online.	Pharmacist can sell them without prescription by providing paper information. Pharmacist also can sell them online if permitted by government.	Pharmacist or registered sales clerks can sell them without prescription by making efforts to provide drug information. If permitted by government, they can be sold by online.	Pharmacist or registered sales clerks can sell them without prescription. If permitted by government, they can be sold by online.

Crude drugs are classified among ethical drugs other than prescription drugs, the second-class over-the-counter (OTC) drugs, and the third-class OTC drugs. Crude drug products and Kampo products are classified among ethical drugs other than prescription drugs, pharmacy-made pharmaceuticals, the second-class over-the-counter drugs, and the third-class over-the-counter drugs

distributed as the ethical drugs. As for Kampo medicines, 294 items are approved as OTC drugs and 148 items are approved as the ethical drugs. And the latter is listed in the National Health Insurance Drug Price Standard. Most of the crude drugs distributed in Japan are used as raw materials for manufacturing Kampo products.

As mentioned above, the classification of crude drugs by the usage in Japan is quite complicated due to many duplications (Fig. 4.1 and Table 4.2).

※Column: Examples of the Same Crude Drugs in Japan and China That Refer to Different Substances Derived from Different Plants [1, 2]

The origin of *toki* (当帰) in Japan is the dried root of *Angelica acutiloba* (Umbelliferae) (*toki* in Japanese), i.e., the term *toki* in Japanese is a polysemous word that refers to both the plant *Angelica acutiloba* and the crude drug derived from this plant. Its official English name in Japanese Pharmacopoeia is Japanese Angelica Root. In China, the origin of Angelica Root (当帰) is the dried root of *Angelica sinensis* (it is distributed under the name *karatoki* in Japan, but it is not approved by Japanese Pharmacopoeia). In Japan, the origin of *boi* (防已) is the dried stem and rhizome of *Sinomenium acutum* (Menispermaceae). In China, the origin of *fanji* 防己 (much similar but slightly different *kanji* (*Han*-letter) from Japanese 防已) is the root of *Stephania tetrandra*. In China, the dried stem and rhizome of *Sinomenium acutum* are distributed as the name of *qingfengteng*青風藤 (*seifuto* in Japanese). Since there are so many examples like these confusions, it is necessary to be careful in the identification of the origin of crude drugs by the differences between Japan and China, which use the same *kanji* (Han-letters).

※Column: Pharmacy-Made Pharmaceuticals

There are two classifications of pharmaceutical products in Japan: over-the-counter (OTC) drugs that consumers can purchase at pharmacies or drug stores without a prescription issued from physicians, and the ethical drugs that can be purchased generally based on the prescriptions. However, among the ethical drugs, the drugs that are not designated as the prescription drugs can be purchased without a prescription issued from physicians. Since OTC drugs are not covered by the health insurance, patients have to bear entire price when they purchase them. While when patients purchase the ethical drugs, they can bear the partial price of the drugs depending on their health insurance qualification (without the prescription issued by physicians, patients have to bear entire price). In addition, OTC drugs are further classified into categories 1, 2, and 3. The OTC drugs of the first category can be sold only by licensed pharmacists, but the products of the second and third categories can also be sold by registered sales clerks as well as licensed pharmacists. Many crude drugs, crude drug products, and Kampo products are classified into the second category of OTC drugs, and even non-pharmacists can sell them if they are qualified as registered sales clerks.

As a drug classification located between ethical drugs and OTC drugs, there are **pharmacy-made pharmaceuticals**. When pharmaceutical products are manufactured, the institutions have to pass the license of the pharmaceutical manufacture to produce pharmaceutical products. Since Kampo products are regulated as the same way, each pharmacy has to pass this license when the pharmacists belonging to the pharmacy opens the crude drug product packages manufactured by pharmaceutical manufacture and prepares the mixture of crude drugs as Kampo prescriptions in order to sell them. However, since extremely complicated procedures are required in order to pass the license, the items of pharmacy-made pharmaceuticals listed in the guideline supervised by the Ministry of Health, Labor and Welfare have been registered. The approval to sell pharmacy-made pharmaceuticals in pharmacy manufactured according to this guideline is easier than that of producing pharmaceutical products. Then, the licensed pharmacists can manufacture and sell Kampo products in pharmacy by this approval. In this guideline, 237 Kampo products have been approved as the pharmacy-made pharmaceuticals, and it is possible to have a business form so-called Kampo consultation pharmacy, where the pharmacists manufacture and sell Kampo products as pharmacy-made pharmaceuticals that suit each patient after consulting.

Pharmacy-made pharmaceuticals are the drug that can be sold at the discretion of the pharmacist without the prescription issued from physicians, but they are classified into the category of "pharmacy drugs" that cannot be sold by registered sales clerks, and the licensed pharmacists keep their usefulness and safety.

1.3 Quality Control of Crude Drugs and Handling of Contained Ingredients

Keywords: Origin, Marker constituents, Active constituents, Major constituents.

Crude drugs are pharmaceutical products and have not only beneficial properties but also the side effects. Therefore, the specialized knowledge is required to use them safely and effectively. Since crude drugs are made from naturally derived materials, it is fundamental that the quality of crude drugs varies depending on the regions where they were harvested and the season of the year. However, as long as they are pharmaceutical products, it is essential to maintain a certain level of quality.

In addition, when crude drugs are viewed as commercial products, their prices are usually higher than those of foods made from naturally derived materials. Since general consumers without specialized knowledge do not have the technique to know the quality of crude drugs, many counterfeit and inferior crude drug products had been distributed in past.

Therefore, when using crude drugs in Japan, the specialists such as licensed pharmacists are supposed to sell pharmaceutical products with a certain quality with the explanation how to use them. Approximately, 280 items of crude drugs (not all of them are used as the raw materials for Kampo products. They include the raw materials for folk medicines and Western crude drugs) are listed in the "Japanese Pharmacopoeia." Then, the quality of each crude drug is specified.

In order to distribute crude drugs as commercial pharmaceutical products conforming to the Japanese Pharmacopoeia, the products have (1) correct origins, (2) correct taste and smell, and (3) passed with various crude drug tests such as confirmation test, purity test, etc., that are specified in each individual crude drug. The **origin** of crude drug is the definition of the raw material of crude drugs, and in the case of animal or plant-derived crude drugs, the origin is defined and expressed as the species name of the organism with the medicinal part.

For example, in order to use ginger, which is also used as food, as crude drug product, the product is derived from the dried rhizome of *Zingiber officinale* (this is called the origin of ginger. The term "ginger" is also polysemy, which refers to both food and crude drug.) (Fig. 4.2). It must have a peculiar smell, an extremely spicy taste, the content of 6-gingerol can be confirmed by thin layer chromatography, and it must be recognized that the amount of heavy metal or other foreign substances are less than the specified amount. On the other hand, in the case of ginger in food market, there is no such quality regulation; therefore, consumers have to judge the quality, cost, and the taste of ginger food products to purchase them.

Although crude drugs contain innumerable chemical compounds, the ingredients used for quality control of crude drugs, such as 6-gingerol contained in ginger, are called the marker constituents defined in Japanese Pharmacopoeia. The marker constituent is a characteristic compound contained in the specific crude drug, and is defined in order to guarantee the quality by quantifying the presence or absence of the compound and to distinguish it from a similar crude drug or a foreign substance that is easily mixed as a fake drug. Therefore, the marker constituents are usually different from pharmacologically active constituents that show medicinal properties.

For example, the marker constituent of *daio* is sennoside A, and this compound is pharmacologically active constituent for its laxative effect, but the pharmacological efficiencies of *daio* cannot be fully explained by sennoside A. *Daio* product which has high content of sennoside A is suitable as a laxative; however, it is an unsuitable product that easily causes the side effect of diarrhea as a blood[TM] stasis-resolving drug in Kampo medicine. It is not enough that the content of the marker constituent is high, but it is important to keep it within a certain range from the viewpoint of quality assurance.

Since the quality of crude drug is not determined only by the content of marker constituent, the quality of crude drug in markets actually varies depending on the producing regions and manufacturers even if the name is the same. When pharmaceutical industries manufacture the Kampo extract preparation products (see p. X), they have the technology to alleviate the variation of such crude drugs by blending them well and to maintain the stable quality of the

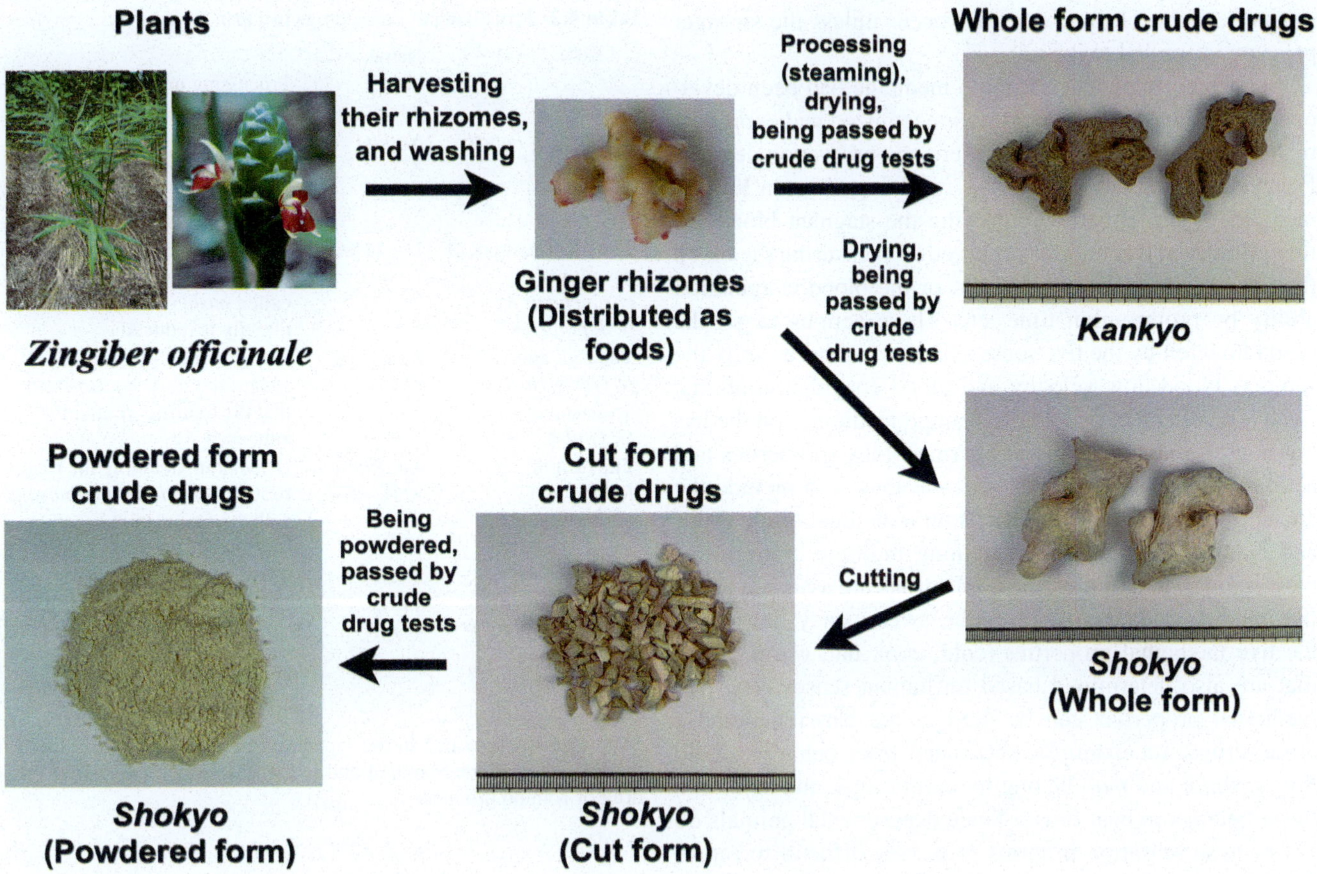

Fig. 4.2 The relationship of plant and crude drugsAs an example, the process from the production of *shokyo* from ginger (plant) is shown. Since *shokyo* is not an "exclusive drug" under the borderline of pharmaceuticals to non-pharmaceuticals (see Chap. 4, Sect. 1.1), its rhizome is also distributed as food. The rhizome of ginger (plant) is dried, and after passing the crude drug tests specified by the Japanese Pharmacopoeia, it becomes *shokyo* and is distributed as pharmaceutical product. The Japanese Pharmacopoeia stipulates three types of forms: whole form (raw), cut form (chopped), and powdered form (powder); the chopped and powdered forms are actually used in the preparations of Kampo medicine (small-sized whole crude drugs can be prepared without cutting). In addition, the crude drug processed ginger *kankyo* is the one that has been produced (see Chap. 4, Sect. 1.5) by steaming the rhizome of raw ginger (plant), drying it, and passing the crude drug test. *Shokyo* and *kankyo* are made from the same origin, but are expected as the different effects in Kampo medicine

final product. However, since this process is possible only when a large amount of preparation is produced, a pharmacist's connoisseur is required when dispensing crude drugs for decoction in a pharmacy according to the symptoms of individual patients.

※Column: Expression of the Ingredients of Crude Drugs

The term "main component," which is often used in general, is not used in current pharmacognosy. The term "main" includes the meaning of high content. For example, the compound (main component) with the highest content in rhubarb is starch, which the plant itself stores as a nutrient source, but starch is not an important constituent when using rhubarb as a crude drug. What is important as a drug is a marker constituent that proves quality control or the pharmacologically active constituent that shows medicinal properties, and these are sometimes expressed as the premiere component.

1.4 Modern Pharmacology (*Yakuri*) and Traditional Pharmacology (Properties and Actions, *Yakuno*) of Crude Drugs

Since crude drugs are pharmaceutical products, they naturally have some useful effects on the living body. When describing the action of pharmaceutical products on a living body, there is the term pharmacology. In modern Western medicine, where pharmacology has developed, the pharmacological action of a drug refers to the content that can be reproduced and proved by experiments. For example, when a rabbit is infected with a certain virus, the body temperature of the rabbit rises. When a drug having an antipyretic effect is administered to a rabbit, the increased body temperature decreases. When a drug having a diuretic effect is administered to a rat, the urine volume increases. When a drug with an analgesic effect is administered to mice, the escape reaction of mice does not occur unless the stronger pressure is applied to the tail.

In ancient times when Kampo medicine had been developed, the efficacy of all drugs was recognized and expressed by human senses because there were no observation devices. For example, the blood[TM1] stasis-resolving effect in Kampo medicine is the effect of improving the stagnant blood[TM1] flow. However, it cannot be observed by measuring the blood flow using a laser Doppler meter, or the blood coagulation ability by prothrombin time, etc. These actions target the blood flow felt by the five senses, and are not necessarily the same as blood flow velocity and blood coagulation ability. Such kind of action peculiar to Kampo medicines on the living body is called traditional pharmacology (properties and actions, *yakuno*). Sometimes, *yakuno* may also include the ancient pharmacological ideas. Both individual crude drugs and Kampo prescriptions containing multiple crude drugs have *yakuno*. In addition, the crude drugs are assigned to the five medicinal flavors (acid, bitter, sweet, spicy, salty) and the five medicinal properties (cold, cool, flat, warm, heat), that are also determined based on human senses. The five medicinal properties can be used as the classification for crude drugs, for example, *sekko* and *oren* belong to cold drugs, *ninjin* and *mao* belong to warm drugs, and *kojin* and *bushi* belongs to heat drugs. Since experimental animals do not express sensation in terms, it is very difficult to reproduce *yakuno* of crude drugs and Kampo prescriptions in the experiments, and the clinical trials using human beings who expressed their sensitivities as terms are the only way to clarify *yakuno* scientifically.

Crude drugs contain innumerable chemical compounds, and some specific compounds of them act on the living body as the pharmacologically active ingredients. However, since it is difficult to carry out the experiments to reproduce *yakuno*, the active ingredients that indicate *yakuno* of crude drugs have usually been unknown. On the other hand, digitalis, a Western crude drug, has a pharmacology called cardiotonic action, and as a result of the pharmacological experiments, it has been clarified that its active ingredient is digoxin. Digoxin, which can ensure the quality with a numerical value such as 99% purity, is easier to use as a pharmaceutical product than crude drug digitalis, having variations about the contents of compounds. Therefore, digitalis, a crude drug, has now been deleted from the Japanese Pharmacopoeia. The term "digitalis" is used only as a classification term for cardiotonics in current medicine. In this way, that the active ingredients are still unknown is one of the reasons for continuing to use crude drugs in Kampo medicine. The ingredients contained in the crude drugs listed in Chap. 9 are sometimes not pharmacologically active ingredients but just as marker ingredients.

Table 4.3 Processing of crude drugs in Japan

Origin	Name before processing	Processing method and the name after processing
The root of *Panax ginseng*	*Ninjin* (人参)	Dried after steaming the fresh root of *Panax ginseng* is called *Kojin* (紅参). It is said that the tonic effect is enhanced
The tuberous root of *Aconitum carmichaeli* or *A. Japonicum*	*Uzu* (烏頭)[a]	Dried after autoclaving the dried root of aconite root is called *bushi* (附子). The toxicity is reduced
The root and stolon of *Glycyrrhiza uralensis* or *G. Glabra*	*Kanzo* (甘草)	Baked using fire is called *shakanzo* (炙甘草). It is said that the tonifing-*qi* effect is enhanced
The root of *Rehmannia glutinosa*	*Jio, Kanjio* (地黄, 乾地黄)	Dried after steaming the fresh root of *Rehmannia glutinosa* is called *jukujio* (熟地黄). It is said that the tonifing-blood[TM1] effect is enhanced
The rhizome of *Zingiber officinale*	*Shokyo* (生姜)	Dried after steaming the fresh rhizome of *Zingiber officinale* is called *Kankyo* (乾姜). It is said that the interior-warming effect is enhanced

[a]Although not specified in the Japanese Pharmacopoeia, it is listed in the NHI Drug Price Standard and is used as a raw material for crude drug or Kampo products

1.5 Processing of Crude Drugs

Processing is the technique for crude drugs to modify the pharmacological actions such as increasing effectiveness or reducing toxic action by performing other processing techniques other than drying and cutting, though the origin of crude drug is the same part of the same plant species as a raw material. In traditional Chinese medicine, processing is often conducted, but not as much in Japan, and the following five items are registered in Japanese Pharmacopoeia (Table 4.3).

Column: Processing in Traditional Chinese Medicine
Chukajimminkyowakokuyakuten 中華人民共和国薬典 *(Pharmacopeia of the People's Republic of China)* specifies various processing methods for crude drugs by establishing general rules. In Japan, only processing in crude drugs are used by heating or steaming, but in China, the processing supplements such as honey, ginger juice, Shaoxing wine, wheat bran (wheat seed coat), and river sand are often used. For example, the Japanese Pharmacopoeia registers processed licorice (*shakanzo*, 炙甘草) as roasted one, but the Chinese Pharmacopoeia registers 炙甘草 as roasted one soaked in honey. Therefore, 炙甘草 refers to the different substances in the Japanese and Chinese Pharmacopoeia. In addition, *hange* (半夏), which has a unique irritating taste, is

considered to be a poison in China, and is often used as processed 半夏 where the irritating taste is removed by dipping it in ginger juice or alum. (The irritating taste of *hange* disappears by preparing the decoction by boiling it in water, so no toxicity appears when *hange* is used as the hot water decoction.) The processing methods of crude drugs are also one of the differences between Japanese Kampo medicine and traditional Chinese medicine.

2 Theory for Combining Crude Drugs to Make Kampo Formulas

Toshiaki MakinoTatsuhiko Suzuki, Yoshiharu Tobina and Kazuyoshi Kawazoe

2.1 Combination Theory for Crude Drugs

Regardless of Western or Oriental medicines, it is rare to use a single drug when performing pharmacotherapeutics; typically multiple drugs are mixed and prescribed according to the patient's symptoms. In ancient Chinese medicine, which is the origin of Kampo medicine, many formulas have already been created for various pathological conditions since before the Common Era. The original formulae for the current Kampo medicines (Kampo formulas, Kampo prescriptions) were introduced from ancient China to Japan. These were given unique names as promised prescriptions after modifying the ingredients in the development of Japanese Kampo medicine.

The theory for combining pairs of crude drugs is called **drug pairs** (*yakutui*). Drug pairs have been described in classical pharmacopeia texts. The change in pharmacology (*yakuno*) when a pair is combined is called **seven relations** (*shichi-jo*). Today, the seven relations are explained as the following six relations (the seven relations combines the six relations with the effect of a drug used singly).

①. Combination that enhances drug efficacy

Mutual promotion: By combining crude drugs, they enhance each other's actions.

Mutual enhancement: One drug enhances the efficacy of another main crude drug.

②. Combination that diminishes toxic effects

Incompatibility: One drug weakens the toxicity of another main crude drug.

Counteract toxicity of another drug: One main crude drug weakens the toxicity of another drug.

③. Contraindications

Mutual inhibition: By combining crude drugs, their actions are canceled out.

Clashing antagonism: Combining crude drugs causes new toxicity.

The theory for understanding the combination of crude drugs in Kampo formula, or for assembling Kampo formula, is called Sovereign, Minister, and Assistant and Guide. These terms are likened to the ancient government system. In the early textbooks of herbalism, crude drugs were classified into three groups, upper, middle, and lower. Classical texts describe the roles of these three groups related to the groups of Sovereign, Minister, and Assistant and Guide, respectively. The rule for composing a formula in the Shinsen style was "one Sovereign, two Ministers, and five Assistants and Guides" or "one Sovereign, three Ministers, and nine Assistants and Guides." In this system, each crude drug was classified into the abovementioned three groups, and this classification had not been changed over time.

The 74th chapter *(Zhizhenyaodalun)* of "*Somon* 素問 *(Basic Questions)*" suggests "one Sovereign and two Ministers," "two Sovereigns and three Ministers," "two Sovereigns and four Ministers," or "two Sovereigns and six Ministers." Thus the rule of combination was broader and physicians could understand the role of Sovereign, Minister, and Assistant and Guide in a formula. After this, the roles of each crude drug belonging to the groups of Monarch, Minister, and Assistant and Guide were changed depending on the era.

The roles of Sovereign, Minister, and Assistant and Guide are recognized as follows:

Sovereign drugs: The drug with main action of the formula.

Minister drugs: They play a role in assisting Sovereign drugs and regulating the action.

Assistant and guide drugs: They treat the accompanying symptoms or relieve the effects of other drugs when they are too strong.

Although the classification of Sovereign, Minister, and Assistant and Guide drugs were derived from ancient herbalism and not all the formulas were created with this system, this system can be used for interpreting formulas.

Later, the group Assistant and Guide were separated, and this four-group system was applied to consider which meridians the crude drugs acted on.

In classical Kampo medicine, the principle is to assemble and administer Kampo prescription that suits each patient's condition as in Western medicine. In Japan today, however, it is popular to use prescriptions created by predecessors as is, without modification. The use of ethical or medical Kampo products follows this precedent.

2.2 Classification of Kampo Medicines

Various combinations of crude drugs comprise Kampo prescriptions, and one prescription is indicated for multiple pathological conditions. Therefore, it is difficult to comprehensively classify these prescriptions without duplication. Even in classic texts of prescriptions, it is common to classify the prescriptions by diseases and to arrange the applicable prescriptions, so that one prescription is often listed in several categories. Under these circumstances, Japanese traditional Kampo medicine classifies the prescriptions described in *Shokanzatsubyoron* (Treatise on Cold Damage Diseases) by focusing on the basic prescriptions and organizing similar prescriptions of the crude drugs' components in consideration of the pathology (classification using related formulas). This was the method often adopted throughout the Edo and Showa era [3, 4].

2.2.1 The Method Focusing on the Major Prescriptions (Classification Using Related Formulas)

The classification using related formulas, which is categorized by the main prescription, was found in medical texts of *Koho* school in the Edo period, and was also adopted by the classicist school. It was also mainly adopted in *Koho* school in the Showa period, and had been partially adopted by *Gosei* school. In particular, the prescriptions described in *Shokanzatsubyoron* (Treatise on Cold Damage Diseases) changes the prescription according to the disease pattern, so the classification using related formulas contribute to the understanding of the prescription. In Japan, there are relatively few prescriptions that are covered by health insurance, and most of them are prescriptions from *Shokanzatsubyoron*. Therefore, the classification using related formulas is easy to use.

The following are examples of classifications of related formulas in the Edo and Showa period.

Formulas in keishito group, Maoto-group, Kakkonto-group (Fig. 4.3a), Saikoto-group (Fig. 4.3b), formulas in jokito group, formulas in shashinto group, *Goreisan* group, formulas in ninjinto group, Hangeto-group, Kanzoto-group, Shishito-group, Kyukito-group, formulas in shigyakuto group, Kososan-group, Heiisan-group, Nizhinto-group, Shikunshito-group, *Jinkigan* group, Byakkoto-group.

Today, the classification is often combined with the characteristic crude drugs in the prescription and the classification using related formula, such as the formulas with Ephedra Herb, the formulas with Bupleurum root, the formula including *ogon* and *oren*, the formulas with Rhubarb, the formulas with Gypsum, the formulas with Ginseng and Astragalus root, the formulas with Rehmannia root, and the formulas with Processed Aconite root. The classification method based on one or two crude drugs has a different principle from the classification using related formula based on the disease pattern, and there is a difference in the classification.

2.2.2 Classification Using the Effect of Kampo Formulas

In addition to the classification using related formula, the prescriptions are sometimes classified using the expressions that indicate the effect and properties of the prescription. As mentioned above, Kampo prescriptions are often used for the multiple disease patterns, and some crude drugs in the prescription play various roles, and the prescriptions are composed by combining them. Therefore, it is difficult to make a solid classification without any duplication by belonging to only one category. The following are examples of widely accepted categories.

Tonic formulas are formulas to tonify the body and restore the weaken body. Tonic formulas are further classified as follows according to the object to be tonified.

Qi tonifying formulas: Tonic formulas for qi deficiency. Sometimes called spleen[TM1] tonifying formulas (e.g., Shikunshito, Hochekkito, etc.)

Blood[TM1] tonifying formulas: Tonic formulas for blood[TM1] deficiency (e.g., Shimotsuto, Tokishaykuaykuysan, etc.)

Yin tonifying formulas: Tonic formulas for yin, fluid[TM1], and blood[TM1] deficiencies. Sometimes called yin nourishing formulas (e.g., Jiinkokato, Jiinshihoto, etc.)

Kidney[TM1] tonifying formulas: Tonic formulas for kidney[TM1] deficiency (e.g., Rokumigan, Hachimijiogan, Goshajinkigan, etc.)

Warming and tonifying formulas: Tonic formulas for deficiency cold patterns (e.g., Shinbuto, Maobushisaisinto, Hachimijiogan, etc.)

Draining formulas are formulas to expel pathogens (e.g., Orengedokuto, etc.). Draining formulas are further classified as follows according to the object to be drained.

Qi regulating formulas: Formulas to treat qi stagnation, qi depression. Formulas to treat qi counter flow in particular are called qi descending formulas (e.g., Hangekobokuto, etc.)

Blood[TM] stasis resolving formulas: Formulas to remove static blood[TM] (e.g., Keishibukuryogan, Tokisyakuyakusan, Tokaujokito, Daiobotanpito, etc.)

Fluid[TM1] regulating formulas: Formulas to treat fluid[TM1] retention (e.g., Goreisan, Ryokeijukkanto, Boiogito, etc.)

Exterior releasing formulas: Formulas to treat exterior patterns and to release pathogens on the body surface by sweating. Sometimes called sweat inducing formulas (e.g., Maoto, Kakkonto, etc.)

Purgative formulas: Formulas to relieve constipation (e.g., Daiokanzoto, Daojokito, etc.)

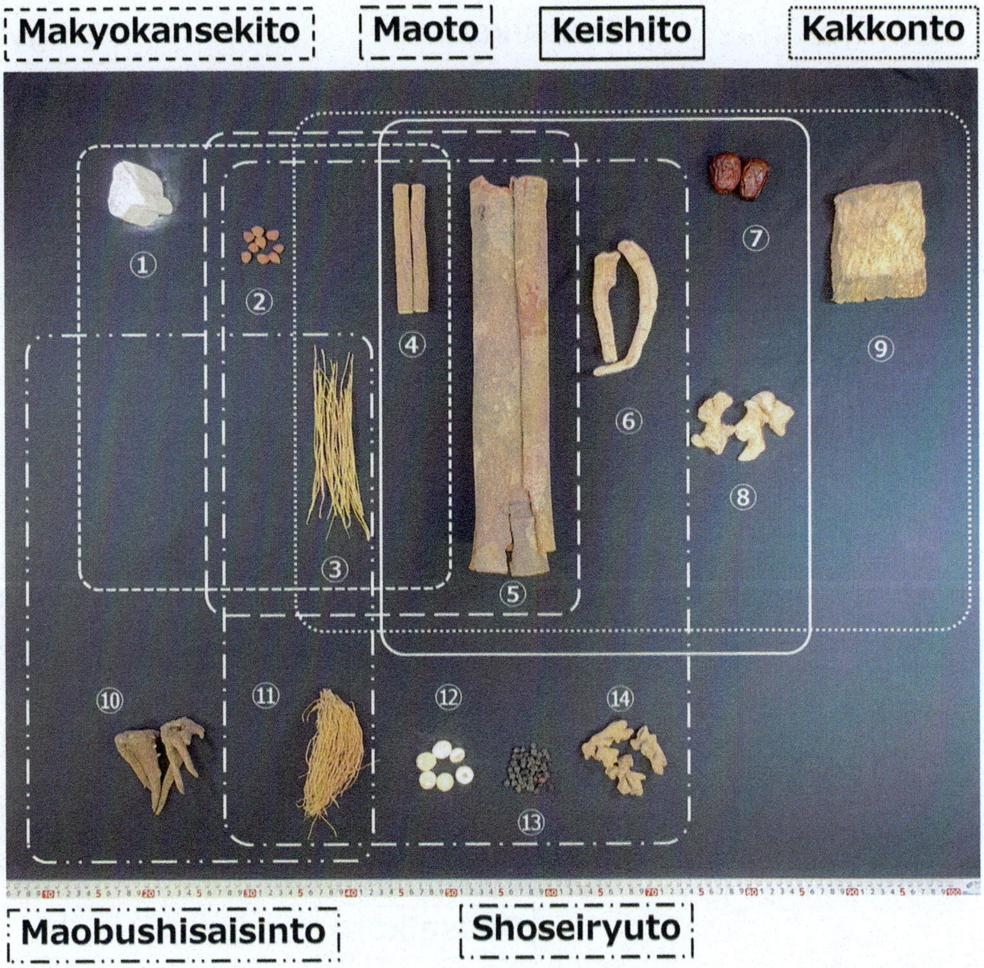

Fig. 4.3a Formulas in Keishito and Maoto groups During the early yang stage pattern period, a formula containing ⑤ Cinnamon Bark and ③Ephedra Herb (exterior releasing formulas) is used to induce sweating. If the patients have strong heat patterns, use ① Gypsum, which has a heat-clearing effect. if the patients have strong cold patterns and the disease has progressed to the middle yin stage pattern, use Processed Aconite Root, that has a warming effect, ② Apricot Kernel, ④ Glycyrrhiza, ⑥ Peony Root, ⑦ Jujube, ⑧ Ginger, ⑨ Pueraria Root, Asiasarum Root, Pinellia Tuber, Schisandra Fruit, Processed Ginger

Heat clearing formulas: Formulas to treat heat patterns with cooling crude drugs (e.g., Orengedokuto, Byakkokaninjinto).

Harmonizing formulas: Formulas to eliminate pathogens in the body by harmonizing the organs, without the actions of sweating, vomiting, and purgation (e.g., Shosaikoto, etc.)

Column: Why Does the Formula Keishito Contain Keihi and Not Keishi?

The current "Japanese Pharmacopoeia" and "non-Pharmacopoeial crude drugs"define the origin of *keihi* (桂皮) as the dried bark of *Cinnamomum cassia* and the origin of *keishi* (桂枝) as its twigs (see Chap. 9). On the other hand, in the current Chinese Pharmacopoeia, the crude drug whose origin is the bark of *C. cassia* is *rougui* (肉桂), and the crude drug whose origin is the twig of *C. cassia*. That is, Japanese keihi (桂皮) and Chinese *rougui* (肉桂) are synonymous, and桂枝 refer to the same substance in Japan and China. In China, the term 桂皮 refers to the spice made from the bark of other plants such as *C. tenuifolium* and *C. tamala*. However, what the crude drug named 桂枝 refers to has been changed depending on the periods and is quite confusing.

In mainland China, in the early Qing dynasty, *Bencaochengyabanji* (1647), both the twig and bark of *Cinnamon* sp. is 桂枝, thin trunk skin of *Cinnamon* sp. is 桂皮, and thick trunk skin of *Cinnamon* sp. is 肉桂. In the latter half of the Qing dynasty, in *Bencaoshugouyuam* (1833), 桂皮 is a general term for 肉桂, 桂皮, etc., and the bark is 肉桂, finely chopped bark is 桂枝. That is, all 桂枝, 桂皮, 肉桂 referred to the bark of *Cinnamon* sp. In *Bencaobiandu* (1887), the name of 桂皮 disappeared, 肉桂 was the bark, and 桂枝 was the twig, and then, this classification had been continued in the current Chinese Pharmacopoeia.

On the other hand, in Japan, in *Honsobenmei* (1772), 桂皮 as the name of crude drug did not appear, and the thick bark of *Cinnamon* sp. was 肉桂and the thin bark was 桂枝. In the late Edo period, Ono Ranzan's *Honzokomokukeimo* 本草綱目啓蒙 *(Elucidation of Compendium of Materia Medica)* (1803–05) stated that the thick bark of *Cinnamon* sp. was 肉桂, and that the bark of thin branches of *Cinnamon* sp. was both 桂枝 and 桂皮. After that, the Japanese Pharmacopoeia first edition (1886) edited with reference to

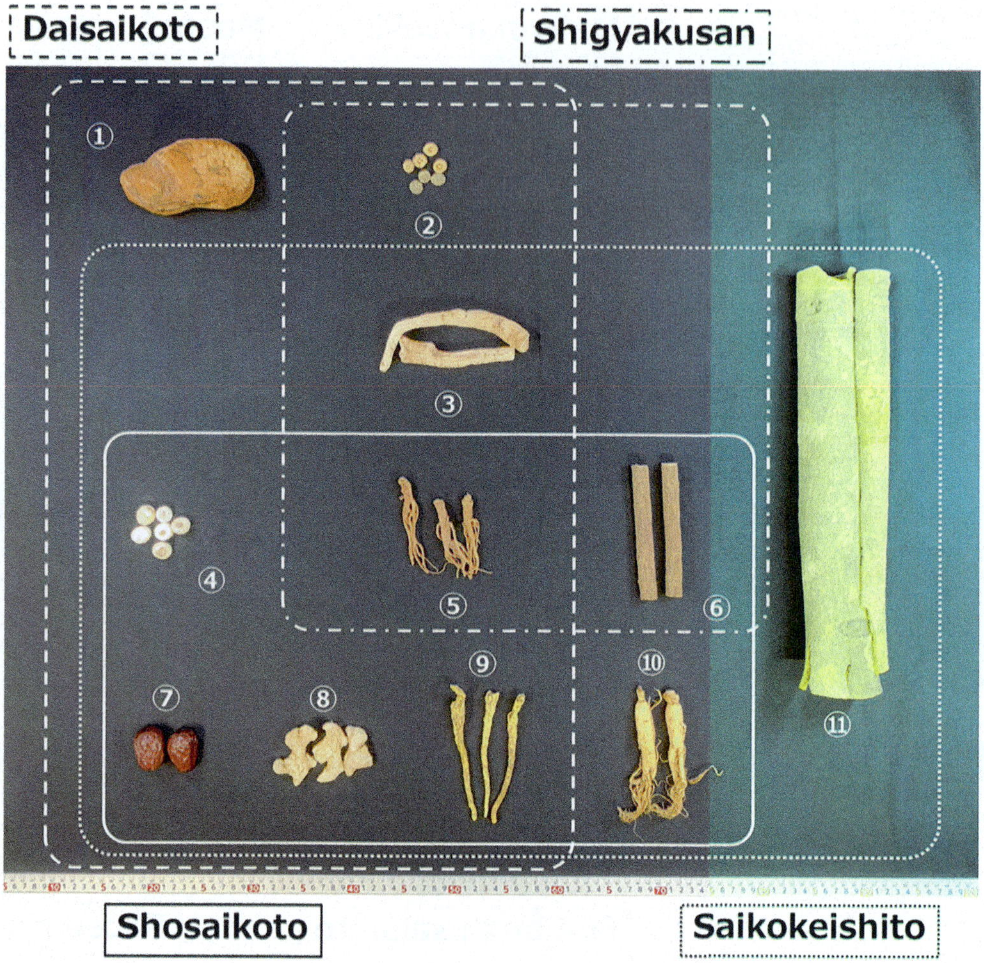

Fig. 4.3b Formulas containing Bupleurum Root During late yang stage pattern, harmonizing formulas, containing ⑤ Bupleurum Root and ⑨ Scutellaria Root, are used to harmonize pathogenic qi that has invaded into half-exterior, half-interior in the body. Bupleurum Root is also prescribed in the formulas to eliminate qi stagnation① Rhubarb, ② Immature Orange, ③ Peony Root, ④ Pinellia Tuber, ⑥ Glycyrrhiza, ⑦ Jujube, ⑧ Ginger, Ginseng, Cinnamon Bark

the Dutch Pharmacopoeia, 桂皮 was listed as a Western crude drug (see Chap. 4, Sect. 1.2), and it was defined as the bark of *C. cassia* as it is today. This definition has held until now.

By the way, in medicinal texts before the Song dynasty such as *Shanhalun* (*Shokanzatsubyoron,* Treatise of Cold Damage), the term 桂 or 桂心 was used. When this text was revised in the Song dynasty, it was uniformly rewritten as 桂枝. However, crude drugs made from the bark of *Cinnamon* sp. had been continued to be used, and crude drug names such as 桂心 continued to be used. Therefore, it is thought that the relationship between the crude drug name and what it refers to had been confused.

From the above, *keishi* (桂枝) obviously should be included in Keishito (桂枝湯), but it is clear that it depends on the historical period whether the term 桂枝 refers to the bark or the twig of *Cinnamon* sp. Currently in Japan, most pharmaceutical companies manufacture and sell Kampo products using *keihi* according to the Japanese Pharmacopoeia, and other pharmaceutical companies use *keishi* as a raw material. Even if the names of Kampo medicines are the same, the raw materials used are different for each pharmaceutical company because they reflect a complicated historical background.

Column: The Classification Method of the Formulas in Traditional Chinese Medicine

The classification method of the Qing Dynasty text, *"Ihoshukai 医方集解 (Collected Exegesis of Prescriptions)"* was accepted in both China and Japan. Traditional Chinese Medicine today uses a classification method that has been further developed from "*Ihoshukai* 医方集解 *(Collected Exegesis of Prescriptions).*" This system have become established not only in China but as an international standard. Some of these can be applied to the formulas in Kampo medicine. Only the classification names of formulas in traditional Chinese medicine are listed below.

Exterior-releasing formulas (pungent warm exterior-releasing formula, pungent cool exterior-releasing formula, exterior-interior dual releasing formula), purgative formulas (cold purgative formula, warm purgative formula, lubricant laxative formula, water[TM1]-expelling formula), harmonizing formula (lesser yang harmonizing formula, liver[TM1] and spleen[TM1] harmonizing formula, gastrointestinal harmonizing formula), heat clearing formula (qi aspect heat clearing formula, nutrient aspect clearing and blood[TM]-cooling formula, heat-clearing toxin-releasing formula, heat-clearing hotness dispelling formula), warming interior formula (center-warming and cold-dispelling formula, returning yang and counterflow-stopping formula, channels-warming and cold-dissipating formula), tonifying formula (qi-supplementing formula, blood[TM1]-tonifying formulas, qi and blood-tonifying formulas, yin-supplementing formula, yang-supplementing formula, yin and yang dual supplementation formula), astringent formula, tranquillizing formula, resuscitative formula, qi-regulating formulas (qi-moving formula, qi-descending formula), blood[TM1]-regulating formula (blood[TM1]-moving and stasis-dispelling formula, blood[TM1]-stanching formula), wind-relieving formula, dryness-relieving formula, dampness dispelling formula (dampness-drying and stomach harmonizing formula, heat-clearing and dampness-dispelling formula, water[TM]-disinhibiting and dampness-percolating formula, cold dampness warming and transforming formula), phlegm expelling formula (dampness-drying and phlegm-transforming formula, heat-clearing and phlegm-transforming formula), digestive formula, anthelmintic formula, emetic formula.

3 Clinical Pharmacognosy

Crude drugs (herbs) are distributed as pharmaceutical products individually, but they are processed, combined, and distributed as herbal products and Kampo products. This chapter summarizes the knowledge and precautions required when using them in the clinical setting.

3.1 Pharmaceutics in Crude Drugs and Kampo Medicines

Toshiaki MakinoTatsuhiko Suzuki, Yoshiharu Tobina and Kazuyoshi Kawazoe

Dosage forms of Kampo medicines include (1) decoction, (2) powder, (3) pills, and (4) ointment. These each correspond to the terms of *to*, *san*, *gan*, and *ko* at the end of the names of Kampo formulas (Fig. 4.4). In rare cases, there may be something other than these four terms at the end of the formula name (XX-in, XX-ho, etc.), but in these cases, the formula is often prepared as a decoction. For each mixture of cut crude drugs, (1) put the mixture in water and boil them (decoction), (2) make the mixture into powder and mix them, (3) knead the mixed powder with concentrated honey and shape into a ball, (4) put in an ointment base that is a mixture of vegetable oil and animal fat; heat and then cool and harden to create the product. Furthermore, only (1) is prepared at the time of use, and as will be described later in the next section, the pharmacy provides the patient with a mixture of cut crude drugs (corresponding to the tea preparation in the Japanese Pharmacopoeia) as a drug prescription, after which patients brew the decoction on their own.

Since it is a burden for the patient to prepare the decoction on their own, the extract preparation has been developed in Japan as the standard dosage form. These extract preparations are further processed by adding an excipient such as lactose and a binder such as starch to produce granules, tablets, capsules, etc. for ease of use. These dosage forms are called Kampo extract products (in general, the expression "extract preparation" is often used as an abbreviation for Kampo extract products. Strictly speaking, however, they are different concepts). Since the Kampo extract products have many advantages over the decoction, it greatly contributed to the spread of Kampo medicine (Table 4.4). At present, Kampo extract products prepared from decoctions are commercially available for items that are not in their original dosage forms, such as Tokishakuyakusan and Hachimijiogan. In such cases, the term of *ryo* is added at the end of the formula name *san* or *gan*, when prepared as decoction. Depending on the pharmaceutical company, the term *ryo* is omitted even if it is an extract preparation.

3.2 Pharmacy in Crude Drugs and Kampo Medicines

Toshiaki MakinoTatsuhiko Suzuki, Yoshiharu Tobina and Kazuyoshi Kawazoe

3.2.1 Storage and Management of Crude Drugs and Kampo Products

Raw materials for ethical crude drugs are distributed in cut form with a size that is easy to dispense, or in powdered form. These are packaged in plastic bags of 500 g units from pharmaceutical industries and delivered to pharmacies. In this state, since the inside of the bag is replaced with nitrogen with oxygen scavenger, it can be stored relatively stable in a dark place. Once the bag is opened and transferred to the druggist's chest of drawers (*hyakumi* chest), however, crude drugs sometimes absorb moisture, pests sprout, mold grows, and essential oil components are lost due to volatilization with extended storage periods. In principle, they should be used promptly after opening the package, and if possible, they should be stored in a sealable container such as Tupperware®.

At present, the price of raw materials for crude drug for ethical use is rising, and the drug prices of crude drugs covered by health insurance are lower than the prices of crude drugs purchased by pharmacies from wholesalers. This may result in a deficit for pharmacies (Table 4.5). Furthermore, it

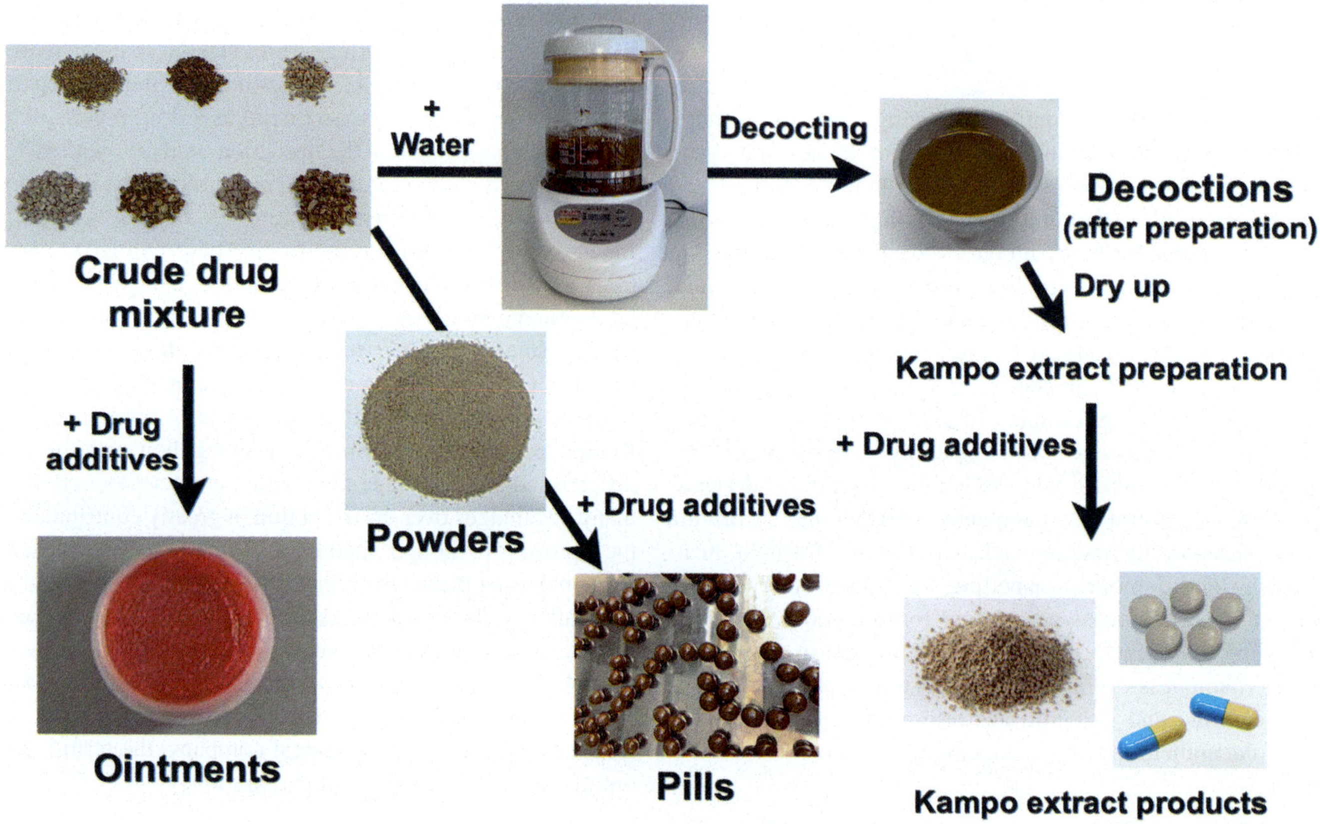

Fig. 4.4 Various dosage forms of Kampo medicines. In OTC Kampo products, various dosage forms such as granules, tablets, capsules, drinks, chewables, or jelly forms made from the extracts are commercially available

becomes difficult for pharmacies to accept the prescriptions calling for crude drugs because it costs a lot of money for pharmacies to maintain and dispense ethical crude drugs, including maintaining the quality of crude drugs and the labor involved in dispensing [5, 6].

At pharmacies, when charging for the crude drugs alone will result in a deficit, this is covered by dispensing technical fees, etc. Additional technical fees are not billable for prescriptions of 28 days or more. This is why long-term prescriptions should be avoided. It is necessary to devise ways to maintain use of crude drugs by the decoction method, which is the original form of Kampo medicinal practice. This can be done by cooperation between doctors, pharmacists, wholesalers of crude drugs, and patients. One way is to get patients to purchase crude drugs that are sold as foods out of pocket, and not include these on the prescription sheet.

In general, Kampo extract products are highly hygroscopic. When they are stored in an unsealed state, they will absorb moisture and solidify. Most Kampo extract products delivered from pharmaceutical companies are packed in heat-sealed plastic sheets to prevent absorbing moisture. When pharmacists dispense the granule form of Kampo extract products to prepare pharmacy packages, consumers are advised to keep them in a sealable container with a desiccant or in a refrigerator. Even in the case of herb mixtures (teabag preparations) for preparing decoctions, insect damage can be prevented by storing them in a refrigerator.

3.2.2 Preparation of Decoctions

If physicians want to prescribe Kampo products that are not approved for medical usage or to adjust the dose of crude drugs according to the patient's condition, they can write in individual crude drugs on the prescription sheet; pharmacists then prepare a decoction (tea prescription) by it.

When pharmacists prepare a decoction (tea preparation), the cut herbs for the required number of days are weighed together and then packaged in wrapping paper (Fig. 4.5). Since the shape and weight of each piece of herb is different, the blending of cut herbs is not as good as that of powdered herbs. Therefore, it is desirable to place each cut herb in a packaging machine and keep the herbs separate. Particular attention should be paid to the packaging of heavy herbs such as *sekko*, light herbs such as *hakka*, and highly toxic ones like *uzu*.

If the packaging is Japanese paper or non-woven fabric, it can be set in a decoction pot just like a tea bag, which simplifies the work performed by the patient. In this case, it is better to use a larger size package so that the herbs spread in the

Table 4.4 Advantages and disadvantages of extract products and decoctions in Kampo medicines

	Extract products	Decoction
Advantages in extract products	Can be taken immediately	Takes time to prepare
	Convenient to carry	Requires a water bottle to carry it
	Good compliance	Patients may stop taking due to cumbersome preparation
	The taste can be masked by formulation	Difficult to drink due to bitterness depending on formulas
	Quality is stable	The quality of the final dose varies since it is prepared by individual patients
	It will not get damp easily if the package is not opened. (the expiration date is fixed for each company)	The crude drug mixture before pre-decoction can have problems such as insect damage or mold due to long-term storage. It should be taken immediately after decocting
	Placebo can be made for clinical trials	Difficult to make a placebo
Disadvantages in extract products	For ethical use, it is limited to 148 formulas. Physicians or pharmacists cannot change the prescription	The dosages of crude drugs can be changed (portions can be adjusted) according to the patient's symptoms
	When used in combination, there may be overdose due to crude drug duplication	When prescribing a combined formula, the amount of overlapping crude drugs can be adjusted
	Even with the same formula name, the efficacy and prescription content of the products approved by the government are sometimes different	Since there is no specific disease name for the approved indication, it can be prescribed relatively freely according to the patient's symptoms
	Low volatile component content in the formulation	Volatile components tend to remain even in the final state
	Lactose used as an excipient may sometimes cause gastrointestinal disorders	–
	Prescriptions that originally came as powders and pills are also supplied as extracts	–

Table 4.5 Examples where the prices of NHI Drug Price Standard are lower than the wholesale prices (yen per 10 g)

	Wholesale price	NHI Drug Price Standard (as of July 2020)
Saiko (made in China)	80	45.3
Kanzo (made in China)	35	20.9
Ninjin (made in Japan)	420	176.4
Mao (made in China)	21	12.3

package when decocting. Nevertheless, Japanese paper has the disadvantage being opaque and hard to check the contents after dispensing. In that case, transparent plastic packaging is also possible. If there is no automatic herb packaging machine, it has to be literally hand packed, which is a lot of work.

After the pharmacist dispenses the herbs (tea preparation), patients must decoct it on their own. Since the manner of decoction varies greatly by the patient [7], it is important for the pharmacist to explain the procedure. When preparing a decoction, 400–600 mL of tap water is usually added to the daily dose of crude drugs and then boiled for 30–50 min. The decoction is squeezed and strained while still hot. It is then taken in 2 to 3 divided doses.

Aside from this, to produce decoctions for standard granular extracts specified by the Ministry of Health, Labor and Welfare, 10–20 times of the amount of tap water to the weight of the daily herb dosage is added and this mixture is decocted for 30–40 min. The heat and time of decoction are adjusted so the volume of decoction fluid is reduced to about half after being boiled. To decoct herbs, decocting machines are commercially available from several manufacturers. It is desirable to reduce the variation in the procedure of the decoction by using decocting machines. If the heat and time of decocting are kept consistent, however, it is fine to decoct herbs in a regular pot.

After decocting, remove the crude drug residue with a tea strainer, etc. while it is still hot. The decoction is taken in 2–3 doses, but the remaining solution should be stored in a sealed container and warmed in a microwave oven immediately just before drinking. The decoction can be stored at room temperature for about one day (preferably stored in the refrigerator), but mold may sometimes grow in the refrigerator, so

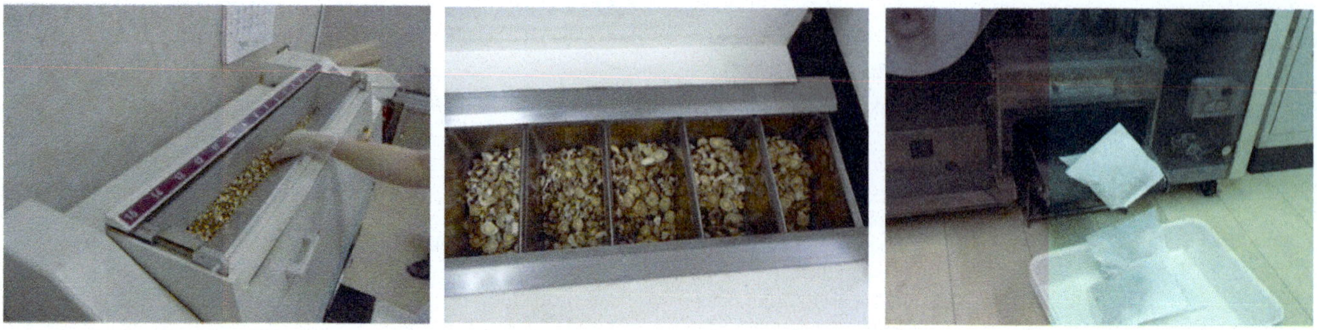

Fig. 4.5 Packaging using automatic herb packaging machine

storage for more than two days should be avoided in the liquid state. To keep longer, it is necessary to freeze it in a freezer.

Depending on the prescription, patients may be instructed to add individual herbs to boiling water instead of decocting the herb mixture at the same time. The action of *chotoko* diminishes when it is boiled for a long time [8]. The decoction time of *daio* is also adjusted to regulate the elution of its laxative active ingredients [9]. These herbs are sometimes to be added after decocting other crude drugs, and to be decocted only for the last 5–15 min. This is called post-decocting. *Hakka*, *soyo*, and *keihi*, which contain a large amount of essential oil components, that are volatilized and lost by the decoction when the decoction time is long [10], so post-decocting is sometimes recommended. For *akyo*, and *koi*, the other herbs are decocted and dissolved directly in the decoctions after removing the residue. For *uzu*, if the decocting time is short, the decomposition of highly toxic alkaloids will be insufficient [11]. Therefore, decocting time needs to be adjusted strictly to control the balance between efficacy and toxicity.

Column: Interactions Among Crude Drugs During the Decoction Process

The instruction in the *Shokanron* (Treatise of Cold Damage) for preparing a prescription containing *mao* is to first put the *mao* in water and decoct, then remove the froth, and then other herbs are added to decoct the mixture further. That is, *mao* required pre-decoction. When *mao* is decocted in water, however, it actually doesn't produce froth, so the meaning of the above instruction had been a mystery. Fueki et al. revealed that the difference lay in water quality between Japan and mainland China. Froth was produced when herbs were decocted with tap water in Beijing. The hardness components of water used for decoction there (Ca^{2+}, Mg^{2+}, etc.) affects the occurrence of froth [12]. In fact, this froth adsorbs ephedrine alkaloids, and this froth is discarded when the herbal residue is filtered, and this reduces the extraction efficiency. By decocting *mao* and *taiso* at the same time, citric acid contained in Jujube chelates the hardness component, softens the water, and makes it less likely to froth, thereby improving its extraction efficiency.

It is also known that the elution of alkaloids from herbs into the decoction varies depending on the pH of the decoction. Since *taiso*, *kanzo*, and *gomishi* acidify the decoction, decocting at the same time as *mao* and *bushi* increases the elution of alkaloids from these herbs into the decoction [13]. Since the elution of alkaloids from *mao* and *bushi* is associated with the probability of side effects, when formulating a prescription by combining multiple herbs, one must consider not only the actions of each crude drug simply adding up, but also the elution of ingredients from other herbs.

Column: Decoction Packaging Machine

In order to save the patient the trouble of decocting the herbs on their own, the pharmacy can take over the operation of decocting by the patient's request. Automatic crude drug decocting and packaging machines are sold by several manufacturers. When a mixture of herbs for the specified number of days is set in this device, it is collectively extracted with hot water, filtered, and then packaged in a plastic or aluminum bag as a liquid for the specified number of doses. Since it is packaged airtight as hot water, it does not easily spoil and can be stored at room temperature for about a week (Fig. 4.6).

3.2.3 Preparation of Powder Preparations

In powder preparations, the pharmacist weighs powdered herbs according to the prescription or the guidelines, mixes it, and dispenses it as single doses. When powdered crude drugs are not listed in the NHI Drug Price Standard list, such as *chorei* in goreisan, the pharmacist grinds cut herbs for dispensing in a mill, passes this through a sieve, and prepares the powdered formula. The same packaging machine as Western medicine can be used for packaging powders in Kampo medicine, In principle, however, herbs in powder form are highly hygroscopic and should be used immediately after preparation (or stored in the refrigerator).

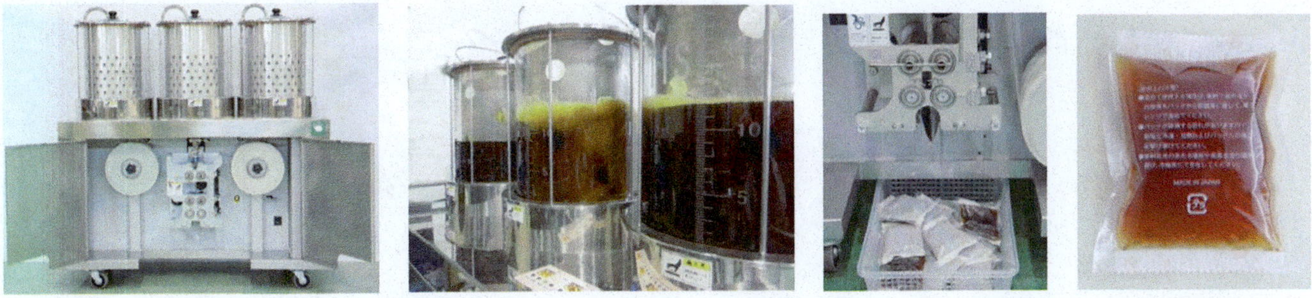

Fig. 4.6 Example of packaging using herb decocting and packaging machine

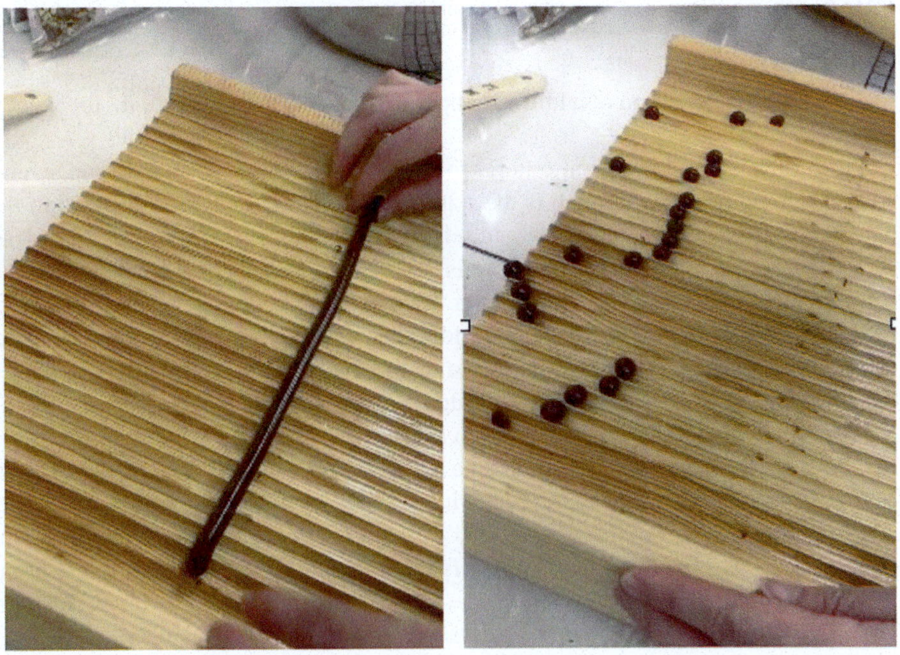

Fig. 4.7 Preparation of Keishibukuryogan using a pill maker

The dose of powder is often about one quarter to a half of the dose of decoction because it does not produce crude drug residue.

3.2.4 Preparation of Pills

Compared to powder prescriptions, pills are more stable, store better, easier to take, and more convenient to carry. About same weight of honey as the raw herb material is used as the binder. The honey is boiled down to remove water, and the powder is mixed with the honey. This is formed in a clay shape, stretched into a stick shape, cut into a certain size, rolled into a spherical shape, and then dried to make pills (Fig. 4.7).

3.2.5 Preparation of Ointments

The softness of an ointment is determined by adjusting the mixture of sesame oil (liquid at room temperature) and beeswax (solid at room temperature) as the ointment base. The specified amount of ointment base is heated in an appropriate container to make it liquid, and then the cut herbs are added into this for extraction. Next, the herb residue is filtered, and then cooled to room temperature while kneading to make Shiunko (Fig. 4.8). For some ointments, herb powder is added to a liquid base and kneaded (Chuoko).

3.3 Drug Informatics in Crude Drugs and Kampo Medicines

Toshiaki MakinoTatsuhiko Suzuki,
Yoshiharu TobinaKazuyoshi Kawazoe and Tatsuya Nogami

Below is the outline of information on the package insert of Kampo products [14, 15].

3.3.1 Composition and Description

This description sheet item usually contains the information on the daily dosage of herb, the amount of dried extract

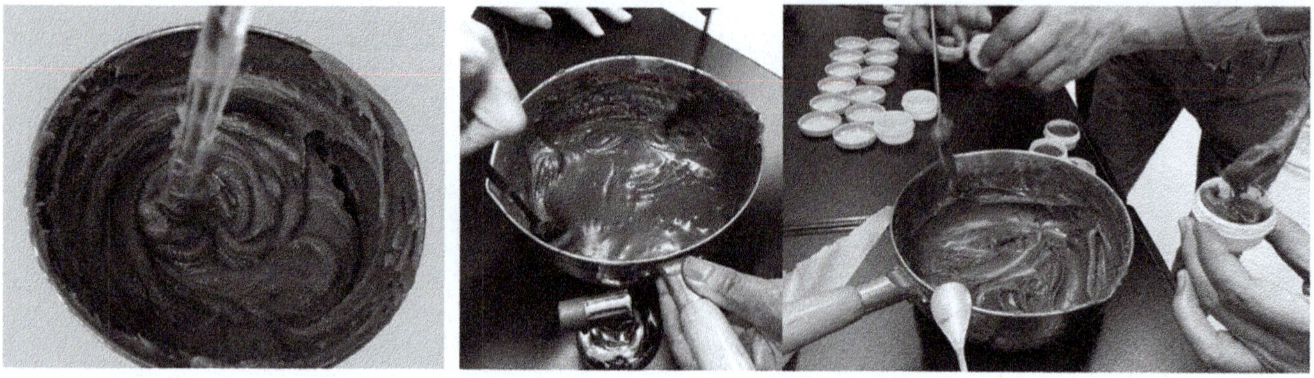

Fig. 4.8 Shiunko prepared as pharmacy-made ointment

obtained, the composition of additives, and the dosage form, color, odor, and taste.

According to the "Approval criteria for over-the-counter (OTC) Kampo products," which is the standard for pharmaceutical companies to manufacture and sell Kampo products issued by Japanese Government, there is a range of crude drug contents used as raw materials for Kampo products. Since each pharmaceutical company decides the contents of crude drugs according to these criteria and received approval for each product, the contents of crude drugs in Kampo products sold in Japan will be different even when the product names are the same. For example, the ethical kakkonto extract products in Japan have the following five patterns:

Company A: *Kakkon* 8 g, *mao* 4 g, *taiso* 4 g, *keihi* 3 g, *shakuyaku* 3 g, *kanzo* 2 g, *shokyo* 1 g.
Company B: *Kakkon* 4 g, *mao* 3 g, *taiso* 3 g, *keihi* 2 g, *shakuyaku* 2 g, *kanzo* 2 g, *shokyo* 1 g.
Company C: *Kakkon* 4 g, *mao* 3 g, *taiso* 3 g, *keihi* 2 g, *shakuyaku* 2 g, *kanzo* 2 g, *shokyo* 2 g.
Company D: *Kakkon* 4 g, *mao* 4 g, *taiso* 3 g, *keihi* 2 g, *shakuyaku* 2 g, *kanzo* 2 g, *shokyo* 1 g.
Company E: *Kakkon* 4 g, *mao* 3 g, *taiso* 3 g, *keishi* 2 g, *shakuyaku* 2 g, *kanzo* 2 g, *namashokyo* 3 g.

Even if the daily dosage of crude drugs is the same, the amount of dried extract and the amount of additives obtained may differ depending on the pharmaceutical company. Therefore, there are no generic drugs in Kampo products. Physicians have to issue the prescription with not only the name of Kampo formula but also the name of the pharmaceutical company (it is true that the official Kampo formula names contain the name of pharmaceutical companies). Thereby, pharmacists can dispense Kampo products to the patients according to the prescription. Although these Kampo products have the disadvantages that the herbs contained cannot be adjusted according to the condition of each patient as with prescription as decoctions, it may be possible to adjust it to some extent by choosing pharmaceutical companies.

In addition, even if the ingredients are the same as mentioned in Section 4-A (see p. XX), there are variations in crude drugs used as raw materials, and the standards for blending them to maintain stable quality of the products differ for each pharmaceutical company. It can be said that the quality of Kampo products is consistent within the same company, but there may be differences in quality among products manufactured by different companies.

3.3.2 Indications, Dosage, and Administration

The effect of Kampo formulas with the same product names may differ depending on the times when each individual pharmaceutical company received approval from Japanese Government. For example, Maoto manufactured by Tsumura can only be prescribed for influenza, and Kamishoyosan product manufactured by Kotaro Pharmaceutical can only be prescribed to men.

These effects expressed in the indication are the translations of *yakuno* in Kampo medicine into the term of Western medicine, but since this translation is not complete, similar effects sometimes are not approved even if the usage is correct in Kampo medicine. Using health insurance for medical treatment, it is a principle to use drugs according to the approved indications; therefore, prescriptions containing non-approved indications should be avoided. Since the effects differ depending on the pharmaceutical company, it is possible to choose the ethical Kampo products depending on the approved effects of each pharmaceutical company. When pharmacists find an indication not approved in the prescription, they can suggest the products from different companies that have proper indications to physicians.

All Kampo formulas are designated to be taken before or between meals. Therefore, when pharmacists receive the prescriptions requiring Kampo formulas to be taken after meal, pharmacists have to make an inquiry to physicians. The rationale for taking Kampo products on an empty stomach is not highly justified, either classically or scientifically. In general, the absorption of drugs in the gastrointestinal tract is faster when food is not contained in the stomach. It is therefore presumed that Kampo medicines were supposed to be taken before or between meals so that they could be absorbed well. When taking them on an empty stomach causes stomach problems like stomach upset, or if patients tend to forget taking their medicine, it is thought to be fine if Kampo formulas are taken after meals, since this is not an important issue. In that case, after the inquiry to the physician, it will be explained to the patient at the time of medication instruction that it is okay to take it after meals.

The dosage is specified as the daily dosage for adults, but this can be adjusted according to the patient's age, body weight, and symptoms.

With some exceptions, the indications and dosage of herbs for ethical use are "dispensing for the prescription in Kampo formula" without specific disease names and dosages. Therefore, unless the herb is named specifically in a prescription sheet, the combination of crude drugs can be freely chosen according to the patient's symptoms. Some herbs are approved as single herb product with specific indications, and physicians can note these herbs alone in the prescription sheet. For example, *daio* and *bushi* have been approved as the herb products with the indications of "laxative" and "cardiotonic, analgesic, and diuretic," respectively.

Column: Reasons Why Kampo Products Are Administered Before and Between Meals

In the past, one reason why Kampo products are administered before or between meals was explained as follows: The molecular type of alkaloids, which have relatively strong effect under acidic conditions, became cations in empty acidic stomach and based on the pH-distribution hypothesis alkaloids are absorbed slowly. Another reason given was that glycosides contained in herbs are not absorbed as their original form, and that they can be absorbed after hydrolyzed into aglycones by intestinal bacteria. Therefore, they should be quickly transported to the large intestine where there are intestinal bacteria [16]. However, there is almost no difference in the absorption speed of alkaloids between the range from acidic to neutral. Also, it is well known that since the absorption mechanism by active transport of drugs by various transporters whose transport capacity changes depending on pH [17], the pH-distribution hypothesis alone cannot explain the absorption of drugs. In addition, many studies have revealed that glycosides contained in herbs are hydrolyzed to aglycone by lactase-phlorizin hydrolase expressed in the epithelium of small intestine [18], and that glycosides are detected with the original form in blood [19]. Therefore, these reasons are not always correct.

According to the classics, pre-meal and post-meal administration of Kampo medicines is decided according to how the drug works. Also, many Chinese patent medicines in China (preparations made from herbs) are post-meal administration. The instruction that Kampo medicine was to be administered before meals first appeared in *"Kamposhinryonojissai* 漢方診療の実際 *(Standard Practice of Kampo Medicine)"* published by Otsuka et al. in 1954. In general, Kampo medicines does not contain stimulating ingredients that damage the gastric mucosa, and the drugs are absorbed from the digestive tract faster when food is not contained in the stomach. Therefore, it is presumed that instruction was given in this text that Kampo medicines should be taken on the empty stomach so that they could be absorbed as well as possible.

Column: Should Kampo Extract Products Be Taken After Dissolving in Hot Water?

Kampo extract products are sometimes likened to instant coffee because they are prepared by removing the water in the decoction. Since the taste and aroma of Kampo medicines are considered to be part of the medicinal effects (except for Kampo powdered prescription such as Tokishakuyakusan and Keishibukuryogan), it is said that it is more effective to take Kampo extract products dissolved in hot water than to take them in the form of granules or tablets.

When there is a possibility that compliance may decrease by requiring even bitter formulas, such as Orengedokuto, to be dissolved in hot water, it is not necessary to require this. In addition, when Kampo medicine is prescribed to warm the body, such as formulas containing *mao* or *bushi*, taking them with hot water will strengthen their effect. On the other hand, it may be better to take Kampo formulas containing herbs to clear heat, such as *sekko*, with cold water. Furthermore, granules or tablets may not dissolve completely in hot water. Instruction must be given to scrape the undissolved residue and to take the entire product in such cases.

3.3.3 Precautions

Adverse Reactions (Side Effects) [20]

In the past, there was no concept of side effects in Kampo medicine. It was said that side effects were mistakes in diagnosis and they were called "mistreatment." It was also said that side effects would not occur unless the "pattern" was wrong. In modern times, however, it is considered natural that substances with some pharmacological action could have side effects. Therefore, it is becoming understood that the view that Kampo medicines have no side effects is clearly mistaken.

In addition, it is known that Kampo medicines cause a temporary response called *mengen* or healing reaction in which symptoms temporarily worsen after the administration of the drug before the disease is completely cured. In some cases, the formula is continued regardless. This, however, is not acceptable today, and side effects should be suspected if any abnormal reaction is observed, and Kampo medicines should be discontinued (see Chap. 1, Sect. 6.1, Chap. 3, Sect. 3.1.7).

- **Pseudoaldohypersteronism due to Glycyrrhiza-containing Kampo medicines**

Pseudohyperaldosteronism is a relatively common serious side effect of Kampo medicine, and is a condition in which symptoms similar to primary aldosteronism are observed in spite of the absence of hyperaldosteronism. It is characterized by hypertension, hypokalemia, hypernatremia, metabolic alkalosis, low plasma renin activity, low or normal plasma aldosterone, malaise, and weakness/numbness. In severe cases, it causes rhabdomyolysis, renal failure, heart failure, and sometimes even death. It is known that this side effect depends to some extent on the intake of *kanzo*. The frequency of pseudohyperaldosteronism in patients who used 1 g of *kanzo* daily is 1.0% on average. The frequency for daily dosages of 2 g, 4 g, and 6 g was 1.7%, 3.3%, and 11.1%, on average respectively [21]. Special care should be taken when prescribing Kampo medicines containing 2.5 g or more of *kanzo* in a daily dose. Since *kanzo* is contained in many Kampo formulas, it is necessary to pay attention to the duplication of *kanzo* when using multiple Kampo formulas at the same time. In addition, since *kanzo* is added to foods as a sweetener, it may be ingested by patients without being aware of it. Physical findings such as elevated blood pressure and edema should always be noted, and blood tests should be performed on a regular basis.

The pathogenic mechanism is suggested as follows: glycyrrhetinic acid, which is a metabolite of the major component glycyrrhizinic acid in *kanzo*, and its sulfate conjugate inhibit type 2 11β-hydroxysteroid dehydrogenase (11β-HSD2) in renal tubular epithelial cells. This causes cortisol to accumulate, and cortisol stimulates mineral corticoid receptors to induce the expression of sodium/potassium channels in the tubular epithelium, promoting renal reabsorption and potassium excretion from the renal tubules (Fig. 4.9) [22, 23].

Known factors that increase the risk of pseudohyperaldosteronism include the concomitant use with diuretics or steroids that cause hypokalemia, [24] hypoalbuminemia, and aging [25]. For high-risk cases, it is necessary to exercise caution even when small doses of *kanzo* are being administered. When pseudohyperaldosteronism occurs, the use of

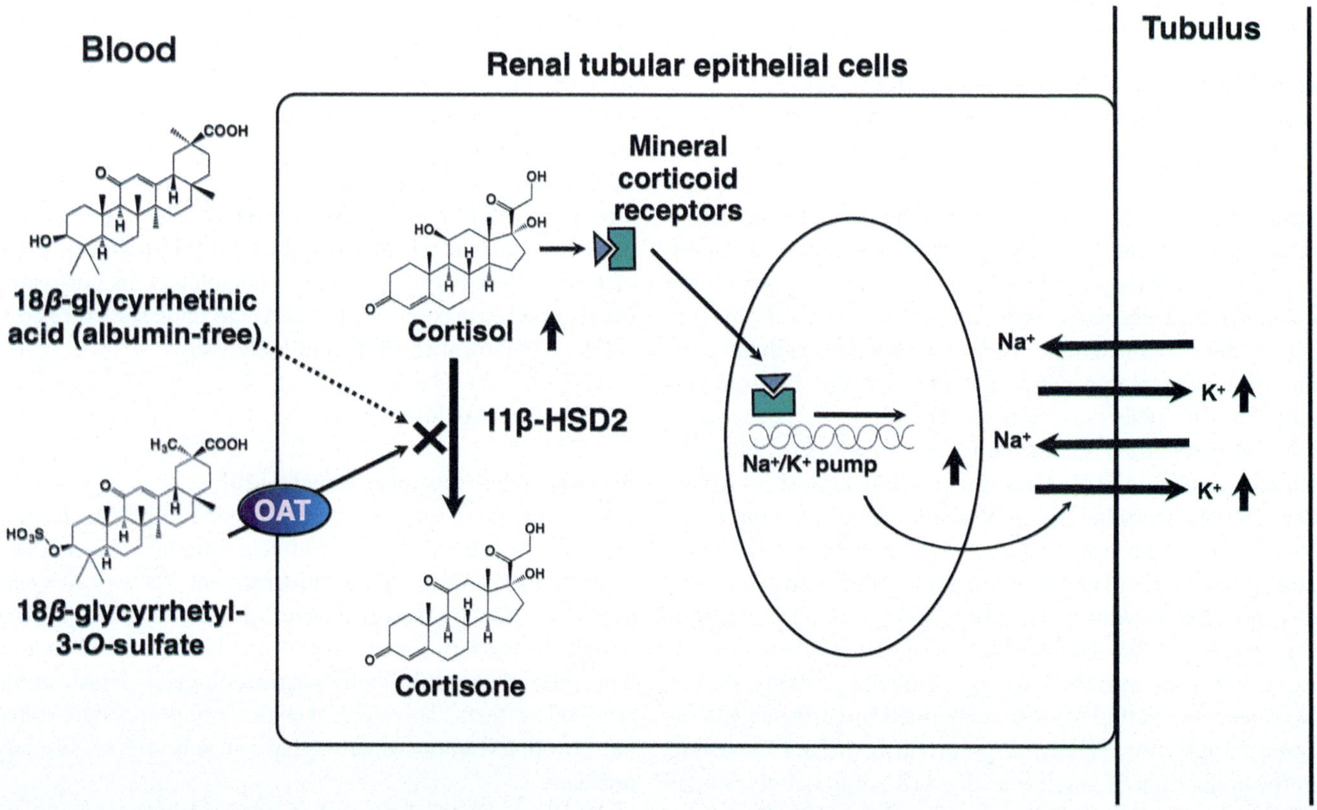

Fig. 4.9 Schematic diagram of the onset mechanism of pseudohyperaldosteronism caused by *kanzo*

kanzo must be stopped immediately, potassium should be supplemented, and aldosterone antagonists administered, or appropriate treatment must be given for hypertension, heart failure, or kidney failure. When pseudohyperaldosteronism is discovered early by rise in blood pressure or edema, it does not present such a big problem. If discovery is delayed, however, this condition can be fatal, so it is necessary to track the patient's progress carefully.

- **Drug-induced liver injury**

The frequency of drug-induced liver injury caused by Kampo medicines is said to be 0.1% or less, but it is one of the side effects that require attention. From a pharmacoepidemiological point of view, it is known that the frequency of drug-induced liver injury is high with drugs containing *ogon* [26]. It has been reported that about 1% of patients with *ogon* had drug-induced liver injury [27]. Hepatic dysfunction has been reported, however, even with formulas that do not contain *ogon*, so caution is required. Drug-induced liver injury rarely presents clinical symptoms in the early stage, but it is often advanced in the stage when symptoms such as jaundice and malaise appear, so it is important to detect it early in blood tests.

The onset of drug-induced liver injury caused by Kampo medicines is assumed to be an allergic mechanism, and in many cases, it develops 1 to 2 months after the start of administration. Therefore, especially when prescribing a Kampo medicine containing *ogon*, it is advisable to perform a blood test 1 to 2 months after the start of administration to determine the presence or absence of liver dysfunction. In the treatment of drug-induced liver injury, it is most important to discontinue the causative drug promptly. In many cases, drug-induced liver injury caused by Kampo medicines is improved relatively quickly by discontinuation. The Kampo prescriptions for ethical use in which liver dysfunction and jaundice are described as side effects in the attached sheet are shown below. Prescriptions containing *ogon* are underlined.

Bakumondoto, <u>bofutsushosan,</u> boiogito, daikenchuto, <u>daisaikoto</u>, goreisan, goshajinkigan, goshuyuto, <u>hangeshasinto,</u> hochuekkito, inchinkoto, <u>junchoto,</u> juzentaihoto, kakkonto, kamishoyosan, <u>keigairengyoto</u>, keishibukuryogan, maobushisaishinto, ninjinyoeito, <u>nijutsuto, nyoshinsan, orengedokuto</u>, <u>otsujito</u>, rikkunshito, <u>ryutanshakanto, saibokuto</u>, <u>saikokaryukotsuboreito, saikokeishikankyoto, saikokeishito, saireito, san'motsuogonto, san'oshashinto, seihaito, seijobofuto, seishinrenshiin</u>, shakuyakukanzoto, <u>shi'iseihaito</u>, shoseiryuto, <u>shosaikoto, shosaikotokikyosekko, unseiin</u>, yokukansan (by March 2021).

- **Drug-induced lung injury (drug-induced interstitial pneumonia)**

Drug-induced lung injury sometimes occurs as a side effect of Kampo medicines. The most serious case is drug-induced interstitial pneumonia. Currently, there have been reports of drug-induced interstitial pneumonia with approximately 30 kinds of Kampo prescriptions, and there have been reports of deaths [28]. It is said to be relatively common in the elderly, but it may also occur in young people. An allergic mechanism is assumed, as with drug-induced liver injury, but the mechanism of onset is not clear, and it is difficult to predict the onset. It is important to respond in the early stage, and physicians and pharmacists have to instruct patients that they must stop taking the medicine immediately when symptoms such as fever, coughing, and shortness of breath occur after starting to take Kampo medicines. They must also promptly consult a medical clinic. For early detection of drug-induced lung injury, the measurement of percutaneous arterial oxygen saturation is convenient and useful. If interstitial pneumonia is suspected, it is necessary to promptly perform imaging tests such as chest X-rays and chest CT scans as well as blood tests to make a diagnosis. The serum marker KL-6 is higher in interstitial pneumonia than infectious pneumonia and this is useful for auxiliary diagnosis [29]. Since the causes of interstitial pneumonia are diverse, in order to diagnose drug-induced interstitial pneumonia due to Kampo medicines, allergies to environmental antigens, infectious diseases, connective tissue disease, and non-Kampo medicines should be determined by careful history and various tests. Interstitial pneumonia from other causes should be carefully ruled out.

Among the herbs that cause drug-induced interstitial pneumonia, *ogon* is suspected by pharmacoepidemiological analysis, as is the case with drug-induced liver injury [26]. Occasionally, there is a combination of drug-induced interstitial pneumonia and drug-induced liver injury. It has been reported that 0.27% of patients who received *ogon* developed drug-induced interstitial pneumonia, so special care should be taken when administering *ogon* [30]. It should be noted, however, that the onset of interstitial pneumonia has also been reported with Kampo formulas without *ogon*.

To treat drug-induced interstitial pneumonia with Kampo formulas, it is important to first discontinue the causative formula. In mild cases, discontinuation of the formula can improve the condition. In severe cases, systemic management including the administration of steroids and immunosuppressants is required. Since drug-induced lung injury often recurs due to reingestion of the causative formula, guidance should be given to the patient to prevent reingestion of the causative formula and of the causative herb (especially *ogon*).

The Kampo prescriptions for ethical use in which interstitial pneumonia is described as the side effect in the attached sheet are shown below. Prescriptions containing *ogon* are underlined.

Bakumondoto, bofutsushosan, boiogito, daikenchuto, daisaikoto, gorinsan, hangeshasinto, hochuekkito, junchoto, keigairengyoto, nijutsuto, orengedokuto, otsujito, ryutanshakanto, saibokuto, saikokaryukotsuboreito, saikokeishikankyoto, saikokeishito, saireito, san'motsuogonto, seihaito, seishinrenshiin, shakuyakukanzoto, shi'iseihaito, shoseiryuto, shosaikoto, shosaikotokikyosekko, unseiin, yokukansan (by March 2021).

- **Drug eruptions**

Drug eruptions sometimes occur by Kampo medicines. Various types of drug eruptions may occur, such as eczema-type, erythema multiforme-type, and disseminated erythema-papules-type; also cases of Stevens-Johnson syndrome have been reported. Clinically, drug eruption is often experienced with prescriptions containing *keihi*, *mao*, *ninjin*, and *ogi*. In recent years, there have been reports of pigmented drug eruption caused by *sanshishi* and other Kampo medicines.

- **Drug-induced cystitis**

Kampo medicines sometimes cause drug-induced cystitis. It has been reported that frequent urination, pain during urination, hematuria, etc. occurred, and the pathological findings of eosinophil cystitis were observed. It has been reported that shosaikoto, saireito, saibokuto, saikokaryukotsuboreito, unseiin, and shin'iseihaito were used. In many cases, the condition is relieved by discontinuing medication.

- **Gastrointestinal symptoms (stomach heaviness, anorexia, diarrhea, etc.)**

Prescriptions containing *jio*, *sekko*, *mao*, etc. sometimes cause stomach discomfort such as stomach heaviness. Kampo medicines are basically administered before meals, but such symptoms may be avoided by administering them after meals.

Daio has a laxative effect, and overdose causes abdominal pain and diarrhea. In addition, long-term continuous use of rhubarb may cause melanosis coli in which lipofuscin is deposited on the intestinal wall (Fig. 4.10). It should be noted that melanosis coli may cause intestinal peristalsis at a high level, and that the frequency of colorectal adenomas is high in cases of melanosis coli [31]. This can be alleviated within a few years by discontinuing intestinal stimulant laxatives such as rhubarb. In addition, taking *daio* sometimes causes redness of urine, but this doesn't cause any problem. Physicians and pharmacists can provide this drug information to the patients when prescribing formulas with rhubarb.

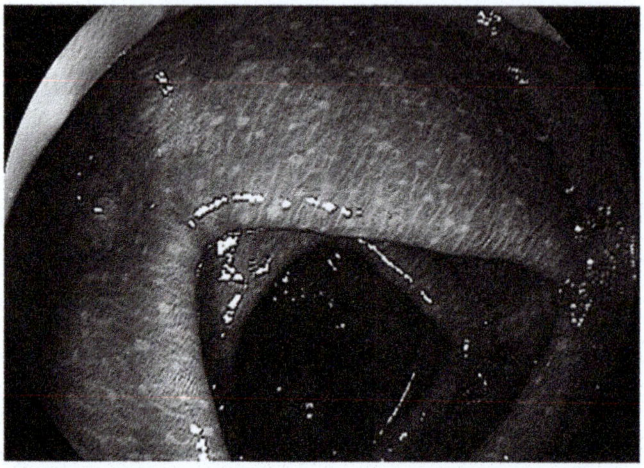

Fig. 4.10 Colonoscopic findings of colorectal melanosis. Extensive dark brown pigmentation in the large intestine

Since *bosho* is also a salt laxative, overdose may cause diarrhea and abdominal pain.

Some Kampo extract products contain lactose as an excipient and others do not. Taking a preparation containing lactose may cause diarrhea in lactose intolerant patients. Diarrhea due to lactose intolerance may be improved by the combined use of lactose-degrading enzyme preparations.

- **Idiopathic mesenteric venous sclerosis (abdominal pain, diarrhea, constipation, abdominal distension, etc.)**

Idiopathic mesenteric venous sclerosis is the side effect that is thought to be related to *sanshishi* (Fig. 4.11). According to a national survey conducted by Shimizu et al., surveying 222 cases of mesenteric venous sclerosis, 169 patients had been taking Kampo medicines, and among them, 147 (87%) cases took prescriptions containing Gardenia Fruit, 14 cases (9.5%) were unknown, and another 14 cases (9.5%) took *sanshishi*-free prescriptions [32]. Symptoms at the time of onset were abdominal pain 45%, diarrhea 17.3%, abdominal distension 16.8%, intestinal obstruction 16.8%, nausea/vomiting 10.5%, constipation 7.7%, bloody stool 7.3%, and others 7.7%. However, it is expected that a considerable number of asymptomatic cases exist because no medical institution will scrutinize the disease if it is completely asymptomatic. The average duration of administration of Kampo prescriptions containing *sanshishi* was 13.6 years, distributed from 3 to 51 years, with 92.6% of patients taking 5 years or more and 69.5% taking prescriptions for 10 years or more. However, it is reported

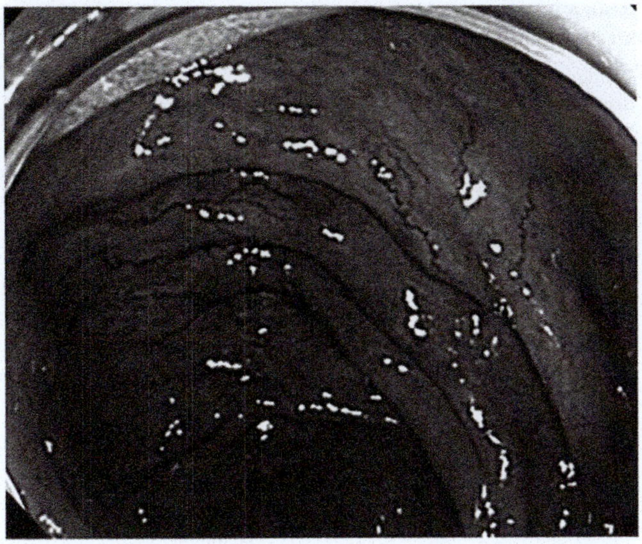

Fig. 4.11 Colonoscopic findings: Bronze pigmentation is observed in the ascending colon

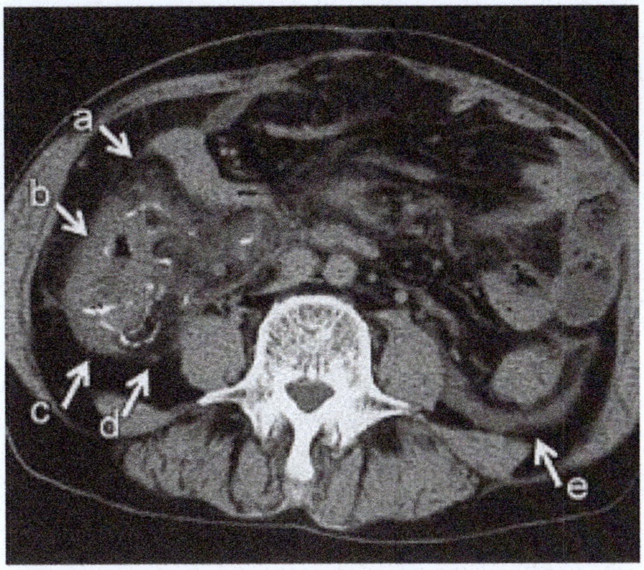

Fig. 4.12 Simple abdominal CT findings in a 70-year-old male case with severe mesenteric venous sclerosis. A total of 8119 g of Gardenia Fruit had been taken. Findings such as increased peri-ascending colon fat tissue concentration (**a**), thickening of the ascending colon wall (**b**), calcification in the ascending colon (**c**), calcification of the mesenteric vein around the ascending colon (**d**), and ascites retention (**e**) were observed, and right hemicolectomy was required

that the total dose is more important than the administration period, and the number of cases increases when the total dose of *sanshishi* is 5 g [33].

The pathogenic mechanism is geniposide contained in *sanshishi* being hydrolyzed to genipin by the intestinal bacteria in the large intestine. Genipin is absorbed from large intestine and reaches the liver through the mesenteric vein, where it reacts with amino acids and proteins.

The cause is thought to be the formation of a blue pigment, which at the same time causes fibrous thickening and calcification of the mesenteric vein wall. However, as mentioned above, there are cases in which Gardenia Fruit has not been taken, and in these cases, the pathogenic mechanism is not clear.

As mentioned above, mesenteric venous sclerosis often progresses asymptomatically, so in order to detect it early, abdominal X-ray examination, abdominal CT, and colonoscopy are performed on patients who have been receiving *sanshishi* for a long period of time. It can be said that examinations such as endoscopy should be actively carried out. Abdominal X-ray examination and abdominal CT show findings of linear and punctate calcification along the large intestine wall centering on the right abdominal colon or the mesenteric vein (Fig. 4.12). Abdominal CT scans are more sensitive. Colonoscopy reveals dark purple, bronze mucosal color changes, edema, loss of vascular transparency, swelling of the crescent folds, poor extension, luminal narrowing, erosion/ulcer, etc. In severe cases of mesenteric venous sclerosis, cases leading to intestinal resection have also been reported [34], so it is important to detect this condition as early as possible to avoid this disease. It is important not to administer Kampo medicines containing *sanshishi* for an extended period. Kampo prescriptions for ethical use that contain *sanshishi* include the following:

Bofutsushosan, gorinsan, inchinkoto, kamikihito, kamishoyosan, keigairengyoto, orengedokuto, saikoseikanto, seijobofuto, seihaito, shin'iseihaito, shishihakuhito, unseiin.

- **Food allergies**

In patients with allergies to certain foods, Kampo prescriptions containing herbs that have similar origins as those foods may cause hypersensitivity. Skin symptoms are common, and various symptoms such as respiratory, mucosal and gastric symptoms, and shock occur in food allergy. The origins of *keihi*, *kobei*, *san'yaku*, *shobaku* are the same as cinnamon, rice, Japanese yam, and wheat, respectively. Therefore, it is advisable to thoroughly check for food allergies before giving Kampo prescriptions. For example, Kambakutaisoto or Shokenchuto should be avoided for the patients with wheat allergy and rice allergies, respectively.

- **Other Side Effects**

Kampo formulas containing *mao* sometimes cause insomnia, palpitation, mental agitation, and dysuria associated with sympathetic nerve stimulation by ephedrine. It should be used with caution for patients with angina, myocardial infarction, severe hypertension, dysuria, and hyperthyroidism.

Kampo formulas containing *bushi* sometimes cause neurotoxic side effects such as palpitations, headache, and tongue numbness due to the aconitine-type alkaloids. However, this side effect is greatly diminished by heat-processing. The susceptibility to this side effect varies greatly among individuals, and caution is required. When using *bushi* or *uzu* in a decoction, without processing, it is important to infuse it for a sufficient period of time before taking. In addition, since the amount of aconitine-type alkaloids increases when the decoction becomes acidic (C-1 column), it is necessary to pay attention to other herbs prescribed together that are decocted at the same time (Table 4.6).

Column: Side Effects of Kampo Medicines and Drug Lymphocyte Stimulation Test (DLST)

The drug-induced lymphocyte stimulation test (DLST) is a test for diagnosing drug allergies, and is used when there is drug-induced liver injury, drug-induced interstitial pneumonia, drug eruption, etc. Also this test is often used when side effects from Kampo medicines are suspected. However, Kampo medicines and herbs sometimes have mitogen activities, and DLST tends to be positive regardless of the presence or absence of drug allergies. Therefore, DLST for Kampo medicines and herbs sometimes produce false positive, and may confuse the diagnosis of drug-induced liver injury, interstitial pneumonia, and drug eruption, and leads to misdiagnosis. When performing DLST in the diagnosis of allergies with Kampo medicines, the characteristics should be understood and the results should be interpreted carefully [35].

- **Administration to pregnant and lactating women**

Herbs to Be Careful with in Pregnancy

In the 11th chapter of "*Fujintaizenryoho* 婦人大全良方 *(Complete Collection of Effective Prescriptions for Women)*" published in the Song dynasty, herbs contraindicated for use during pregnancy, are presented as a mnemonic song. Among these herbs, those currently used in Japan are as follows:

Bushi, *gooh*※, *goshitsu*, *yokuinin*, <u>*bosho*</u>, *botampi*, *keihi*, *keishi*, *kengoshi*※, *tonin*, *hange*, *tennansho*, *shokyo*

The 2020 edition of the Chinese Pharmacopoeia describes herbs that should be used with caution during pregnancy. Among these herbs, those currently used in Japan are as follows:

Contraindications: *Uzu*※, *gajutsu*※, *kengoshi*※

Careful administration: Aloe※, *kikoku*, *kijitsu*, *keihi*, *keishi*, *koka*, *gooh*※, *goshitsu*, saffron※ *sanshichininjin*※, Musk, *senso*※, senna leaf※, *soboku*, *daio*, *tennansho*, *temma*, *tonin*, *bushi*, *bosho*, *botampi*, *yakumoso*, *yokuinin*, *ryuno*※

Note at the bottom of the page:

Since the following crude drugs are not included in Kampo prescription used in Japan, and not included in the list of crude drugs on Chap. 9. Their origins and usages are described here. [JP] means registered in the Japanese Pharmacopoeia 18th edition, 2020, and [non-JP] means regis-

Table 4.6 List of crude drugs that have to be attention to cause side effects and their clinical symptoms

Crude drug name	Side effects	Clinical symptoms
Ogi	Drug eruption	Various exanthema
Ogon	Drug-induced liver injury Drug-induced lung injury Drug-induced cystitis	Sense of fatigue, jaundice, liver dysfunction Cough, shortness of breath, fever, difficulty breathing Frequent urination, urination pain, hematuria
Kanzo	Pseudohyperaldosteronism	Edema, weakness, sense of fatigue, hypertension, hypokalemia, hypernatremia, metabolic alkalosis
Keihi, keishi	Drug eruption Allergy to cinnamon	Various exanthema, difficulty breathing, anaphylaxis
Kobei	Allergy to rice	Exanthema, difficulty breathing, anaphylaxis
Sanshishi	Mesenteric venous sclerosis Drug eruption	Abdominal pain, diarrhea, abdominal distension, bloody stools, intestinal obstruction Hyperpigmented drug eruption
San'yaku	Allergy to Japanese yam	Exanthema, difficulty breathing, anaphylaxis
Jio	Upper gastrointestinal symptom	Stodginess, loss of appetite, stomachache
Shobaku	Allergy to wheat	Exanthema, difficulty breathing, anaphylaxis
Sekko	Upper gastrointestinal symptom	Fullness in stomach , anorexia
Daio	Lower gastrointestinal symptom Melanosis coli	Diarrhea, abdominal pain Decreased intestinal peristalsis, increased colorectal adenoma
Ninjin	Drug eruption	Various exanthema
Bushi, uzu	Poisoning to aconitine	Palpitations, headache, numbness of the tongue, arrhythmia
Bosho	Lower gastrointestinal symptom	Diarrhea, abdominal pain
Mao	Drug eruption Upper gastrointestinal symptom Sympathomimetic symptom	Various exanthema, anorexia, stodginess Asomnia, palpitations, mental agitation, dysuria

tered in the Japanese standards for non-Pharmacopoeial crude drugs in 2018.

Aloe[JP]: The dried juice of the leaves mainly of *Aloe ferox*. It is used as purgative formulas.

Uzu, Raw Aconite Root: The dried the tuberous root of *Aconitum carmichaeli* or *Aconitum japonicum*. It is the substance before the processing of *bushi*[JP].

Gajutsu, Crucuma Rhizome[JP]: The dried rhizome of *Curcuma zedoaria*. It is used as aromatic stomachic.

Go-oh, Oriental bezoar[JP]: The dried stone formed in the gall sac of *Bos taurus* var. *domesticus*. It is prescribed in Japanese traditional pharmaceutical products such as Rokushingan.

Kengoshi, Pharbitis Seed[JP]: The dried seed of *Pharbitis nil*. It is prescribed in OTC Kampo product Hachimisenkiho, which components are *keihi*, *mokutsu*, *engosaku*, *tonin*, *uyaku*, *kengoshi*, *daio*, and *botampi*, and this formula is used for back or menstrual pain.

Saffron[JP]: The dried stigma of *Crocus sativus*. It is used as the additive components of Kampo prescriptions to strengthen the effect of resolving blood[TM1] stasis.

Sanshichininjin, Panax notoginseng Root[non-JP]: The dried root of *Panax notoginseng*. It is used for hemostasis and resolving to resolve blood[TM] stasis.

Musk: The dried secretions in the seminal vesicle of *Moschus moschiferus*. It is prescribed in Japanese traditional pharmaceutical products such as *Rokushingan*.

Senso, Toad Cake[JP]: The dried parotoid secretion of *Bufo bufo gargarizans* or *Bufo melanostictus*. It is prescribed in Japanese traditional pharmaceutical products such as Rokushingan.

Senna leaf[JP]: The dried leaflets of *Cassia angustifolia* or *Cassia acutifolia*. It is used as cathartic.

Ryuno, Dryobalanops aromatica resin: Crystals formed in the gaps of the trunk of *Dryobalanops aromatic*. It is prescribed in Japanese traditional pharmaceutical products such as *Rokushingan*.

The current package insert for Kampo products states that "the safety of administration of Kampo medicines during pregnancy has not been established," and in principle, it should be administered only when it is judged that the therapeutic benefit outweighs the risk for women who may be pregnant. Nevertheless, shohangebukuryoto, which contains *hange*, which is included in the song of "*Fujintaizenryoho* 婦人大全良方 *(Complete Collection of Effective Prescriptions for Women)*," is often used for hyperemesis gravidarum (morning sickness), and no health hazard to the fetus has been reported. Some formulas have the traditional efficiency of "calming fetus," and Tokishakuyakusan, a typical Kampo prescription that is often used to calm fetus and to maintain health of pregnant women.

A study analyzing clinical data from a large number of 121,287 pregnant women found no significant difference in safety with or without taking Kampo medicines. Also, unplanned hospitalization for pregnant women with hyperemesis gravidarum (odds ratio 0.80, 95% confidence interval 0.69 ~ 0.92) and total cost (factor [US $] 12.8, 95% confidence interval − 23.2 ~ −2.4) in the Kampo medication group were significantly lower than those without Kampo medication [36]. This suggests that the use of Kampo medicines for pregnant women is beneficial.

Kampo medicines are the drugs that have undergone extensive field testing on humans to begin with, while the mechanism of action has only been elucidated in animal experiments in recent years. Laxative herbs or those for blood[TM1] stasis, dredging channels were contraindicated or carefully administered over the long history due to concerns about the effects on fetal growth and the possibility of uterine bleeding. The classical descriptions and indications cannot be completely ignored without clear evidence.

The package insert of Kampo products approved in Japan states that "it is desirable not to administer to pregnant women or women who may be pregnant" for the preparations containing rhubarb, sodium sulfate, safflower, peach kernel, and Moutan bark. Typical prescriptions containing them include Daiobotanpito, Choijokito, Daijokito, Tokakujokito, Tsudosan, Keishibukuryogan, Unkeito, Kamiyoyosan, and Bofutsushosan.

Column: Should Yokuinin Not Be Used in Pregnant Women?

In the classics, *yokuinin* is said to soften hardness and eliminate edema (dissolve the mass formed in the body), and there was concern about it eliminating fetuses. It is also contraindicated in the abovementioned contraindication rhyme for pregnant women. It has been pointed out that *yokuinin* should not be used in pregnant women due to its teratogenicity. According to the results of animal experiments, fetal reabsorption and post-implantation fetal mortality significantly increased. Also, spontaneous contractile force when the uterus was removed was also significantly increased after the administration of *yokuinin* hot water extract to rats at approximately 25 times dosage of human [37]. Opinion was divided because another study revealed that contractile force did not changed when *yokuinin* powder had been administered at approximately 50 times the dosage of humans to rats from the 0th day of pregnancy to the delivery. The raw material of *yokuinin* is *Coix lacryma-jobi* var. *ma-yue*. It has been pointed out that the origin of this contraindication could have been miscarriage by uterine contractions caused by ergot alkaloids produced by *Claviceps purpurea* infecting *Coix lacryma-jobi* var. *ma-yuen*. From the above, it is thought that there is no problem with the use of *yokuinin* for pregnant women, as long as the normal dosage is used when necessary.

- **Crude drugs to be careful with while breastfeeding**

The package insert for Kampo products for ethical use containing rhubarb states "Be careful in use for lactating women," and the OTC Kampo products or herbal products containing rhubarb states "Do not take this drug while breastfeeding; otherwise avoid breastfeeding while taking this drug." The reason is that anthraquinone derivatives in rhubarb may transfer to breast milk and cause diarrhea in infants.

Column: Should Daio Not Be Used while Breastfeeding?
The article pointing out the risk of diarrhea in infants, who ingest anthraquinone derivatives when they are transferred into breast milk published in 1937, is very old. The anthraquinone derivative used in this study was senna leaf, which isn't used in Kampo prescriptions. Then, in 1963, clinical trials using senna leaf preparations containing anthraquinones and placebo (Senna Leaf preparation group and placebo group was 50 patients each) showed no abnormal diarrhea in infants between the two groups [38]. In 1973, it was reported that senna leaf-derived compounds were not detected in milk [39]. Then in 1983, the article describing that very low concentrations of anthraquinones were detected in the milk of 20 women who took senna leaf preparation, but this was far from the level at which a laxative effect appeared even when ingested by infants. Also, no abnormal diarrhea was observed in infants that were actually breastfed by these mothers [40]. Based on the above, the American Academy of Pediatrics stated in 2001 that there was no problem with the use of senna during lactation [41], and the package insert for senna leaf preparations marketed only in the United States states that physicians or pharmacists should be consulted before use during lactation [42]. The package insert of senna leaf products approved as a purgative formula in Japan, however, states that "This drug should not be taken during lactation or otherwise breastfeeding should be avoided while taking this herb," or "It is desirable to avoid breastfeeding" [43]. There are few reports about the transfer of components into milk when lactating women take *daio*. Also senna, which contains sennosides, the same laxative active ingredient as *daio*, is considered a laxative that can be used during lactation in the United States. Even though it is prudent to use medicines with caution, it seems that there is no problem if *daio* is used during lactation.

Contraindications/Cautions

The package inserts sometimes list the cases that should never be administered as contraindications, and serious side effects are noted as cautions.

Shosaikoto is contraindicated in patients receiving interferon preparations, patients with liver cirrhosis/liver cancer, and patients with hepatic dysfunction in chronic hepatitis with a platelet count of 100,000/mm^2 or less.

A preparation containing 2.5 g or more of Glycyrrhiza per day is contraindicated in patients with aldosteronism, myopathy, and hypokalemia.

In addition, Shiunko is contraindicated in patients with a history of hypersensitivity to this product or its ingredients. Also, patients with severe burns/trauma, those with high fever due to purulent wounds, and severe wetness and soreness of the affected area are contraindicated.

Shosaikoto has been cited with the possibility of interstitial pneumonia as a serious side effect.

Drug Interaction Between Kampo Medicines and Western Medicines

- **Preferred drug interaction**

Kampo medicine has an important role to play in contemporary medicine by complementing the limits of the symptomatic aspect of Western medicine. Generally, the interactions between both medicines tend to be positive.

- **Combination of anticancer drug and Kampo medicines**

It has been pointed out that the combined use of Juzentaihoto with chemotherapy using anticancer drugs reduces the side effects of anticancer drugs and prevents the interruption of chemotherapy [44]. In addition, using Hangeshashinto in combination with irinotecanis is recommended in order to prevent and improve delayed diarrhea—a side effect of irinotecan (see Chap. 4, Sect. 4.2.8).

- **Combined use of Sansoninto or Hangeshashinto with anxiolytics**

There are clinical reports that the combined use of Sansoninto or Hangeshashinto and benzodiazepine anxiolytics worked synergistically with the anxiolytic effects of both, resulting in a reduced dose of Western drugs.

- **Unfavorable drug interaction**

When grapefruit juice has been reported to increase blood levels of Ca antagonists [45], it was suspected that similar interactions might occur with *kijitsu* and *chimpi*, because their source is citrus fruit. Later, however, it became clear that the causative component was furanocoumarins [46], which is not contained in *kijitsu* and *chimpi*. There are trace amounts of franocoumarins in *byakushi* and *kyokatsu*, but the level is not enough to cause a drug interaction.

This type of unfavorable drug interactions where there are drug interactions between Kampo medicines and Western medicines are described below.

- **Kampo medicines containing *kanzo* and loop diuretics, thiazide diuretics, or glycyrrhizin preparations**

Loop diuretics and thiazide diuretics have the side effect of hypokalemia, and when these are used in combination with *kanzo*, the side effects overlap and hypokalemia is likely to occur. Glycyrrhizin contain the causative substance in *kanzo* that causes the side effect, so their combined use results in overdose.

- **Kampo medicines containing *mao* and monoamine oxidase inhibitors, thyroid preparations, catecholamine preparations, or xanthine-based preparations**

All of these have the effect of exciting the autonomic nervous system, and side effects such as insomnia, excessive sweating, tachycardia, palpitation, and mental excitation are likely to occur. The combination of ephedrine and caffeine, which was once done in the United States for dieting, causes many serious health hazards. So this is now contraindicated in the United States. There is no problem with the amount of caffeine contained in coffee and tea consumed on a daily basis, but more caution is required for the pharmaceutical products for the common cold or beverages called energy drinks, since these contain relatively high amounts of caffeine.

- **Interferon preparation and Shosaikoto**

The combined use of these increases the risk of interstitial pneumonia, which is a side effect of both drugs.

- **Kampo medicines including *sekko* and tetracyclines and new quinolones antibiotics**

Tetracyclines antibiotics and new quinolones antibiotics generate chelates with calcium ions and magnesium ions to suppress their gastrointestinal absorption [47]. Therefore, they should be avoided in combination with dietary supplements and pharmaceuticals containing calcium and magnesium. The main component of *sekko* is calcium sulfate, and it is advisable to avoid the combined use of the above antibiotics with Kampo formulas containing *sekko*.

Column: Crude Drug and Cytochrome P450

Cytochrome P450 (CYPs) are known as drug-metabolizing enzymes and are important when considering in vivo drug interactions. In many crude drugs, the inhibitory effects on CYP2C9, CYP2D6, or CYP3A4 were reported in vitro using human liver microsomes. However, the concentrations were too high compared to the clinical doses, and there is a limit to linking experimental results to clinical practice (p. XX, 4-D-1, Limitations of basic pharmacological tests of crude drugs). In clinical studies, there were a few reports that the blood concentration of the drug that is the substrate for CYP changed by taking Kampo medicines. In a clinical study, when midazolam, which is the substrate for CYP3A4, was orally administered after the treatment of Anchusan extract three times a day for 6 consecutive days, the maximum blood concentration increased 1.36 times. However, the change in blood concentration after oral administration of midazolam 2 h after administration of Anchusan extract three times a day was not changed. Therefore, these clinical studies reported that Anchusan extract is unlikely to cause CYP3A4-mediated drug interactions. It can be said that, at this time, among Kampo products approved in Japan, the effect on CYPs in human beings is probably very low with normal doses, but further studies are required.

Banned Drugs in Doping

Banned drugs in doping are not described in package insert of drugs, but this is necessary information for the safe and effective use of drugs.

The World Anti-Doping Agency, which aims to prevent doping to uphold the spirit sports, has designated many compounds as banned drugs [48]. Banned drugs are classified into three types: (1) substances that are always prohibited, (2) substances that are prohibited during competitions, and (3) substances that are prohibited in specific competitions. Among the substances contained in Kampo medicine, higenamine, contained in *goshuyu*, *saishin*, and *bushi*, is described as a prohibited substance in (1), and ephedrine and pseudoephedrine, contained in *mao*, are described as applicable substances in (2). (There is a text stating that higenamine is contained in *choji* and ephedrine, in *hange*. Both of these are denied as a result of analysis of currently circulating commercial *choji* and *hange* [49].) In addition, synephrine contained in *chimpi* and *kijitsu* is regulated as a monitored substance. When athletes are using Kampo medicines containing these herbs, they should avoid using them at least 1 week before testing.

4 Pharmacology of Crude Drugs and Kampo Medicines

Toshiaki Makino

In order to clarify the scientific evidence of the efficacy of crude drugs and Kampo medicines, clinical trials using medicinal products derived from herbs (crude drugs) and Kampo formulas with proper quality control are required. Under such circumstances, the guidelines published from clinical medical societies and groups of experts have presented the standard treatment policies for various diseases using medicinal products derived from herbs and Kampo formulas that have shown certain levels of evidence. Though it is possible through clinical trials to statistically clarify whether the target drugs are effective, the mechanism of their actions is not clarified. For that purpose, pharmacological studies of formulas and Kampo medicines with basic pharmacological methods using lab animals and cultured cells are required.

4.1 Limitations of Basic Pharmacological Tests Using Crude Drugs and Kampo Medicines

4.1.1 Not All Compounds Contained in Herbs and Kampo Formulas Are Absorbed in the Digestive Tract

The simplest basic pharmacological test is to detect the change in cell activity that occurs when cultured cells are prepared from human or experimental animal tissue and the cells are cultured in a medium containing drug samples. That is, metabolites in the medium or cells are measured to analyze the expression levels of specific proteins and mRNAs extracted from the cells. At this time, when a test sample consisting of a pure substance is used as a research material, the test sample is dissolved in the medium by referring to the blood concentration obtained when it is actually used by humans. Then the results of the pharmacological test can be translated into the effect on human beings. In the case of herbs or extracts of crude drugs and Kampo formulas, however, myriad of compounds are ingested orally when people take them. Some of these compounds are rapidly absorbed in the digestive tract and appear in the blood, some appear slowly as the digested compounds are metabolized by the intestinal bacteria in the colon, while others are not absorbed at all in the digestive tract. This is therefore significantly different from compounds in the dissolved or suspended state. Therefore, the results of pharmacological tests from such studies cannot be translated into effects on humans without adjustments. In order to apply the results of pharmacological tests on cultured cells to humans, the results of the experiments are used as an index to separate and purify substances that show effectiveness by various chromatographies for the compounds contained in the extracts of herbs or Kampo formulas. It is necessary to obtain these substances and confirm that these pure substances appear in the blood when human beings take herbs or Kampo formulas orally.

4.1.2 Limitations of Animal Experiments

It is difficult to translate the results of pharmacological experiments obtained by suspending the extracts of herbs or Kampo formulas in physiological saline and by injecting them intraperitoneally or intravenously into mice or rats for the reasons mentioned above.

In addition, since lab animals such as mice and rats have a faster drug metabolism rate than humans, animal experiments need to be conducted administering 10–20 times the dose of the normal dose of the drugs in humans in terms of body weight. There are, however, no established methods for converting the dose set in animal experiments for humans. In addition, there are non-negligible species differences not only in drug reactivity but also in drug-metabolizing enzyme expression patterns and substrate affinity between test animals and humans. Therefore, translating the results of animal experiments to humans is done on a case-by-case basis. When judging the usefulness in humans from the results of pharmacological tests conducted in animal experiments using herbs or Kampo formulas, it is judged that a dose of 25 times or more compared to the normal dose for humans will be excessive amounts for the translation. Animal experiments should be aimed at estimating the mechanism of pharmacological action and exploring the active ingredients of herbs or Kampo formulas.

4.2 Examples of Basic Pharmacological Research Results Using Kampo Medicines Published in Various Guidelines

4.2.1 Anti-Allergic Effect of Shoseiryuto [50–52]

Shoseiryuto is a prescription that is strongly recommended for perennial allergic rhinitis in the clinical practice guidelines for nasal allergy. The usefulness of shoseiryuto has also been reported in some animal experiments. Oral administration of shoseiryuto extract significantly suppressed the number of sneezes and ovalbumin (OVA)-specific IgE concentration in the blood for an allergic rhinitis model created by intranasally administered OVA into the nasal cavity of mice. The helper T (Th) 1/Th2 balance of cytokines produced when CD_4^+ cells in lung tissue cultured shifted to the Th1 side. Significant symptom suppression was observed by oral administration of shoseiryuto extract in the passive skin cutaneous anaphylaxis (PCA) reaction model. This is a type I allergy model that develops after intradermal administration of anti-OVA serum to normal rats and intravenous administration of OVA. Among the constituent herbs, shoseiryuto, *saishin*, *hange*, and *kanzo* contributed to the effect of suppressing the PCA reaction of shoseiryuto in mice. Another constituent herb *shaykuyaku* suppressed the effect of the abovementioned herbs in shoseiryuto. Mudanpioside E has been isolated and identified as the counteracting component.

4.2.2 Effects of Tokishakuyakusan, Keishibukuryogan, and Kamishoyosan on Gynecological Diseases [53–57]

Obstetrics and gynecology have the highest usage rate of Kampo medicines among clinical departments, and Kampo medicines are often the first-line drugs for women-specific diseases such as menopause and dysmenorrhea. According to the obstetrics and gynecology practice guidelines, tokishakuyakusan, keishibukuryogan, kamishoyosan, and tokakujokito are recommended to use for menopausal disorders, functional dysmenorrhea, premenstrual syndrome, premenstrual dysphoric disorders, etc.

Oral administration of tokishakuyakusan extract showed a significant effect on anemia symptoms including the improvement of the serum transferrin and erythropoietin levels, and an increase in erythroblast count in bone marrow cells in rats reared with iron-deficient diet.

When calcitonin gene-related peptide (CGRP) was intravenously administered to the rats that had been subcutaneously administered with gonadotropin-releasing hormone (GnRH) derivative, menopause symptoms and increased skin temperature equivalent to hot flashes appeared. Those symptoms were significantly suppressed by oral administration of keishibukuryogan.

In the behavioral observation of normal mice, the time of social interaction was significantly increased in the mice to which kamishyosan extract was orally administered, and an anxiolytic effect was observed. Its action was inhibited by $GABA_A$ receptor blockers and antiandrogens, suggesting that kamishoyosan is useful for anxiety in menopause. Furthermore, *hakka* and *sanshishi* contribute to this effect among the herbs contained in kamishoyosan.

4.2.3 Effect of Saireito on IgA Nephropathy [58–61]

Saireito is a weakly recommended prescription for pediatric IgA nephropathy in clinical practice guidelines. In animal experiments, when saireito extract was administered to spontaneous IgA nephropathy model mice, mesangial cell proliferation and glomerular sclerosis score were significantly improved without affecting glomerular deposition of IgA. In a model of nephritis caused by intravenous administration of anti-glomerular basement membrane antibody to rats, oral administration of saireito extract improved proteinuria, crescent formation, adhesion to Bowman's capsule, and macrophage infiltration. Furthermore, the expression of various adhesion molecules in glomeruli was significantly suppressed. In addition, in a model of mesangial proliferative nephritis caused by intravenous administration of anti-thymus cell antigen to rats, oral administration of saireito extract significantly suppressed proteinuria, cell proliferation, macrophage infiltration, and intraglomerular transforming growth factor (TGF)-β and connective tissue growth factor (CTGF) expression in glomeruli.

4.2.4 Effect of Yokukansan on the Concomitant Symptoms of Dementia [62–65]

According to the dementia disease treatment guidelines, yokukansan is recommended to be used for behavioral and psychological symptoms of dementia (BPSD) and sleep disorders accompanying with dementia with Lewy bodies (DLB). It is stated that yokukansan may be considered for use in frustrated excitement, hallucinations, and delusion.

It has been reported that yokukansan extract significantly improved the occurrence of aggressive behavior and the decrease in memory score in social behavior tests caused by administration of amyloid β into the ventricles of mice. Mechanism of action is associated with the improvement of neurotransmitter secretion in the acetylcholine nerve system. In addition, it has been reported that the increase in aggressive behavior and anxiety behavior caused by breeding mice and rats on a thiamine-deficient diet was suppressed by the administration of yokukansan extract. Its mechanism of action is associated with the suppression of spongy astrocyte formation in the brain stem nerve loss in hippocampus and cerebral cortex, vacuole formation of astrocytes in the cerebral cortex, and dendrite swelling and glutamate uptake damage.

4.2.5 Effect of Daikenchuto on Ileus [66–72]

Ileus due to impairment of intestinal peristalsis frequently develops when open abdominal surgery is performed. It has become widely known that the onset of ileus can be prevented with daikenchuto, and positive results have been obtained in various clinical trials. Although it is not yet listed in the clinical practice guidelines as of 2021, many surgeons have started to use the ethical daikenchuto extract preparation. This not only improves the QOL of patients, but also reduces medical expenses by significant shortening of the length of hospital stay after surgery and the starting time of meal intake.

Oral administration of daikenchuto extract to anesthetized rats caused a transient increase in blood flow. The increase in gastrointestinal motility caused by the administration of the cholinergic drug carbachol to mice was significantly suppressed by the oral administration of daikenchuto extract. For each effect, it has been shown that the former is associated with *kankyo*, and the latter is associated with *kankyo* and *ninjin*. The decrease in gastrointestinal tract transporting capacity observed in a rat model produced by opening the abdomen under anesthesia, mechanically stimulating the gastrointestinal tract, and closing the abdomen was significantly recovered by the administration of daikenchuto extract. This effect is associated with *sansho*. In addition, the postoperative adhesion disorder observed in the model of abdominal closure after spraying talc on the gastrointestinal tract was relieved by the administration of daikenchuto extract. This activity was associated with serotonin-mediated cholinergic nerve and temperature-sensitive TRP channel TRPV1. Daikenchuto extract has also been reported to improve blood flow by releasing adrenomedulin via the TRPA1 channel in the gastrointestinal epithelium. It is therefore presumed that the positive effects of daikenchuto on ileus were related to above mechanisms (Fig. 4.13).

Fig. 4.13 Blood flow increasing effect of daikenchuto extract in anesthetized rats Oral treatment of daikenchuto extract (DKCT), cilostazol, a vasodilator, or scissors, a serotonin receptor agonist to anesthetized rats, and the changes in blood flow in the small intestine were traced. Mean ± standard error ($n = 7–8$). $^*p < 0.05$, $^{**}p < 0.01$ vs. vehicle-1; $^{\dagger}p < 0.01$ vs. vehicle-2

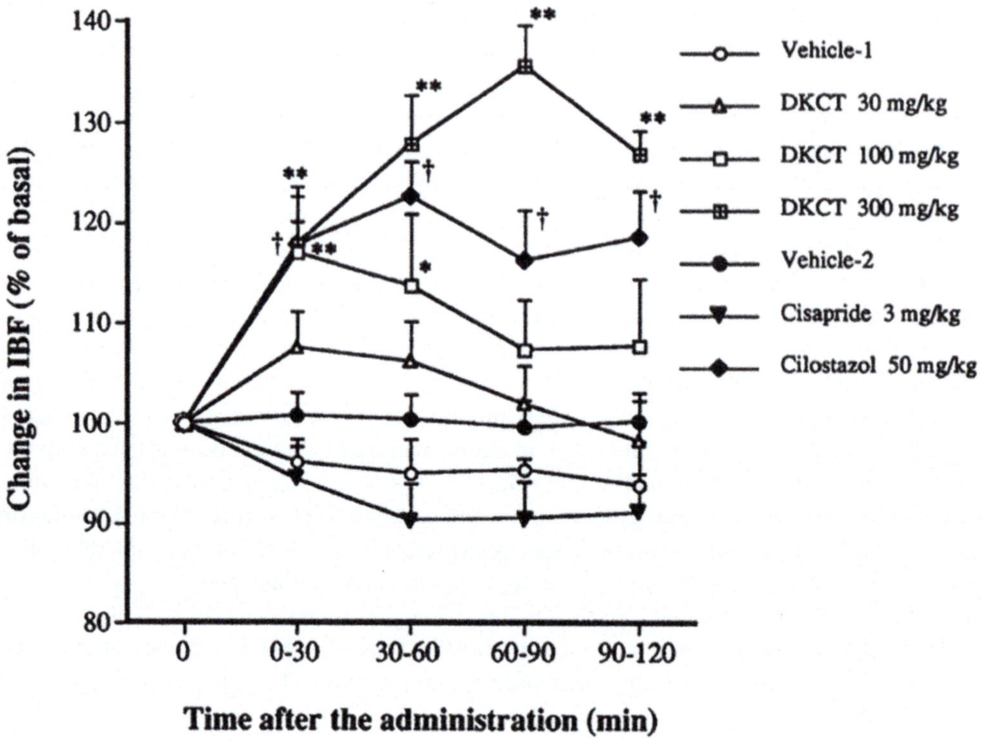

4.2.6 Effect of Rikkunshito on Functional Dyspepsia [73–76]

Clinical trials have revealed that rikkunshito has a palliative effect on functional dyspepsia (FD), and the guidelines issued by the Japanese Society of Psychiatry and Physical Medicine and the Japanese Society of Gastroenterology recommend the use of rikkunshito on FD. In addition, the results of clinical trials showed the usefulness of rikkunshito for a similar condition of the upper gastrointestinal tract, gastroesophageal reflux disease (GERD), which causes mucosal damage in the lower esophageal mucosa due to the reflux of stomach contents, causing symptoms such as dysphagia and heartburn.

The decrease in gastric emptying rate was suppressed by the administration of rikkunshito extract when serotonin was intraperitoneally administered to rats, and this effect was abolished by the administration of atropine. Rikkunshito extract did not affect the decrease due to dopamine. This suggests that rikkunshito improves anorexia by antagonizing the cholinergic nervous system that activates serotonin receptors. In addition, the decrease in food consumption caused by intraperitoneal administration of cisplatin to rats was suppressed by the administration of rikkunshito extract. This activity was inhibited by the administration of ghrelin receptor blocker. The decrease in acylgrelin, the activated form of grelin, concentration and the amount of ghrelin in the hypothalamus was recovered by the administration of rikkunshito extract. Therefore, it was speculated that the mechanism of action of rikkunshito is through the stimulation of ghrelin secretion in the hypothalamus via the suppression of serotonin nervous system.

4.2.7 Effect of Hochuekkito on the Immune System [77, 78]

Hochuekkito is a prescription that is expected to have an effect of enhancing immunity, and its usefulness against pulmonary nontuberculous mycobacterial infection has been reported in clinical trials. Oral administration of hochuekkito extract restored the decrease in the number of white blood cells in the blood, the lethal activity of natural killer cells in the spleen cells, the suppression of antibody production, and the decrease in the number of hematopoietic stem cells in the bone marrow cells in immunodeficiency models developed by administering the immunosuppressant cyclophosphamide and in models due to old age or to restraint stress.

Although hochuekkito is not indicated for the insurance medical treatment, its use for atopic dermatitis is weakly recommended in the treatment guidelines. In animal experiments, various pharmacological actions have been reported such as the suppression of scratching behavior, the suppression of blood concentrations of antigen-specific IgE antibody and inflammatory cytokine, the suppression of antibody production and inflammatory cytokine from cultured spleen cells collected from murine allergy models using hapten or OVA as antigens, and spontaneous atopic dermatitis model, etc. For details, refer to the review by Takayama et al. [78].

4.2.8 Effect of Hangeshashinto on Late-Onset Diarrhea, a Side Effect of Irinotecan [79–81]

Side effects of irinotecan, an anticancer drug, include early diarrhea that develops within 24 hours after the start of its administration and late diarrhea that develops several days after administration. To prevent this delayed diarrhea, a regimen using hangeshashinto has been established. Hangeshashinto has been shown to significantly improve grade 3 or higher diarrhea by a randomized, double-blind clinical trial.

The onset of delayed diarrhea induced by intravenous administration of irinotecan to rats, decreased water absorption capacity, and increase in prostaglandin E_2 level in the large intestine mucosa were significantly suppressed by oral administration of hangeshashinto extract. The mechanism of the side effects of irinotecan is that after the glucuronide conjugate of SN-38, the metabolite of irinotecan is excreted into bile. SN-38 appears after digestion by intestinal bacteria in the colon, and stimulates colonic peristaltic movement. It has been suggested that hangeshashinto and baicalin, which is contained in abundance in *ogon*, prevent the side effects of irinotecan by inhibiting its digestion of deglucuronide-conjugation.

4.2.9 Effect of Juzentaihoto on the Side Effects of Anticancer Drugs, Such as Compromised Immunity and Hematopoietic Function [82]

The combined use of fluorouracil and juzentaihoto in gastric cancer patients has been shown a strong effect in improving anorexia, general malaise, and leukopenia that develop as side effects, as well as extending survival time.

In animal experiments, it has been reported that the decrease in white blood cell count and hematopoietic stem cell count that occurs with administration of the anticancer drug TS-1 was suppressed by the combined use with juzentaihoto extract in mice.

4.2.10 Effect of Goshajinkigan on Neuropathic Pain as a Side Effect of Paclitaxel or Oxaplatin [83–88]

The use of anticancer drugs paclitaxel and oxaliplatin frequently causes sensory-impaired peripheral neuropathy (numbness) and neuropathic pain (hyperalgesia) in the extremities. These side effects are often severe and may even cause termination of chemotherapy. The usefulness of oshajinkigan is expected for these side effects, and some clinical trials have reported improvements. However, clinical trials have been reported that deny the effect on peripheral neuropathy caused by oxaliplatin, and administration is not recommended.

Neuropathic pain caused by intraperitoneal administration of paclitaxel to mice or oxaliplatin to rats was suppressed by oral administration of goshajinkigan extract, and it is speculated that its mechanism of action was involved in the suppression of the temperature-sensitive TRP channels TRPM8 and TRPA1. In an experiment in which paclitaxel or oxaliplatin was intraperitoneally administered to mice, the herb *bushi* contained in goshajinkigan, and one of its constituents neoline, are presumed to be the active ingredients (Fig. 4.14).

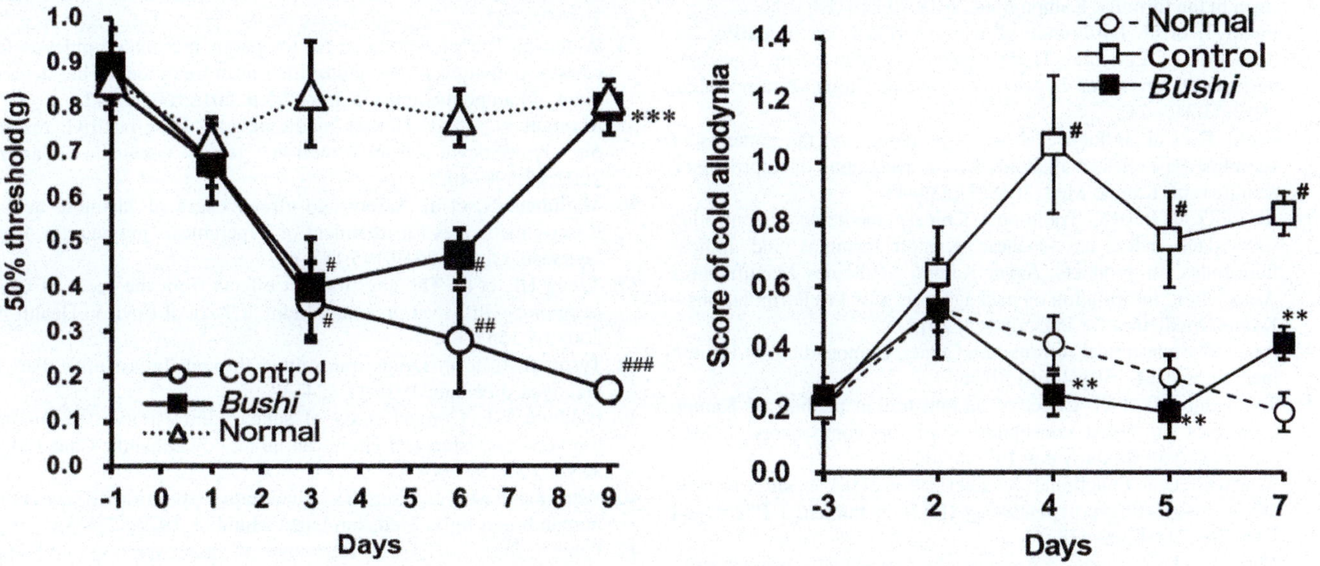

Fig. 4.14 Protective effect of *bushi* against neuropathic pain after administration of paclitaxel (left) or oxaliplatin (right) to mice. On day 0, the mice were administered paclitaxel (left) or oxaliplatin (right), and then bred with oral treatment of *bushi*. Subsequent mechanical allodynia (left) and cold hyperalgesia (right) were evaluated by von-Fray test (the lower the value, the more hyperalgesia) and the acetone test (the larger the value, the more hyperalgesia), respectively. The data are shown as mean ± standard error (n = 6–7). $^{\#}p < 0.05$, $^{\#\#}p < 0.01$, $^{\#\#\#}p < 0.001$ vs. normal group; $^{**}p < 0.01$, $^{***}p < 0.001$ vs. paclitaxel or oxaliplatin (control) group

References

1. ISO/TR23021:2018. Traditional Chinese medicine – controlled vocabulary on Japanese Kampo crude drugs.
2. Makino T, Yasui H, Namiki T. Comparison of the names and origins of crude drugs used in ethical Kampo extract formulation and listed in the Western pharmacopoeias with those in the pharmacopoeias in east Asian countries. Kampo Med. 2021;72:402–14.
3. Sakai Y, et al. Kampo formulae classifications in Kenzo Okuda's Kampo Koho Yoho Kaisetsu – the historical positioning of classifications in Japan and future issues. Kampo Med. 2012;63:340–6.
4. Hiraji H, et al. The development for the classification of formula based on the main crude drug and its background; consideration of the relationship between the classification of formulae based on the main crude drugs in Japan and formulae on Shang Han Za Bing Lun. Kampo Med. 2018;69:407–16.
5. Mitsuma T, et al. Assessment of the appropriate fee for dispensing herbal medicine. Kampo Med. 2005;56:211–20.
6. Ohno K, et al. The present status and problems of dispensing herbal medicine by the analysis of questionnaire survey to insurance pharmacies. Kampo Med. 2009;60:595–605.
7. Iwai T, et al. Evaluation of Xiao-chai-hu-tang prepared by patients. Kampo Med. 1989;39:49–53.
8. Sakakibara I, et al. Evaluation of Gou-teng (hooks and stems of Uncariae plants) III. Hypotensive principle from *Uncaria rhynchophylla* and alteration of its content on extraction process. Nat Med. 1999;53:308–12.
9. Doui M, et al. Study on decocting time for rhubarb from ancient times. Kampo Med. 2010;61:282–8.
10. Fueki T, et al. Development of quick and high-yielding method for the preparation of decoctions, inspired by the "zhu san fa" of the song period (part 2 – easy method to separate muddy residue from decoction). Kampo Med. 2016;67:114–22.
11. Fueki T, et al. The content of the aconitine-type diester alkaloids in the decoctions of the formula containing unprocessed aconite root in "Songban Shanghanlun" – influence of dried ginger and glycyrrhiza in the formula. Kampo Med. 2019;70:313–23.
12. Fueki T, et al. Difference of water hardness on preparing the decoction of Ephedrae Herba: especially focused on the comparison of tap water between Japan and China. Kampo Med. 2012;63:313–21.
13. Fueki T, et al. Influence of water properties on the contents of aconitine-type diester alkaloids in the decoctions of unprocessed aconite root. Kampo Med. 2018;69:336–45.
14. ISO/TR23022:2018. Traditional Chinese medicine – controlled vocabulary index on Japanese Kampo formulas and indication codes for products. Japan Kampo Medicines Manufactures Association. Information on package inserts of 148 Formulations – Kampo Medicines for Prescription; 2012.
15. Japan Pharmaceutical Information Center. Compendium of Kampo medicines 2014. ISBN4865150196.
16. Tomogane M, et al. Effect of administration method of Kampo medicines on blood concentration of the components. J Med Pharmceu Soc Wakan-yaku. 1991;8:402–3.
17. Nozawa T, et al. Functional characterization of pH-sensitive organic anion transporting polypeptide OATP-B in human. J Pharmacol Exp Ther. 2004;308:438–45.
18. Makino T, et al. Enzymatically modified isoquercitrin, α-oligoglucosyl quercetin 3-*O*-glucoside, is absorbed more easily than other quercetin glycosides or aglycone after oral administration in rats. Biol Pharm Bull. 2009;32:2034–40.
19. Yu K, et al. Absorption, disposition, and pharmacokinetics of Saponins from Chinese medicinal herbs: what do we know and what do we need to know more? Curr Drug Metab. 2012;13:577–98.
20. Shimada Y, et al. Adverse events associated with ethical Kampo formulations: analysis of the domestic adverse-event data reports of the Ministry of Health, labor, and welfare in Japan. Evid Based Complement Alternat Med. 2019;2019:1643804.
21. Mantani N, et al. Relationship between incidence of pseudoaldosteronism and daily dose of Glycyrrhiza: review of the literature. Kampo Med. 2015;66:197–202.
22. Ishiuchi K, et al. 18β-glycyrrhetyl-3-*O*-sulfate would be a causative agent of licorice-induced pseidoaldosteronisum. Sci Rep. 2019;9:1587.
23. Makino T, et al. Exploration for the real causative agents of licorice-induced pseudoaldosteronism. J Nat Med. 2021;75:275–83.
24. Ishida T, et al. Risk factors for pseudoaldosteronism with yokukansan use: analysis using the Japanese adverse drug report (JADER) database. Biol Pharm Bull. 2020;43:1570–6.
25. Shimada S, et al. Liquorice-induced hypokalaemia in patients treated with Yokukansan preparations: identification of the risk factors in a retrospective cohort study. BMJ Open. 2017;2017:e014218.
26. Terada M, et al. Pharmacoepidemiology of interstitial pneumonia and liver dysfunction associated with Kampo medicine. Jap J Pharmaceu Health Care Sci. 2002;28:425–34.
27. Mantani N, et al. Incidence of liver injury related to kampo medicine containing *Scutellaria baicalensis* at our clinic. Kampo Med. 2017;68:377–81.
28. Enomoto Y, et al. Japanese herbal medicine-induced pneumonitis: a review of 73 patients. Respir Investig. 2017;55:138–44.
29. Nakajima N. Diagnosis of drug-induced pneumonia. Kampo Med. 2012;63:81–8.
30. Nogami T, et al. Incidence of kampo medicine-induced interstitial pneumonia: 10 year retrospective study at a university hospital kampo medicine department. Tradit Kampo Med. 2019;6:26–31.
31. Nusko G, et al. Retrospective study on laxative use and melanosis coli as risk factors for colorectal neoplasma. Pharmacology. 1993;47(Suppl 1):234–41.
32. Shimizu S, et al. Involvement of herbal medicine as a cause of mesenteric phlebosclerosis: results from a large-scale nationwide survey. J Gastroenterol. 2017;52:308–14.
33. Nagata Y, et al. Total dosage of gardenia fruit used by patients with mesenteric phlebosclerosis. BMC Complement Altern Med. 2016;16:207.
34. Watanabe T, et al. Screening for idiopathic mesenteric phlebosclerosis in outpatients undergoing long-term treatment at the department of kampo medicine. Kampo Med. 2016;67:230–43.
35. Mantani N, et al. Herbal medicine and false-positive results on lymphocyte transformation test. Yakugaku Zasshi. 2002;22:399–402.
36. Michihata N, et al. Safety and effectiveness of Japanese herbal Kampo medicines for treatment of hyperemesis gravidarum. Int J Gynaecol Obstet. 2019;145:182–6.
37. Tzeng HP, et al. The abortifacient effects from the seeds of *Coix lachryma-jobi* L. var. *ma-yuen* Stapf. J Toxicol Environ Health A. 2005;68:1557–65.
38. Tyson RM, et al. Drugs transmitted through breast milk. Part I: laxatives. J Pediatr. 1937;11:824–32.
39. Baldwin WF. Clinical study of senna administration to nursing mothers: assessment of effects on infant bowel habits. Canad Med Ass J. 1963;89:566–8.
40. Werthmann MW Jr, Krees SV. Quantitative excretion of Senokot in human breast milk. Med Ann Dist Columbia. 1973;42:4–5.
41. Faber P, Strenge-Hesse A. Relevance of rhein excretion into breast milk. Pharmacology. 1988;36(Suppl 1):212–20.
42. American Academy of Pediatrics – Committee on Drugs. The transfer of drugs and other chemicals into human milk. Pediatrics. 2001;108:776–89.
43. Dailymed. https://dailymed.nlm.nih.gov/dailymed/fda/fdaDrugXsl.cfm?setid=ea14be82-1d4d-41fe-9e2f-3f4df9393be5&type=display
44. Ikemoto T, et al. Changes of immunological parameters with administration of Japanese Kampo medicine (Juzen-Taihoto/TJ-48)

in patients with advanced pancreatic cancer. Int J Clin Oncol. 2014;19:81–6.
45. Bailey DG, et al. Interaction of citrus juices with felodipine and nifedipine. Lancet. 1991;337:268–9.
46. Edwards D, et al. Identification of 6′,7′-dihydroxybergamottin, a cytochrome P450 inhibitor, in grapefruit juice. Drug Metab Dispos. 1996;24:1287–90.
47. Ohnishi M, et al. Effect of a Kampo preparation, byakkokaninjinto, on pharmacokinetics of ciprofloxacin and tetracycline. Biol Pharm Bull. 2009;32:1080–4.
48. World Anti-doping Agency. World anti-doping code and international standard framework development and implementation guide for stakeholders. World anti-doping agency. 2021. https://www.wada-ama.org/sites/default/files/resources/files/worldconference-backgrounder_0.pdf
49. Yahagi T, et al. Quality evaluation of Pinellia tuber by LC-TOF/MS targeted to ephedrine. J Nat Med. 2021;75:692–8.
50. Ikeda Y, et al. Possible involvement of suppression of Th2 differentiation in the anti-allergic effect of Sho-seiryuto in mice. Jap J Pharmacol. 2002;90:328–36.
51. Sakaguchi M, et al. Pharmacological characteristics of Sho-seiryu-to, an antiallergic Kampo medicine without effects on histamine H1 receptors and muscarinic cholinergic system in the brain. Methods Find Exp Clin Pharmacol. 1996;18:41–7.
52. Tsukamoto K, et al. Counteractive effect of Paeonia lactiflora root constituent mudanpioside E against suppressive effect of Shoseiryuto-extract on passive cutaneous anaphylaxis reaction in mice. J Ethnopharmacol. 2014;153:884–9.
53. Akase T, et al. A comparative study of laboratory parameters and symptoms effected by Toki-shakuyaku-san and an iron preparation in rats with iron-deficiency anemia. Biol Pharm Bull. 2004;27:871–8.
54. Akase T, et al. Efficacy of tokishakuyakusan on the anemia in the iron-deficient pregnant rats. Biol Pharm Bull. 2007;30:1523–8.
55. Noguchi M, et al. Skin temperature rise induced by calcitonin gene-related peptide in gonadotropin-releasing hormone analogue-treated female rats and alleviation by Keishi-bukuryogan, a Japanese herbal medicine. Life Sci. 2005;76:2079–90.
56. Mizowaki M, et al. Anxiolytic effect of kami-Shoyo-san (TJ-24) in mice: possible mediation of neurosteroid synthesis. Life Sci. 2001;69:2167–77.
57. Toriizuka K, et al. Anxiolytic effect of Gardeniae Fructus-extract containing active ingredient from kamishoyosan (KSS), a Japanese traditional Kampo medicine. Life Sci. 2005;77:3010–20.
58. Hattori T, et al. Effect of saireito (TJ-114) on adhesion molecule expression in glomeruli of anti-GBM nephritis rats. Jap J Nephlol. 1995;37:373–83.
59. Hattori T, et al. Saireito probably prevents mesangial cell proliferation in HIGA mice via PDGF-BB tyrosine kinase inhibition. Clin Exp Nephrol. 2007;11:275–82.
60. Liu N, et al. Suppressive effects of Sairei-to on mesangial proliferation in a rat model of glomerulonephritis. Clin Exp Nephrol. 2004;8:216–22.
61. Ono T, et al. Suppressive mechanisms of Sairei-to on mesangial matrix expansion in rat mesangioproliferative glomerulonephritis. Nephron Exp Nephrol. 2005;100:e132–42.
62. Sekiguchi K, et al. Effects of yokukansan, a traditional Japanese medicine, on aggressiveness induced by intracerebroventricular injection of amyloid beta protein into mice. Phytother Res. 2009;23:1175–81.
63. Sekiguchi K, et al. Effects of yokukansan and donepezil on learning disturbance and aggressiveness induced by intracerebroventricular injection of amyloid beta protein in mice. Phytother Res. 2011;25:501–7.
64. Uchida N, et al. Cholinergic involvement and synaptic dynamin 1 expression in yokukansan-mediated improvement of spatial memory in a rat model of early Alzheimer's disease. Phytother Res. 2013;27:966–72.
65. Ikarashi Y, et al. Effects of yokukansan, a traditional Japanese medicine, on memory disturbance and behavioral and psychological symptoms of dementia in thiamine-deficient rats. Biol Pharm Bull. 2009;32:1701–9.
66. Satoh K, et al. Dai-kenchu-to enhances accelerated small intestinal movement. Biol Pharm Bull. 2001;24:1122–6.
67. Murata P, et al. The herbal medicine Dai-kenchu-to and one of its active components [6]-shogaol increase intestinal blood flow in rats. Life Sci. 2002;70:2061–70.
68. Tokita Y, et al. The pharmacological effects of Daikenchuto, a traditional herbal medicine, on delayed gastrointestinal transit in rat postoperative ileus. J Pharmacol Sci. 2007;104:303–10.
69. Tokita Y, et al. Possible involvement of the transient receptor potential vanilloid type 1 channel in postoperative adhesive obstruction and its prevention by a kampo (traditional Japanese) medicine, daikenchuto. J Pharmacol Sci. 2011;115:75–83.
70. Hosaka M, et al. Efficacy of daikenchuto, a traditional Japanese Kampo medicine, for postoperative intestinal dysfunction in patients with gastrointestinal cancers: meta-analysis. Int J Clin Oncol. 2019;24:1385–96.
71. Kono T, et al. Epithelial transient receptor potential ankyrin 1 (TRPA1)-dependent adrenomedullin upregulates blood flow in rat small intestine. Am J Phys. 2013;304:G428–36.
72. Hiraishi K, et al. Daikenchuto (Da-Jian-Zhong-tang) ameliorates intestinal fibrosis by activating myofibroblast transient receptor potential ankyrin 1 channel. World J Gastroenterol. 2018;24:4036–53.
73. Tominaga K, et al. The traditional Japanese medicine rikkunshito promotes gastric emptying via the antagonistic action of the 5-HT3 receptor pathway in rats. Evid Based Complement Alternat Med. 2011;2011:248481.
74. Takeda H, et al. Rikkunshito, an herbal medicine, suppresses cisplatin-induced anorexia in rats via 5-HT2 receptor antagonism. Gastroenterol. 2008;134:2004–13.
75. Yakabi K, et al. Rikkunshito and 5-HT2C receptor antagonist improve cisplatin-induced anorexia via hypothalamic ghrelin interaction. Regul Pept. 2010;161:97–105.
76. Yakabi K, et al. Reduced ghrelin secretion in the hypothalamus of rats due to cisplatin-induced anorexia. Endocrinology. 2010;151:3773–82.
77. Enomoto Y, et al. Pilot quasirandomized controlled study of herbal medicine Hochuekkito as an adjunct to conventional treatment for progressed pulmonary Mycobacterium avium complex disease. PLoS One. 2014;9:e104411.
78. Takayama S, et al. Basic pharmacological mechanisms and clinical evidence of the efficacy of hochu-ekkito against infectious diseases and its potential for use against COVID-19. Trad Kampo Med. 2021;8:3–21.
79. Kase Y, et al. Preventive effects of Hange-shashin-to on irinotecan hydrochloride-caused diarrhea and its relevance to the colonic prostaglandin E2 and water absorption in the rat. Jpn J Pharmacol. 1007;75:407–13.
80. Stoh T, et al. Inhibitory effects of baicalein derived from Japanese traditional herbal medicine on SN-38 glucuronidation. J Pharm Pharm Sci. 2018;21:195–206.
81. Mori K, et al. Preventive effect of Kampo medicine (Hangeshashin-to) against irinotecan-induced diarrhea in advanced non-small-cell lung cancer. Cancer Chemother Pharmacol. 2003;51:403–6.
82. Ogawa K, et al. Protective effect of the Japanese traditional medicine juzentaihoto on myelosuppression induced by the anticancer drug TS-1 and identification of a potential biomarker of this effect. BMC Complement Altern Med. 2012;12:118.

83. Andoh T, et al. Effects of goshajinkigan, hachimijiogan, and rokumigan on mechanical allodynia induced by paclitaxel in mice. J Trad Complement Med. 2014;4:293–7.
84. Kato Y, et al. Gosha-jinki-Gan reduced oxaliplatin-induced hypersensitivity to cold sensation and its effect would be related to suppression of the expression of TRPM8 and TRPA1 in rats. Anti-Cancer Drugs. 2014;25:39–43.
85. Mizuno K, et al. Goshajinkigan, a traditional Japanese medicine, prevents oxaliplatin-induced acute peripheral neuropathy by suppressing functional alteration of TRP channels in rat. J Pharmacol Sci. 2014;125:91–8.
86. Suzuki T, et al. Processed aconite root and its active ingredient neoline may alleviate oxaliplatin-induced peripheral neuropathic pain. J Ethnopharmacol. 2016;186:44–52.
87. Tanimura Y, et al. Neoline is the active ingredient of processed aconite root against murine peripheral neuropathic pain model, and its pharmacokinetics in rats. J Ethnopharmacol. 2019;241:111859.
88. Kono T, et al. Goshajinkigan oxaliplatin neurotoxicity evaluation (GONE): a phase 2, multicenter, randomized, double-blind, placebo-controlled trial of goshajinkigan to prevent oxaliplatin-induced neuropathy. Cencer Chemother Pharmacol. 2013;72:283–1290.

5 Therapy Details

Shin-ichi Muramatsu, Akira Saito, Toru Kaneko, Tatsuya Ishige, Hiroshi Odaguchi, Koichiro Tatsumi, Takashi Ito, Shuji Yakubo, Tetsuro Oikawa, Hirokuni Okumi, Makoto Fujimoto, Tadamichi Mitsuma, Takao Ikeuchi, Takahisa Ushiroyama, Koji Watanabe, Kako Watanabe, Mayumi Tamada, Toshiaki Kogure, Yutaka Shimada, Masaru Natsuaki, Hironobu Iguchi, Eiichi Tahara, Shinji Nishida, Kenshu Lai, Takaaki Kosuge, Motoko Fukuzawa, Hideaki Yamaguchi, Akito Hisanaga, Ikuro Wakayama, Toshihiro Togo, Takashi Seki, Yoshiharu Motoo, and Makoto Arai

1 Head

1.1 Headache

Shin-ichi Muramatsu

1.1.1 Overview of Disease

Headache is a frequent symptom, and the 1-year prevalence of tension-type headache, the most common type of headache, is regarded as 11–45% [1]. The International Headache Society has classified headaches (ICHD-3), indicating the various diagnostic criteria for primary headache and secondary headache [2]. Primary headache includes migraine and tension-type headache. Secondary headache is caused by trauma or injury to the head and/or neck, cranial and/or cervical vascular disorder, intracranial neoplasia, infection, or psychiatric disorders.

The prodromal symptoms of migraine include yawning, irritability, hunger sensation, and edema. In typical cases, signs of scintillating scotoma are found as visual aura. An intense pulsatile headache follows, accompanied by nausea and vomiting, which may continue for several hours up to 72 h. Symptoms are exacerbated with sound or light stimulation, movement, or posture change. Since walking, ascending/descending stairs, and other daily activities may exacerbate symptoms, patients often remain still in a darkened room.

S.-i. Muramatsu · T. Ikeuchi
Division of Oriental Medicine, Center for Community Medicine, Jichi Medical University, Shimotsuke, Japan

A. Saito
Wako-ent Clinic, Saitama Medical University, Wako, Japan

T. Kaneko
Kaneko Otolaryngology Clinic, Utsunomiya, Japan

T. Ishige
Kobushi ENT Clinic, Yashio, Japan

H. Odaguchi
Kitasato University Kitasato Institute Hospital, Tokyo, Japan

K. Tatsumi
Department of Respirology, Graduate School of Medicine, Chiba University, Chiba, Japan

T. Ito
Akashi Clinic Kanda, Tokyo, Japan

S. Yakubo
Department of Medicine, The Nippon Dental University School of Life Dentistry, Tokyo, Japan

T. Oikawa
Center for Kampo Medicine, Tokyo Medical University Hospital, Tokyo, Japan

H. Okumi
Ihoukai Medical Association Okumi Clinic, Osaka, Japan

M. Fujimoto
Department of Japanese Oriental Medicine, Graduate School of Medicine and Pharmaceutical Sciences(School of Medicine), University of Toyama, Toyama, Japan

T. Mitsuma
Department of Kampo Medicine, Aizu Medical Center Hospital, Fukushima Medical University, Aizuwakamatsu, Japan

T. Ushiroyama
Osaka Medical and Pharmaceutical University Health Science Clinic, Takatsuki, Japan

Kampo Medical Literature Editorial Committee, The Japan Society for Oriental Medicine (ed.), *Complete Japanese Traditional (Kampo) Medicine*, https://doi.org/10.1007/978-981-96-7143-4_5

1.1.2 Indications for Kampo Therapy

Primary headache—migraine and tension-type headache—is a good indication for Kampo medicines.

The drug of first choice in the treatment of migraine is triptan formulations, serotonin receptor ($5\text{-}HT_{1B/1D}$) agonists. Triptans, however, do not reduce the frequency of attacks and are ineffective in one-third of cases. Kampo medicines are indicated even for medication overuse headache (MOH) caused by overuse of triptans or various anti-inflammatory analgesics.

There are not many options among Western drugs that can be used for symptomatic treatment of tension-type headaches. Anti-anxiety agents and muscle relaxants are problematic because of drowsiness, lightheadedness, and other side effects. Kampo medicines increase treatment options remarkably.

Kampo medicines may be tried for secondary headaches associated with organic diseases, particularly sensations of heavy-headedness associated with chronic subdural hematoma or brain tumors.

1.1.3 Frequently Used Formulas (Table 5.1a, b)

Migraine

The edema preceding migraine, vomiting during attacks, and excess urination during recovery are considered to be the results of fluid[TM1] retention. Therefore, it is most appropriate to use fluid[TM1]-regulating formulas containing jutsu, bukuryo, and takusha. At the onset of a migraine attack, the typical Kampo medicines to be administered are goreisan and goshuyuto. Many women suffer from migraines, which are often worse during menstruation. In this case, the use of blood[TM1] stasis resolving formulas containing toki and tonin may be helpful.

- **Goreisan**: Widely used mainly for patients with medium (excess, deficiency) patterns. Indications include thirst, decreased urine volume, vomiting by counterflow of water, and teeth marks. However, not all these symptoms need to be present. It is effective for patients who suffer headaches before rain. Goreisan is also used for hangover and chronic subdural hematoma [3].
- **Goshuyuto**: Used for migraine with vomiting in patients with a slight deficiency pattern who are prone to fatigue and suffer from coldness of limbs. This formula is considered to be effective for patients who suffer menstruation-related migraine, shoulder, and neck stiffness before migraine attacks, or epigastric fullness from counterflow during migraine attacks.
- **Keishininjinto**: Used for headache in slight deficiency ninjinto-pattern patients with interior cold, characterized by a weak digestive system, chronic indigestion, and tendency to have diarrhea. These patients often have epigastric stuffiness.
- **Tokishakuyakusan**: Normally used for slight deficiency pattern patients to treat heavy sensation in the head. Administration in between attacks of menstruation-related migraines, however, can also reduce the frequency of attacks and severity of pain. This medication is effective for women who have poor complexion and poor circulation and complain of dizziness and shoulder stiffness.

K. Watanabe
Watanabe Sanfujinka, Hiki-gun, Japan

K. Watanabe
Obiyama Central Hospital, Kumamoto, Japan

M. Tamada
Institute of Oriental Medicine Tokyo Women's Medical University, Tokyo, Japan

T. Kogure
Maebashi Fueki Clinic, Maebashi, Japan

Y. Shimada
Osawano Clinic, Toyama, Japan

M. Natsuaki
Department of Dermatology, Hyogo Medical University, Nishinomiya, Japan

H. Iguchi
Sawa Memorial Hamamatsu Hospital, Hamamatsu, Japan

E. Tahara
Department of Kampo Medicine, Aizu Medical Center, Fukushima Medical University, Aizuwakamatsu, Japan

S. Nishida
Nishida Clinic, Sakai, Japan

K. Lai
Kampo Lai Clinic, Tokyo, Japan

T. Kosuge
Kosuge Clinic Yokohama Suzaku Kampo Medical Center, Yokohama, Japan

M. Fukuzawa
Omotesando Fukuzawa Clinic, Tokyo, Japan

H. Yamaguchi
K Children's Clinic, Nagoya, Japan

A. Hisanaga
Department of Psychiatry, Hospital Bando, Bando, Japan

I. Wakayama
Kansai University of Health Sciences, Sennan-gun, Japan

T. Togo
Meiji University of Integrative Medicine, Nantan, Japan

T. Seki
The Integrative Medicine Center, Fuji Toranomon Orthopedic Hospital, Gotenba, Japan

Y. Motoo
Department of Internal Medicine, Fukui Saiseikai Hospital, Fukui, Japan

M. Arai (✉)
Department of Kampo Medicine, Tokai University School of Medicine/Department of General Internal Medicine, St. Marianna University School of Medicine, Kawasaki, Japan
e-mail: office@jsom.or.jp

Table 5.1 (**a**) Frequently used formulas for headache (excess pattern). (**b**) Frequently used formulas for headache [medium (excess, deficiency) patterns]

(a) Excess pattern	
High blood pressure—Facial redness	San'oshashinto Orengedokuto
Shoulder stiffness and posterior cervical tightness	Kakkonto
Shoulder stiffness—Insomnia	Daisaikoto
Agitation—Oversensitivity	Yokukansan
Hot flashes—Blood stasis Dizziness	Tokakujokito Tsudosan
Insomnia—impatience—palpitation	Saikokaryukotsuboreito
(b) Medium (excess, deficiency) pattern	
Pulsatile headache—Vomiting	Goreisan
Dizziness—Hot flashes	Ryokeijutsukanto
High blood pressure—Shoulder stiffness—Dizziness	Chotosan
Hot flashes—Dizziness—Shoulder stiffness	Nyoshinsan
Nervousness	Shigyakusan
Common cold	Senkyuchachosan
Trigeminal autonomic cephalalgias (TACs)	Seijokentsuto

- **Tokakujokito**: Used to treat headaches in slight excess to excess patterns in women with a good physique who suffer from irregular menstruation and constipation. The characteristic abdominal pattern is lower abdominal cramps.

Tension-Type Headache

Tension-type headache sufferers complain of heaviness of the head, as though wearing something heavy on the head. In Kampo medicine, this symptom is termed "hat-wearing sensation," and many known formulas are used. Differentiation is made by consideration of coexisting symptoms, including hypertension, dizziness, shoulder stiffness, and coldness, in the deficiency, medium (excess, deficiency), and excess patterns.

(a) **Headache associated with shoulder stiffness and occipital pain**

- **Kakkonto**: Used in medium to slight excess pattern patients with physical strength and whose digestive system is not weak. In cases of sinusitis, shin'i, senkyu, sekko, and/or kikyo are added.
- **Daisaikoto**: Appropriate for headache in excess pattern patients with good physique and tight abdominal muscles. Other symptoms include shoulder stiffness, insomnia, and excitability.
- **Saikokaryukotsuboreito**: Preferable to daisaikoto for headache in patients with the slight excess pattern. Other symptoms include palpitations, shortness of breath, and psychoneurotic symptoms such as irritability, insomnia, excessive dreaming, impatience, depression, and flightiness. In addition, there can be fullness and discomfort in the chest and hypochondrium and palpitation in the para-umbilical region.
- **Shigyakusan**: Good for medium to slight excess pattern patients with a nervous, introverted character and a tendency of anxiety and/or depression.
- **Kamishoyosan**: Appropriate for patients with slight deficiency pattern. Used when there are many fluctuating complaints, including headache, dizziness, tinnitus, palpitation, shoulder stiffness, low back pain, and insomnia.
- **Yokukansan**: Used for slight excess pattern patients with tension-type headaches with oversensitivity such as irritability and short temper, or excitability and insomnia. In chronic cases, if the abdomen is soft and aortic pulsation is palpable, yokukansankachimpihange is preferable.

(b) **Headache with dizziness**

- **Ryokeijutsukanto**: Broadly used for fluid[TM1] retention in patients with slight deficiency pattern and frequently used for chronic dizziness, including the sensation of unsteadiness and orthostatic dizziness. Typical cases are characterized by decreased urination, cold limbs, and a deep and tight pulse. Abdominal examination reveals splashing sounds and epigastric distension (epigastric fullness from counterflow). It may be used as the combined formula renjuin, along with shimotsuto.
- **Hangebyakujutsutemmato**: Used for dizziness and headache in patients with slight deficiency pattern and constitutional gastrointestinal weakness. It is also good for vertigo, the feeling of unsteadiness, and lightheadedness upon standing. Low blood pressure is common.
- **Nyoshinsan**: Good for the sensation of heaviness or hat-wearing on the head, dizziness, hot flashes, and shoulder stiffness in medium to slight excess pattern women with menopausal disorders. The primary indications are hot flashes and dizziness.

(c) **Headache with high blood pressure**

- **Orengedokuto**: For slight excess to excess pattern patients with facial redness and conjunctival congestion. Other symptoms include hot flashes, anxiety and uneasiness, insomnia, and nasal bleeding.

- **San'oshashinto**: Used for slight excess to excess pattern patients with orengedokuto pattern with pronounced epigastric stuffiness and constipation.
- **Shichimotsukokato**: Used for slight deficiency pattern patients with high blood pressure. Considered to be good for patients with proteinuria and those with high diastolic blood pressure.
- **Chotosan**: Used for hypertensive patients with medium pattern, associated with headache, hot flashes, conjunctival hyperemia, shoulder stiffness, dizziness, or tinnitus. The skin is dry with less luster; the abdomen is weaker and slacker than that of yokukansan-pattern patients. It is considered good for patients who suffer headaches in the morning.
- **Tsudosan**: Used for patients with excess pattern, associated with epigastric distress, insomnia, anxiety and other neuropsychiatric symptoms, dysmenorrhea, constipation, hot flush, and hypertension.

(d) **Headache with sensitivity to cold**

- **Goshakusan**: Used for coldness in the lower body and hot flashes in the upper body, or upper heat and lower cold. Effective for anemia as well as headache or low back pain with sensitivity to cold in patients with slight deficiency to medium pattern.
- **Tokishigyakukagoshuyushokyoto**: Used for patients with deficiency pattern who have strong coldness of extremities and are prone to frostbite.

Other Headache: Facial Pain

Cluster headaches and closely related conditions consisting of autonomic symptoms such as clustering of severe headaches, conjunctival congestion, epiphora, nasal obstruction, and palpebral edema are termed trigeminal autonomic cephalalgia (TAC). Kampo medicines may be tried in cases associated with organic diseases, including cerebellopontine angle tumors.

- **Senkyuchachosan**: Used for medium pattern patients with headaches in general, but is particularly good for headaches following the common cold.
- **Seijokentsuto:**[1] Used for medium pattern patients with headaches or trigeminal neuralgia not relieved by other formulas.

[1] Not available as a medically approved Kampo extract formulation.

1.2 Dizziness/Vertigo: Tinnitus [4–6]

Akira Saito

1.2.1 Overview of Disease

Dizziness/Vertigo

The origins of dizziness/vertigo vary and include inner ear disorders (such as Meniere's disease and benign paroxysmal positional vertigo), central nervous system diseases (such as cerebellar infarction), autonomic nervous system abnormalities, and aging-related changes. In quite a few cases, hearing and equilibrium function tests or brain MRIs show no abnormality, and psychogenic elements such as stress can contribute to the dizziness. Many drug therapies are available, but in some cases, psychotherapy or therapeutic exercise may be effective, while in others, surgery is required. Improvement of daily living habits is also important.

Tinnitus

The origins of tinnitus may often lie in the regions of the acoustic pathway from the outer ear to the central nervous system, in addition to the inner ear. Tinnitus associated with conduction hearing loss may improve with otological treatment or surgery. Drug therapies using vitamins, circulation-improving agents, and anti-anxiety drugs are widespread. Treatment may include counseling or sound therapy. When patients are told that tinnitus does not heal, their resistance to therapy increases. It is, therefore, important to explain that although the tinnitus itself will not disappear, it is possible to lead daily life without being bothered by it. Improvement of daily living habits is also important.

1.2.2 Indications for Kampo Therapy

Western medical therapies are favored when drinking formulas is difficult in the acute phase, the dizziness/vertigo is life-threatening, or tinnitus is associated with acute sensory hearing loss. In all other cases, dizziness/vertigo and tinnitus are good candidates for Kampo therapy.

Fundamentally there is no problem in combining Kampo therapy with Western drugs. Such combination therapy should be proactively considered when symptoms get worse. For example, if Meniere's disease is being treated with Kampo medicines and attacks occur with increased hearing loss, administration of steroids or an osmotic diuretic may be required.

The potential of Kampo medicines having a direct effect on the inner ear cannot be denied, but mostly they are considered to alleviate dizziness/vertigo and tinnitus by improving insomnia, psychological agitation, shoulder stiffness, and hot flashes.

1.2.3 Frequently Used Formulas (Fig. 5.1)

Although it is often said that the pathologic condition of dizziness is fluid[TM1] retention, dizziness is caused by abnormalities of qi or blood[TM1] as well as fluid[TM1]. In blood[TM1] stasis or fluid[TM1] retention, the smooth flow of qi and blood[TM1] to the brain is inhibited. Qi deficiency and blood[TM1] deficiency mean nutrients are lacking, while qi counter flow means excessive qi is being supplied to the brain. Qi stagnation means qi is stagnant and does not circulate to the brain. Similarly, tinnitus can arise because of an abnormality of qi, blood[TM1], or fluid[TM1].

Most Kampo medicines prescribed for dizziness/vertigo are also used for tinnitus.

- **Juzentaihoto:** Used for deficiency pattern with dizziness associated with orthostatic dysregulation or fatigue. Symptoms include anemia, fatigue and malaise, anorexia, poor complexion, and lusterless skin.
- **Shimbuto:** Used for orthostatic dysregulation, dizziness with intense coldness in the upper and lower limbs, and dizziness in elderly people. Patients are fragile and weak and also have general malaise, diarrhea, and abdominal pain.
- **Kamishoyosan:** Used for dizziness coinciding with the estrous cycle or menopause, in addition to highly psychogenic dizziness and tinnitus. Used for slight deficiency-pattern patients with anxiety, irritability, insomnia, shoulder stiffness, paroxysmal sweating, and burning sensation.
- **Shimotsuto:** Used for dizziness related to dysmenorrhea or delivery in women with slight deficiency pattern with anemia and skin dryness. Frequently used in combination with ryokeijutsukanto.
- **Ninjin'yoeito:** Used for dizziness in slight deficiency pattern patients with a stronger tendency toward anxiety, depression, and palpitation than patients with *juzentaihoto* pattern.
- **Tokishakuyakusan:** Effective for menopausal dizziness as well as dizziness coinciding with the estrous cycle. Patients have a slight deficiency pattern with coldness and anemia.
- **Hachimijiogan—Goshajinkigan:** Used for lightheadedness and tinnitus due to age-related changes. Frequently used in elderly patients. Patients have a slight deficiency pattern with coldness in the lower back and legs, numbness, and a feeling of weakness, along with nocturia and blurred vision.
- **Hangebyakujutsutemmato:** Used for inner ear dizziness and tinnitus, orthostatic dysregulation, and shoulder stiffness, as well as dizziness after eating. Patients have a slight deficiency pattern and poor digestive function, anorexia, coldness, and heavy-headedness.
- **Hochuekkito:** Effective for dizziness associated with orthostatic dysregulation or fatigue-related lightheadedness. Patients have a slight deficiency pattern with symptoms including weak constitution, strong general malaise, reduced digestive function, low energy, tendency to fatigue, postprandial sleepiness, spontaneous sweating, quiet voice, and headache.
- **Yokukansankachimpihange:** Used for patients with slight deficiency pattern and weaker than those of yokukansan-pattern patients. Effective for tinnitus and dizziness associated with depressive tendency.
- **Ryokeijutsukanto:** Used for inner ear dizziness and tinnitus, orthostatic dysregulation, and dizziness associated with palpitation. Patients have a slight deficiency pattern and also have coldness in the limbs, palpitations, anxiety, shortness of breath, and decreased urine output.
- **Rokumigan:** Used for patients with slight deficiency pattern with tinnitus and dizziness associated with aging. Compared with *hachimijiogan* and *goshajinkigan*, *rokumigan* is appropriate for patients with less severe coldness but a heat sensation in the limbs.
- **Kamikihito:** Used for highly psychogenic tinnitus and dizziness. Also effective for tinnitus related to the patulous Eustachian tube. Patients have slight deficiency to medium patterns with poor complexion, anemia, insomnia, and mental instability.
- **Goreisan:** Widely effective for dizziness in slight deficiency to medium pattern patients who have medium physical strength with edema, thirst, decreased urine output, and diarrhea.
- **Saireito:** Used for most types of dizziness (including inner ear disorder dizziness) and tinnitus associated with low-tone sensory-neural hearing loss. Patients have medium pattern, thirst, decreased urine output, and edema. Also appropriate for Meniere's disease unsuccessfully treated with an osmotic diuretic.
- **Takushato:**[2] Used for most types of dizziness, including inner ear disorder dizziness, in patients who have medium physical strength and decreased urine output.
- **Chotosan:** Frequently used for tinnitus as well as dizziness associated with high blood pressure and arteriosclerosis. Patients are middle-aged or older and have a medium pattern. They complain of headaches early in the morning or upon waking, hot flashes, and bulbar conjunctiva congestion.
- **Keishibukuryogan:** Used for dizziness coinciding with the estrous cycle or menopause. Patients have a medium to slight excess pattern along with hot flashes and coldness in the feet. Other indications include resistance and

[2]Not available as a medically approved Kampo extract formulation.

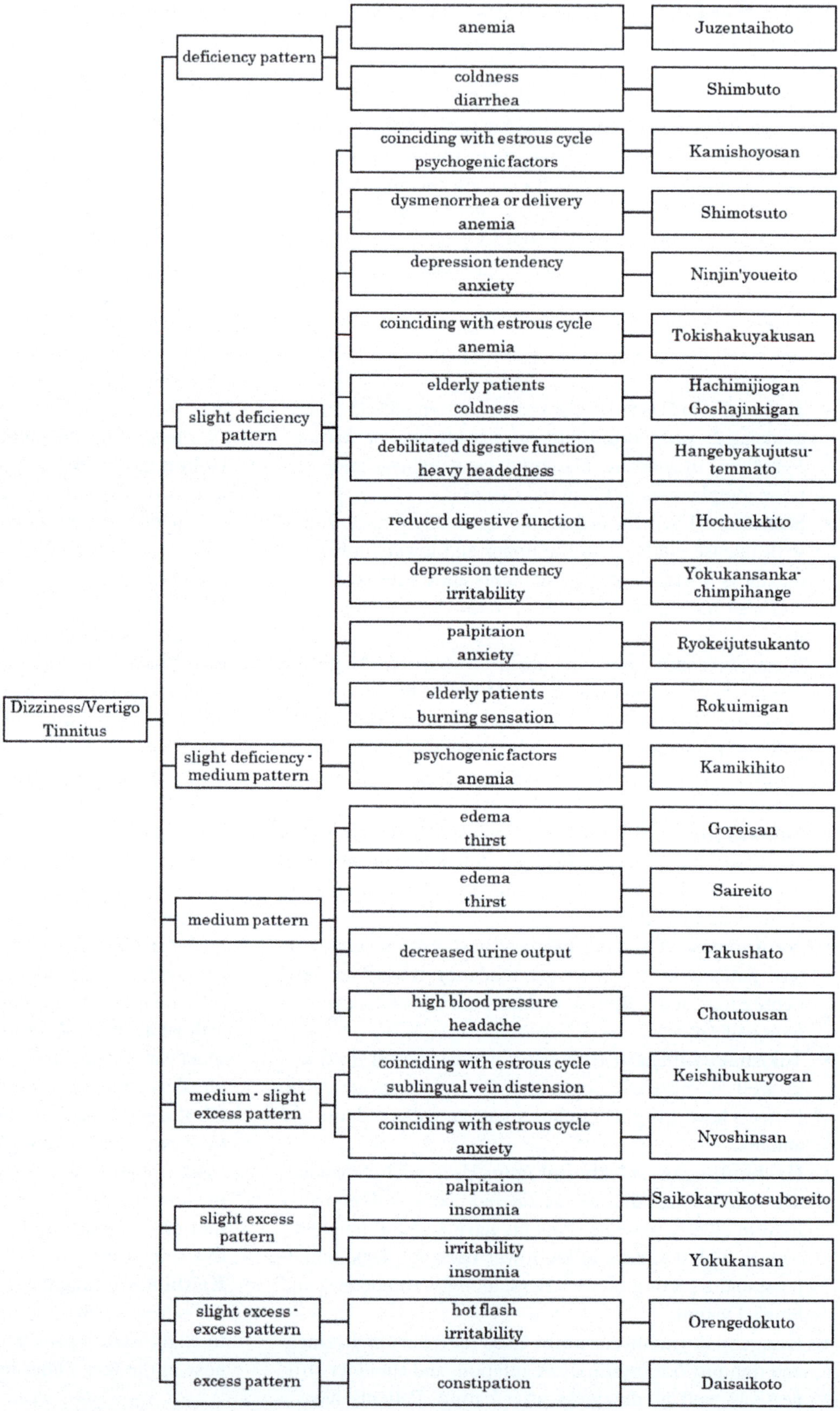

Fig. 5.1 Frequent formulas prescribed for dizziness/vertigo and tinnitus

tenderness in the lower abdomen and sublingual vein distension.

- **Nyoshinsan:** Used for dizziness coinciding with estrous cycle or menopause. Patients have a medium to slight excess pattern along with anxiety, hot flashes, and palpitations.
- **Saikokaryukotsuboreito:** Good for highly psychogenic tinnitus and dizziness, along with shoulder stiffness and high blood pressure. Patients have a slight excess pattern and also have hypersensitivity symptoms such as palpitations, insomnia, irritability, and a tendency to be startled.
- **Yokukansan:** Good for psychogenic dizziness and autonomic imbalance. Patients have a slight excess pattern; they are nervous, short-tempered, and irritable, and they complain of insomnia. Some patients also have twitching in their eyelids.
- **Orengedokuto:** Used for slight excess to excess pattern patients with psychogenic or hypertension-related dizziness. Also used for patients with hot flash tendencies, facial redness, and psychoneurotic symptoms such as insomnia and irritability.
- **Daisaikoto:** Used for excess pattern patients with dizziness, shoulder stiffness, and high blood pressure. Patients also have constipation, headaches, irritability, and distended painful sensations in the upper abdomen. Since this formula contains herbs with a purgative effect, including *daio*, it should not be used for patients with weak abdominal strength or those with chronic diarrhea or gastrointestinal weakness.

1.3 Sneezing, Nasal Discharge, Nasal Obstruction, and Postnasal Drip

Toru Kaneko

1.3.1 Overview of Disease

In Western medical thinking, acute diseases that cause sneezing, nasal discharge, nasal occlusion, and postnasal drip include the common cold, acute rhinitis, seasonal allergic rhinitis, and acute sinusitis. The chronic causative diseases include chronic rhinitis, perennial allergic rhinitis, and chronic sinusitis. Whether the cause is an allergy or an infection is determined on the basis of the properties of the nasal discharge. Sneezing, watery nasal discharge, and nasal obstruction are referred to as the three main signs of allergic rhinitis. If the nasal discharge is purulent, infectious sinusitis may be present. Unlike rhinorrhea, postnasal drip is often responsible for cough, laryngopharyngeal discomfort, hoarseness, etc. Some elderly patients complain of watery nasal discharge only (particularly postnasal drip). A common cause is said to be fluid absorption disorder in the nasal mucosa due to nasal mucosal atrophy or reduced nasal mucosa temperature.

In Western medicine, the main treatments for allergic rhinitis are oral medication (typically antihistamines) and steroid nasal sprays. Radical therapies include hyposensitization. The acute-phase treatment of sinusitis is antibacterial therapy, chiefly using quinolones for adults (who show a good response) and quinolones and carbapenems (which have started to be used recently), as well as the relatively new cephems (which are generally considered helpful) for children. For chronic-phase treatment in both adults and children, long-term therapy using low-dose macrolide antibiotics is recommended.

In Kampo medicine, sneezing (or sternutation) is interpreted as a response of the body involving ciliary movement to eject the inhaled foreign matter via exhalation. It occurs with a cold sensation and is associated with heat production. Nasal discharge is necessary for mucosal protection, warming, moistening, and dust removal, but when it becomes imbalanced, fluid[TM1] retention can occur. Nasal obstruction involves fluid stagnation with edematous change in nasal mucosa (fluid[TM1] retention) and proliferation of secretion glands, followed by nasal discharge. Postnasal drip is a symptom of sinusitis. It is a condition of fluid[TM1] retention and may also involve psychological factors (qi stagnation).

1.3.2 Indications for Kampo Therapy

In classical Kampo thinking, nasal diseases are classified as *bikyu* (allergic rhinitis) or *bien* (sinusitis), and nasal discharge is categorized as *seitei* (clear snivel) or *dakutei* (turbid snivel). The putative diseases for *bikyu* include present-day allergic rhinitis. The associated thin nasal discharge, including sputum, is termed *seitei*. On the other hand, *bien* can be considered as the present-day sinusitis with the associated purulent yellow nasal discharge termed *dakutei*.

In principle, Kampo therapy is used for unpleasant subjective symptoms. In both modern medicine and Kampo medicine, it is critical in the treatment of rhinitis to subdivide the disease according to the properties of nasal discharge. When symptoms are severe, treatment with Kampo medicines alone is difficult, and concomitant use of Western drugs is often required.

Sublingual immunotherapy for dust mites and pollen allergy has been introduced as a treatment for allergic rhinitis. The concept of this therapy is an attempt to change the immune system's response. This point of view is consistent with the basic thinking in Kampo of constitution improvement. Kampo therapy is used to suppress allergic exacerbation or to relieve allergic symptoms in sublingual immunotherapy [7–8].

1.3.3 Frequently Used Formulas (Fig. 5.2)

Watery Nasal Discharge

Commonly found in the early stage of allergic rhinitis and the common cold. The principal formulas in the acute phase are formulas with ephedra herb, such as *kakkontokasenkyushin'i* and *shoseiryuto*. Formulas with processed aconite root, such as *maobushisaishinto,* may be selected for patients with more intense cold sensations and those having white nasal mucosa.

When symptoms are severe owing to cedar pollen allergy and the like, the quantity of *mao* may be increased. For example, *gokoto* may be added to *shoseiryuto*, or *eppikajutsuto* may be used. During the high-pollen season, treatment with Kampo medicines alone is difficult. Concomitant use of Western drugs, such as oral antihistamines and steroid nasal sprays, is frequently required. The combined use of formulas with ephedra herb on such occasions not only alleviates the symptoms but can also be expected to reduce the adverse effect of drowsiness caused by the antihistamines. Naturally, attention must be paid to the adverse effects of formulas with ephedra herb (palpitation, stomach pain, etc.).

If nasal discharge is accompanied by cough, *shoseiryuto* is helpful in mild cases, while *makyokansekito*, *gokoto*, or *shimpito* is often required in severe cases. *Bakumondoto* and *jiinkokato* are used either singly or jointly in patients with a strong tendency to dryness in the oral cavity.

The treatment of chronic-phase nasal obstruction is often very difficult in Western medicine as well. In this case, root treatment according to pattern is required rather than symptomatic treatment.

- **Kakkonto:** Effective for rhinitis in the early stage of the common cold, particularly in patients also having headaches and stiffness in the neck and back, with medium to slight excess pattern. If systemic pain is present or symptoms are severe, *maoto* is more helpful.
- **Kakkontokasenkyushin'i:** Consists of *kakkonto* with *senkyu* and *shin'i*. Effective for severe nasal obstruction or discharge, as well as the target symptoms for *kakkonto* in patients with medium to slight excess pattern. An important formula for sinusitis and allergic rhinitis associated with viscous nasal discharge. Combined use with long-term low-dose macrolide antibiotics is also effective.
- **Shoseiryuto:** Effective for fluid disturbance symptoms such as watery nasal discharge, sneezing, and cough in patients with slight deficiency pattern. Considered the first choice for allergic rhinitis.
- **Maobushisaishinto:** Target patients must have a Yin pattern or cold pattern, comprising coldness and poor complexion. Effective for early stage common cold and allergic rhinitis in elderly patients and patients with weak constitutions.

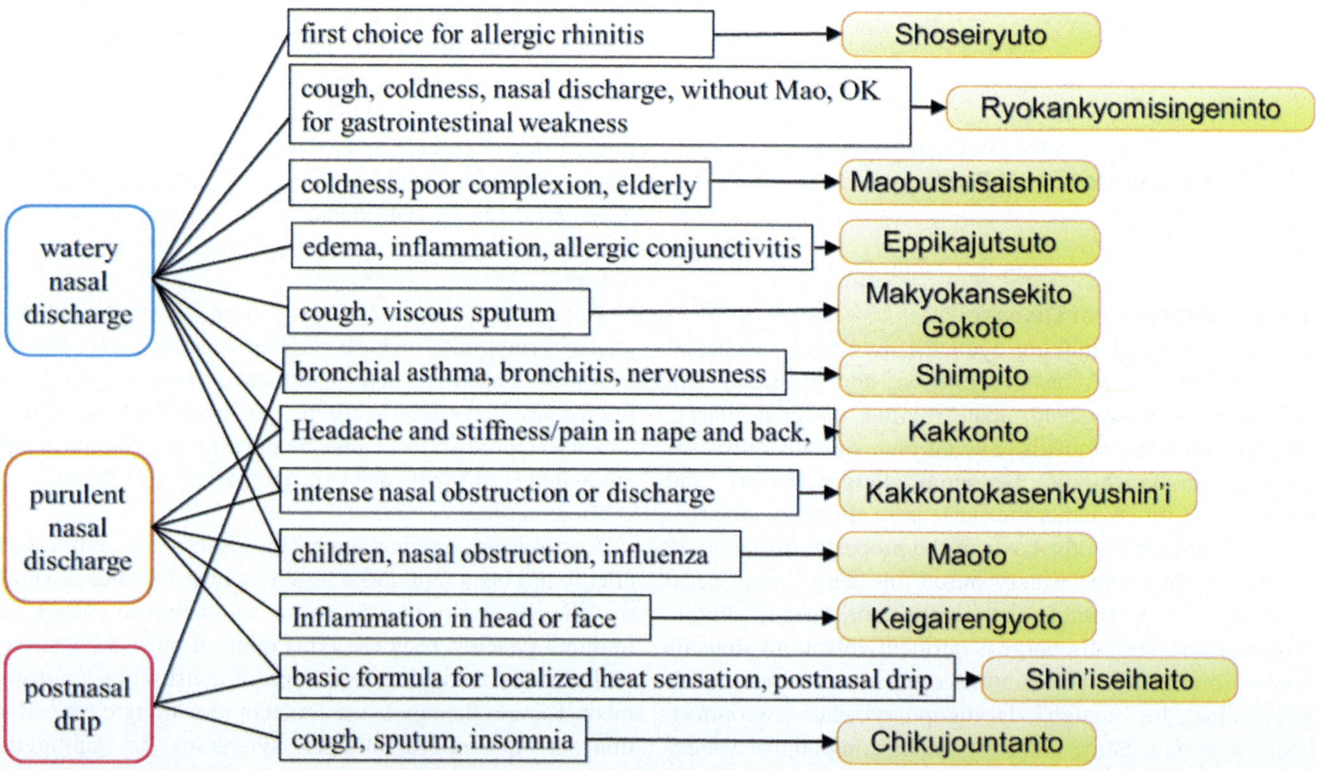

Fig. 5.2 Kampo therapy for rhinitis and sinusitis

- **Makyokansekito:** Effective for cough-associated rhinitis and viscous sputum accompanied by bronchitis or pneumonia in patients with slight excess pattern.
- **Gokoto:** Consists of *makyokansekito* with *sohakuhi*, which enhances the antitussive effect of the former in patients with slight excess pattern.
- **Maoto:** Effective for watery nasal discharge associated with headache, fever, chill, myalgia, and/or arthralgia in patients with slight excess pattern to excess pattern. Often offered to children with severe nasal obstruction. Frequently used for the early stage of influenza.
- **Shimpito:** Effective for allergic rhinitis accompanied by bronchial asthma or bronchitis in patients with medium pattern.
- **Eppikajutsuto:** A formula for facial, limb, and joint edema and inflammation. Also appropriate for allergic rhinitis with palpebral edema or conjunctivitis.
- **Ryokankyomishingeninto:** Used for allergic rhinitis in patients who are not indicated for formulas with ephedra herb due to gastrointestinal weakness. This formula has a relatively mild effect, different from formulas with ephedra herb.

Purulent Nasal Discharge

Many patients with acute-phase sinusitis complain of pain and tension in the face, neck, and back. For these signs and symptoms, formulas with ephedra herb including *kakkontokasenkyushin'i,* are effective. Following that, the use of formulas such as *shin'iseihaito* containing *sekko* is common. For patients with concomitant pimples or tonsillitis, *keigairengyoto* is frequently used. Combined use with antibacterial drugs is effective, and this alleviates symptoms more rapidly than administration of either Kampo medicines or antibacterial drugs alone.

- **Kakkonto and Kakkontokasenkyushin'i:** (See above.)
- **Shin'iseihaito:** Appropriate for patients with localized inflammation and intense heat sensation in patients with medium to slight excess pattern. Since this formula doesn't contain *MAO*, it can be used for patients susceptible to the adverse effects of *MAO*. Also helpful when used as a basic formula for postnasal drip. It can also be used for allergic rhinitis and is effective when used concomitantly with low-dose and long-term macrolide antibiotics.
- **Keigairengyoto:** Effective for dermatological inflammatory diseases of the head and face, but also effective for otorhinological inflammatory diseases in patients with slight excess pattern. Concomitant use with macrolides is effective.

Postnasal Drip

Treatment is administered for cases in which the causative disease is clear. When the cause is not clear, even treatment with Western medicine is difficult.

- **Shin'iseihaito:** (See above.)
- **Chikujountanto:** Used for symptoms such as copious coughing and sputum, insomnia, and mental anxiety in patients with medium pattern. Can be effective when combined with *shin'iseihaito.*

1.4 Oral Discomfort

Tatsuya Ishige

1.4.1 Overview of Disease [9]

Intraoral complaints include tongue and mouth pain, dysgeusia, and a feeling of dryness in the mouth and are often encountered in routine practice. Representative diseases involving oral discomfort include stomatitis, xerostomia, glossalgia, dysgeusia, and persistent idiopathic facial pain, which are often encountered as comorbidities. Stomatitis is characterized by the formation of flares, swelling, ulcers, bullae, etc., on the oral mucosa; its causes varying widely from dental caries stimulation to radiation, anticancer medications, and viral and bacterial infections. Xerostomia is relatively common among elderly women, and its causes include aging, systemic diseases such as Sjogren's syndrome, diabetes, chronic renal insufficiency, and the use of drugs contributing to salivation suppression, such as hypotensives and anti-anxiety drugs. Glossalgia is a form of burning mouth syndrome (BMS). Glossalgia in its narrower definition is characterized by persistent complaints of spontaneous pain and foreign sensation in the tongue and the absence of corresponding organic changes; it is necessary to rule out oral candidiasis, lingual cancer, etc. It is relatively common among middle- to old-aged women, induced by perimenopausal hormonal changes, stress, etc. This condition is differentially diagnosed as secondary glossalgia when caused by decreased salivation due to conditions like Sjogren's syndrome or organic factors such as zinc, iron, and vitamin B12 deficiencies. While dysgeusia occurs from a wide variety of causes, including zinc deficiency, drug use, the common cold, and psychogenic factors, the sense of taste usually decreases with aging. Cases of dysgeusia can be divided into two types: quantitative and qualitative. Quantitative forms include hypogeusia and ageusia, and qualitative forms include spontaneous dysgeusia and heterogeusia. Spontaneous dysgeusia is defined as a condition where a particular taste, such as bitterness or sweetness, is perceived even without taking anything. Persistent idiopathic facial pain is an intractable pain in the facial and oral regions that is not due to organic or functional lesions. It is relatively common among women and is associated with psychiatric symptoms at a high percentage.

1.4.2 Indications for Kampo Therapy

Although Kampo therapy may be applied to all these diseases, Kampo treatments are well indicated for patients who do not respond to or cases that are difficult to manage with only Western medical treatment. This includes glossalgia and unspecific oral complaints, which depend largely on psychological factors, systemic diseases such as Sjogren's syndrome and diabetes, and dry mouth due to side effects of Western drugs. Dysgeusia is treated mainly by zinc adjunctive therapy [10]. Kampo treatments are indicated if this is ineffective, and in other cases, dysgeusia of unknown cause, psychogenic dysgeusia, and aging-related hypogeusia. Kampo formulas are used to improve quality of life (QOL) in patients with stomatitis who suffer recurrent or multiple onsets, concurrent gastrointestinal symptoms such as diarrhea and stomach distension, or side effects of chemotherapy or radiation in cancer management. Persistent idiopathic facial pain may be treated with antidepressants, but no standard treatment has been established, so Kampo treatments are also attempted.

1.4.3 Frequently Used Formulas

Stomatitis (Fig. 5.3)

In stomatitis, it is important to determine whether the condition is excess heat or deficiency heat. Focus on formulas containing *oren* and *sanshishi*, which have heat-clearing effects, to treat excess heat patterns in the acute stage. To treat deficiency patterns in the chronic stage, use formulas containing *kanzo* and *jio*, which supplement fluids by tonifying the spleen[TM1] and kidney[TM1]. The pattern should be identified by referring to bowel movement status, tongue findings, etc.

- **Orengedokuto**: Slight excess pattern to excess pattern patients with signs such as ruddy face, hot flashes, eye hyperemia, insomnia, intense irritation, red tongue body, and yellow coating.
- **Inchinkoto**: Widely used for damp-heat conditions in patients with medium to slight excess pattern. Findings include thirst, decreased urine volume, constipation, red tongue body, and yellow coating. Applicable to pruritic rashes such as urticaria.
- **Hangeshashinto** [11]: Medium pattern patients with findings such as nausea, epigastric stuffiness, borborygmus, diarrhea, epigastric resistance, and hardness in the abdominal examination, and white coating. For oral mucositis caused by anticancer medication or radiotherapy, direct anti-inflammatory and analgesic effects are obtained not only by drinking the formula but also by gargling.
- **Orento**: Medium pattern patients with symptoms such as heartburn, nausea, stomachache, and anorexia, often accompanied by a white to yellow coating on the tongue. Contains a higher Coptis rhizome content and has a greater heat-clearing effect than *hangeshashinto*.
- **Jiinkokato**: Used in patients with slight deficiency pattern with relatively healthy stomachs and intestines who have symptoms such as dry skin, constipation, and coughing. This condition is relatively common among elderly persons, with severe loss of fluid[TM1] and obvious oral dryness.
- **Seinetsuhokito**[3]: Used in patients with impaired digestive function, such as chronic gastritis, manifesting with lingual papilla atrophy, little tongue coating, fissured tongue, and geographical tongue. This is a formula that mitigates spleen[TM1]/stomach[TM1] deficiency and ameliorates fluid[TM1] consumption or depletion. Since no useful extract formula is available, instead *hochuekkito* or *shikunshito* and *bakumondoto* are used together.

Xerostomia (Fig. 5.4)

Xerostomia can occur in two forms: thirst and dry mouth. Thirst refers to a state in which the patient feels dry in the mouth and wants to drink water, whereas dry mouth refers to a state in which the patient feels dry in the mouth but does not want to drink water. Candidate formulas include *goreisan*, *byakkokaninjinto*, and *hachimijiogan* for thirst, and formulas with Bupleurum root and blood stasis resolving formulas for dry mouth. In reality, this condition is relatively common among elderly persons, and tonic formulas are often indicated. These conditions are distinguished with reference to water consumption, sweating status, urination frequency, and presence/absence of nocturia.

- **Byakkokaninjinto**: For the medium pattern to slight excess pattern patients with severe thirst, water consumption exceeding 2 liters/day in some cases. This is accompanied by hot flashes on the body and massive sweating.
- **Goreisan**: Used for thirst, decreased urine volume, vertigo, and headache, mainly for medium pattern patients. Vertigo and headache tend to get worse in bad weather. Teeth marks, tongue, and lower limb edema are noted.
- **Bakumondoto**: A formula used for slight deficiency pattern to medium pattern as the first choice drug for xerostomia. Given the evidence available for salivation improvement in patients with Sjogren's syndrome, this formula is applied as a moisturizing agent.

[3]Not available as a medically approved Kampo extract formulation.

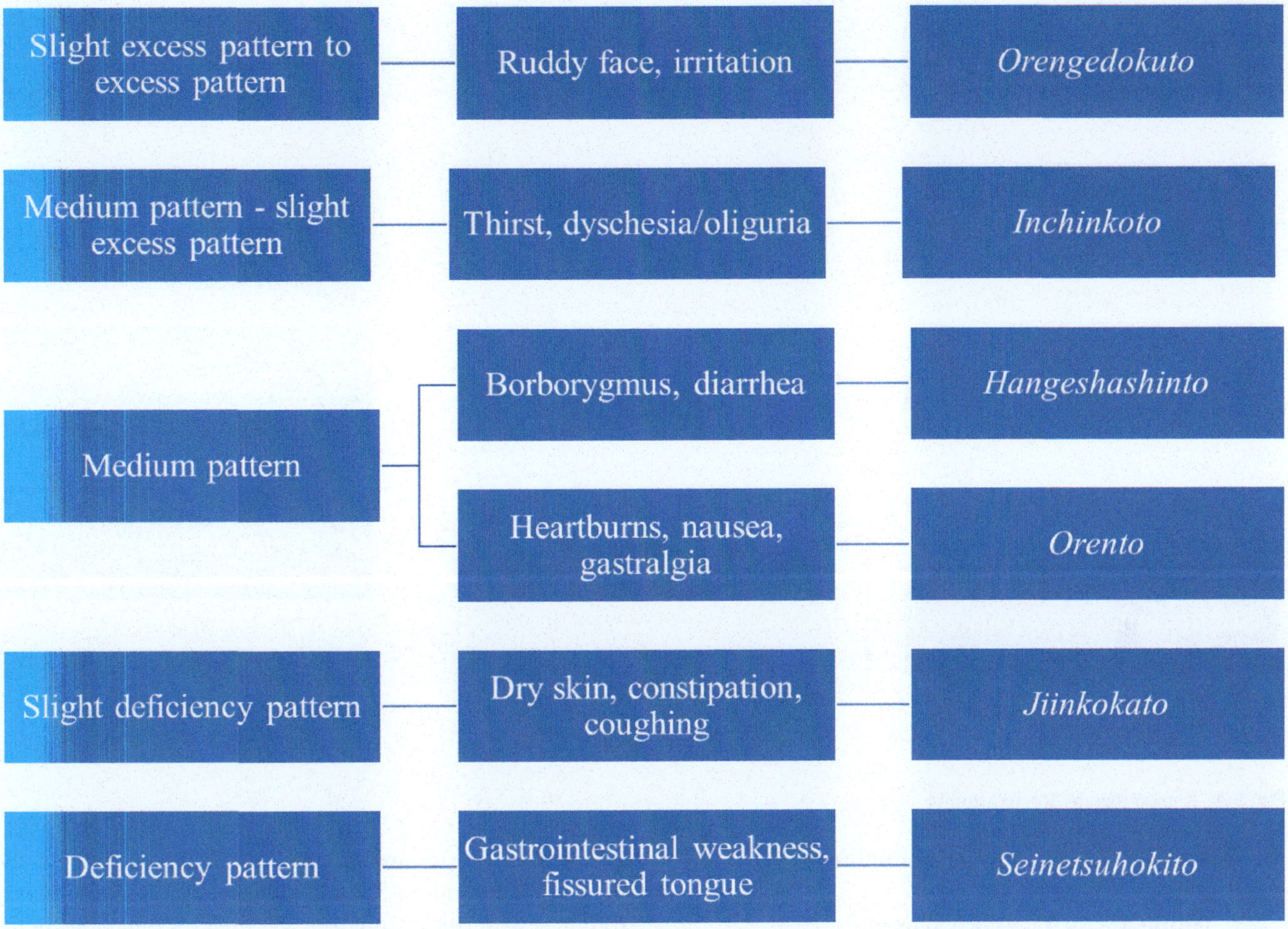

Fig. 5.3 Kampo therapy for stomatitis

- **Hachimijiogan**: Used basically for polydipsia and polyuria without the thirst indicated by *byakkokaninjinto*. Indicated for kidney[TM1] deficiency conditions and administered mainly to middle-aged to elderly patients with slight deficiency pattern. Fatigue and malaise, lumbago, feeling cold in the feet, and nocturia are noted along with weakness of the lower abdominal region in the abdominal examination.
- **Ninjin'yoeito**: Used in cases of patterns with both qi and blood[TM1] deficiency, seen relatively commonly in chronic wasting diseases such as malignant tumors and postpartum malaise. Often, the patient has a slight deficiency pattern, accompanied by symptoms such as hair loss, dry skin, nail deformation, insomnia, and frequent forgetfulness.

Glossalgia (Fig. 5.5)

For glossalgia in its narrower definition, when associated strongly with psychological stress, treatment is chosen mainly from among formulas with Bupleurum root and *oren* and qi-tonifying formulas. For secondary glossalgia with severe dry mouth findings, the use of yin tonifying formulas is also considered.

(a) Cases with a Strong Association with Psychological Stress

- **Orengedokuto** (described above).
- **Saikokaryukotsuboreito**: Used in nervous, easily startled patients with slight excess pattern. Indicated for psychosomatic symptoms such as palpitations, insomnia, excessive dreaming, and fullness and discomfort in the chest and hypochondrium, as well as pulsations above the umbilicus as found in the abdominal examination.
- **Kamishoyosan**: Used in patients with slight deficiency pattern with vertigo, tinnitus, palpitations, stiff shoulders, menstruation irregularity, and irritation, sometimes accompanied by constipation. Patients typically have multiple complaints. Abdominal findings include mild fullness and discomfort in the chest and hypochondrium, tender points in the lower abdomen, and the tongue body is red.
- **Kososan**: Used for thin patients with gastrointestinal weakness with deficiency pattern. Treatment targets symptoms like anorexia, melancholy, and anxiety.

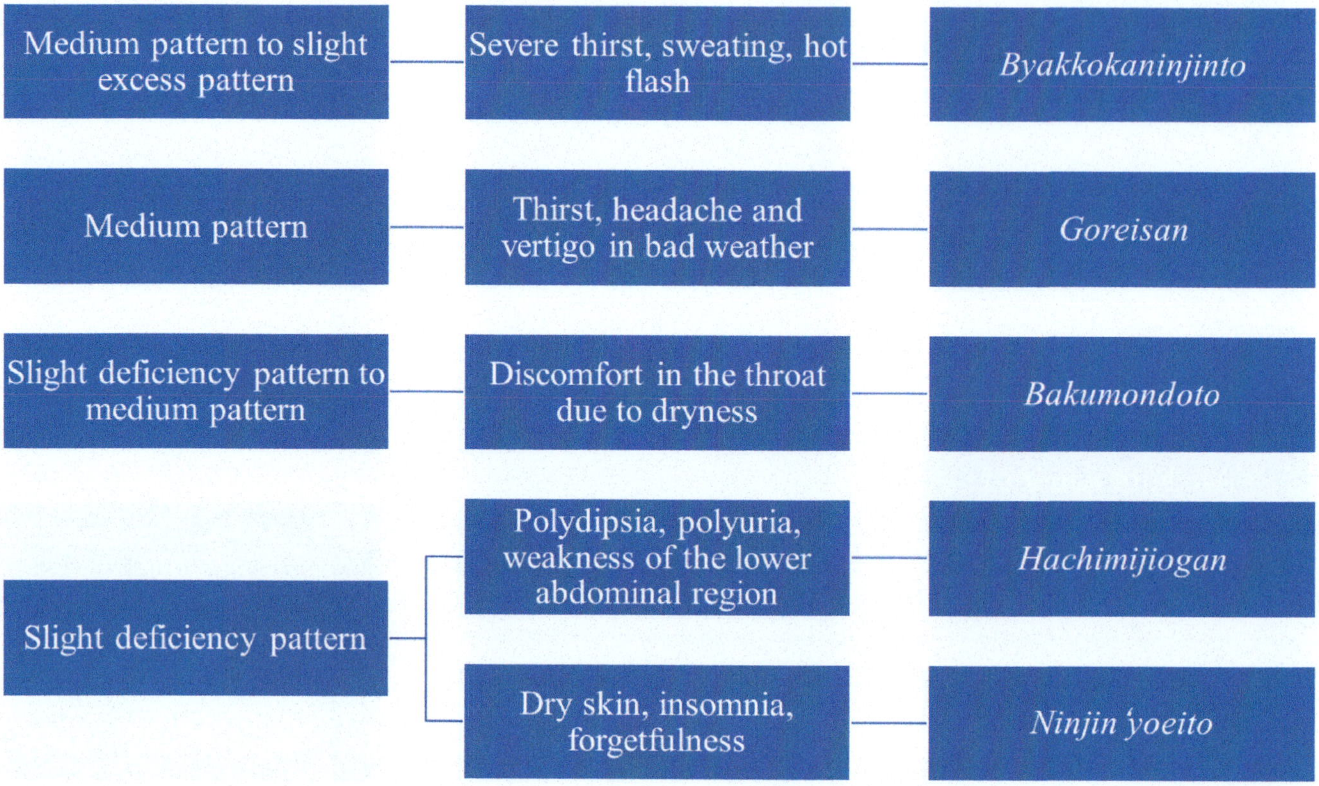

Fig. 5.4 Kampo therapy for xerostomia

(b) **Cases with Severe Dry mouth Findings**

- **Ninjin'yoeito** (described above)
- **Seinetsuhokito**[4]: (described above)

(c) Others

- **Rikkosan:** Can be used without strictly taking patterns into account. Its constituent herbs include *ryutan* and *shoma*, which are effective in clearing heat and pain relief. It also contains *saishin* and *bofu*, which are effective in eliminating wind and pain relief. It should be swallowed only after being kept in the mouth for a while. It may be used by gargling in cases of stomach distention.

Dysgeusia (Fig. 5.6)

The classical literature has a range of descriptions for dysgeusia, including "bitter taste, weakness of the mouth, ageusia, and inability to taste food." These may be associated with late yang stage to middle yang stage patterns of the six stages, and in terms of the five zang organs, with the liver[TM1], heart[TM1], spleen[TM1], and kidney[TM1] are involved.

Formulas are chosen aiming for improvements in the function of the spleen[TM1] and kidney[TM1]. These are mainly formulas with Bupleurum root and *oren* for infections in the late yang stage for cases having a strong association with psychological stress. Otherwise, yin tonifying formulas for marked dry mouth and tonic formulas are used for chronic hypogeusia associated with loss of physical strength.

- **Orengedokuto** (described above)
- **Saikokaryukotsuboreito** (described above)
- **Byakkokaninjinto** (described above)
- **Shosaikoto**: Used for medium pattern patients with oral discomfort such as bitter taste and stickiness in the mouth, anorexia, nausea, slight fever, red tongue body, and dry white coating. Also, abdominal examination shows fullness and discomfort in the chest and hypochondrium.
- **Hangeshashinto** (described above)
- **Hochuekkito**: The aim of treatment is general malaise, anorexia, slight fever, night sweating, and susceptibility to common colds. For slight deficiency pattern patients with weak abdominal strength and pulsation next to the navel.
- **Hachimijiogan**: (described above)

Persistent Idiopathic Facial Pain

This condition is differentiated mainly on the basis of heat and cold and qi, blood[TM1], and fluids[TM1]. Candidate formu-

[4]Not available as a medically approved Kampo extract formulation.

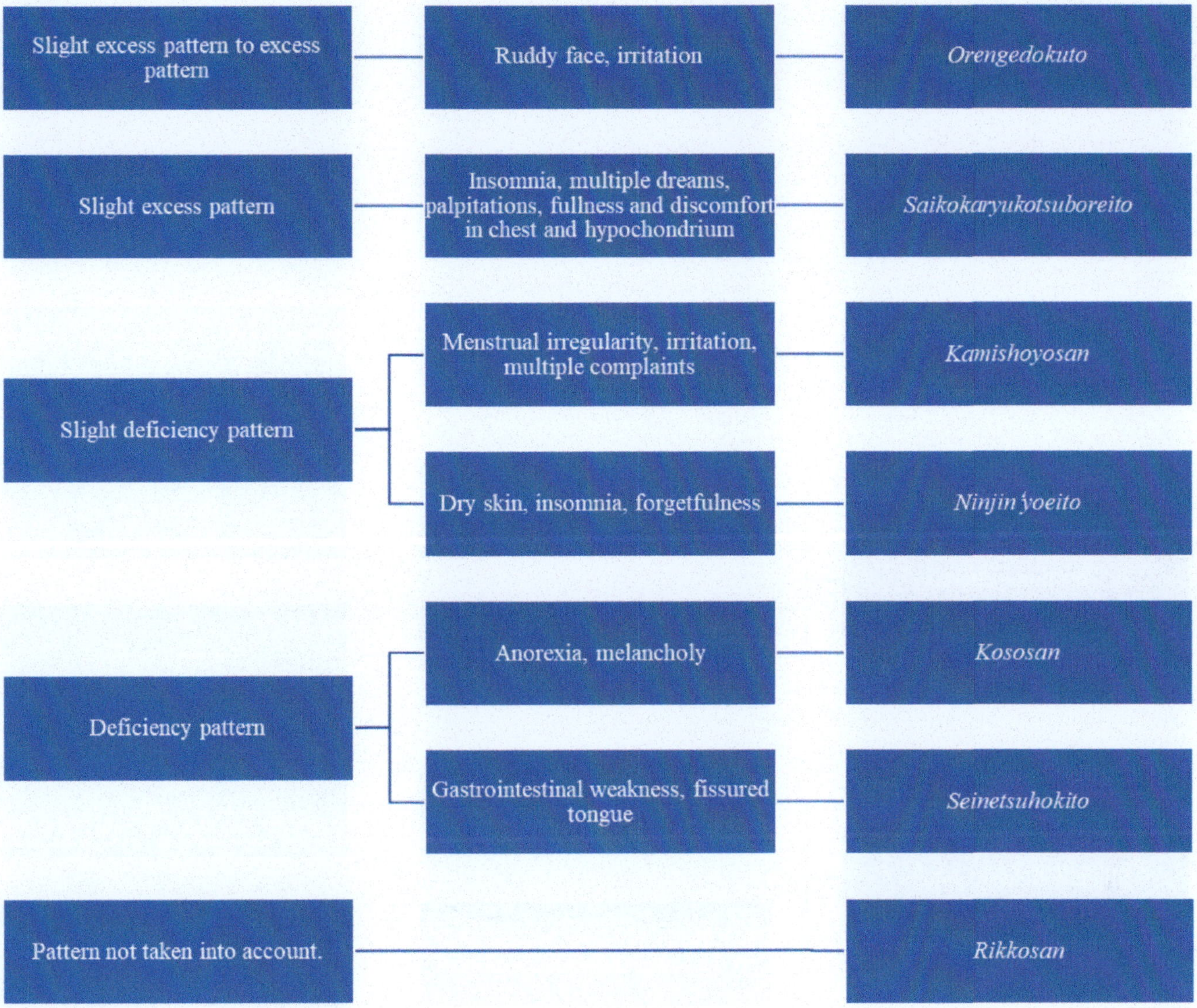

Fig. 5.5 Kampo therapy for glossalgia

las are *hangekobokuto* and *saikokaryukotsuboreito* for qi stagnation and qi counter flow; *kamishoyosan* for static blood[TM1]; and *goreisan* for fluid[TM1] retention. *Rikkosan* can be used without taking patterns into account. A decoction known as *keikyososooshinbuto*[5] is also useful.

2 Chest

2.1 Common Cold Syndrome

Hiroshi Odaguchi

2.1.1 Outline of the Disease

The common cold syndrome is characterized by acute inflammation in the upper airway from the nasal cavity to the pharynx and larynx, and it is usually caused by rhinovirus, coronavirus, adenovirus, etc. Influenza is an acute febrile infection caused by an influenza virus. COVID-19 and SARS-CoV-2 are usually managed separately because they involve severe systemic symptoms such as fever and muscle pain, along with serious pneumonia, etc., as complications. In this section, however, these are included in the differentiation of the common cold syndrome for the sake of convenience.

The common cold develops when a pathogen such as a virus attaches to the airway mucosa, enters the airway tissue, and proliferates there. The presence/absence of onset depends on environmental and host factors. Common symptoms are mainly in the nose (nasal discharge, nasal obstruction) and throat (pharyngeal pain) and may also include headache, general malaise, and slight fevers. If inflammation affects the lower airway, from the trachea, bronchus, and lung, lower airway symptoms (coughing and sputum) will also develop.

[5]Not available as a medical Kampo extract preparation.

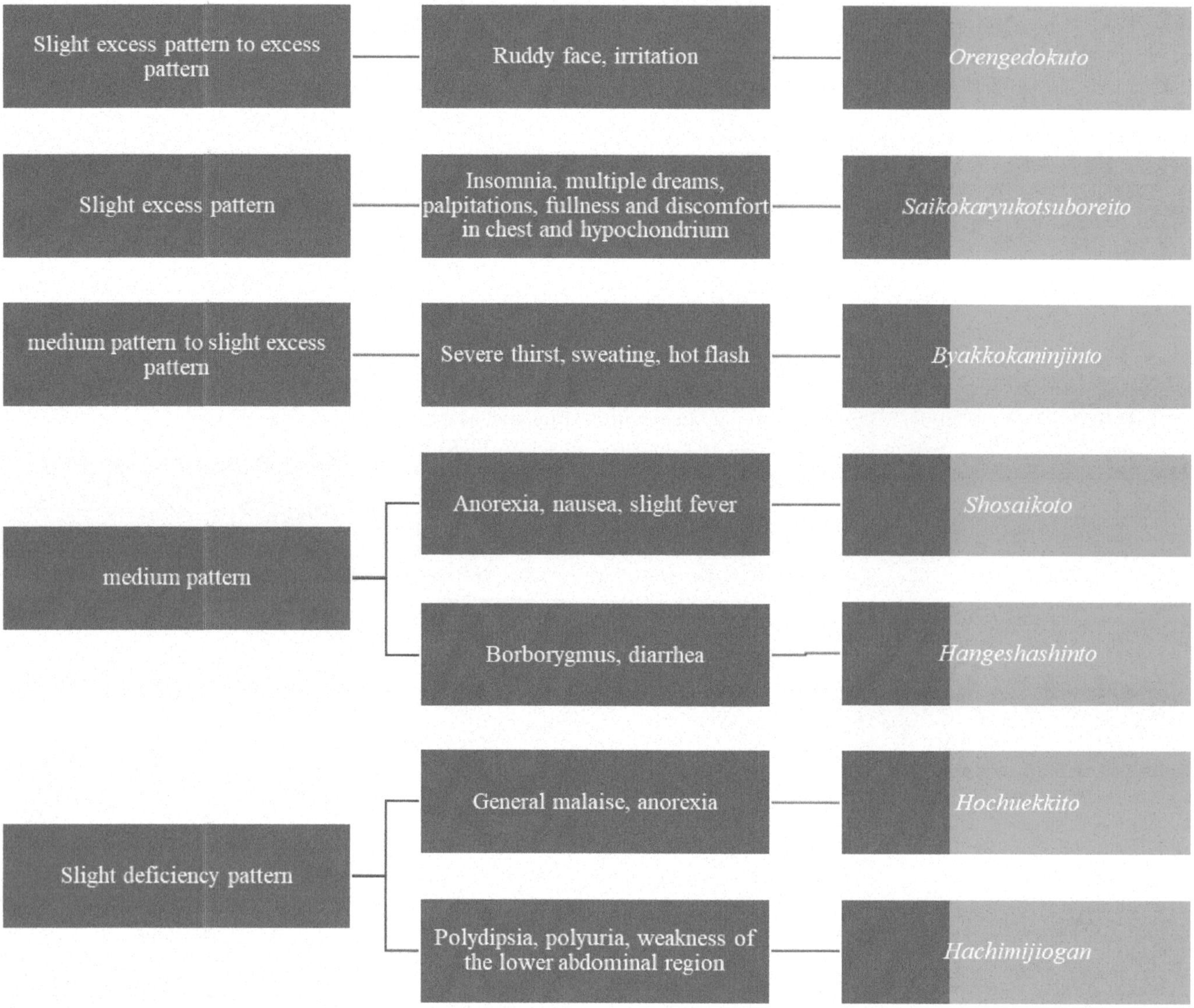

Fig. 5.6 Kampo Therapy for Dysgeusia

No Western medical treatment is available specifically for the common cold syndrome. Usually, it resolves spontaneously with rest, hydration, etc., Although antihistamines, antipyretics, etc. are administered according to symptoms, antibacterials need not be administered unless bacterial infections are present as complications.

2.1.2 Indications of Kampo Treatments [12]

In acute infections such as the common cold, the concept of the six-stage patterns in Kampo medicine is helpful. The first stage is described in the ancient Chinese medical text *Shanghanlun* as "the disease in the early yang stage is characterized by floating pulses, severe headache and neck stiffness, and chills." The early yang stage usually corresponds to the beginning of common cold syndrome. Specifically, the common cold syndrome is characterized mainly by the feeling of cold, which can be accompanied by a wide variety of symptoms such as headache, nuchal stiffness, fever, nasal discharge, and joint pain, depending on the patient's condition. An early yang stage pattern normally persists for 3–4 days, but if it doesn't resolve, it transitions to the late yang stage. The late yang stage pattern is described in the *Shanghanlun* as a "condition with a bitter taste in the mouth, dry throat, and vertigo." Typically, alternate chilling and fevers occur in the afternoon on consecutive days, with stickiness in the mouth and discomfort, tenderness, and resistance below the costal arch. Also, coughing symptoms due to lower airway inflammation develop in this stage. Usually, the condition proceeds to a resolution through the late yang stage. On rare occasions, however, it progresses from the late yang stage to the next stage, the middle yang stage, accompanied by abdominal distention and constipation. Here we refer generically to all three yin stages (early yin stage pattern, middle yin stage pattern, and late yin stage pattern) as "yin stage pattern." These are the last three of the six-stage patterns, and the "yin stage pattern" is positioned as the stage next to the middle yang stage. The common cold syndrome, however, seldom follows a course from the middle yang stage pattern to "yin stage pattern." Even in patients with a deficiency pattern and those with an excess pattern, the common cold syndrome associated with exhaustion can develop initially as a yin stage pattern. In yin stage patterns, cold symptoms are the main feature, with diarrhea often noted in addition to upper airway symptoms.

2.1.3 Frequently Used Formulas (Table 5.2)

Basic View Based on the Six-Stage Patterns

(a) **Early Yang Stage**

The most important thing in determining whether a condition is an early yang stage pattern is to know whether the pulses are floating. A floating pulse, however, is a finding that isn't specific to the early yang stage pattern. When symptoms such as headache, chilling, nuchal stiffness, and joint pain are present, an early yang stage pattern can be diagnosed without a floating pulse. Above all, chilling is considered an essential symptom. Chilling in the early yang stage pattern, unlike that in the yin stage pattern, is accompanied by fevers. A fever, as mentioned herein, is not an elevation of body temperature but is a sensation of heat. In summary, the presence of headache, nuchal stiffness, and joint pain, in addition to chilling with heat sensation and a floating pulse, supports the diagnosis of an early yang stage pattern.

- **Kakkonto** [13]: Indicated for medium to slight excess pattern patients with strong floating pulse, chilling with heat sensation, and stiffness from neck to back, without spontaneous sweating.
- **Maoto:** Used for slight excess to excess pattern patients with strong floating pulse, chilling with heat sensation, headache, and joint pain, without spontaneous sweating.
- **Daiseiryuto:**[6] Indicated for persons with *maoto* indications and dysphoria (a symptom of interior heat that causes limb thrashing due to agonizing heat).
- **Keimakakuhanto (keishimaokakuhanto):** Indicated slight deficiency pattern patients with a floating pulse, chilling with severe heat sensation, and complaints of throat pain, along with headache, without spontaneous sweating.
- **Keishinimaoitto:**[4] Used for patients indicated for *keimakakuhanto* with slight sweating.
- **Keishinieppiitto:**[7] Used for patients indicated for *keishinimaoichito* with thirst.
- **Keishito:** Used for slight deficiency pattern patients with a weak floating pulse, chilling with heat sensation, headache, and nuchal stiffness. May be used in both cases with spontaneous sweating and cases without (absence of sweating).
- **Keishikakakkonto:** Used for slight deficiency pattern patients with the same symptoms as above, but with spontaneous sweating. This formula can be used in the absence of sweating, but in this case, it is distinguished from *kakkonto* by a weaker pulse strength.

(b) **Late Yang Stage**

The illness intensifies as one enters the late yang stage, and the body in response manifests various signs and symptoms. First, a bitter taste in the mouth, dry mouth, and vertigo are noted. The above-described alternating chills and fever are also typical in the late yang stage. Tongue examination reveals a white or yellow coating, and abdominal examination reveals fullness and discomfort in the chest and hypochondrium.

- **Daisaikoto:** Used for patients with complaints of nausea, vomiting, neck stiffness, upper abdominal distention, and constipation, along with a dry, thick, white, or yellow tongue coating. Abdominal examination reveals strength in the upper abdomen (excess pattern), fullness and discomfort in the chest and hypochondrium, and epigastric stuffiness and resistance.
- **Shosaikoto:** Indicated for cases with medium pattern with complaints of nausea, vomiting, neck stiffness, and upper abdominal distention. The tongue coating is dry and white, and abdominal examination reveals fullness and discomfort in the chest and hypochondrium and epigastric stuffiness resistance.
- **Saikokeishito:** Used in slight deficiency to medium pattern patients for whom *shosaikoto* is indicated, with headache, joint pain, heat sensation, etc. (exterior pattern). Abdominal examination reveals abdominal muscle tension in the upper abdomen.

[6]Not available as a medical Kampo extract formulation nor as an OTC Kampo extract formulation.

Daiseiryuto: mao 6.0, kyonin 5.0, keihi 3.0, taiso 3.0, kanzo 2.0, shokyo 2.0, sekko 10.0.

Keishinimaoitto: keihi 4.5, shakuyaku 3.0, taiso 3.0, mao 1.5, kyonin 1.5, kanzo 2.5, shokyo 1.0.

[7]Not available as a medical Kampo extract formulation.

Table 5.2 Classification of Kampo medicine for the common cold

Early yang stage pattern Floating pulse Headache Nuchal stiffness Chilling with heat sensation	Excess pattern	**Kakkonto**	Absence of sweating, stiffness down the back
		Maoto	Absence of sweating, joint pain
		Daiseiryuto*	Absence of sweating, joint pain, dysphoria
	Medium pattern	**Keimakakuhanto**	Absence of sweating, throat pain
		Keishinimaoitto*	Spontaneous sweating, throat pain
		Keishinieppiitto*	Spontaneous sweating, throat pain, thirst
	Deficiency pattern	**Keishito**	Spontaneous sweating or absence of sweating
		Keishikakakkonto	Spontaneous sweating or absence of sweating, stiffness down the back
Late yang stage pattern Alternating chills and fever White tongue coating Fullness and discomfort in chest and hypochondrium	Excess pattern	**Daisaikoto**	Nausea, neck stiffness, constipation
	Medium pattern	**Shosaikoto**	Nausea, neck stiffness
		Saikokeishito	Nausea, neck stiffness, headache, hot sensation
	Deficiency pattern	**Saikokeishikankyoto**	Thirst, head sweating, abdominal pulsations
Yin stage pattern Sunken pulse Chilling	Deficiency pattern	**Maobushisaishinto**	Hot sensation, headache, throat pain
		Shimbuto	Abdominal pain, diarrheal symptoms

*Not available as a medically approved Kampo extract formulation

- **Saikokeishikankyoto:** Used for patients with a bad complexion who feel coldness and complain of thirst, palpitations, and head sweating. Abdominal examination reveals slightly weak abdominal strength (slight deficiency pattern), mild fullness and discomfort in the chest and hypochondrium, and pulsations above the umbilicus.

(c) **Yin Stage**

In yin stage patterns the disease dominates the patient's physical strength. If pulses are deep, body temperature is high but heat sensation is absent and the patient feels chilled, signs of cold limbs are objectively noted, and diarrheal symptoms are present, in principle the condition may be diagnosed as a yin stage pattern.

- **Maobushisaishinto:** Indicated for cases with a deep pulse, together with indications like those of *keishito* (headache, throat pain, and chilling accompanied by heat sensation), which is indicated for the initial stage of a common cold. A condition in which a yin stage pattern (middle yin stage pattern) develops immediately, without following a normal progression through yang stage patterns (early, late, and middle yang stage patterns), may be referred to as "direct strike into the middle yin stage." This is relatively common among patients with deficiency pattern and is occasionally accompanied by heat sensation even though it is a yin stage pattern.
- **Shimbuto:** Used in cases where abdominal pain and diarrheal symptoms are present, in addition to upper airway symptoms accompanied by chilling.

Kampo Treatments Based on Other Concepts

Not just the common cold syndrome, but other kinds of diseases can be treated with Kampo treatments without adhering to concepts in the *Shanghanlun*. It is appropriate to use not only the concept of the six stages but also other Kampo formulas proposed in texts other than the *Shanghanlun* to treat a range of cases, including cases where the abovementioned formulas fail to achieve a cure and cases where recovery is slow even after a cure.

- **Kososan:** Covers a wide range of cases of common cold syndrome, including deficiency patterns for which various Kampo drugs are not appropriate. This formula is preferably taken as soon as possible when the patient complains of headache, chilling, and a slight fever. It can be safely prescribed for elderly patients and those with gastrointestinal weakness.
- **Shomakakkonto:** Indicated for medium pattern in the early stage of common cold with throat pain.
- **Jinsoin:** Indicated for slight deficiency pattern in elderly patients and those with gastrointestinal weakness with prolonged symptoms of the common cold.
- **Seihaito:** Indicated for a medium pattern with coughing accompanied by large amounts of viscous sputum.
- **Chikujountanto:** Indicated for medium pattern patients who are unable to sleep well due to coughing and sputum expectoration in prolonged cases of the common cold.
- **Jiinshihoto:** Indicated for slight deficiency pattern patients with large amounts of easily clearable serous sputum, complaints of anorexia, and night sweats. Abdominal examination reveals mild fullness and discomfort in the chest and hypochondrium.

- **Bakumondoto:** Used for slight deficiency to medium pattern patients whose common cold symptoms have almost healed. They don't have sputum or difficult-to-clear viscous sputum and tend to have fits of coughing that can cause facial flushing.
- **Jiinkokato:** Used for slight deficiency pattern patients with indications for *bakumondoto* with dry skin and constipation. This is relatively common among physically weak or elderly patients.

2.2 Persistent Cough, Chronic Cough, and Expectoration

Koichiro Tatsumi

2.2.1 Overview of Disease [14]

Cough Categorization According to Its Duration

Coughing is distinguished according to its duration: 3 weeks or less (acute cough), 3–8 weeks (persistent cough), and 8 weeks or more (chronic cough). The causes of acute cough mostly lie in respiratory tract infections. Noninfectious mechanisms are largely responsible for persistent or chronic cough, in contrast to acute cough. Administration of an antibacterial drug is necessary for a cough due to bacterial infection, and Kampo therapy alone should be avoided. The combined use of antibacterial drugs and Kampo medicines is not considered problematic.

Cough Categorization According to the Presence or Absence of Expectoration

Coughing is categorized as either nonproductive or productive, according to the presence or absence of expectoration. The key point in Kampo therapy for productive cough is whether the cough is infectious or not. Prior to the initiation of Kampo therapy, it is similarly necessary to categorize the causal pathophysiologic condition as either infectious or noninfectious.

2.2.2 Indications for Kampo Therapy [15–16]

The causal pathologic conditions must be considered. Western medical therapy may be preferred, concurrent use of Western medical therapy and Kampo therapy may be helpful, or Kampo therapy alone may be effective based on the above consideration. Frequent formulas are listed below according to pathophysiologic conditions.

2.2.3 Frequent Formulas

1. **Persistent Cough Following Bronchitis** (Fig. 5.7)

In cases of acute bronchitis that are not cured within a short period, coughing may persist. Eppikahangeto[8] and makyokansekito are the formulas of choice for persistent violent cough.

- **Eppikahangeto**[6]: Eppito[6] is used for exterior fluid retention, often associated with thirst. In addition, hange has an expectorant effect. Combined use of eppikajutsuto with hangekobokuto or shohangekabukuryoto extract formulations is a possible alternative.
- **Makyokansekito:** Indicated for patients presenting with a somewhat excess pattern. Makyokansekito is appropriate for a cough that is not as violent as the cough for which eppikahangeto[9] is used but does not respond well to bakumondoto. Combined use with shosaikoto extract formulation is effective.
- **Gokoto:** Indicated for patients presenting with a somewhat excess pattern. Gokoto is makyokansekito with sohakuhi, which has anti-inflammatory and antitussive actions. Accordingly, gokoto gives a slightly stronger antitussive effect than makyokansekito.

Persistent Cough with Chronic Respiratory Disease (Fig. 5.8).

- **Saibokuto:** Indicated for patients presenting a medium pattern. Saibokuto is a combined formula of hangekobokuto, which improves qi stagnation, and shosaikoto, which has an anti-inflammatory action. In cases of bronchial asthma in which adequate Western drug therapy does not eliminate coughing or expectoration, concomitant use of saibokuto may offer a reduction in the dose of steroid inhalers.
- **Shimpito:** Indicated for patients presenting a medium pattern. Shimpito appears to be a combination of formu-

[8]Not available as a medical Kampo extract formulation nor OTC Kampo extract formulation.

[9]Not available as a medical Kampo extract formulation nor as an OTC Kampo extract formulation.

Eppikahangeto: mao 6.0, sekko 8.0, taiso 3.0, kanzo 2.0, shokyo 1.0, hange 4.0.

Eppito: mao 6.0, sekko 8.0, taiso 3.0, kanzo 2.0, shokyo 1.0.

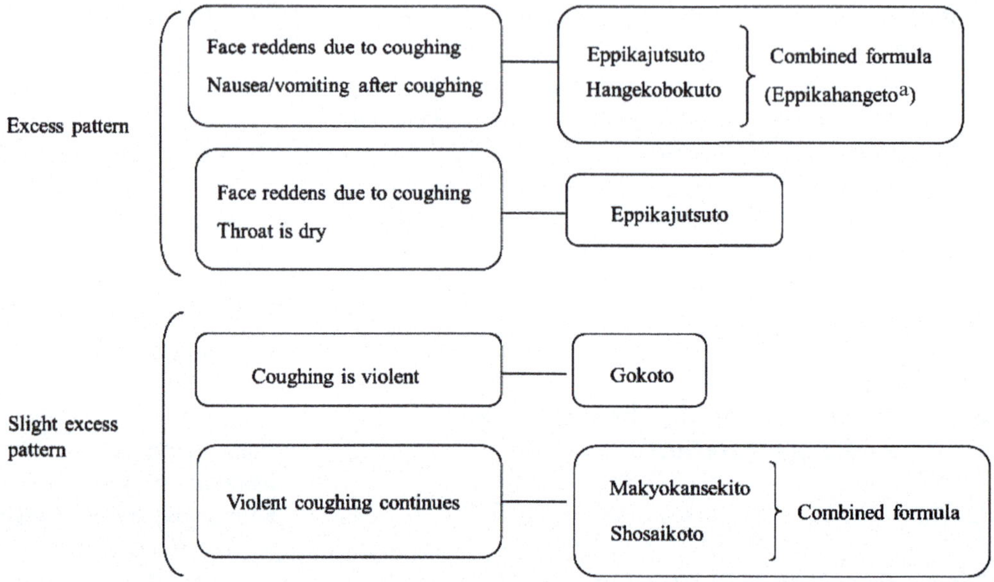

Fig. 5.7 Frequent formulas for persistent cough following bronchitis
[a]Not available as a medical Kampo extract formulation nor OTC Kampo extract formulation

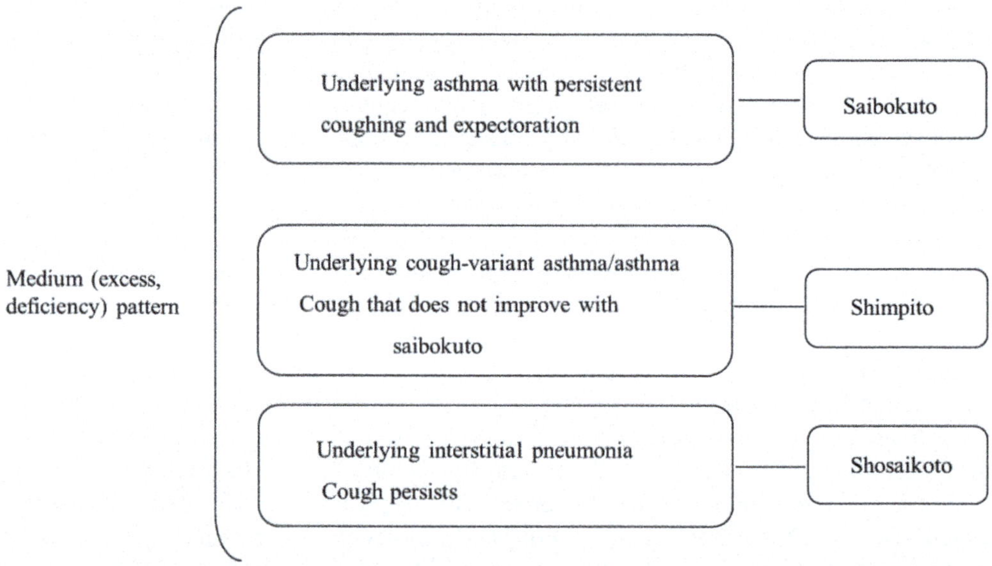

Fig. 5.8 Frequent formulas for persistent cough with chronic respiratory disease

las with Bupleurum root and formulas with Ephedra Herb. This formula can be tried if *saibokuto* shows no effect.

- **Shosaikoto:** Indicated for patients presenting a medium pattern. Shosaikoto can be tried at an early stage for idiopathic pulmonary fibrosis after patient consent is obtained. Results cannot be expected for late-stage honeycomb lung. Use concurrently with keishibukuryogan if blood[TM1] stasis signs are present.

Persistent Cough (Fig. 5.9)

Formulas are used for mild coughs, regardless of the presence or absence of underlying disease.

- **Bakumondoto:** Indicated for patients presenting medium to slight deficiency pattern. Bakumondoto can be used instead of expectorant if the throat and nasal meatus are mildly dry. Effective for violent dry cough. It can be expected to moisten the airway, improve sputum expectoration, and soothe coughing and dry mouth, so it is effective as a basic therapeutic medicine for chronic respiratory tract disease.
- **Hangekobokuto:** Indicated for patients presenting a medium pattern. Using this formula for patients with a medium pattern with laryngopharyngeal paresthesia (obstructive discomfort in the throat) is an approach based on the classical Kampo texts. This formula been shown to

Fig. 5.9 Frequent formulas for persistent cough

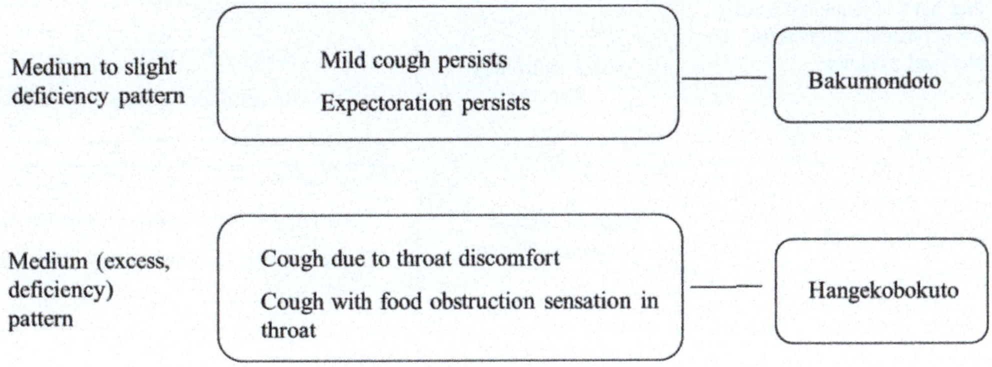

Fig. 5.10 Frequent formulas for persistent cough associated with sinusitis

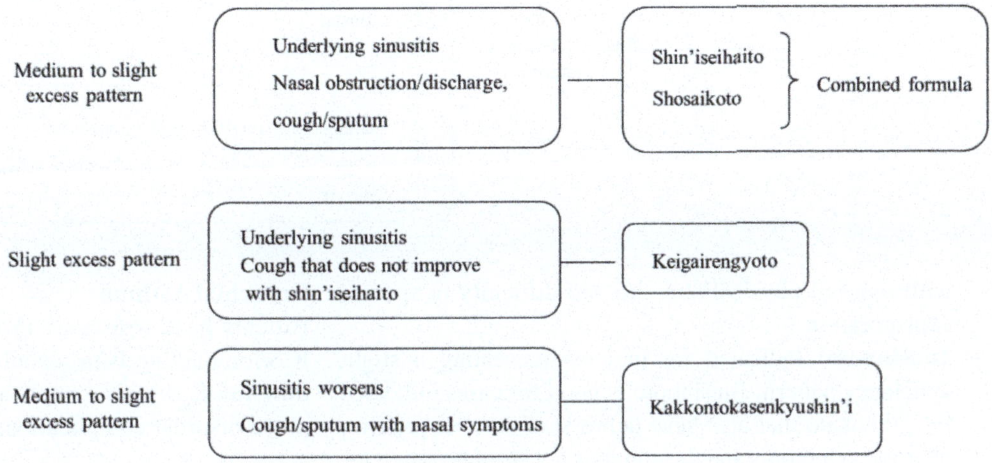

increase substance P in the laryngopharynx, improve swallowing and cough reflexes, and prevent aspiration pneumonia in elderly people.

Persistent Cough Associated with Sinusitis (Fig. 5.10).

- **Shin'iseihaito:** Indicated for patients presenting medium to slight excess pattern. Shin'i is effective for nasal occlusion. Combination with shosaikoto may be helpful if the use of shin'iseihaito alone doesn't have the sufficient effect.
- **Keigairengyoto:** Indicated for patients presenting a slight excess pattern. Keigairengyoto may be used if shin'iseihaito and shosaikoto are not effective.
- **Kakkontokasenkyushin'i:** Indicated for patients presenting a medium to somewhat excess pattern. A formula consists of kakkonto, in addition to senkyu, which improves blood flow, and shin'i, which improves nasal obstruction. Used for short periods when sinusitis symptoms are severe.

Persistent Cough with Physical Weakness (Deficiency Pattern) (Fig. 5.11)

- **Hochuekkito** [17, 18]: Indicated for patients presenting a slight deficiency pattern. Hochuekkito does not have a direct effect on coughing or expectoration but improves the general condition. This results in effective reduction of common cold symptoms, improvement of respiratory infection conditions, and a decrease in coughing and expectoration.
- **Chikujountanto:** Indicated for patients presenting a medium pattern. Chikujountanto is used for its expectorant and tranquilizing effects when mild cough and expectoration continue with the onset of intense psychoneurotic symptoms such as insomnia, depression, and irritability.
- **Jiinkokato:** Indicated for patients presenting a slight deficiency pattern. Jiinkokato is a basic tonifying formula for blood deficiency. It is a nourishing tonic using shimotsuto as blood[TM1] tonic as its base. It is better than bakumondoto in patients whose overall condition is extremely dry (blood deficiency), including the skin,

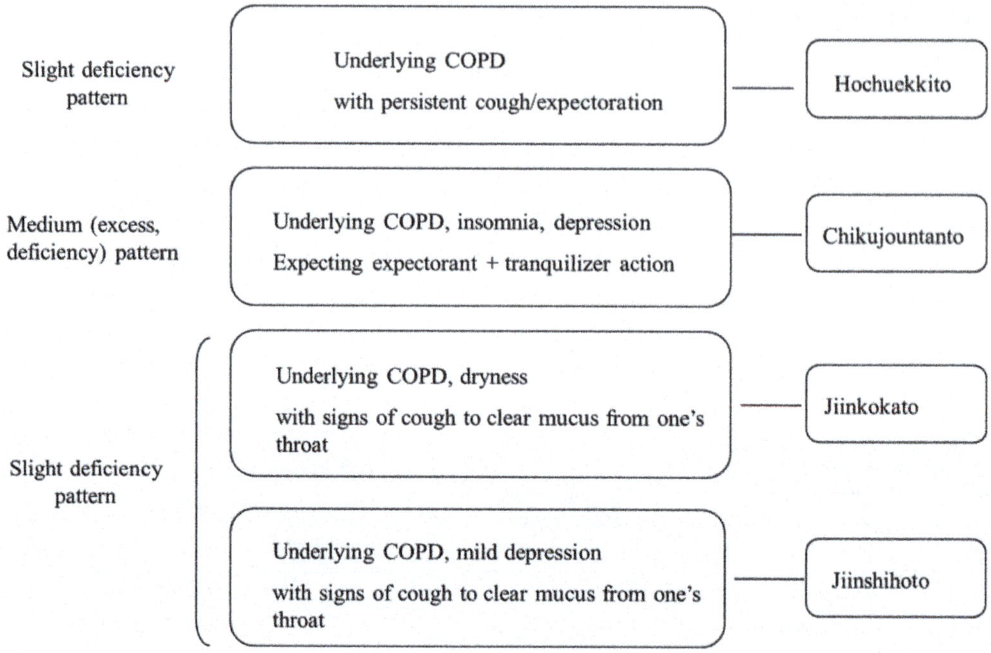

Fig. 5.11 Frequent formulas for persistent cough with physical weakness

with reduced physical strength and difficulty in sputum expectoration.

- **Jiinshihoto:** Indicated for patients presenting a slight deficiency pattern. Jiinshihoto is good for cases indicated for jiinkokato that also have depression or other psychoneurotic symptoms and the cough is not strong enough for expectoration.

2.3 Wheezing and Dyspnea

Takashi Ito

2.3.1 Overview of Disease

The primary or underlying diseases for dyspnea are asthma, chronic obstructive pulmonary disease (COPD), asthma and COPD overlap (ACO), interstitial pneumonia, and chronic respiratory failure of the respiratory disease. With heart disease, cardiac insufficiency could be an underlying condition. In the treatment of these diseases, priority is given to Western medicine, at least in Japan. In intractable cases, however, Kampo medicines are important for their complementary role.

2.3.2 Indications for Kampo Therapy

Cases in which kampo medicines are useful are listed below. In each case, Western medicine should be seriously considered but need not be used in all cases.

Bronchial Asthma

Patients have resistance to inhaled corticosteroid (ICS) or ICS/long-acting $beta_2$ agonists (LABA) therapy, low peak-flow value, rhinitis complication, susceptibility to infection, mood disorder complication, and allergy to Western drugs.

COPD, Chronic Respiratory Failure

Patients have severe shortness of breath despite LABA and long-acting muscarinic antagonist therapy, recurrent lower respiratory tract infection despite long-term use of macrolide antibiotics, anorexia, susceptibility to infection, and heart failure complications.

2.3.3 Frequently Used Formulas

In the 2015 guidelines for the treatment of asthma, the Kampo therapy guidelines outline the general principles of Kampo formulas for dyspnea and wheezing dyspnea (Fig. 5.12). More specifically, formulas with ephedra herb are used in attacks, formulas with bupleurum root between attacks, and tonic formulas in patients with weakness. The formulas with Ephedra Herb include *makyokansekito* for heat patterns, *shoseiryuto* for cold patterns, and *bakumondoto* for severe dry coughs. Formulas with Bupleurum root are appropriate for prevention of attack. Combined formulas of *Saiko*-containing formula and *hangekobokuto* are helpful in patients with throat discomfort. Tonic formulas offered to patients with weakness include *hochuekkito* for spleen deficiency and *hachimijiogan* for kidney deficiency. Differentiated use of formulas during attacks (or when symptoms worsen) and between attacks is important.

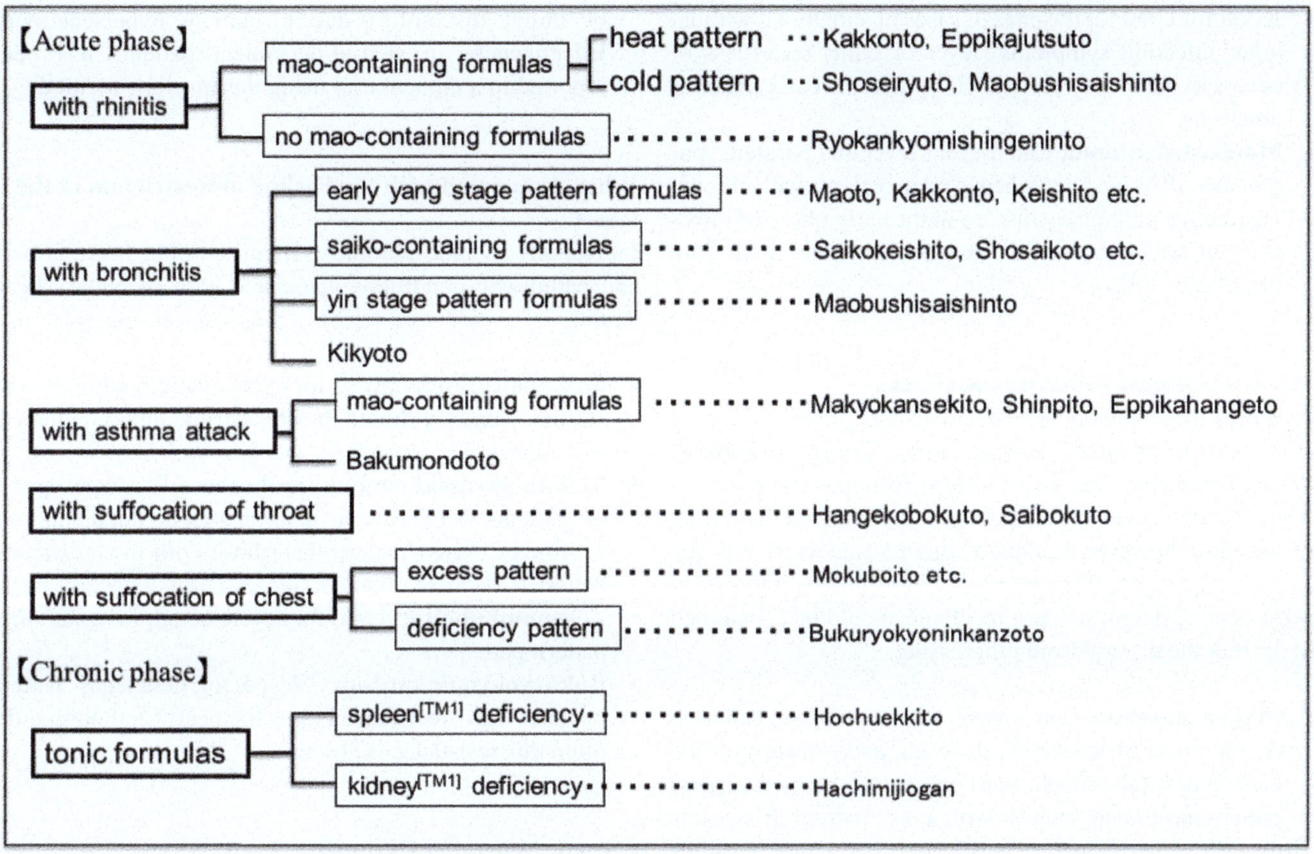

Fig. 5.12 Kampo medicine administration guidelines for wheezing and dyspnea

In Japan today, the treatment of asthma focuses on ICS or ICS/LABA, and Kampo therapy during attacks is generally considered unimportant. Kampo specialists are expected to successfully prevent asthma attacks as well as aggravation of lower respiratory tract symptoms following viral infection, using not only standard Kampo formulas but also special formulas containing *keishi* and *mao* during attacks.

Dyspnea Associated with Rhinitis

It has been pointed out that respiratory distress can occur along with rhinitis.

- **Kakkonto:** Helpful when used in medium to slight excess pattern in patients having chronic sinusitis, neck and back stiffness, and little sweating.
- **Eppikajutsuto:** For patients having intense sneezing and nasal discharge. Helpful if mucous membrane redness and swelling are present.
- **Shoseiryuto**: Used for slight deficiency pattern patients with slight facial pallor and the tendency for edema. Effective for allergic rhinitis and asthma. It seems, however, that increased severity of pollen allergy symptoms in Japan recently has decreased the number of effective cases.
- **Ryokankyomishingeninto:** Although target symptoms are almost the same as for *shoseiryuto*, this is used for patients who can't tolerate *MAO*. Patients often have rhinitis that persists all year, along with coldness and edema.
- **Maobushisaishinto:** Good for patients with poor complexion and chills.

When Associated with Airway Infection

Viral infection readily induces asthma attacks, exacerbation of COPD, and aggravation of respiratory failure. If fever is present, formulas with ephedra herb for early yang stage pattern are often prescribed. If the illness is persistent, formulas with Bupleurum root for late yang stage pattern are recommended.

- **Early yang stage pattern formulas:** Used within one to 3 days after infection. See "Common Cold Syndrome" for details.
- **Formulas with Bupleurum root:** Used from the fourth day after infection in cases of alternating chills and fever and fullness and discomfort in the chest and hypochondrium. Includes *shosaikoto*, *saikokeishito*, and *saikokeishikankyoto*. See "Common Cold Syndrome" for details.

- **Kikyoto:** Used for dyspnea in cases of sore throat without other infection symptoms (fever or chill) regardless of excess or deficiency pattern. Helpful in the early phase of tonsillitis.
- **Maobushisaishinto:** Can prevent fever and purulent sputum as well as dyspnea when used in patients with chronic obstructive pulmonary disease in the early phase of infection, in which bronchitis aggravation starts with sore throat and chills.

When Associated with Asthma Attacks

As a rule, the following formulas with ephedra herb are used at the time of an attack. In Japan today, priority is given to Western medicine. The use of Kampo formulas is considered when the effects are unsatisfactory. Depending on the timing of their use, however, Kampo medicines may exert efficacy equal or superior to Western drugs. Nevertheless, if improvement is not evident, modern medicine should be considered to prevent the disease from progressing.

- **Makyokansekito**: Can control asthma attacks when used on the onset of wheezing, dyspnea, and sweating in the early stage of the attack. Most patients with a slight excess pattern have facial redness with a heat pattern. If sweat is absent, dehydration is suspected, and this requires caution.
- **Eppikahangeto**[10]: Effective for attacks with severe coughing (as if the eyes were going to pop out) and vomiting at the peak of the attack.
- **Shimpito**: For patients with medium pattern. Target symptoms are persistent cough with fullness and discomfort in the chest and hypochondrium. Also effective for rather severe coughs.

When Associated with the Feeling of Restriction in the Pharynx

- **Hangekobokuto:** Appropriate for obstructive discomfort in the throat to the chest. Patients with medium pattern commonly have background mental health issues, including anxiety and depression. Frequently used for laryngopharyngeal neurosis.
- **Saibokuto:** A combined formula of *hangekobokuto* and *shosaikoto*. Used for medium pattern patients with asthma or throat discomfort due to airway hypersensitivity. Effectiveness in steroid-dependent patients has been reported in a clinical trial using the envelope method.

When Associated with the Feeling of Restriction in the Chest

Indications include chronic asthma, chronic heart failure, and pathologic conditions associated with secondary heart strain.

- **Mokuboito:** Appropriate for excess pattern patients with stuffiness and rigidity in the epigastrium along with thirst and edema.
- **Mokuboikyosekkokabukuryoboshoto:**[11] Appropriate for patients who have constipation with no thirst and have a stronger excess pattern than those with the *mokuboito* pattern.
- **Zosonmokuboito:**[8] Used for severe cough in *mokuboito*-pattern patients.
- **Bukuryokyoninkanzoto:**[12] Used for deficiency pattern patients with "resistance below the heart," although quite often this resistance is absent.

Chronic Wheezing Dyspnea

- **Hachimijiogan:** Appropriate for slight deficiency pattern patients with kidney deficiency; specifically, weakness of the lower abdominal region, nocturia, lower body pain, numbness, and weakness. Effective in cases of low peak-flow value, but efficacy cannot be expected in severe cases of 250 L/min or less [19].
- **Hochuekkito**: The main indication is qi deficiency (spleen deficiency), specifically, weak eyes, loss of spirit, loss of vigor, anorexia, low-grade fever tendency, susceptibility to colds, etc. In slight deficiency pattern patients with chronic obstructive pulmonary disease, improvement of QOL, reduced incidence of common cold syn-

---

[10] Not available as a medical Kampo extract formulation.

[11] Not available as a medical Kampo extract formulation nor an OTC Kampo extract formulation.

Eppikahangeto: *mao* 6.0, *sekko* 8.0, *taiso* 3.0, *kanzo* 2.0, *shokyo* 1.0, *hange* 4.0.

Mokuboikyosekkokabukuryoboshoto: *boi*・*bukuryo* 4.0, *keihi*・*ninjin* 3.0, *bosho* 5.0.

Zosonmokuboito: *boi* 4.0, *sekko* 10.0, *keihi*, *ninjin*, *sohakuhi* 3.0, *shokyo* 1.0, *shisoshi* 5.0.

[12] Not available as a medical Kampo extract formulation.

drome, and improvement in nutritional condition have been reported [20].

2.4 Palpitation and Shortness of Breath

Shuji Yakubo

2.4.1 Overview of Disease

This overview deals with palpitation and shortness of breath by distinguishing that associated with heart failure and other types of palpitation.

Symptoms of Heart Failure

Treatment must be carried out in consideration of the pathological condition and underlying diseases of heart failure.

For mild heart failure, treatment aims to avoid reductions in quality of life (QOL) by using diuretic, digitalis, catecholamine, and vasodilator drugs.

For severe heart failure, a catheter is inserted to measure cardiac index and pulmonary capillary wedge pressure. If the cardiac index is low, treatment should take pulmonary capillary wedge pressure into account with cardiac pumping ability maintained.

In cases of valve disease, hypertensive heart disease, cardiomyopathy, and ischemic heart diseases (such as cardiac infarction) that impair cardiac function, the necessary drug therapy, interventions, and surgical management should be carried out.

Palpitations

Treatment plans will differ according to the presence or absence of palpitation-linked arrhythmia and underlying diseases that cause arrhythmia. Arrhythmia is either tachycardia arrhythmia (tachyarrhythmia) or bradycardia arrhythmia (bradyarrhythmia).

Dangerous tachyarrhythmia includes ventricular fibrillation and ventricular tachycardia. If these conditions are identified, or if long QT syndrome, Brugada syndrome, or late ventricular potential on signal-averaged electrocardiogram is found, aggressive treatment with anti-arrhythmic drugs should be given. Dangerous bradyarrhythmia requires therapy using a pacemaker.

Tachyarrhythmia that reduces QOL includes paroxysmal atrial fibrillation and paroxysmal supraventricular tachycardia, both also treated with anti-arrhythmic drugs.

Excluding dangerous arrhythmias and QOL-reducing arrhythmias, arrhythmias that aren't dangerous or associated with underlying diseases are generally not treated with anti-arrhythmic drugs. Tranquilizers are administered for subjective symptoms such as palpitations. However, anti-arrhythmic drugs may be administered in cases in which significant subjective symptoms coincide with arrhythmia events.

2.4.2 Indications for Kampo Therapy

Symptoms of Heart Failure

Modern intensive medical treatment is required for acute and severe life-threatening heart failure. Kampo therapy is used for chronic and non-severe pathologic conditions, which include New York Heart Association (NYHA) Functional Classification Class II and Class III heart failure involving the appearance of heart failure symptoms even with daily activities or light work.

Palpitations

Priority is given to modern medical treatment for dangerous arrhythmia.

Kampo medicines such as shakanzo-to are used for paroxysmal atrial fibrillation and paroxysmal supraventricular tachycardia, which reduce QOL. Mokuboito is used for bradyarrhythmia.

Aggressive treatment with Kampo medicines may be considered for arrhythmia with strong subjective symptoms that do not require therapy with the anti-arrhythmic drugs of Western medicine.

2.4.3 Frequently Used Formulas

Kampo therapy for heart failure symptoms such as shortness of breath, palpitation, and edema includes the use of Kampo prescriptions using herbs with a fluid-regulating effect combined with herbs with a qi-tonifying effect.

Herbs with a heat-clearing effect, or antifebrile effect, are appropriate for palpitations not associated with heart failure. For palpitations associated with blood deficiency, prescriptions containing herbs with a blood stasis resolving effect are recommended.

Symptoms of Heart Failure (Fig. 5.13).

- **Mokuboito** [21, 22]: Used for heart failure symptoms such as respiratory distress, cough, and edema, associated with abdominal distension, thirst, and reduced urination. Specifically useful for patients with signs of blue-blackish complexion, wheezing, dyspnea, and abdominal swelling. The pulse is deep *and tight. Patients tend to have* a slight excess pattern, and regardless of abdominal strength, the abdomen presents a stuffiness and rigidity in the epigastrium. There are reports that serum concentration of B-type natriuretic peptide (BNP), a heart failure marker, has been reduced with moku-boi-to.
- **Ryokeijutsukanto**: Used for palpitation, shortness of breath, and dizziness. Indicated for slight deficiency pattern patients who have coldness in the lower limbs and

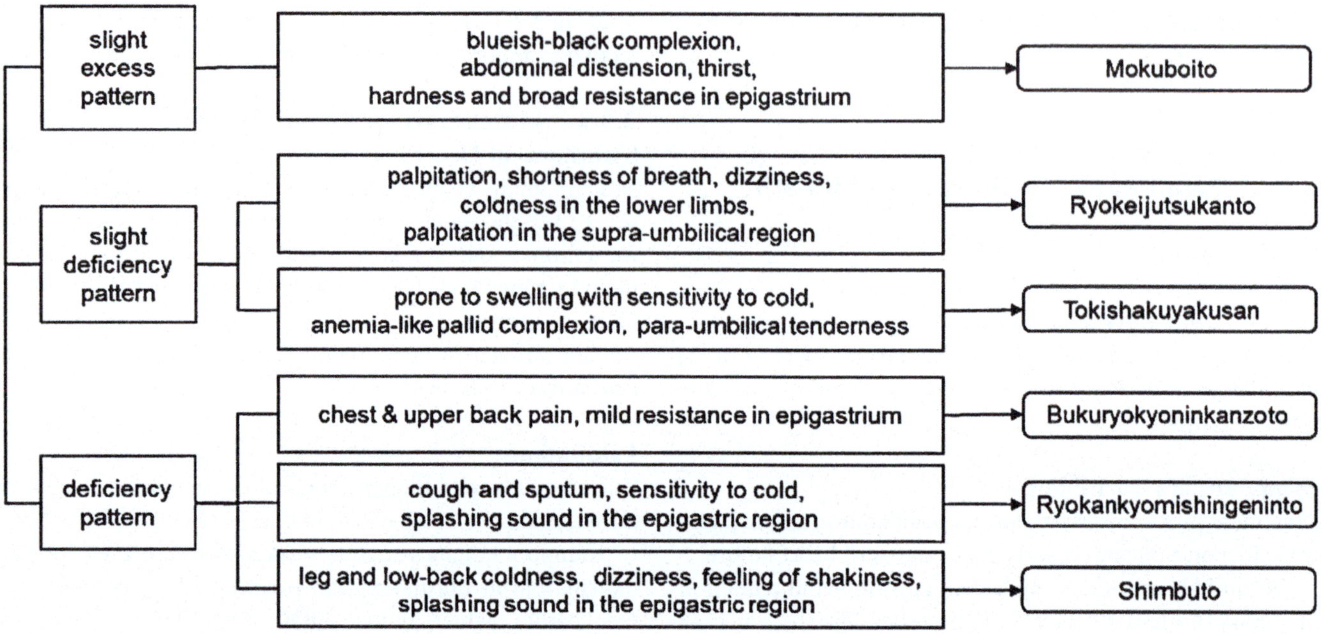

Fig. 5.13 Frequent Kampo formulas for cardiac insufficiency

reduced urination. The pulse is deep and tight. Abdominal examination shows abdominal strength is intermediate or weaker. The abdomen has palpitation in the supra-umbilical region and splashing sounds.

- **Tokishakuyakusan**: Specifically used in swelling-prone patients with sensitivity to cold and other symptoms such as palpitation. They are slight deficiency pattern patients who are prone to fatigue and suffer from general malaise. They have anemia-like pallid facial color with soggy, slack skin; their pulse is deep and weak. Abdominal examination shows weak abdominal strength, splashing sounds in the stomach, and para-umbilical tenderness and resistance.
- **Bukuryokyoninkanzoto**:[13] Indicated for patients with fullness in the chest and signs of dyspnea, palpitation, and radiating chest or back pain; sometimes accompanied by respiratory distress and edema. They have a deficiency pattern with a deep and faint pulse. Abdominal examination shows the abdomen is weak with soft resistance in the epigastric region. Thirst is absent.
- **Ryokankyomishingeninto**: Contains the constituent herbs of *bukuryo-kyonin-kanzo-to*. Used for palpitation, shortness of breath, cough, and sputum, specifically in deficiency pattern patients with fatigue and sensitivity to cold. They are also characterized by poor complexion, wheezing, and edema. The pulse is deep and weak. Abdominal examination often shows weakness with splashing sounds in the epigastric region.

[13] Not available as a medical Kampo extract formulation.

- **Shimbuto**: Specifically indicated for deficiency pattern patients who have reduced metabolism and poor peripheral circulation. These patients complain of general malaise and coldness in the legs and lower back. Also, in addition to palpitations, they have dizziness, a feeling of shakiness, edema, and reduced urination. The pulse is deep and weak. Abdominal examination shows a thin abdominal wall and reduced abdominal strength with splashing sounds. Occasionally there may be slight tension in the rectus abdominis muscles.

Palpitation (Fig. 5.14)

- **Orengedokuto**: Indicated for patients who are easily aroused and have palpitations and tachycardia when aroused. They have excess or slight excess pattern patients and show signs of hot flashes with facial redness as well as psychoneurotic symptoms of anxiety and irritability. Abdominal examination shows distension in the abdomen; abdominal strength is intermediate or stronger. There is a soft epigastrium.
- **Saikokaryukotsuboreito** [23]: Used for stress-induced hypertension and palpitation. Used in slight excess pattern in patients who are irritable, prone to anger, and anxiety. Abdominal examination shows intermediate or stronger abdominal strength. There is fullness and discomfort in the chest and hypochondrium and epigastric stuffiness and resistance along with pulsation in the supra-umbilical region. The pulse is a string-like pulse.

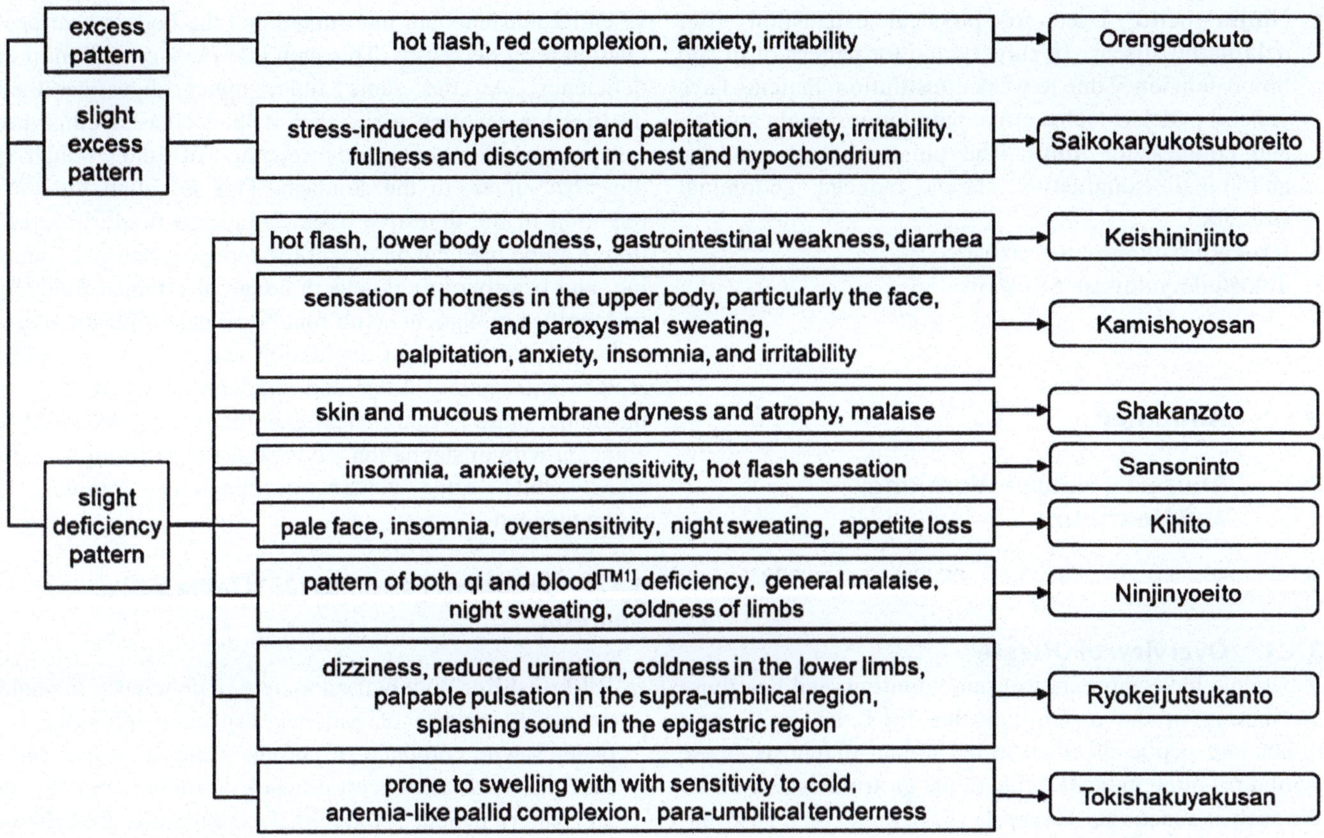

Fig. 5.14 Frequent Kampo formulas for palpitation

- **Keishininjinto**: Effective for hot flashes and palpitations. Administered to slight deficiency pattern patients with lower body coldness who have gastrointestinal weakness and are prone to diarrhea. Abdominal examination shows slight weakness in the abdomen; abdominal strength is intermediate or weaker. Epigastric discomfort, resistance, and splashing sound are also present. Occasionally there is palpable tightness in a thin abdominal wall. The pulse is floating and weak.
- **Kamishoyosan**: Indicated for slight deficiency pattern patients who suffer coldness and have palpitation, anxiety, insomnia, and irritability; sometimes associated with a sensation of heat in the upper body, particularly the face, and paroxysmal sweating. The pulse is deep and thin. Abdominal strength is intermediate or weaker. Slight resistance and tenderness in the epigastric region and slight fullness and discomfort in the chest and hypochondrium are present. Also associated with para-umbilical tenderness and resistance.
- **Shakanzoto**: Also called *fukumyakuto*. Used for palpitation and shortness of breath in slight deficiency pattern patients, who have skin and mucous membrane dryness and atrophy; burning sensation in the limbs; thirst and other blood deficiency symptoms; as well as constipation and malaise. They are also prone to fatigue. The pulse is weak, sometimes frequent, irregular, and intermittent.
- **Sansoninto**: Used for insomnia in mentally and physically fatigued patients with slight deficiency pattern. They may have decreased physical strength, chest pains, and palpitations. Also associated with psychoneurotic symptoms such as anxiety and oversensitivity, as well as dizziness, burning sensation in the limbs, and hot flashes. The skin tends to be dry. Abdominal examination shows reduced abdominal strength. Pulsation in the supra-umbilical region is not present.
- **Kihito**: Used for tachycardia, palpitation, insomnia, and psychoneurotic symptoms (including anxiety, oversensitivity, overanxiety, and forgetfulness) in slight deficiency pattern patients with anemia and pale faces. Sometimes associated with fever, night sweating, and loss of appetite. Abdominal examination shows a soft and weak abdomen with reduced abdominal strength.

- **Ninjin'yoeito**: Used for physical exhaustion after debilitating disease or surgery and for pattern of qi and blood deficiency due to weak constitution. Patients have general malaise, tachycardia, palpitations, night sweats, and coldness of limbs. The pulse is weak, and an abdominal examination shows reduced abdominal strength.
- **Ryokeijutsukanto**: See above
- **Tokishakuyakusan**: See above

3 Abdomen

3.1 Anorexia, Nausea, Vomiting, and Heartburn

Tetsuro Oikawa

3.1.1 Overview of Disease

If patients have anorexia, nausea, vomiting, and heartburn originating in the upper digestive tract, and malignant tumor and peptic ulcer are ruled out in diagnosis, these symptoms often indicate a functional gastrointestinal disorder such as functional dyspepsia (FD). Functional gastrointestinal disorders are complex pathologic conditions. Western medicine with a singular locus of action is often not completely effective. For these pathologic conditions, Kampo medicines considered to have multiple loci of action are as effective as, or more effective than, Western drug therapies. Actually, *rikkunshi-to,* effective for chronic indigestion symptoms, has been shown to have a variety of actions, including improvement of gastric emptying function and adaptive relaxation, as well as stimulation of secretion of ghrelin, which has an appetite-increasing effect [24]. Also, among gastroesophageal reflux diseases (GERD) with heartburn as the main complaint, intractable esophageal reflux, non-erosive reflux disease (NERD), reflux disease reflux hypersensitivity, and functional heartburn, which don't respond well to proton pump inhibitors (PPIs), are designated as refractory GERD. Among refractory GERD that is receiving attention as being resistant to treatment, it has been reported that the combination of PPIs and *rikkunshito* is effective for NERD. When the limitations of Western medical approaches become apparent, the value of complementary Kampo medicines comes to the forefront.

3.1.2 Indications for Kampo Therapy

In Kampo medicine, anorexia, nausea, vomiting, and heartburn tend to be associated with qi deficiency. When anorexia, nausea, vomiting, and heartburn occur because of upper digestive tract dysfunction, digestion and absorption of essential nutrients are interrupted and the body's heat production level decreases. This then leads to a condition of qi deficiency. At the same time, upper digestive tract dysfunction is often associated with decreased emptying function, which results in the retention of fluid[TM1]such as digestive juices, in the stomach. This is called fluid[TM1] retention in the digestive tract, or phlegm-fluid[TM1] retention. Kampo medical treatment for anorexia, nausea, vomiting, and heartburn facilitates drainage of retained fluid[TM1] and tonifies qi. Patients with functional gastrointestinal disorders also suffer from depression and anxiety and often receive anti-anxiety drugs and antidepressants. In Kampo medicine, these psychological conditions are considered to coincide with qi stagnation, and active use of Kampo medicines, which often contain qi-regulating formulas, is recommended.

3.1.3 Frequent Formulas [25] (Table 5.3)

Anorexia

- **Rikkunshito**: Widely used mainly in deficiency to slight deficiency pattern of patients. Especially effective for patients who complain of chronic indigestion and early satiety. Expected to exert efficacy on these symptoms in any pattern patients. Abdominal examination often shows epigastric stuffiness and resistance and splashing sound. This formula is one of the Kampo medicines whose action mechanisms have been intensively elucidated, and there is a range of evidence for FD treatment and alleviation of adverse effects of psychoactive drugs.
- **Shikunshito**: This is rikkunshito without *chimpi* and *hange*. The removal of these ingredients weakens the efficacy of chronic indigestion and other symptoms due to phlegm-fluid[TM1] retention.
- **Ninjinto**: Patients have a slender build (deficiency pattern) and mostly have epigastric stuffiness and resistance. They may also have plywood-like hardness in the upper abdomen. The combination of *kanzo* and *kankyo* eliminates interior cold and reduces coldness in the feet and body.
- **Hangeshashinto**: Patients often have subjective symptoms of gastric stuffiness and discomfort, with objective findings of epigastric stuffiness and resistance. Patients may also have symptoms such as abdominal rumbling and diarrhea. Effective for so-called stress gastritis in young patients.
- **Orengedokuto**: Patients often have gastric stuffiness and discomfort, with the abdominal pattern of epigastric stuffiness and resistance. Used in patients with increased secretion of gastric acid who complain of heartburn and other symptoms such as gastric stuffiness and discomfort. *Orengedokuto* is similar to *rikkunshito* and *hangeshashinto* in that patients' abdominal findings include epigas-

Table 5.3 Kampo Formulas for anorexia, nausea, vomiting, and heartburn

Excess pattern	Anorexia/heartburn	Facial redness Epigastric stuffiness and resistance Stomach swelling after eating	Orengedokuto Heiisan
	Nausea/vomiting	Fullness and discomfort in chest and hypochondrium Constipation	Daisaikoto
Medium (excess, deficiency) pattern	Anorexia	Epigastric stuffiness and resistance Abdominal rumbling	Hangeshashinto
	Nausea/vomiting	Tongue fur Fullness and discomfort in chest and hypochondrium	Shosaikoto
		Obstructive discomfort in the throat Qi stagnation	Hangekobokuto
		Thirst Decreased urine volume and urination frequency Edema	Goreisan
		Epigastric stuffiness and resistance Abdominal rumbling	Hangeshashinto
	Heartburn	Obstructive discomfort in the throat Qi stagnation	Hangekobokuto
		Epigastric stuffiness and resistance Abdominal rumbling	Hangeshashinto
		Tongue fur Stomach pain	Orento
		Fullness in the chest Indescribable pain and agony around the chest	Shishishito[a]
Deficiency pattern	Anorexia	Chronic indigestion Splashing sound	Rikkunshito
		Poor complexion	Shi-kunshito
		Epigastric stuffiness and resistance Coldness	Ninjinto
		Enlarged tongue Atony	Hochuekkito
	Nausea/vomiting	Chronic indigestion Splashing sound	Rikkunshito
		Splashing sound Hyperemesis gravidarum Epigastric stuffiness and resistance Coldness	Bukuryoin Shohangekabukuryoto Goshuyuto
	Heartburn	Chronic indigestion Splashing sound	Rikkunshito
		Coldness Stomach pain	Anchusan

[a]Not available as medical Kampo extract formulation

tric stuffiness and resistance, but the above formula is more appropriate for excess to slight excess pattern patients. It is also effective for facial redness and hot flashes.

- **Hochuekkito:** This is a typical qi-tonifying formulas and is widely used for anorexia. It is especially effective in slight deficiency pattern patients who have atonic constitution, characterized by gastroptosis, anal prolapse, and the like. Tongue diagnosis shows an enlarged tongue, and slight fullness and discomfort in the chest and hypochondrium are evident in the abdominal examination. Pulse diagnosis reveals a unique pulse called dissipated large.
- **Heiisan**: This formula is used for dyspepsia symptoms such as stomach distension after eating. It's more suited to excess pattern patients than *rikkunshi-to.*

Nausea and Vomiting

- **Shohangekabukuryoto**: Often used for hyperemesis gravidarum. Also effective for slight deficiency pattern patients with similar symptoms. When symptoms are severe, taking the formula cold facilitates dosing.
- **Rikkunshito**: See Section 3.1.3, Anorexia.
- **Hangekobokuto:** A typical qi-regulating formula. Appropriate for patients with neurotic tendencies or digestive tract symptoms involving stress. Effective in patients with abdominal distension or laryngopharyngeal discomfort called "obstructive discomfort in the throat." Often tongue diagnosis shows scalloped tongue or white tongue coating, and abdominal examination reveals abdominal fullness.

- **Bukuryoin:** This formula drains phlegm/fluid[TM1] retention and is more effective than *shohangekabukuryoto* against strong feelings that food does not digest normally. Abdominal examination often reveals a splashing sound. *Bukuryo-in* is often used as a combined formula with *hangekobokuto*.
- **Goreisan**: A standard fluid[TM1]-regulating formula. The main indications are thirst, a tendency to sweat, decreased urine volume, and urinary frequency. Widely used for nausea, vomiting, and diarrhea in acute gastroenteritis.
- **Shosaikoto**: A typical formula for the late yang stage, but nausea and vomiting are also indications. Often patients have a medium pattern, and an abdominal examination reveals fullness and discomfort in the chest and hypochondrium, and tongue diagnosis shows a white coating. Given this, this formula may be used for various chronic digestive diseases.
- **Daisaikoto**: More effective than *shosaiko-to* in patients with excess pattern who have intense fullness and discomfort in the chest and hypochondrium, nausea, vomiting, and other symptoms associated with a tendency of constipation.
- **Hangeshashinto**: See 3.1.3 Anorexia.
- **Goshuyuto**: Known as a formula used for headaches in patients with slight deficiency pattern, but this formula is highly effective for nausea and vomiting associated with headaches and coldness in the limbs. Often, there is coldness in the limbs, and abdominal examination reveals epigastric stuffiness and resistance.

Heartburn

- **Rikkunshito:** See Sect. 3.1.3 Anorexia and Nausea & Vomiting.
- **Hangekobokuto**: See Sect. 3.1.3 Nausea & Vomiting.
- **Hangeshashinto**: See Sect. 3.1.3 Anorexia and Nausea &Vomiting.
- **Orengedokuto**: See Sect. 3.1.3 Anorexia.
- **Orento**: Good for medium pattern. Berberine contained in *oren* possesses antiulcer, anti-inflammatory, and antibacterial effects. Effective for heartburn; sometimes associated with headache or stomach pain. Patients frequently have the thick white tongue coating as well as epigastric stuffiness and resistance or tenderness in abdominal examination.
- **Anchusan**: A combination of herbs including *keihi* with body-warming effect, *borei* with acid-suppressing effect, and *engosaku* with excellent analgesic effect. Appropriate for deficiency to slight deficiency pattern patients who have coldness and complain of abdominal pain and heartburn.
- **Shishishito**:[14] This formula, containing *sanshishi*, is mainly used for heartburn associated with indescribable pain and agony around the chest.

3.2 Constipation, Diarrhea, Abdominal Pain, and Abdominal Distention [26, 27]

Hirokuni Okumi

3.2.1 Outline of the Disease and Indications of Kampo Treatments

In the treatment of constipation, diarrhea, abdominal pain, and abdominal distention, basically the first step is to identify organic pathology, and Western medical treatment takes precedence in Japan. Kampo treatments, however, are indicated in some cases of infectious gastroenteritis, postoperative intestinal adhesion, and functional gastrointestinal disorders (FGIDs), which often involve psychosomatic issues. Kampo prescriptions are thought to ameliorate not only the primary complaints but also benefit the foregoing or accompanying mental symptoms as well as decreased energy and malaise.

3.2.2 Frequently Used Formulas

Constipation (Fig. 5.15)

The aim in treating excess pattern constipation is to obtain regular bowel movements using formulas containing rhubarb (*daio*), immature orange (*kijitsu*), and mirabilite (*bosho*), which have strong qi-regulating effects. When abdominal distention and pain are present, formulas other than the above, containing peach seed (*tonin*) and safflower (*koka*) (resolving blood[TM1] stasis), and angelica root (*toki*) and peony root (*shakuyaku*) (tonifying blood), are considered. To treat deficiency pattern constipation, formulas containing herbs that balance gastrointestinal function and soften feces, such as ginseng (*ninjin*) and hemp fruit (*mashinin*), are used. The use of strong purgatives, such as rhubarb, can aggravate abdominal pain and cause severe diarrhea. In cases of constipation accompanied by abdominal distention, abdominal pain, and cold, in addition to qi-regulating formulas, those that promote both fluid[TM1] and qi-regulation with phlegm-dispelling herbs like pinellia tuber (*hange*), citrus unshiu peel (*chimpi*), and poria sclerotium (*bukuryo*) are considered.

[14]Not available as a medical Kampo extract formulation.

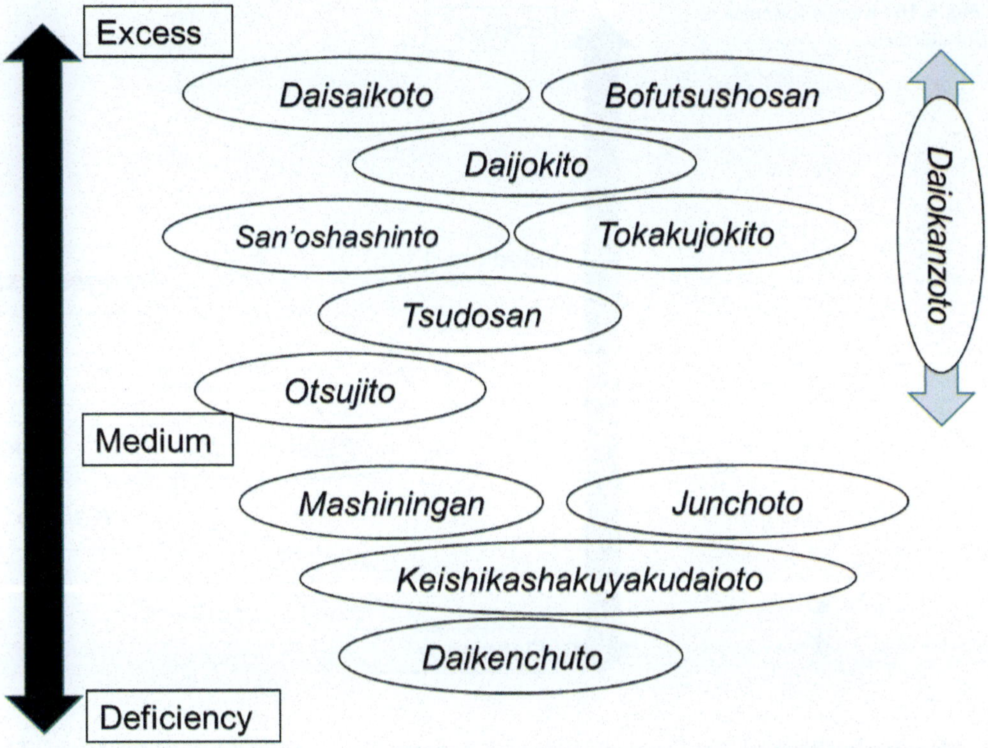

Fig. 5.15 Kampo formulas for constipation

- **Daiokanzoto:** Used generally for constipation in medium to excess pattern.
- **Daisaikoto:** For excess pattern with severe fullness and discomfort in chest and hypochondrium, epigastric distress, and complaints of stiff shoulders and depressed mood.
- **Daijokito:** For slight excess to excess pattern with distension and elasticity in the abdomen and tendency of gas retention.
- **•San'oshashinto:** For slight excess to excess pattern with epigastric stuffiness and resistance, hot flash, irritation, insomnia, and head heaviness.
- **Tokakujokito:** For slight excess to excess pattern patients with strong physiques and signs of blood[TM1] stasis. Before menstruation, patients complain of mental symptoms such as irritation, hot flashes, and insomnia. Lower abdominal cramp.
- **Tsudosan:** For patients inclined toward slight excess to excess pattern with a tendency of blood[TM1] stasis, such as dysmenorrhea and constipation accompanied by lower abdomen tenderness.
- **Bofutsushosan:** Used for excess pattern patients who are solid but overweight with a firm abdomen around the umbilicus, so-called potbelly.
- **Otsujito:** For medium to slight excess pattern with hemorrhoids.
- **Mashiningan:** Used for elderly patients and those with weak constitutions with slight deficiency to medium pattern who pass hard, round scybala.
- **Junchoto:** Used for slight deficiency to medium pattern patients with dry skin. The dry skin is more severe than in those for which *mashiningan* is indicated.
- **Keishikashakuyakudaioto:** Used for slight deficiency to medium pattern patients who complain of abdominal distention and pain and tenesmus.
- **Daikenchuto:** Used for slight deficiency to deficiency pattern patients with constipation and gas retention or unstable peristalsis in the abdomen.

Diarrhea (Fig. 5.16)

Cases of diarrhea with tenesmus accompanied by abdominal pain, hematochezia, and mucous and bloody stool are caused by intestinal mucosal inflammatory conditions such as infections, inflammatory bowel disease, and dietary intemperance. The main formulas used contain scutellaria root (*ogon*), Coptis rhizome (*oren*), and rhubarb (*daio*), which have heat-clearing effects, or Angelica root (*toki*), peony root (*shakuyaku*), and moutan bark (*botampi*), which have blood[TM1] regulating effects. In cases of frequent soft to watery feces without tenesmus caused by external pathogens, dietary intemperance, chronic disease, or aging, the main formulas used contain Atractylodes lancea rhizome (*sojutsu*) and poria sclerotium (*bukuryo*) (fluid[TM1] regulating effects), magnolia bark (*koboku*) and Citrus unshiu peel (*chimpi*) (qi-regulating effects), Atractylodis rhizome (*byakujutsu*), ginseng (*ninjin*), and processed ginger (*kankyo*) (qi-tonifying effects).

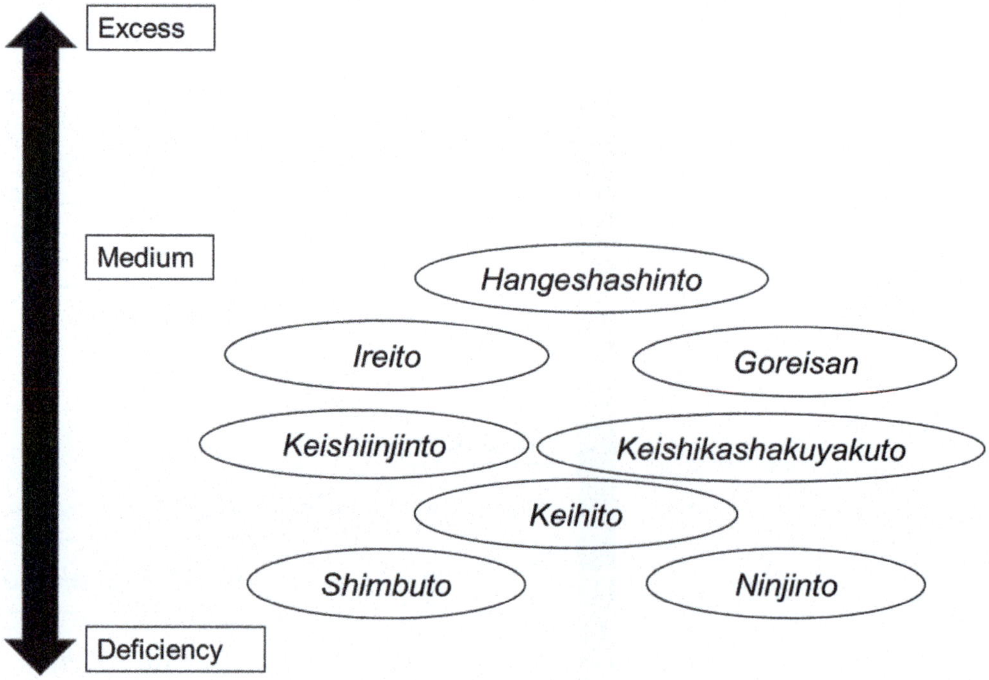

Fig. 5.16 Kampo formulas for diarrhea

- **Hangeshashinto:** Used for medium pattern patients with epigastric stuffiness and resistance and borborygmus.
- **Ireito:** Used for medium pattern with acute gastroenteritis, etc., which manifest as abdominal pain and diarrhea.
- **Keishikashakuyakuto:** Used for functional diarrhea in slight deficiency pattern patients with abdominal pain and tenesmus.
- **Goreisan:** Used for medium pattern with fluid[TM1] retention symptoms such as thirst, lightheadedness, and edema.
- **Shimbuto:** Used for deficiency pattern with a weak, soft abdomen and weak pulse, without cold or tenesmus, and with only mild gastric symptoms and abdominal pain.
- **Ninjinto:** Used for deficiency pattern similar to the *shimbuto* pattern, except there are many additional gastric symptoms such as decreased appetite and stomach distension.
- **Keishininjinto:** Used for slight deficiency pattern with signs resembling *ninjinto* pattern, accompanied by hot flash, headache, and chilling.
- **Keihito:** Can be tried for slight deficiency pattern patients with frequent watery feces for whom *shimbuto* and *ninjinto* are ineffective.

Abdominal Pain (Fig. 5.17)

For upper abdominal pain, primarily in the epigastric region, so-called formulas of involving Bupleurum radix with a qi-regulating effect are frequently used. For upper abdominal pain accompanied by anorexia and epigastric distension, formulas are selected that contain qi-regulating herbs including bupleurum root and immature orange (*kijitsu*); fluid-regulating herbs with phlegm-dispelling effects such as pinellia tuber (*hange*) and poria sclerotium (*bukuryo*); qi-tonifying herbs such as rhizomes of Atractylodes spp. (*jutsu*), ginseng (*ninjin*), and processed ginger (kankyo); as well as blood[TM1] tonifying herbs such as angelica root (*toki*) and peony root (*shakuyaku*). For swelling in the epigastric region accompanied by pain, formulas are selected that contain herbs with qi-regulating effects, such as Crataegus fruit (*sanzashi*), malted rice (*shingiku*), immature orange (*kijitsu*), and pinellia tuber (*hange*); herbs with pain, relieving effect, such as Corydalis tuber (*engosaku*) and fennel fruit (*uikyo*); and herbs with qi-tonifying effects.

For lower abdominal and umbilical pain, on the other hand, formulas in the keishito group containing peony root (*shakuyaku*) alone or in combination with cinnamon twig (*keishi*) are mainly used. In cases tending toward deficiency with abdominal distention and fatigability, formulas in the kenchuto group, such as *shokenchuto* (prepared by adding malt sugar (*koi*), which has a nutritive effect), as well as *keishikashakuyakuto* and *daikenchuto*, with a slightly different intent, are used. In cases of chronic lower abdominal pain induced or worsened by cold stress, formulas containing herbs with strong warming and tonifying effects, such as evodia fruit (*goshuyu*) and ginger, are chosen. If the condition involves dysmenorrhea, a blood[TM1] regulating formula such as *tokishakuyakusan* or *keishibukuryogan* is prescribed.

- **Anchusan:** Used for deficiency to slight deficiency pattern with chronic dull epigastric pain; effect for heartburn symptoms and menstrual pain can be expected.

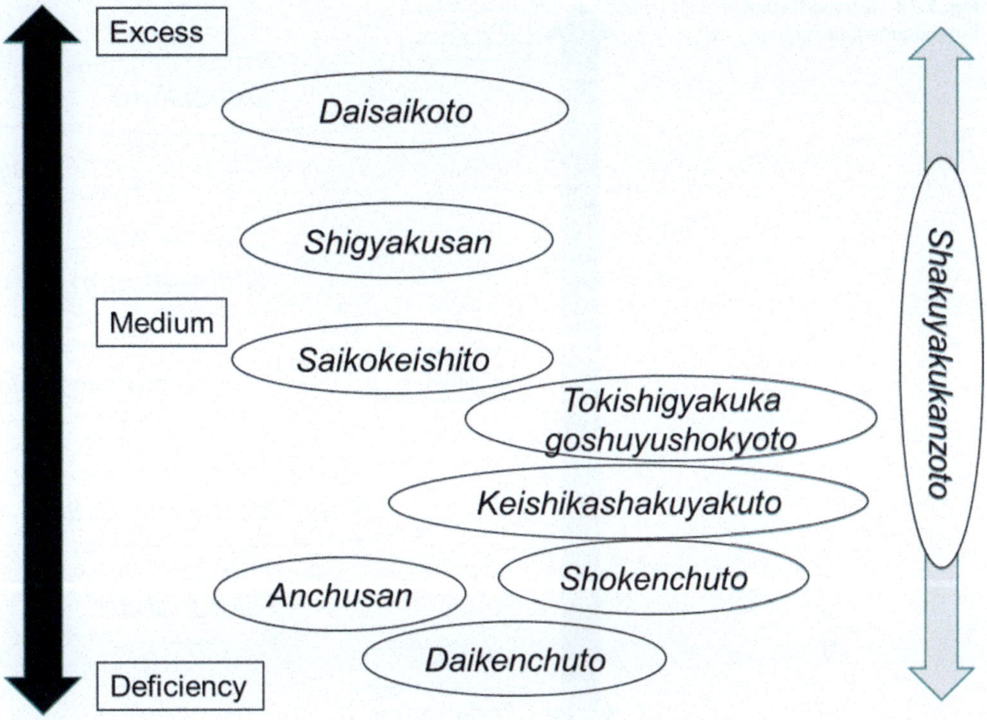

Fig. 5.17 Kampo formulas for abdominal pain

- **Daisaikoto:** Used for upper abdominal pain in excess pattern patients with high abdominal elasticity and marked fullness and discomfort in the chest and hypochondrium.
- **Saikokeishito:** Used for slight deficiency to medium pattern patients with fullness and discomfort in the chest and hypochondrium and upper abdominal muscle tension. Also commonly used for upper abdominal pain.
- **Shigyakusan:** Used for medium to slight excess pattern patients with signs similar to those for *daisaikoto* patterns, but with mild constipation and rectus abdominis tension.
- **Keishikashakuyakuto:** Used for slight deficiency pattern patients with colic pain around the umbilicus to the lower abdomen due to gastrointestinal distress.
- **Shokenchuto:** Used for slight deficiency patterns with more weakness than *keishikashakuyakuto* patterns.
- **Daikenchuto:** For deficiency to slight deficiency pattern patients with a thin abdominal wall through which increased peristalsis is visible, along with abdominal distention due to gas retention.
- **Shakuyakukanzoto:** Effective in pain relief for abdominal pain attacks when used on demand, alone or in combination with *anchusan,* etc. Widely used for deficiency pattern to excess pattern.
- **Tokishigyakukagoshuyushokyoto:** A representative formula used for cold abdominal colic in slight deficiency pattern.

Abdominal Distention (Fig. 5.18)

In Kampo medicine, upper abdominal to epigastric distention reported as stomach distension is called epigastric stuffiness and resistance. When epigastric stuffiness is accompanied by anorexia and is caused by environmental factors (high humidity or coldness) and dietary intemperance, etc., the following formulas are indicated: for excess pattern formulas in shashinto group such as *hangeshashinto*; for deficiency pattern formulas in ninjinto group such as *ninjinto* and *shikunshito*, and also *rikkunshito*, which contains qi-tonifying herbs such as pinellia tuber (*hange*) and Citrus unshiu peel (*chimpi*).

For the treatment of lower abdominal distention, the abdomen is warmed and tonified mainly with formulas in jokito group such as *daijokito* for excess patterns (elasticity and swelling in the entire abdomen), or with formulas in kenchuto group such as *daikenchuto* and *shokenchuto* for the weak constitution, postoperative ileus, etc., in which there is abdominal pain and fatigability. These formulas are prescribed in combination with qi-regulating formulas like magnolia bark (*koboku*), immature orange (*kijitsu*), and small amounts of rhubarb (*daio*).

- **Rikkunshito:** First choice formula for deficiency to slight deficiency pattern patients with stomach stuffiness and upper abdominal distention.

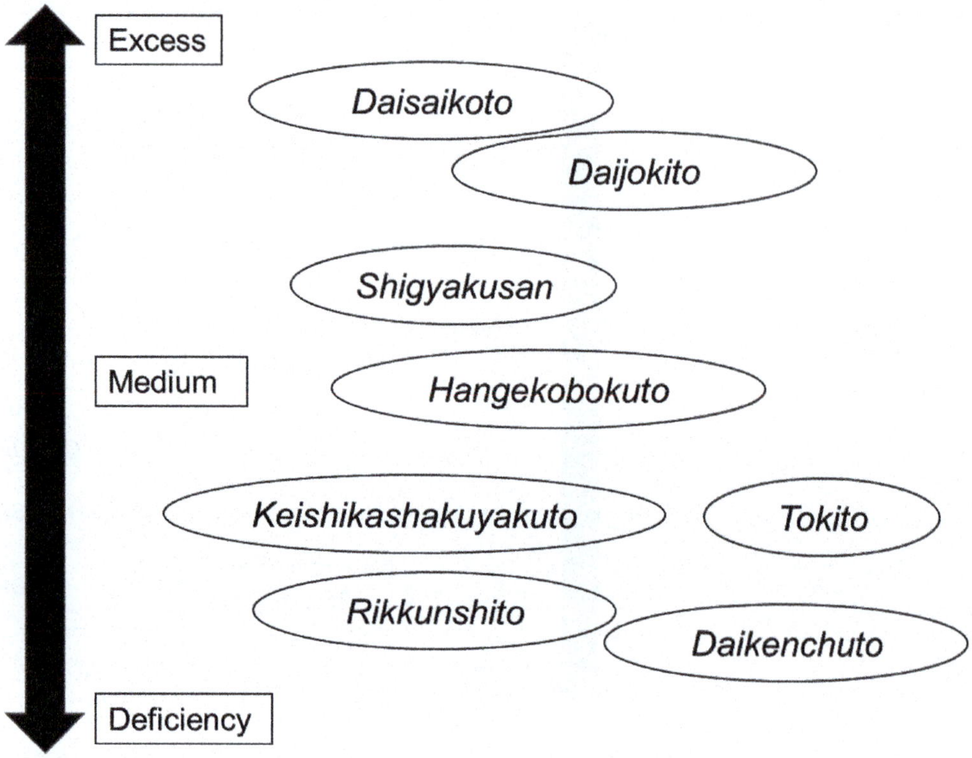

Fig. 5.18 Kampo formulas for abdominal distention

- **Hangekobokuto:** Effective for medium pattern not only for obstructive discomfort in the throat to chest, but also for stomach stuffiness.
- **Daisaikoto:** Used for abdominal pain in excess to slight excess pattern patients with constipation tendency and severe fullness and discomfort in chest and hypochondrium.
- **Shigyakusan:** Used for medium to slight excess pattern patients with signs similar to those of *daisaikoto* patterns, but with mild constipation and rectus abdominis tension.
- **Keishikashakuyakuto:** Used for abnormal bowel movement in slight deficiency pattern patients with abdominal pain.
- **Daikenchuto:** Used for deficiency to slight deficiency pattern patients with abdominal distention with unstable peristalsis. Also used frequently for abdominal distention due to postoperative intestinal adhesion. If it is not sufficiently effective, *daikenchuto* may be used in combination with *keishikashakuyakuto* (*chukenchuto*).
- **Tokito:** Containing both ginseng (*ninjin*) and astragalus root (*ogi*), this formula is used for slight deficiency pattern, with the aims of *daikenchuto*, *keishikashakuyakuto*, and *hangekobokuto*.
- **Daijokito:** Used for slight excess to excess pattern patients with constipation and a generally distended elastic abdomen.

3.2.3 Kampo Treatments for Functional Gastrointestinal Disorders (FGIDs) as Defined by Rome Classification IV (Table 5.4)

FGIDs are attracting attention in terms of psychosomatic associations, of which the best-known conditions are functional dyspepsia (FD) and irritable bowel syndrome (IBS). In Rome IV as revised in 2016, FD is divided into two forms: postprandial distress syndrome (PDS) with postprandial gastric distention and early satiation as chief complaints, and epigastric pain syndrome (EPS) with complaints of epigastric pain and epigastric heat sensation not related to meals. Appropriate formulas are determined based on these differences.

IBS, on the other hand, was previously defined with abdominal pain or abdominal discomfort as the chief complaint. At present, however, lower abdominal pain alone is included in the definition; therefore, a formula for lower abdominal pain and a formula for diarrhea or constipation are combined according to the classification.

Table 5.4 Kampo treatments for FGIDs as defined by Rome IV

Postprandial dyspepsia syndrome (PDS): Postprandial stomach distension, early satiation
Excess pattern: *Daisaikoto, saikokaryukotsuboreito, shigyakusan* Medium pattern: *Hangekobokuto, heiisan, nichinto, orento, bukuryoin, goreisan* Deficiency pattern: *Rikkunshito*
Epigastric pain syndrome (EPS): Pain and heat sensation in the epigastric region
Excess pattern: *Shigyakusan* Medium pattern: *Saikokeishito* Deficiency pattern: *Anchusan, rikkunshito, saikokeishikankyoto*
Diarrhea-type irritable bowel syndrome (IBS-D): Abdominal pain, diarrhea, soft feces
Medium pattern: *Hangeshashinto* Deficiency pattern: *Keishikashakuyakuto, tokishigyakukagoshuyushokyoto, ogikenchuto, shimbuto*
Constipation-type irritable bowel syndrome (IBS-C): Abdominal pain, constipation, hard feces
Excess pattern: *Tokakujokito, tsudosan* Deficiency pattern: *Daikenchuto, keishikashakuyakuto, keishikashakuyakudaioto, shokenchuto, mashiningan*
Mixed irritable bowel syndrome (IBS-M): Abdominal pain, diarrhea, constipation
Deficiency pattern: *Keishikashakuyakuto, shokenchuto, ogikenchuto, tokikenchuto*

3.3 Hepatic Dysfunction

Makoto Fujimoto

3.3.1 Outline of the Disease

The diseases that cause hepatic dysfunction include some types of viral hepatitis, such as chronic hepatitis B and chronic hepatitis C, alcoholic liver disorders, autoimmune hepatitis, primary biliary cholangitis, nonalcoholic fatty liver disease (NAFLD), and associated conditions such as liver cirrhosis and drug-induced liver disorders. Diseases involving hepatic dysfunction in blood biochemistry also include cholecystitis and cholangitis. In chronic hepatitis C, treatments with direct antiviral drugs enable viral elimination (markedly effective) in almost all cases. In chronic hepatitis B, nucleic acid analogue preparations and pegylated interferon (PEG-IFN) α-2a preparations are used as standard treatments to increase the negative conversion rate for HBs antigen. NAFLD is a hepatic phenotype of metabolic syndrome, in which the first priority should be given to lifestyle improvements, such as dietary therapy and exercise therapy.

3.3.2 Indications of Kampo Treatments

Acute Hepatitis and Active Stages of Chronic Hepatitis

Inchinkoto is used for moderate or severe jaundice with thirst, oliguria, constipation, and chest discomfort. *Inchingoreisan* is used for mild jaundice with thirst and oliguria. In cases where fullness and discomfort in the chest and hypochondrium are evident and accompanied by epigastric stuffiness and nausea, formulas containing Bupleurum root (*saiko*) as a constituent crude drug, such as *daisaikoto* and *shosaikoto*, are chosen based on the pattern.

Chronic Hepatitis B and C

No hepatitis virus of any type can be eliminated by Kampo treatment. Kampo formulas are rarely used alone for treatment. The common approach is to use Kampo treatment to assist in standard treatment. A study reported that *maoto* ameliorated general malaise and joint pain when prescribed for influenza-like symptoms resulting from interferon (IFN) treatment [28]. During the course of IFN treatment or combination therapy with IFN and ribavirin, symptoms indicative of qi deficiency pattern or blood[TM1] deficiency pattern (such as decreased appetite, susceptibility to infections, and anemia) can develop. This can make continued treatment difficult. In such cases, treatment can be continued with a combination of tonic formulas such as *rikkunshito*, *hochuekkito*, *ninjin'yoeito*, and *juzentaihoto*. As liver fibrosis progresses in the course of hepatitis, static blood[TM1] findings such as the development of small collateral vessels/thread-like collateral vessels on the skin, sublingual vein distention, and palmar erythema are manifested. For this, blood[TM1] stasis resolving formulas such as *keishibukuryogan* and *tokishakuyakusan* are used.

Alcoholic Liver Disorders

The basic approach to the treatment is drinking abstinence/reduction. In Kampo medicine, qi abnormalities like qi deficiency and also blood[TM1] abnormalities are suspected as an outcome of fluid[TM1] retention from drinking and poor nutrition due to an unbalanced diet. In addition to *goreisan*, *inchingoreisan*, *orengedokuto*, and *rikkunshito*, formulas of involving Bupleurum radix may be used alone or in combination with blood[TM1] stasis resolving formulas.

Autoimmune Hepatitis

Generally, prednisolone (PSL) is the first choice drug; however, its prolonged administration can cause problematic side effects because this disease often follows a chronic course. Azathioprine is used in patients who experience repeated relapses or who are unable to use PSL due to side effects. Among Kampo formulas, *saireito* was reported to be effective in reducing or discontinuing commonly used oral steroids, so it may be useful in long-term maintenance therapy with PSL.

Primary Biliary Cholangitis

Generally, ursodeoxycholic acid (UDCA) is the first choice drug and, as a rule, is used in all patients diagnosed with this disease. In Kampo medicine, *inchinkoto* is used concomitantly with UDCA with anticipation of a choleretic effect.

Nonalcoholic Fatty Liver Disease (NAFLD, NASH)

The basic approach to the treatment is body weight reduction by dietary therapy and exercise therapy. Although fatty liver can be ameliorated only by a body weight loss of about 3% to 5%, liver fibrosis cannot be ameliorated without a body weight reduction of 10% or more. In fact, some patients have difficulty losing weight. Weight reduction surgery may be indicated in cases of severe obesity. Any comorbid lifestyle-related disease (dyslipidemia, diabetes, hypertension) should be treated if requiring drug therapy. Although the mechanism of progression to nonalcoholic steatohepatitis (NASH), the severe form of NAFLD, remains unclear, suggested factors include oxidative stress, endoplasmic reticulum stress, mitochondrial functional abnormalities, autophagy, and activated spontaneous immunity due to changes in intestinal bacterial flora. At present, no drugs are available to specifically treat NAFLD and NASH. Kampo formulas used for NAFLD and NASH with obesity and a constipation tendency include *bofutsushosan*, *daisaikoto*, and *tsudosan*. Another study reported that *keishibukuryogan* improved serum ALT levels [29].

Liver Cirrhosis

This is the terminal stage of chronic liver disease. Liver cell functional impairment and portal hypertension produce jaundice, ascites, edema, hepatic encephalopathy, esophageal and gastric varix hemorrhage, and idiopathic bacterial peritonitis. In Kampo medicine, liver cirrhosis is often diagnosed with patterns including both qi and blood[TM1] deficiency, fluid[TM1] retention, and blood[TM1] stasis. Formulas used include *Hochuekkito*, *juzentaihoto*, *goreisan*, *inchingoreisan*, *keishibukuryogan*, *kamishoyosan*, and *tokishakuyakusan*.

Cholecystitis and Cholelithiasis

The basic treatment for the early stage of acute cholecystitis comprises infusions, antibacterial medications, and analgesic administration. In Kampo medicine, hypochondrial fullness and resistance/tenderness due to cholecystitis are classified as "fullness and discomfort in chest and hypochondrium." Formulas of involving Bupleurum radix are often used, including *daisaikoto*, *saikokeishito*, and *shigyakusan*, with *inchinkoto* and *inchingoreisan* also used for accompanying jaundice. *Shakuyakukanzoto* is sometimes used concomitantly for colic attacks. *Daisaikoto* was reported to be possibly useful for the treatment of cholelithiasis with hypertriglyceridemia by ameliorating abnormalities in hepatic lipid metabolism and biliary lipid hydrophobicity [30].

3.3.3 Frequently Used Formulas (Fig. 5.19)

Attention should always be paid to the possible onset of drug-induced liver disorders with the use of Kampo formulas.

- **Daisaikoto:** Used for patients with an excess pattern with strong abdominal strength, constipation, and marked fullness and discomfort in chest and hypochondrium and epigastric stuffiness and resistance. Pulses tend to be deep and excess, and the tongue often has a somewhat dry yellow coating to white-yellow coating. Used for various hepatic dysfunctions, including NAFLD, as well as acute cholecystitis.
- **Shosaikoto:** Used for patients with medium pattern, moderate abdominal strength, fullness and discomfort in chest and hypochondrium, and epigastric stuffiness and resistance. Pulses are wiry, and the tongue often has a white coating which is dry but sometimes slightly wet. Heat in hands and feet with agitation can occur as a symptom. Used for various chronic hepatic dysfunctions but contraindicated for liver cirrhosis and hepatic dysfunction with a platelet count of ≤100,000/mm [3]. Also contraindicated for concomitant use with IFN.
- **Shigyakusan:** Used for patients with medium pattern to slight excess pattern, fullness and discomfort in chest and hypochondrium, and severe abdominal muscle tension. Pulses are wiry, and a white coating is often found on the tongue. Palm sweating is another indication for use. Used for gallstone attacks and cholecystitis.
- **Hochuekkito:** A representative formula for qi deficiency, used to treat general malaise, anorexia, and night sweating in the course of liver disease. Patients have a slight deficiency pattern and slightly weak abdominal strength, and they often experience mild fullness and discomfort in the chest and hypochondrium along with epigastric stuffiness.
- **Juzentaihoto:** Used for patients with deficiency pattern: qi deficiency symptoms such as general malaise and night sweating; blood[TM1] deficiency symptoms such as bad complexion, anemic tendency, skin dryness, and limb coldness. Abdominal strength is weak, with pulses often deep and weak. These symptoms often manifest in compensated cirrhosis.
- **Keishibukuryogan:** This is a representative formula used for blood[TM1] stasis in medium to slight excess pattern patients. In the course of chronic liver disease, blood[TM1] stasis symptoms such as skin capillary dilation, lip and gum dark-reddening, and palm erythema are often observed. Blood[TM1] stasis resolving formulas are commonly used. Rather than being used alone, it's more often used in combination with formulas of involving Bupleurum radix, targeting fullness and discomfort in chest and hypochondrium.
- **Kamishoyosan:** Having a nuance of formulas of involving Bupleurum radix and blood[TM1] stasis resolving formulas, it is used in cases with heat rather than cold. Effective in middle-aged and older patients with slight deficiency pattern and relatively many complaints.

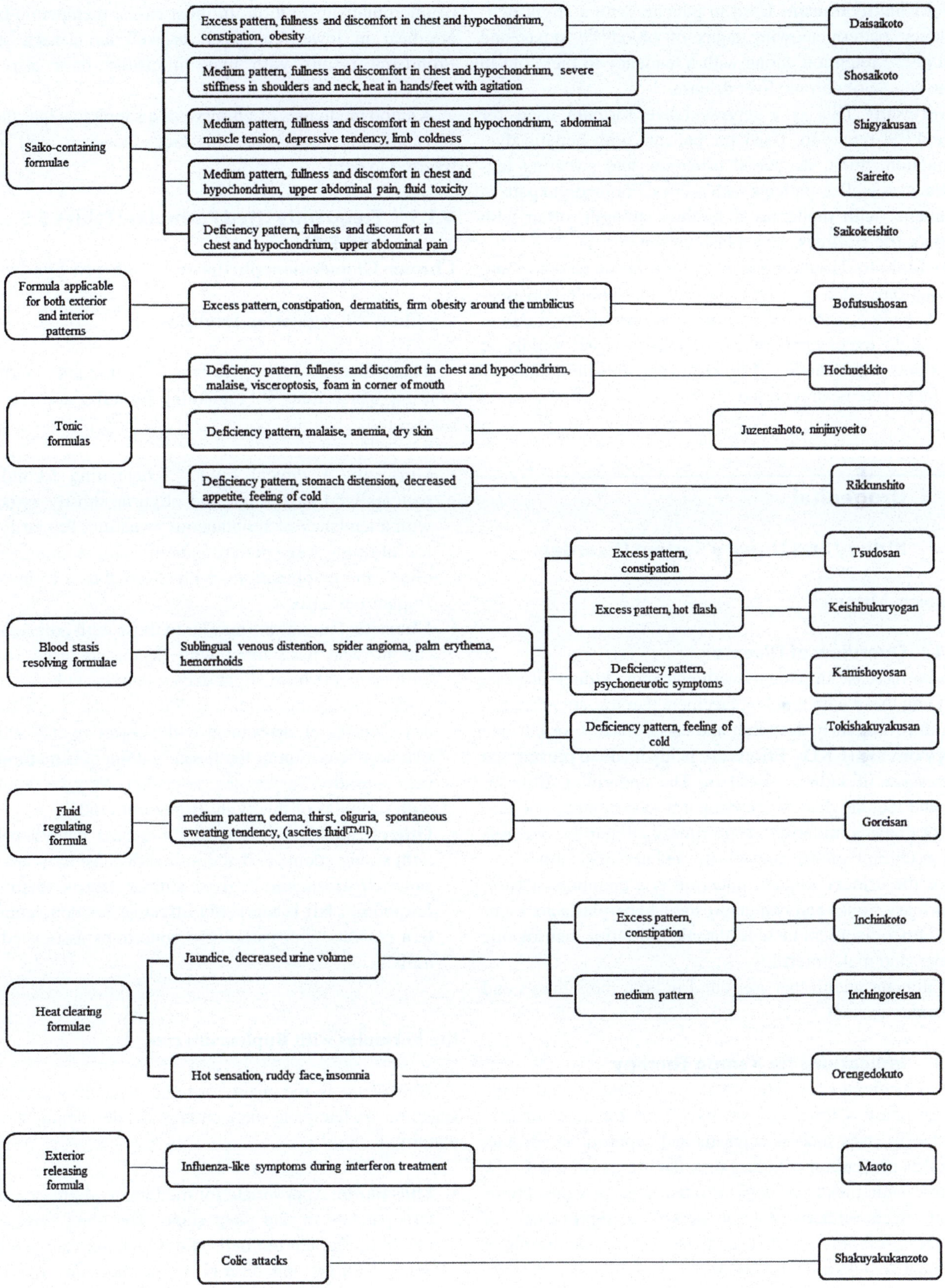

Fig. 5.19 Frequent formulas for liver dysfunction

- **Tokishakuyakusan:** Used in patients with a slight deficiency pattern showing signs of blood[TM1] stasis and fluid[TM1] retention, along with a tendency to feel cold in the course of chronic liver disease.
- **Goreisan:** This is a representative formula used for fluid[TM1] retention. Used for patients with hepatic dysfunction, thirst, decreased urination, and sweating tendency, as well as patients with ascites. For medium pattern patients with moderate abdominal strength, often with epigastric stuffiness and splashing sound.
- **Inchinkoto:** Used for patients with a febrile tendency and symptoms such as a bitter taste in the mouth, constipation, nausea, and chest discomfort. A formula for medium to slight excess pattern, but it may be used widely in patients with jaundice. Choleretic and anti-inflammatory effects have been reported.

4 Urogenital

4.1 Kidney and Urinary System Disorders

Tadamichi Mitsuma

4.1.1 Overview of Disease

With an increase in patients with end-stage kidney disease, including those with renal replacement therapy, attention has been drawn to early detection and early therapy for chronic kidney disease (CKD). Efforts are being made to prevent the progression of kidney disorders. The underlying diseases vary and include diabetic nephropathy (the number one reason for dialysis initiation), and primary glomerular diseases such as chronic glomerulonephritis and nephrosclerosis.

For the urinary system, infection is a common disease, and urinary stones and benign prostatic hyperplasia are common. Other disorders include chronic prostatitis, neurogenic bladder, and male infertility.

Malignant neoplasms are found in both the kidneys and the urinary system.

4.1.2 Indications for Kampo Therapy

Kampo medicines for kidney disease are chiefly used in the chronic phase. Clinical effects have been reported for glomerular diseases such as nephritis and nephrotic syndrome, as well as prevention of kidney disorder progression in CKD. Kampo medicines have demonstrated inhibition and elimination effects on active oxygen as well as improvement of various symptoms in advanced-stage CKD. Acute-phase treatment centers around Western medical therapies.

Kampo medicines exert an immediate effect on urinary infections, even in the acute phase. They are effective for prevention in chronic and recurrent infection, posing no risk of microbial substitution. In most cases, therapeutic targets are heat in lower energizer as well as urinary stones. Promising results with male infertility have also been reported.

Kampo medicines often serve as a supplementary therapy for malignant neoplasms; this facet, however, will not be referred to here.

4.1.3 Frequently Used Formulas (Tables 5.5 and 5.6)

Chronic Glomerulonephritis and Nephrotic Syndrome

(a) **Fluid[TM1] regulating formulas**

These diseases often give rise to edema and overhydration, for which fluid[TM1] regulating formulas are frequently used.

- **Goreisan**: A typical fluid[TM1] regulating formula for patients who have thirst and oliguria, mostly associated with a tendency of spontaneous sweating. Primarily used for late yang stage pattern patients with medium pattern, often in combination with formulas of involving Bupleurum radix.
- **Choreito**: Patients are similar to those with *goreisan* indications who have thirst with decreased urine volume. Often patients have slight excess pattern with mild spontaneous sweating tendency. Patients also have heat in lower energizer, associated with subjective and/or objective heat sensation in the lower abdomen, hematuria, and heat sensation in the genital region. May be combined with formulas of involving Bupleurum radix.
- **Others**: *Bunshoto*[15] is used for excess pattern patients with severe edema and abdominal distension in late yang stage. *Hokikenchuto*[12] gives similar effects to those of *bunshoto*[12], but is markedly effective for deficiency pattern patients with pathologic conditions associated with ascites.

(b) **Formulas with Bupleurum root**

Shosaikoto is the main formula. The chief criteria for selection are late yang stage pattern and deficiency or excess pattern.

- **Shosaikoto**: Appropriate for medium to slight excess pattern patients in late yang stage. The chief formulas of involving Bupleurum radix, for which the therapeutic target is fullness and discomfort in chest and hypochondrium. Often used in combination with other prescriptions

[15] Not available as a medical Kampo extract formulation

Table 5.5 Main formulas for kidney and urinary system disorders

		Main disease			
Formulas group	Formula	CGN/NS	CKD	Urinary tract disorders	Comments
Fluid[TM1]-regulating	Goreisan	○	SCr<4.0		Thirst, oliguria
	Choreito	○		○	Heat sensation in the lower abdomen
Blood[TM1] stasis resolving	Keishibukuryogan	○	○		For typical blood stasis
	Tokishakuyakusan	○	○		Blood stasis+fluid retention
Saiko-containing	Shosaikoto	○			Often combined with other formulas
	Other saiko formulas	○			
Ogi-containig	Hochuekkito	○	○		Saiko and ogi containing
	Juzentaihoto		○		
	Astragalus root		○		
Kidney[TM1]-tonifying	Hachimi(jio)gan	○	SCr<4.0	○	Coldness especially legs
	Goshajinkigan	○		○	Prominent edema in the lower limbs
Daio-containing	Bushirichuto added daio		○		Use for unpito
	Daiokanzoto		○		
	Rhubarb(poeder, cut)		○		
Others	Seishinrenshiin			○	Nervous pollakiuria
	Ryutanshakanto			○	Strong lower-region heat

CGN/NS chronic glomerulonephritis/nephrotic syndrome
SCr serum creatinine level, g/dL

Table 5.6 Main formulas for dialysis complaints

	Main complaint				Comments
Formula	Muscle cramp	Pruritus	Shunt trouble	Restless leg synd.	
Shakuyakukanzoto	○				
Shakuyakukanzobushito	○				For cold if any
Tokiinshi		○			With dryness
Orengedokuto		○			With heat symptoms
Unseiin		○			With both heat & dryness
Keisibukuryogan			○		
Hachimi(jio)gan				○	Coldness especially legs

for late yang stage pattern. There are many reports of multi-center trials using *saireito*, combined with *goreisan*, mainly for nephrotic syndrome. In addition, clinical results for recurrent upper respiratory infection, using *saibokuto* combined with *hangekobokuto*, have been reported. This formula is often combined with blood[TM1] stasis resolving formulas.

- **Other formulas of involving Bupleurum radix**: Used according to pattern. *Daisaikoto* and *saikokaryukotsuboreito* are used for excess pattern patients, and *saikokeishito* and *saikokeishikankyoto* for deficiency pattern patients. Also combined with other formulations.

(c) **Blood[TM1] stasis resolving formulas**

Used for patients with blood[TM1] stasis findings, including dark red tongue and lips, swelling of sublingual vein, small collateral vessels/thread-like collateral vessels, and resistance and tenderness in the lower abdomen. Blood[TM1] stasis rapidly gets worse with steroid use. This formula can improve peripheral blood flow and may be used concurrently with antiplatelet agents or anticoagulation therapy. Often used in combination or concomitantly with formulas of involving Bupleurum radix or other formulations.

- **Keishibukuryogan**: A typical blood[TM1] stasis resolving formula widely used mainly for excess pattern patients in late yang stage. Primary abdominal sign is tenderness along with induration two finger-widths diagonally below the umbilicus (mostly on the left side).
- **Tokishakuyakusan**: Appropriate for pathologic conditions associated with fluid retention in deficiency pattern patients in late yang stage or early yin stage. Patients have chief symptoms of coldness in the limbs and edema, while abdominal signs include poor abdominal strength, abdominal muscle tension, splashing sound in the epigastric region, and tenderness diagonally below the umbilicus

(mostly on left side). Often used together with other formulations; for example, in combination with formulas of involving Bupleurum radix for deficiency pattern.

(d) **Kidney[TM1] tonifying formulas**

- **Hachimijiogan** (Hachimigan): Used for Yin pattern patients. Not recommended for patients with gastrointestinal weakness. Appropriate for patients who have weakness of the lower abdominal region, coldness below the low back (especially below the knees), and lower limb edema. More frequently used in the elderly and often used together with formulas of involving Bupleurum radix or blood[TM1] stasis resolving formulas. *Hachimijiogan* contains *bushi*, which is a warming herb, and is therefore useful for pathologic conditions with cold.
- **Goshajinkigan**: Often effective for *hachimijiogan* pattern patients with pronounced edema in the lower limbs.

Chronic Kidney Disease (CKD)

There are numerous research papers, from basic to clinical, concerning the effect of Kampo medicines for chronic renal impairment. In patients with nondialysis-dependent chronic kidney disease (NDD-CKD) (serum creatinine level 4.0 mg/dL or more), caution is required because *hachimijiogan,* a fluid[TM1] regulating formula containing *bukuryo,* often accelerates renal impairment.

(a) **Daio containing formulas**

Daio containing formula has a laxative effect and, in Kampo medicine, is said to improve metabolism by eliminating toxins in the alimentary canal. In effective cases, a decrease in BUN is evident within 2 weeks of administration.

- **Unpito[16] (Shigyakukaninjinto with daio)**: Consisting of *shigyakuto*[12] (good for severe cold with deficiency pattern), *ninjin* (enhances vigor by enriching fluids[TM1] and activating stomach function), and *daio* (reported to have an anti-uremic effect). Appropriate for deficiency pattern patients. Found to improve the various symptoms of advanced-stage CKD and to effectively control the progression of renal dysfunction. When anorexia as well as epigastric stuffiness and resistance are severe, depending on the severity, *daio* can be added to *bushirichuto* which is *ninjinto* with *bushi*. Although no *unpito*[13] extract preparations are available, *bushirichuto* with *daio* can be prescribed as extract preparations of two kinds. The quantities of *bushi* and *daio* can be adjusted for coldness and bowel movement, respectively.
- **Daiokanzoto**: *Daio* is used for its effect on renal impairment, but the effect of this formula on cold and anorexia is often insufficient. Its inhibitory effect on the progression of kidney disorder is recognized.

(b) **Ogi containing formulas**

Ogi containing formulas have been reported to lower serum creatinine levels in patients with nondialysis-dependent chronic kidney disease (NDD-CKD) [31].

- **Hochuekkito**: This formula contains *saiko* and is appropriate for yang stage in deficiency pattern patients. The therapeutic target is qi deficiency. Patients also have swollen tongues with mottled white fur, a pulse that is dissipated and large (tendency to be floating, large, and weak), and fragile skin (an indication to use *ogi*). Even if other formulas of involving Bupleurum radix may be effective, *hochuekkito* is used in many cases of advanced-stage CKD, and its efficacy is further enhanced by increasing the quantity of *ogi*. In effective cases, the serum creatinine level tends to decrease after one or two weeks. If skin dryness is severe, the combined use with *shimotsuto* is favorable.
- **Other ogi containing formulas**: One prospective clinical study has reported the combination therapy with *shimbuto* and *boiogito* may improve the renal function in NDD-CKD patients with low proteinuria [32]. There are reported cases in which other *ogi* containing formulas—*juzentaihoto* and *ogikenchuto*—are effective for progressed CKD.

(c) **Others**

- **Hachimijiogan (Hachimigan)**: Effective for patients with NDD-CKD (serum creatinine level of 3.0 mg/dL or less) and for restless leg syndrome in patients with DD-CKD.
- **Blood[TM1] stasis resolving formulas**: Widely used to suppress renal impairment in patients with NDD-CKD and to reduce symptoms in patients with DD-CKD, inde-

[16]Not available as medical Kampo extract formulation nor OTC Kampo extract formulation.

Unpito: daio 0.5–required amount, kanzo 4.0, kankyo 3.0, ninjin 2.0, bushi required amount.

Source: Aizu Medical Center Kampo Medicine Prescription Collection.

pendent of renal function level. *Keishibukuryogan* is also effective in the prevention of shunt troubles. For severe cold, *bushi* is added to *tokishakuyakusan*.
- Dialysis complaints (Table 5.6): There are many reports on the rapid effectiveness of *shakuyakukanzoto* for muscle cramps (or *shakuyakukanzobushito* if there is a cold). For pruritus, *tokiinshi* is appropriate when there is dryness; *orengedokuto*, when heat symptoms are present; and *unseiin*, when both heat symptoms and dryness are present.

Urinary Tract Diseases

Among urinary tract diseases, pathologic conditions including infection, stones, and nervous pollakiuria often generate similar signs and symptoms. Appropriate Kampo prescriptions also overlap.

(a) **When "heat in lower energizer" symptoms are present**

Subjective and objective findings indicating heat in the lower energizer include heat sensation in the lower abdomen and genital region, hematuria, painful urination, burning sensation, and occasionally residual urine sensation as well as urination urgency.

- **Choreito**: Typical formula offered for medium pattern patients with heat in lower energizer. Frequently used for acute and chronic cystitis (including similar conditions) and urinary stones. Used for recurrent urinary tract infections in elderly patients, one or two preventative doses per day are often effective.
- **Ryutanshakanto**: Patients have a yang pattern and a slight excess pattern with more heat in the lower energizer compared to *choreito* pattern patients. Effective for pathologic conditions involving severe heat symptoms.

(b) **Pathologic conditions associated with urinary disorder**

Formulas used for heat in the lower energizer are also offered. Other prescriptions are as follows.

- **Hachimijiogan—Goshajinkigan**: Appropriate for slight deficiency pattern with pollakiuria, prolonged urination, and nocturnal urine. Also frequently used for prostatic hypertrophy.
- **Seishinrenshiin**: Used for urination urgency and nervous pollakiuria in slight deficiency pattern patients. This pattern is similar to the *hachimijiogan* pattern but is associated with gastrointestinal weakness, nervousness, or depression tendency.
- **Others**: *Shakuyakukanzoto* is used for colicky pain related to stones, but dosing is difficult for severe pain. Patients with intractable chronic prostatitis are likely to feel stress and are often neurotic. Treatment with formulas of involving Bupleurum radix or blood[TM1] stasis resolving formulas in accordance with the patterns is effective.

4.2 Urination Disorder

Takao Ikeuchi

4.2.1 Overview of Disease

The lower urinary tract is responsible for two conflicting functions: urine storage over a given period and periodic urination. The associated abnormal symptoms are termed lower urinary tract symptoms, regardless of cause. The symptoms are classified into three types: urine storage symptoms, such as pollakiuria (diurnal pollakiuria, when urinary frequency during waking hours is eight times or more, and nocturnal pollakiuria, when urinary frequency during sleeping hours is twice or more), urge to urinate, and incontinence; urination symptoms, such as dysuria; and post-voiding symptoms, such as residual urine sensation. Other less frequent symptoms include painful urination, bladder (lower abdominal) pain, and indefinite urinary tract complaints.

The diseases that give rise to urinary disorders include overactive bladder, stress urinary incontinence, benign prostatic hypertrophy (BPH), lower urinary tract infection (cystitis), prostatitis syndrome, bladder pain syndrome/interstitial cystitis, and unidentified clinical syndromes of the lower urinary tract such as psychogenic nervous pollakiuria. Furthermore, lower urinary tract symptoms may be associated with aging, sensitivity to coldness, menopausal syndrome, sleep disorder, habitual polydipsia, and adverse reactions to Western drugs. The causes are highly varied.

4.2.2 Indications for Kampo Therapy

Elderly people account for the overwhelming majority of patients with complaints of urinary disorders. Therefore, constitutional weakness, decreased anti-disease response, and impaired biological defense mechanisms are probable underlying factors. Most urinary diseases follow a chronic course, and symptoms tend to become prolonged. Pathological conditions like this (psychogenic symptoms and indefinite complaints that lack corresponding abnormal objective findings) are ideal targets for Kampo therapy, which may offer great benefits. In some cases of advanced disease, however, surgical procedures may be required, or Western drug therapy may be preferred. Physicians need to keep in mind the limitations of Kampo therapy and the fact that Kampo therapy cannot be used for some conditions.

In Kampo medicine, practitioners address each of the varied urinary disorder manifestations as part of a systemic problem, regardless of the disease names in Western medicine. It is essential in Kampo medical practice to ascertain the patient's pattern(s) and then select the Kampo prescriptions suitable to the individual patient's physical strength and constitution [1].

4.2.3 Pathological Conditions in Kampo Medicine

When considering urinary disorders from a Kampo medicine perspective, it is important to take into account innate life force, the cycle of predestined human life changes (growth, reproduction, and aging), and fluid[TM1] metabolism. Reductions in urinary functions occur with the physiological decrease in sex hormones with aging. Moreover, qi, the energy that governs life, may become disordered and may develop into qi deficiency or qi stagnation.

With diseases originating in the renal-urinary system organs, the core pathological condition is fluid[TM1] retention. Abnormal fluid[TM1] distribution underlying urinary disorders suggests fluid[TM1] retention. Since the bladder, the urethra, and the prostate gland (the prime organs that cause urinary disorder) are located within the pelvic cavity, blood[TM1] stasis pattern caused by anatomical changes may be an associated pathological condition. As life force decreases with aging, there is a decrease in physical strength, immunity, and mental activity. These decreases are accompanied by qi abnormalities, including qi deficiency, qi stagnation, and qi counter flow qi counter flow from kidney[TM1] deficiency, which come from aging. Therefore, in Kampo, the pathological condition of urinary disorder is presumed to be a pathological combination of kidney[TM1] deficiency, fluid[TM1] retention, blood[TM1] stasis, and qi abnormalities.

4.2.4 Frequent Formulas (Fig. 5.20)

Overactive Bladder

If urge to urinate and pollakiuria (diurnal and nocturnal) are present, the condition is termed overactive bladder, which is associated with urge incontinence in half of the cases. There are effective treatments in Western medicine. Kampo treatment is very useful, however, because it improves various concomitant symptoms.

- **Goshajinkigan, Seishinrenshiin:** Formulas of first choice [33, 34]
- **Junchoto, Keihito:** Formulas of second choice

In addition, blood[TM1] stasis resolving formulas are used together for interior cold aggravated by cold, and blood[TM1] tonifying formulas are used together when bladder ischemia is suspected.

Incontinence

The prescriptions indicated for urinary incontinence differ because the pathological conditions causing incontinence vary according to the underlying cause. Urge incontinence associated with the urge to urinate is dealt with in the above section on overactive bladder. Stress urinary incontinence, which occurs with sudden increases in abdominal pressure, is caused by muscle weakness and ligamentous laxity in the pelvic floor.

- **Hochuekkito:** Used for slight deficiency-pattern patients. Combined formulas with kakkonto containing mao may also be offered.
- **Maobushisaishin-to:** Formulas combining *mao* and *bushi* are used for yin pattern patients.
- **Goshajinkigan, Hachimijiogan, Rokumigan:** Used for slight deficiency pattern patients. Used when neurogenic overactive bladder is caused by spinal cord disease or nervous system disease sequelae or complications and female GSM (genitourinary syndrome of menopause), which is caused by sex hormone deficiency.

Since overflow incontinence is associated with urinary retention with large residual urine volume in end-stage BPH, it is dealt with in the next section.

Benign Prostatic Hypertrophy (BPH)

The presence of dysuria, nocturia, and residual urine sensation in men first indicates BPH. Kampo medicines are best used at an early stage, and the appropriate prescriptions should be selected with consideration of both constitution (presence or absence of cold sensation in hands and feet) and physical strength (excess pattern, medium pattern, and deficiency pattern).

- **Hachimijiogan, Rokumigan Goshajinkigan:** Kidney[TM1]tonifying formulas are the first choice.
- **Choreito, Ryutanshakanto, Gorinsan:** Heat-clearing and fluid[TM1] regulating formulas are the second choice.

When BPH progresses, it can cause blood[TM1] stasis in the pelvic cavity, so blood[TM1] stasis resolving formulas are jointly administered.

Lower Urinary Tract Infection

The presence of irritable bladder symptoms such as pollakiuria (diurnal and nocturnal) and painful urination indicates cystitis. The best indication for Kampo medicines is protracted chronic cystitis.

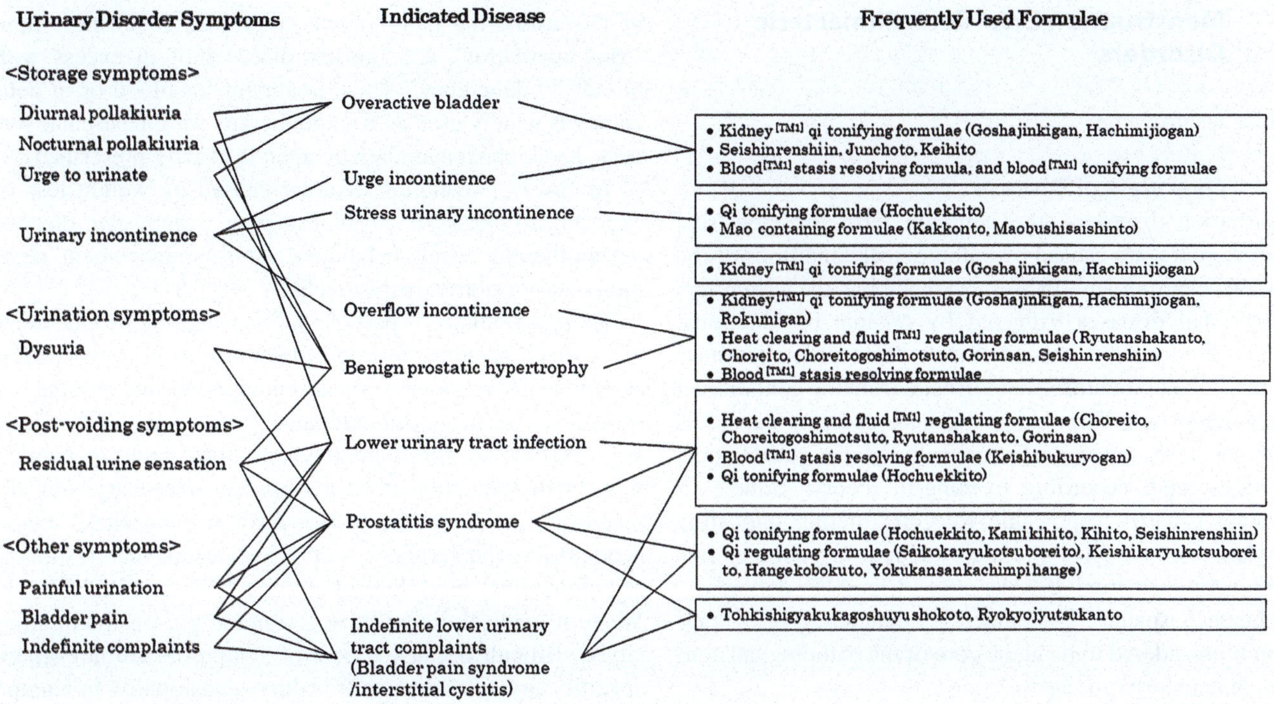

Fig. 5.20 Frequently Used Kampo Formulas for Urinary Disorder

- **Choreito, Choreitogoshimotsuto:** Heat-clearing and fluid[TM1] regulating formulas are the first choice.
- **Ryutanshakanto, Gorinsan:** Second choice.
- **Others:** If the above prescriptions are ineffective, blood[TM1] stasis resolving formulas may be effective for patients whose condition is aggravated by coldness, and qi-tonifying formulas such as *hochuekkito* may be helpful if an underlying factor such as qi deficiency associated with aging is suspected.

Prostatitis Syndrome

Prostatitis syndrome is a number of pathological conditions, including prostatitis and similar diseases. Patients may experience various symptoms aside from urinary disorders and have indefinite complaints. Kampo medicines are most effective in chronic cases that are intractable to Western medical treatment.

- **Keishi-bukuryo-gan:** The most frequent form of prostatitis, intrapelvic venous congestion syndrome, corresponds to blood[TM1] stasis in Kampo medicine [35].

If blood[TM1] stasis resolving formulas are ineffective or disabled, treatment should be administered in accordance with lower urinary tract infections or bladder pain syndrome/ interstitis.

Bladder Pain Syndrome/Interstitial Cystitis and Indefinite Lower Urinary Tract Complaints

The various lower urinary tract symptoms, chiefly consisting of vague complaints, are regarded as a pattern of indefinite lower urinary tract syndrome in Kampo medicine. This pattern covers multiple disease names in Western medicine, such as bladder pain syndrome/interstitial cystitis, nervous pollakiuria, chronic cystitis, urethritis, and prostatitis. In addition, several pathological conditions are also included that originate with sensitivity to cold and climacteric disorders. Accordingly, under Kampo therapy guidelines, a prescription should be selected that matches a Kampo pathological condition (the basis of Kampo therapy). The therapeutic goal for indefinite complaints and psychogenic symptoms involving the lower urinary tract is to improve qi abnormalities (qi deficiency, qi stagnation, and qi counter flow qi counter flow) caused by mental imbalance (psychological function and activity). Accordingly, the practitioner may select the most appropriate qi-tonifying or qi-regulating formulas for the patient's symptoms and pathological condition.

If these are ineffective, heat-clearing and fluid[TM1] regulating formulas or cold treatment agents may also be tried [36].

4.3 Menstruation Disorders: Climacteric Disorders

Naohisa Ushiroyama

4.3.1 Overview of Disease

Menstruation disorders, the common term for menstrual cycle disorders, are caused by pathological conditions of the endocrine environment. In Western medicine, the term refers to functional diseases triggered by organic or functional ovarian abnormality or functional diencephalic/pituitary abnormality, not including hemorrhage from the genital tract due to tumor or inflammation. Kampo medicine considers blood[TM1] stasis the main factor in the above pathological conditions, and, according to zang-fu theory, kidney[TM1] deficiency is partly responsible. Recently, dieting, unhealthy lifestyles, and excessive stress are thought to be major factors in many menstrual disorder cases. Blood[TM1] deficiency, qi deficiency, spleen[TM1]-stomach[TM1] deficiency, or qi stagnation is considered to lie at the core of the pathological condition in a majority of cases.

The climacteric disorder is, in its narrow definition, the endocrine climacteric disorder termed menopausal disorder. The public, however, is likely to think of climacteric disorders as psychosomatic disorders that occur over a period of up to 10 years before and again after menopause. Therefore, the contemporary treatment of climacteric disorders falls within the scope of holistic medicine. Understanding the pathological condition from a Kampo medicine perspective enables the selection of an effective therapeutic approach in many cases. These symptoms have appeared in many classic texts of Kampo medicine for many centuries, and in Japan, they have been treated as blood[TM1] related pattern in Kampo therapy.

Climacteric disorders fitting the strict definition, which consist mainly of autonomic imbalance due to short-term abrupt changes in estrogen or pituitary gonadotropin, account for nearly 30% of cases and are generally indicated for hormone replacement therapy. Psychiatric disorders (depression, anxiety disorder, etc.) account for more than 40% of cases and require psychotropic drugs. Most of the remainder involve psychosocial factors.

4.3.2 Indications for Kampo Therapy

Conditions such as severe ovulation disorder associated with weight loss, menstrual disorder associated with sensitivity to cold, menstrual disorder due to intense psychological stress, and ovulation disorder due to high blood LH level, including polycystic ovary syndrome, respond poorly to Western medications but respond well to Kampo therapy. In particular, *unkei-to* is reported to have a regulatory effect on the pituitary gonadotropin secretory pattern, to stimulate follicle growth and luteal function, and to exert therapeutic effects in all types of menstrual cycle disorders. As mentioned in *Mambyokaishun* 万病回春 *(Restoring Health from Myriad of Diseases)*, the pathological conditions requiring "menstrual regulation" are "mostly diseases of qi excess with blood[TM1] deficiency." Thus, treatment for blood or qi deficiency is widely used as Kampo therapy for menstrual disorders: Kyukichoketsuindaiichikagen is usually prescribed.

In cases of ovulation disorder caused by weight loss or exposure to excessive stress, however, weight-gain diets or psychotherapy using behavioral stress management techniques take priority, respectively.

Kampo medicine is part of a holistic approach to the treatment of climacteric disorder. Obtaining a thorough understanding of the patient's social background and personality traits leads to successful outcomes. Signs of blood[TM1] stasis are observed in approximately one-third, and qi counter flow or qi stagnation in approximately one-quarter, of climacteric disorder patients. Hot flashes, headaches, heavy-headedness, and vertigo/dizziness are various manifestations of pathological conditions of qi, blood[TM1], and fluids[TM1]. In Western medical diagnostics, formulating a treatment strategy is difficult because a host of symptoms are not organ-specific, and syndrome shift occurs occasionally. In Kampo medicine, however, appropriate therapy can be given on the comprehensive diagnosis of individual symptoms.

4.3.3 Frequently Used Formulas

Several kinds of *unkei-to* modifications were frequently used before modern times. In all of these formulas, tonifying blood[TM1], resolving blood[TM1], and activating blood[TM1] are considered the basic therapeutic approaches. These approaches have been carried over to modern formulas, and *tokishakuyakusan, keishibukuryogan*, and *rikkunshito* are used very frequently in modern times, as well as *unkeito* and *kyukichoketsuindaiichikagen*[17].

There is a bias among Western medicine specialties as to which formulas is favored for climacteric disorder.

Gynecologists most frequently prescribe *tokishakuyakusan, kamishoyosan*, and *keishibukuryogan*, which account for half of their Kampo prescriptions. *Tokishakuyakusan* and *keishibukuryogan* are often used for shoulder stiffness, coldness, hot flashes, and numbness in the extremities. These being among the most frequently occurring symptoms in Japanese patients with climacteric disorder. The terms "vexing heat in the chest, palms, and soles; cloudiness and heaviness in the head and eyes; uneasiness and facial redness; menstrual imbalance; and cold and heat like alternating fever and chills disorder," which appear as the indications for *shoyosan*[18], refer to symptoms commonly observed in climacteric disorder and suggest the presence of qi counter flow qi counter flow and blood[TM1] stasis.

Saikokeishikankyoto, hangekobokuto, keishikaryukotsuboreito, saikokaryukotsuboreito, kamikihito, and *yokukansan*

[17]Not available as a medically approved Kampo extract formulation.
[18]Not available as a medically approved Kampo extract formulation.

are being prescribed more frequently in recent times, reflecting the stressfulness of modern society.

Menstruation Disorders [37, 38] (Fig. 5.21)

- **Unkeito:** May be used for all types of menstrual disorders and is sometimes offered to women with high blood LH, polycystic ovarian syndrome, or luteal dysfunction. Appropriate for slight deficiency to medium pattern patients who present with blood[TM1] stasis signs, including lower abdominal tenderness, as well as upper body heat sensation and lip dryness.
- **Kyukichoketsuindaiichikagen:**[19] Patients have a slight deficiency in the medium pattern of both qi and blood[TM1] deficiency and complain of a tendency to fatigue.
- **Tokishakuyakusan:** Used in deficiency pattern patients who have blood[TM1] deficiency and fluid[TM1] retention, as evidenced by anemia and edema.
- **Keishibukuryogan:** Used for medium to slight excess pattern patients with upper heat/lower cold, in addition to lower abdominal tenderness associated with blood[TM1] stasis.
- **Rikkunshito:** Offered to deficiency to slight deficiency pattern patients with decreased appetite and an abdominal pattern of epigastric stuffiness and splashing sound.
- **Kamishoyosan:** Appropriate for slight deficiency pattern patients with qi counter flow and blood[TM1] stasis who have hypochondriac tendencies (including palpitations) as well as coldness in the lower body.
- **Tokakujokito:** Effective for slight excess to excess pattern patients with constipation and intense psychoneurotic symptoms such as irritability, characterized by an abdominal pattern of chafing pain in the left lower abdomen (lower abdominal cramp).
- **Shimotsuto:** A basic formula for blood[TM1] deficiency. Appropriate for patients with slight deficiency pattern. May sometimes be combined with *kamishoyosan*.
- **Tokishigyakukagoshuyushokyoto:** Good for slight deficiency pattern patients with chilblains and intense coldness in the upper and lower limbs.
- **Kyukikyogaito:** Used in deficiency pattern patients for its hemostatic effect. Highly effective for anovulatory cycles.

Climacteric Disorders [39] (Fig. 5.22)

- **Kamishoyosan:** Appropriate for slight deficiency pattern patients but widely prescribed for climacteric disorders. The first choice for patients with pathological conditions mainly consisting of qi counter flow qi counter flow and blood[TM1] stasis and various complaints including irritability, insomnia, shoulder stiffness, and palpitations.
- **Keishibukuryogan:** Appropriate for pathological conditions (including hot flashes) associated with blood[TM1] stasis in medium to slight excess pattern patients. Also effective for deficiency pattern patients as well, because this formula warms the lower body.
- **Tsudosan:** Used for slight excess to excess pattern patients with psychoneurotic symptoms including irritability caused by qi stagnation, as well as facial redness due to blood[TM1] stasis in patients with rather high blood pressure and constipation tendency.
- **Tokishakuyakusan:** Useful for fluid[TM1] retention associated with blood[TM1] stasis in deficiency pattern patients who have coldness in limbs, dizziness, and palpitations.
- **Unseiin:** A typical formula for blood[TM1] deficiency/blood[TM1] heat pattern, or patients with medium constitutions who have hot flashes and coldness and may complain of headache. Their climacteric disorder is associated with high blood pressure and is not well treated with Western medicines.
- **Keishikaryukotsuboreito:** Offered to slight deficiency pattern patients with insomnia, oversensitivity, palpitations, and nervous imbalance, in addition to hair loss due to kidney[TM1] deficiency.
- **Saikokaryukotsuboreito:** Appropriate for slight excess pattern patients with qi stagnation and spleen[TM1] qi deficiency who have psychoneurotic symptoms, including complaints of depression/anxiety and a tendency to insomnia.
- **Hangekobokuto:** Effective for medium pattern patients with anxiety and depression due to qi stagnation. This qi-regulating formulas is offered to patients with obstructive discomfort in the throat as well as palpitations and vertigo.

4.4 Obstetric Diseases

Koji Watanabe

4.4.1 Outline of Diseases

Various symptoms during pregnancy, infertility, recurrent miscarriage, and postpartum disorders are conditions resulting from the female lifecycle. Even normal pregnancy does not always ensure maternal and fetal safety; it is necessary to bear the risks in mind.

4.4.2 Indications of Kampo Treatments

There are many things requiring special caution during pregnancy and treatment for infertility or recurrent miscarriage, including the effects of drugs on the fetus. Kampo treatments

[19] Not available as a medical Kampo extract formulation.

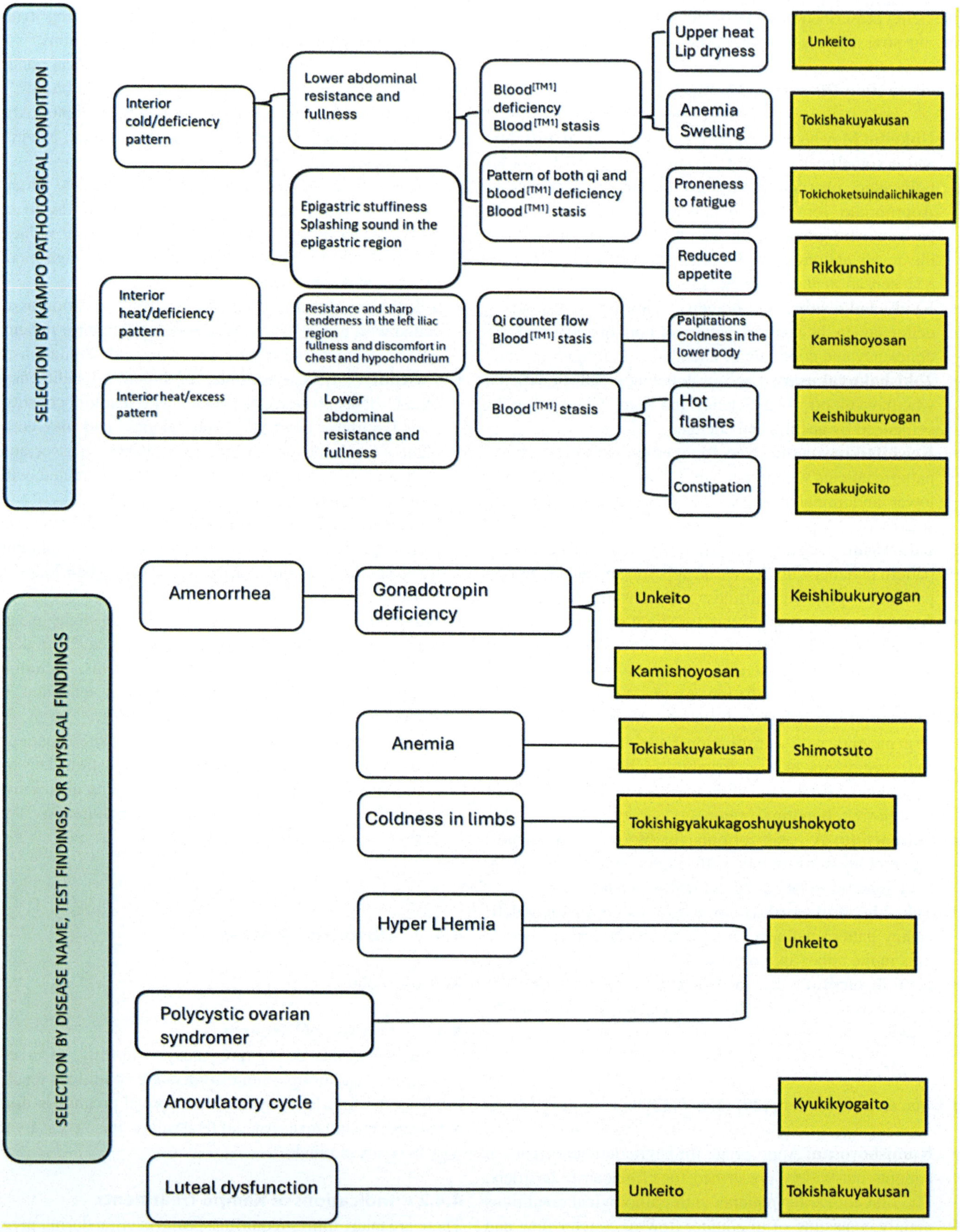

Fig. 5.21 Frequently used formulas for menstruation disorders

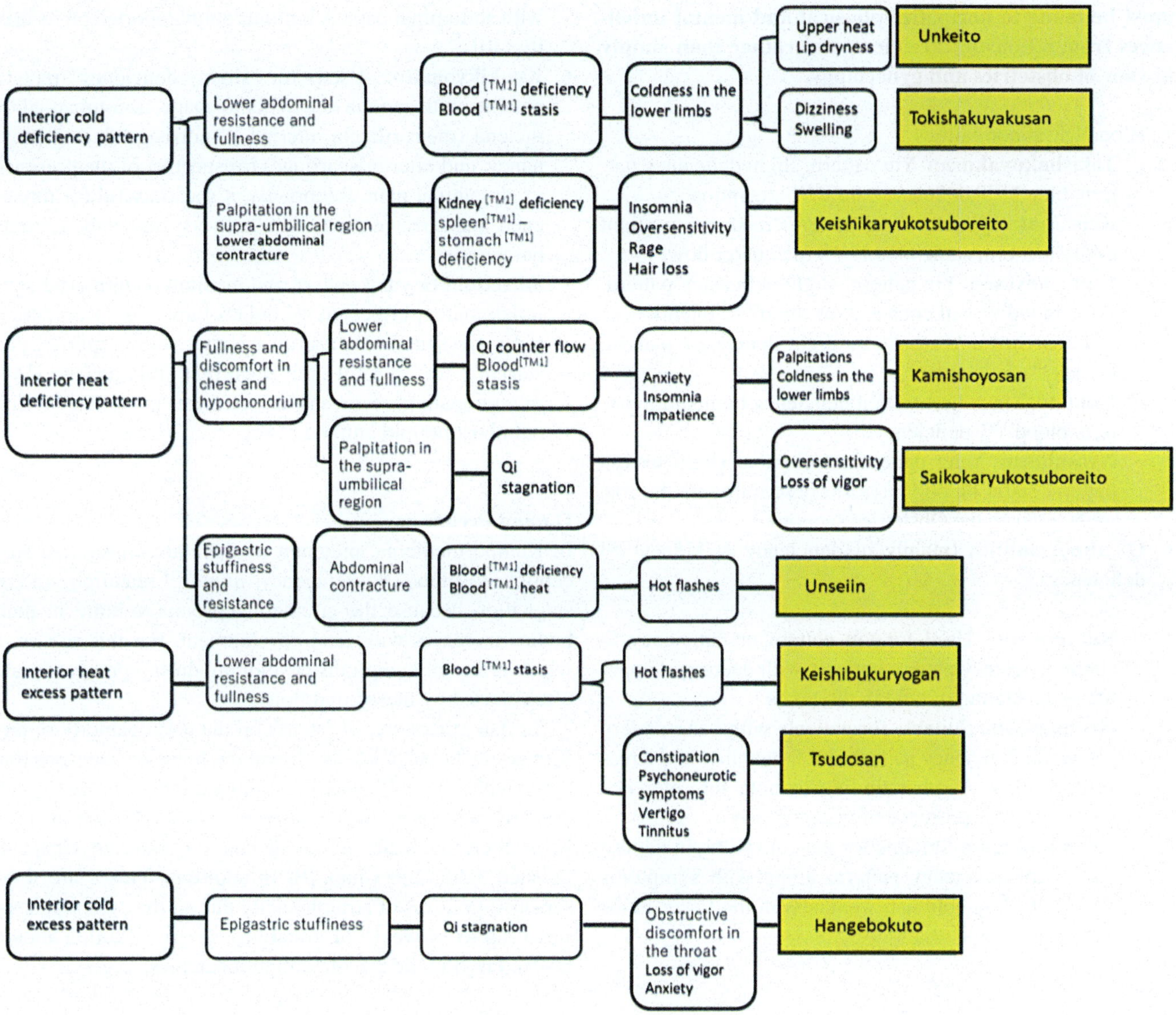

Fig. 5.22 Frequent formulas for climacteric disorders

can also have side effects and should, therefore, be used only when the benefits are considered to outweigh the risks.

Prior to pregnancy, there is a great need for Kampo treatments for infertility and recurrent miscarriage, and Kampo medicines are sometimes used for side effects of hormone treatments. During pregnancy, Kampo medicines are often used as a relatively safe therapy for hyperemesis gravidarum, the common cold, edema, constipation, etc. In the perinatal stage, conditions such as postpartum mastitis, and postpartum depression are good indications of Kampo treatments.

4.4.3 Frequently Used Formulas

During the terms of pregnancy, women often encounter difficulty, both physically and mentally, and this increases the opportunity for using Kampo formulas (taking qi and blood[TM1] deficiencies into account). The constitution is best assessed to be one level closer to a deficiency pattern. Kampo formulas are often sufficiently effective, even at low doses.

Pregestational

(a) **Infertility**

Provided that there is no organic trouble that hampers pregnancy, such as tubal stenosis, Kampo treatments may be attempted.

In the view of Kampo medicine, infertility is often caused by blood[TM1] abnormalities such as blood[TM1] stasis and blood[TM1] deficiency. From the viewpoint of eliminating factors that prevent pregnancy, however, attempts

must be made to normalize physical and mental imbalances from a holistic care viewpoint rather than simply in view of obstetrics and gynecology.

- Blood[TM1] abnormalities
  - **Tokishakuyakusan**: Yin pattern, slight deficiency pattern, blood[TM1] deficiency, fluid[TM1] retention.
  - **Keishibukuryogan**: Yang pattern, medium to slight excess pattern, static blood[TM1], qi counter flow.
  - **Kamishoyosan**: Yin pattern, slight deficiency pattern, static blood[TM1], qi counter flow, fluid[TM1] retention.
  - **Tokikenchuto**: Yin pattern, slight deficiency pattern, blood[TM1] deficiency.
  - **Unkeito**: Yin pattern, slight deficiency to medium pattern, blood[TM1] deficiency.
  - **Nyoshinsan**: Yang pattern, medium to slight excess pattern, static blood[TM1] (for a description of the formula, refer to the Obstetrics section).
- **Qi abnormalities** (mainly qi deficiency & kidney[TM1] deficiency).

  - **Rikkunshito:** Used for yin pattern or deficiency to slight deficiency pattern patients with decreased appetite and a feeling of cold in the limbs.
  - **Hochuekkito**: Suitable for patients with yang pattern and slight deficiency pattern and fatigability and stress susceptibility. Another finding to note for reference purposes is the presence of visceroptosis.
  - **Hachimijiogan**: Suitable for patients with yin pattern and slight deficiency pattern, along with symptoms such as feeling cold and weakness in the lower limbs and frequent nocturia.

(b) **Recurrent miscarriage**

Recurrent miscarriage refers to a condition in which a couple at their reproductive ages wants pregnancy but fails to attain live birth because of repeated miscarriage and/or premature deliveries (stillbirths). While there are a wide variety of causal factors, Kampo medicines can be useful for these conditions, including cases where the cause cannot be identified.

Mothers with recurrent miscarriages tend to have a yin pattern, deficiency pattern, blood[TM1] stasis, blood[TM1] deficiency, or fluid[TM1] retention. In addition to *tokishakuyakusan*, which has long been used to maintain pregnancy as a "miscarriage prevention drug," *shimotsuto* formulas such as *kyukikyogaito* and *saireito* are used.

- **Tokishakuyakusan**: Used for slight deficiency pattern patients with blood[TM1] deficiency and fluid[TM1] retention, who complain of feeling cold. It's also useful in cases with abdominal pain. A big-data study reported on its utility [40].
- **Kyukikyogaito**: Used for slight deficiency pattern patients with anemia due to hemorrhage, accompanied by melena (metrorrhagia, uterine hemorrhage during pregnancy, and after miscarriage) irrespective of the presence of abdominal pain. Reportedly, it's also useful for threatened miscarriage/premature delivery and subchorionic hematoma.
- **Saireito**: For yang pattern and medium pattern. The anti-inflammatory effects of formulas of involving Bupleurum radix are sometimes useful. Another study reported that *saireito* was useful for recurrent miscarriage [41] immunopathic recurrent miscarriage in mothers with antiphospholipid antibody [42].

During Pregnancy

In Kampo medicine, pregnant mothers are considered susceptible to blood[TM1] deficiency, fluid[TM1] retention, and qi stagnation because the circulating plasma volume in their bodies increases with fetal development. For this reason, a wide variety of symptoms developing during pregnancy are often caused by these conditions.

To date, there are no reports on the teratogenicity of any Kampo medicine. Classical literature, however, cautions that herbs with blood[TM1] stasis resolving effects and those with purgative effects should be used carefully. The use of these herbs therefore calls for great caution (refer to Chap. 4, Science 3.3.3, and Chap. 9). In addition, fetuses are most sensitive in terms of teratogenicity during the organogenesis stage (up to 14 weeks of gestation), so great caution should be exercised in the use of Kampo medicines.

(a) **Hyperemesis gravidarum (morning sickness)** (Fig. 5.23)

The frequent vomiting in hyperemesis gravidarum is viewed as a sign of fluid[TM1] retention. Thus fluid[TM1]regulating formulas containing rhizomes of *jutsu* (Atractylodes spp.), *bukuryo* (Poria sclerotium), and *takusha* (Alisma rhizome) are indicated.

Prolonged hyperemesis with no amelioration makes the patient experience mental hardship. Those formulas containing qi-regulating herbs such as *soyo* (Perilla herb) or *koboku* (Magnolia bark) are indicated. Since a scent alone can sicken the pregnant woman and induce nausea in hyperemesis gravidarum, it is necessary to take measures such as cold ingestion and taking little by little.

- **Shohangekabukuryoto**: A basic formula for nausea. Suitable for patients with slight deficiency pattern and early gestational hyperemesis. In case of severe nausea,

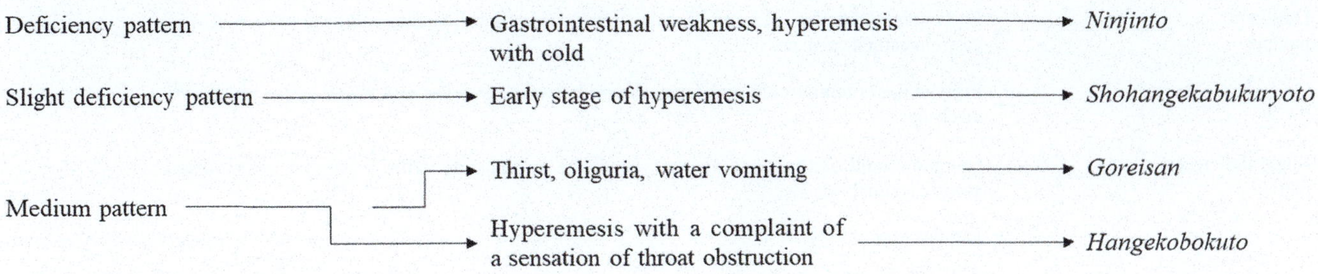

Fig. 5.23 Frequently used formulas for hyperemesis gravidarum

this formula is effective when taken cold little by little with the addition of freshly squeezed ginger juice.

- **Ninjinto**: Indicated for hyperemesis in women with deficiency pattern, with constitutional gastrointestinal weakness, fatigability, and feeling of cold. Such women sometimes complain of increased salivation and a tendency to have soft feces, along with epigastric stuffiness.
- **Goreisan**: A basic formula for fluid[TM1] retention, widely used mainly for medium pattern patients. Primary indications are thirst, oliguria, and vomiting caused by counterflow of water[TM1].
- **Hangekobokuto**: Suitable for nervous persons with medium pattern, hyperemesis, and complaints of sensations of choking and throat obstruction. Such patients have high tendencies for anxiety, insomnia, and depression and sometimes complain of palpitations and vertigo.

(b) **Common cold** (Fig. 5.24)

During pregnancy, treatment should be planned considering the condition to be slightly more deficient compared with the pregestational stage. Hemorrhoids and tooth pain can often be managed by Kampo treatment.

- **Kososan**: Used in the early stage of the common cold in deficiency pattern patients with gastrointestinal weakness. Strongly indicated for patients with anxiety, depressive tendencies, and qi stagnation symptoms.
- **Keishito**: Used for slight deficiency pattern patients in the early stage of the common cold with considerable sweating. Generally useful during pregnancy.
- **Jinsoin**: Suitable for slight deficiency pattern patients with gastrointestinal weakness such that *keishito* and *kakkonto* cause stomach fullness. Also suitable for patients with coughing from the common cold. Generally useful during pregnancy for symptoms including headache and copious expectoration.
- **Ryokankyomishingeninto**: Suitable for slight deficiency pattern patients who took allergy medicines or *shoseiryuto* before pregnancy to treat allergic rhinitis.
- **Bakumondoto**: Strongly indicated for persistent coughing in pregnant women with slight to medium deficiency pattern.

(c) **Edema and pregnancy-induced hypertension**

This was formerly called gestational toxicosis. Cases of hypertension alone developing after 20 weeks of gestation are referred to as pregnancy hypertension. Kampo medicines should be used as a supplement to Western medicines.

– **Candidates** include *goreisan*, *saireito*, *tokishakuyakusan*, and *boiogito*. (refer to Sect. 5.1.2).

(d) **Others**

- **Gastrointestinal symptoms and constipation**

Constipation in pregnant women is often caused by physical compression due to intestinal edema and uterine hypertrophy associated with progesterone. In the classical literature, rhubarb is said to pose a risk of miscarriage and premature delivery. Therefore, formulas with *daio* should be used with due caution.

– Candidates include *keishikashakuyakuto*, *shokenchuto*, and *daikenchuto* (refer to Sect. 3.2.2).

- **Hemorrhoids**

As the fetus grows, the uterus gets larger and compresses the anus and rectum, likely causing venous congestion in the region. In the second trimester and after, pregnant women have difficulty moving and stay seated for a long time. Thus, they are more likely to experience poor blood circulation around the anus.

– **Otsujito**: Used to treat hemorrhoids and anal fissures. For medium to slight excess pattern patients with constipation tendency.

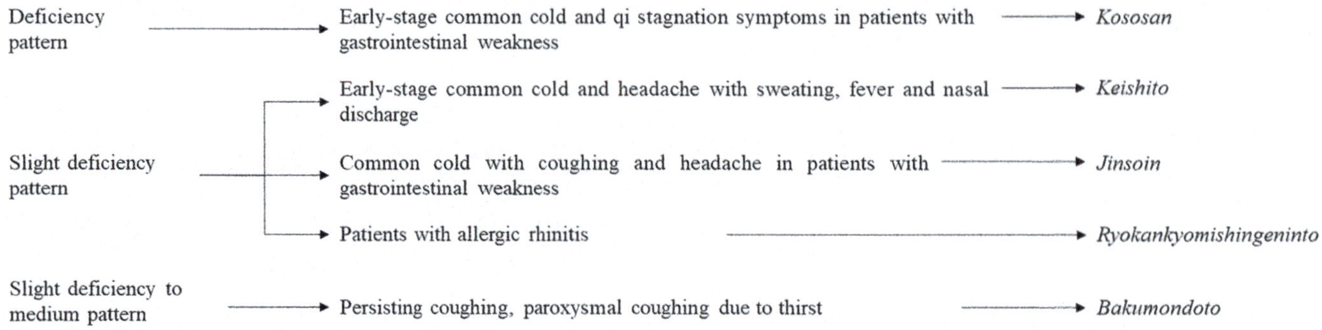

Fig. 5.24 Frequently used formulas for common cold symptoms during pregnancy

- **Hochuekkito**: Used for slight deficiency pattern patients with severe fatigue.
- **Shiunko**: Whether physical strength is in excess or deficient, this formula is considered to be effective for hemorrhoids during pregnancy and after delivery. Stops bleeding and brings relief from pain and swelling. Preferably used in combination with a laxative.

- Tooth pain
  - **Rikkosan**: Used for both excess or deficiency. This formula is taken cold while rinsing the mouth.
- Abdominal distention
  - **Tokishakuyakusan**: Used for patients with slight deficiency pattern, but can be used whether excess or deficient. This formula is also held to be effective for edema and heavy sensation in the body during pregnancy (these are signs of fluid retention).
- Genital bleeding during pregnancy

  - **Kyukikyogaito** (refer to the formulas for recurrent miscarriage).

Perinatal Stage

(a) **Kampo medicines useful in delivery**
- **Cervix-ripening effect**

  A case compilation study reported that *goshakusan* was useful in women with an immature uterine cervix after the estimated date of delivery.
  - **Goshakusan**: Indicated for medium to slight deficiency pattern patients with a feeling of cold. In the past, this was used for difficult labor.
- **Labor promotion**
  - **Keishibukuryogan**: Also known as "*saiseito*" and reportedly effective in labor promotion. This may be prescribed for conditions where some portions of the placenta and villi remain in the uterus after delivery or miscarriage. Its constituent herb, *tonin* (peach kernel), is reportedly effective in enhancing uterine contraction.
  - **Tokakujokito**: Classically reported to be used to promote placenta excretion and treat uterine subinvolution.

(b) **Postpartum mastitis**

Postpartum mastitis involves severe inflammation and heat retention on the body surface early in its onset; therefore, it is managed as an excess pattern of early yang stage. Postpartum mastitis in its subacute stage is handled as a late yang stage and treated with *shosaikoto* and *jumihaidokuto*. If there is abscess formation, *hainosankyuto* and *daiobotampito* are used along with antibiotics.

- **Kakkonto**: Used for the early stage of suppurative mastitis, targeting fever, headache, absence of sweating, swelling and pain of affected sites, and neck stiffness.
- **Shosaikoto**, **jumihaidokuto**, **hainosankyuto**, **daiobotampito**: In cases of severe suppuration, a switch to, or combination of, these formulas will be considered.

(c) **Postpartum depression**

Indicated for pregnant and postpartum women with complications of depression or panic disorder.

- **Kyukichoketsuin**: Used to ameliorate perinatal symptoms in women with deficiency to slight deficiency pattern and blood[TM1] deficiency. They may complain of tinnitus, vertigo, and hot flashes.
- **Hangekobokuto**: Suitable for patients with medium pattern and qi stagnation symptoms such as obstruction in the throat.
- **Kososan**: Suitable for patients with deficiency pattern who have complaints including depressed mood and low energy along with anxiety and restlessness.

- **Yokukansan, yokukansankachimpihange**: Used for patients who are unable to control their outward irritation. The former is used for slight excess pattern, and the latter, for slight deficiency pattern.
- **Kambakutaisoto**: Used in patients with a slight deficiency pattern who are moved to tears with anxiety and have severe nervous excitement.
- **Rikkunshito**: Suitable for patients with deficiency to slight deficiency pattern, decreased appetite, and stomach distension.
- **Hochuekkito**: Used in patients with a slight deficiency pattern with fatigue as the chief complaint.

(d) **Others**

- **Edema**
  - **Goreisan, saireito** (**refer to t**he Edema and Pregnancy-Induced Hypertension sections)
- **Uterine prolapse**
  - **Hochuekkito**: Used in patients with slight deficiency pattern. In addition to its qi-tonifying effects, this formula is effective in uplifting because it contains *shoma* (Cimicifuga rhizome).

5 Limbs, Joints, and Skin

5.1 Edema

Kako Watanabe and Mayumi Tamada

5.1.1 Overview of Disease

Edema is a condition in which the increased volume of body fluid and its abnormal distribution abnormally increase interstitial fluid. Various diseases cause edema, which can be divided into localized and generalized edema.

Localized edema is either unilateral or confined to a specific region. The etiology is categorized as lymphatic, veno-occlusive, allergic, inflammatory, or angioneurotic, including deep vein thrombosis, thrombophlebitis, varix, cellulitis, and lymphedema following surgery or radiotherapy.

Systemic edema is often found bilaterally. In mild cases, edema is readily found in the pretibial region, lateral malleolus, dorsum of the foot, upper eyelids, etc. In severe cases, edema appears as an abrupt increase in body weight, ascites fluid, and pleural effusion. It is categorized as renal, hepatic, cardiac, endocrine, dystrophic, gestational, or idiopathic. Primary diseases include nephrosis, kidney failure, acute glomerulonephritis, liver cirrhosis, congestive heart failure, hypothyroidism, hyperthyroidism, gestosis, and idiopathic edema. Other causes include edema associated with premenstrual syndrome (PMS) and edema due to steroids or nonsteroidal anti-inflammatory drugs (NSAIDs). Otherwise, enhanced activity of the renin-angiotensin-aldosterone system after long-term use of diuretics or laxatives or repetitive intentional vomiting can be causes. Other causes are pseudoaldosteronism as an adverse effect of Kampo medicines (*kanzo*), maintaining the same posture for long periods, or lack of exercise. Edema is commonly induced by drugs and lifestyle.

Treatment consists of treating the primary disease and providing symptomatic therapy for edema, including rest, sodium restriction, fluid[TM1] restriction, physiotherapy, and diuretics.

From the Kampo medicine perspective, edema is perceived as a fluid[TM1] retention, involving generalized or localized retention of water or fluid[TM1] other than blood[TM1]. Symptoms specific to fluid[TM1] disturbance include not only edema but also dizziness, dizziness on standing up, headache, heavy-headedness, tinnitus, watery nasal discharge, sputum, palpitation, thirst, sick feeling, nausea, abdominal rumbling, abdominal distension, diarrhea, coldness, arthralgia, and travel sickness. These symptoms are characteristically aggravated on rainy days and by the approach of low-pressure systems or cold weather. Owing to water's cooling property, patients often complain of cold symptoms such as cold sensation in the edema region.

5.1.2 Indications for Kampo Therapy

If an organic disease is present, treatment of that disease takes precedence. Kampo therapy is considered helpful when the underlying disease is not known and the edema does not resolve despite the disease having been treated, or the swelling sensation is strong despite no edema being found by examination or no abnormality found in tests.

Kampo therapy focuses on fluid[TM1] regulating formulas, which regulate fluid[TM1] distribution in the body. Fluid[TM1] regulating formulas do not simply increase the excretion of urine but are considered to correct uneven distribution of water in the body by regulating fluid[TM1] through sweating as well as in the airway and digestive tract. Most diuretic formulations contain crude drugs such as *bukuryo*, *jutsu*, *takusha*, *chorei*, *mao*, *mokutsu*, *boi*, *ogi*, *hange*, *shokyo*, *kyonin*, *saishin*, *goshuyu*, and *bushi*.

Many of the underlying diseases that cause edema have a long course of illness, as seen in chronic nephritis, chronic hepatitis, and autoimmune diseases, as well as in cases of long-term steroid use. Therefore, in addition to formulas treating fluid[TM1] disturbance only, tonic formulas (such as *hochuekkito*, *juzentaihoto*, *hachimijiogan*, and *goshajinkigan*) are often used either singly or in combination with fluid[TM1] regulating formulas. Also, long-term use of steroids may cause iatrogenic blood[TM1] stasis, so blood[TM1] stasis

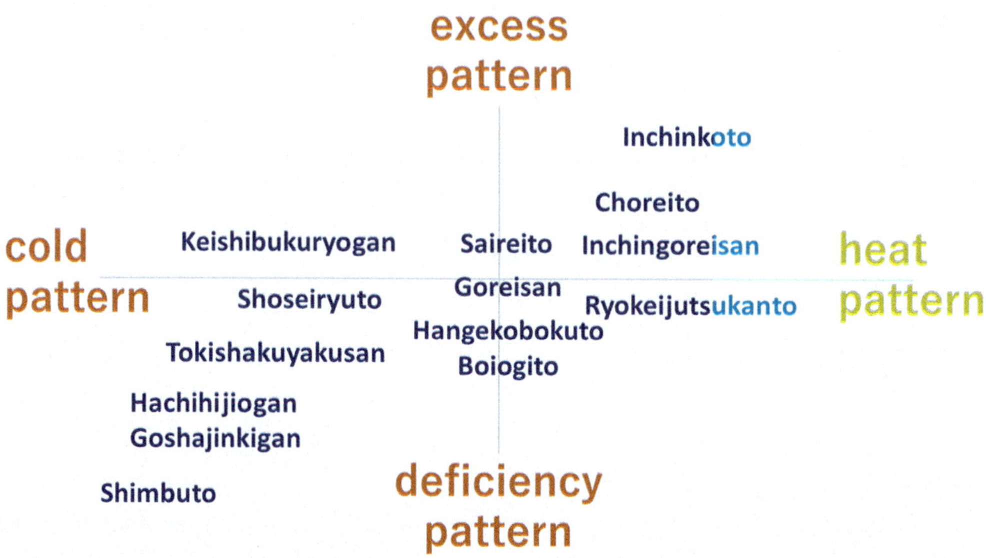

Fig. 5.25 Matrix diagram of frequently used formulas for edema

resolving formulas (such as *tokishakuyakusan* and *keishibukuryogan*) are also used.

Treating edema such as postoperative lymphedema is frequently challenging, but there are reports that *shinko-to*[20] is effective in cases of repeated lymphangitis due to lower limb lymphedema following radiotherapy or after uterine cancer surgery. Kampo medicines may be effective in some cases of edema intractable to modern medical therapy. While the selection of formulas is made on the principle of treatment by pattern identification, they are often prescribed in clinical practice today from a pharmacological standpoint.

5.1.3 Frequently Used Formulas (Fig. 5.25)

- **Goreisan**: Appropriate for medium pattern patients. This is the first choice for edema and a typical fluid[TM1] regulating formulas. Used for nephrosis and other renal diseases as well as nausea-associated headache, dizziness, and diarrhea in patients with thirst and reduced urine volume. In recent years, Gorei-san has been reported to suppress edema by inhibiting aquaporin (AQP), which is one of the water channels, and its use in the field of neurosurgery, such as for mitigating cerebral edema, is increasing [43, 44, 45].
- **Saireito**: Used for medium pattern patients but used widely for edema due to various causes, including renal diseases like chronic nephritis, nephrosis syndrome, and diabetic nephropathy. Originally this formula was used during hot weather when patients have thirst and reduced urine volume, but it is now frequently used to alleviate adverse effects of steroids [46].
- **Choreito**: Frequently used for edema in the lower body associated with cystitis and other urological diseases; symptoms include residual urine sensation, micturition pain, and hematuria. This formula is generally used for medium pattern patients, but it is widely used for other patterns except extreme deficiency pattern patients.
- **Ryokeijutsukanto**: Used for slight deficiency pattern patients with edema associated with palpitation, dizziness, dizziness on standing up, hot flashes, etc. Also frequently used for Meniere's disease (which results from fluid[TM1] retention) and orthostatic dysregulation.
- **Boiogito**: Used for slight deficiency pattern patients with edema associated with excessive sweating, coldness, reduced urine volume, arthralgia, and proneness to fatigue. Used mainly for patients with soft subcutaneous fat and weak muscle tension, or the so-called flabby body type. Also effective for edema localized to the knee joint with osteoarthritis.
- **Shoseiryuto**: Good for slight deficiency pattern patients. This formula corrects uneven distribution of water in the airway. Frequently used for asthma and allergic rhinitis. Also effective for facial edema due to coughing and for edema associated with headache, fever, chill, and cough in patients who have relatively strong digestive systems. It should be noted that caution is advised when using this formula for prolonged edema because it may aggravate the edema.
- **Shimbuto**: Used for deficiency pattern edema associated with diarrhea, dizziness, sensation of shakiness, general malaise, and palpitation in patients having poor complexion and general coldness.
- **Hachimijiogan** and **Goshajinkigan**: Used for slight deficiency pattern edema associated with urinary disorder; coldness, numbness, and pain in the legs and low back; as well as visual and hearing impairment. Often effective for edema in lower limbs in patients with chronic disease and elderly people with kidney[TM1] deficiency.

[20] Not available as a medical Kampo extract formulation.

- **Inchinkoto**: Well known as a jaundice formula, but also has a diuretic effect. Used for medium to slight excess pattern patients with edema with constipation, decreased urine volume, and a feeling of fullness in the epigastrium.
- **Inchingoreisan**: Used for slight excess pattern patients with post-radiotherapy regional edema as well as hepatic cirrhosis and nephrosis in patients with severely decreased urine volume and absence of constipation.
- **Keishibukuryogan**: Appropriate for medium to slight excess pattern patients. This is a typical, blood[TM1] stasis resolving formula used for headache, shoulder stiffness, and hot flashes, but it also improves edema by improving blood flow and eliminating excess fluid[TM1].
- **Tokishakuyakusan**: Used for slight deficiency pattern patients suffering from illness associated with coldness, heavy-headedness, dizziness, and anemia. It has both fluid[TM1] regulating and blood[TM1] tonifying effects and is therefore effective for gestational edema, chronic nephritis, and nephrosis as well.
- **Hangekobokuto**: Frequently used for medium pattern patients as a qi-regulating formula, but in classical terms also has a diuretic effect. It helps patients with frequent complaints such as abdominal distension, anxiety, and obstructive discomfort in the throat.

5.2 Arthralgia and Neuralgia

Toshiaki Kogure

5.2.1 Overview of Disease

Pain is generally classified as acute pain or chronic pain. Kampo therapy is principally used for chronic pain. Chronic pain is defined as pain that persists or recurs repeatedly for 6 months or more, has no clear correlation between pain intensity and the degree of impairment, and is pain that has lost the alarm function of alerting the body to tissue damage. It is known that when inflammation in rheumatoid arthritis (RA) is not controlled and the pain becomes prolonged, a host of psychosocial factors arise that affect the pain. Such a "pain complex" is also considered to be a feature of chronic pain.

Chronic nerve and joint pains are induced by a variety of factors, including inflammation, ischemia, and post-traumatic or degenerative changes. Occasionally chronic pain may be experienced in cases in which intrinsic or psychogenic factors are involved, such as fibromyalgia (syndrome) and complex regional pain syndrome (CRPS), etc.

Before starting treatment, it is essential to gain a clear understanding of the etiology through clinical findings, hematological and serological findings, and diagnostic imaging.

5.2.2 Indications for Kampo Therapy

Kampo medicines are appropriate for simple low back pain, shoulder-arm-neck syndrome, osteoarthritis, RA, and other nociceptive pain; postherpetic neuralgia; thalamic pain; and neuropathic pain, as well as psychogenic pain.

For low back pain (of various causes), shoulder-arm-neck syndrome, and osteoarthritis, non-steroidal anti-inflammatory drugs (NSAIDs), opioid, peripheral circulation improvement agents such as limaprost alfadex, and vitamin E formulations may be tried in addition to physiotherapy. Surgical treatment may be required on occasion, but Kampo medicines are a therapy available throughout the course of the condition. In RA cases, if a thorough understanding of the disease process cannot be obtained to control the inflammation, therapy, including biological drugs and Janus kinase inhibitors (JAK), may be needed. Since some cases respond well to Kampo medicine, however, they can be recommended according to RA medical guidelines, especially for elderly patients and patients with a history of tuberculosis, liver and kidney damage, or interstitial pneumonia. Fibromyalgia is treated with salazosulfapyridine, gabapentin, or anti-anxiety drugs, according to the cluster classification, but Kampo medicines may be appropriate for all clusters.

Postherpetic neuralgia and idiopathic trigeminal neuralgia are both indications for Western medical therapy (neuropathic pain relaxation medicine: pregabalin, mirogabalin; opioids, antidepressants, etc.) as well as Kampo medicines. For central neuralgia, which is intractable, Kampo medicines may be tried to alleviate symptoms and improve the general condition. There are also many opportunities to treat fibromyalgia and CRPS with Kampo medicine in clinical practice. In fact, Kampo therapy is given a recommendation of 2D (weak recommendation) for fibromyalgia in Clinical Practice Guidelines for Chronic Pain in Japan.

5.2.3 Frequently Used Formulas (Table 5.7)

Arthralgia

The section on frequently used formulas is divided here into arthralgia and neuralgia. In Kampo medicine terms, however, both arthralgia and neuralgia occur on the exterior. Accordingly, there is some overlap in indicated Kampo prescriptions. From a Western medical perspective, however, arthralgia occurs in a wide variety of pathological conditions, from inflammatory diseases originating with autoimmune mechanisms such as RA to diseases related to degenerative changes such as osteoarthritis. It is important to consider the underlying pathological condition along with traditional medical approaches.

- **Eppikajutsuto:** Used for severe arthralgia associated with joint swelling in excess and medium pattern patients with fluid[TM1] retention. For postherpetic neuralgia, administration in the stage when vesicles may or may not

Table 5.7 Frequently used formulas for arthralgia

Excess pattern	Arthralgia, joint swelling	Eppikajutsuto
	Early stage peripheral neuralgia, stiffness in the posterior region of neck	Kakkonto
Medium (excess, deficiency) pattern	Various forms of arthralgia and neuralgia, skin dryness	Makyoyokukanto
	Localized heat sensation, chronic pain	Yokuininto
	Frozen shoulders	Nijutsuto
	Blood[TM1] stasis, lower limb pain, sciatica	Sokeikakketsuto
	Varied joint pain and swelling, RA	Keishinieppiitto(karyojutsubu)*
	Neuralgia	Uyakujunkisan*
	Peripheral neuralgia, thirst, reduced urine volume	Goreisan Saireito
Deficiency pattern	Middle-aged overweight, osteoarthritis of the knee	Boiogito
	Chemotherapy related peripheral neuropathy	Ninjin'yoeito
	Anatomical stage advanced RA	Juzentaihoto
	Neuralgia	Shimbuto
	Central and peripheral neuralgia	Shozokumeito*
	Coldness in the back, neuralgia, arthralgia	Bushito**
	Aggravation due to coldness	Keishikajutsubuto
	Joint deformity due to RA	Keishishakuyaku-chimoto
	Joint deformity due to RA, pattern of both qi and blood[TM1] deficiency	Daibofuto
	Low back pain, lower limb coldness, heaviness, edema	Ryokyojutsukanto
	Old age, low back pain, lower limb numbness and coldness, nocturia	Hachimijiogan
	Coldness in the limbs, frostbite	Tokishigyaku-kagoshuyushokyoto
	Intercostal neuralgia	Tokito

*Not available as a medically approved Kampo extract formulation
**Not available as medical Kampo extract formulation nor OTC Kampo extract formulation

be appearing can relieve the pain with recovery from herpes zoster.

- **Makyoyokukanto:** Used for medium pattern patients who have diverse arthralgia and neuralgia and for patients with both skin dryness and blood[TM1] deficiency. RA is referred to as morning stiffness, and the pain intensifies in the early morning but may worsen in the evening. This formula is offered to such RA patients.
- **Boiogito:** Effective for slight deficiency pattern patients with osteoarthritis of the knee with joint swelling. According to qi, blood[TM1], fluid[TM1] theory, joint swelling is considered to be fluid[TM1] retention. This formula is used clinically to resolve fluid[TM1] retention. This formula is indicated for the abdominal finding of "middle-aged obesity."
- **Yokuininto:** Used for medium pattern patients with arthralgia and myalgia associated with heat sensation palpable in the painful part and for patients with not much sign of coldness. Often effective for chronic osteoarthritis pain. May be helpful for RA patients who have somewhat advanced joint deformity but maintain activity of daily living.
- **Keishikajutsubuto:** Appropriate for slight deficiency pattern patients with neuralgia and arthralgia aggravated by coldness and for patients with yin pattern associated with fluid[TM1] retention.
- **Keishinieppiitto**[21]: Often used for RA. Commonly used with the addition of *bukuryo*, *sojutsu*, and *bushi*. It is also commonly used with the addition of *boi* and *ogi*. [47].
- **Juzentaihoto:** Used for pattern of both qi and blood[TM1] deficiency in deficiency pattern patients with wasting diseases.
- **Keishishakuyakuchimoto:** For patients with yin constitution with deficiency pattern patho-condition. Effective for severe degeneration and intense pain in RA patients.
- **Daibofuto:** Used for pattern of both qi and blood[TM1] deficiency in patients with RA. This is similar to the *keishishakuyakuchimoto* pattern, but the condition of both qi and blood[TM1] deficiency is more prominent.
- **Ryokyojutsukanto:** Used for yin pattern patients with slight deficiency pattern, especially those who have coldness in the lower body or complain of heaviness and pain in the low back. Helpful for patients who have a patho-condition of fluid[TM1] retention and complain of swelling of lower limbs in the evening, etc.
- **Hachimijiogan:** Administered to yin pattern patients with slight deficiency pattern, especially targeting low back pain, lower limb numbness, coldness, and nocturia in elderly patients. *Goshajinkigan* is better for the same symptoms when there is a tendency of edema.
- **Tokishigyakukagoshuyushokyoto:** Effective for slight deficiency pattern patients who complain of coldness in the limbs along with chronic low back pain. A history of frostbite in fingers is also an indication. May be effective for patients who complain of chronic headache.
- **Nijutsuto:** Widely used for medium pattern patients with shoulder and upper arm pain (frozen shoulder). Especially effective for shoulder pain accompanied by fluid[TM1] retention signs. *Mao* is added for yang pattern patients and *bushi* for yin pattern patients.

Neuralgia

Yin and Yang differentiation is important in the treatment of neuralgia. Most of the neuralgia patients who receive Kampo

[21] Not available as a medically approved Kampo extract formulation.

therapy have chronic pain, including some who complain of pain over a long period. Among these patients, there are those who have a yang pattern. These patients must be examined very carefully.

- **Kakkonto**: Used in the early stages of peripheral neuralgia of medium to slight excess pattern patients. Often patients also have stiffness in the posterior region of the neck.
- **Uyakujunkisan:**[22] Used for yang pattern neuralgia, particularly effective in cases associated with qi stagnation. [48]
- **Sokeikakketsuto:** Used for blood[TM1] stasis in yang and medium pattern patients. Commonly effective for lower limb pain and sciatica.
- **Goreisan:** Used for medium pattern patients with various forms of peripheral neuralgia. Considered a good formula for patients having pain along with thirst, excessive sweating, and reduced urine volume.
- **Saireito:** Appropriate for medium pattern patients with the same findings as seen for *goreisan* pattern. The presence of fullness and discomfort in the chest and hypochondrium suggests the use of this formula.
- **Tokito:** Formula for slight deficiency pattern patients in early yin stage. Frequently effective for intercostal neuralgia in patients with both qi and blood[TM1] deficiency.
- **Shozokumeito:**[16] Used for Yin pattern neuralgia. Also effective for central neuralgia after cerebral infarction.
- **Bushito:**[23] Offered to patients with middle yin stage and deficiency pattern who have fluid[TM1] retention. Helpful for the complaint of coldness in the back.
- **Ninjin'yoeito:** Good for slight deficiency pattern patients. The efficacy of *ninjin-yoei-to* for the peripheral neuropathy induced by oxaliplatin has recently been demonstrated in randomized controlled trials [49].

5.3 Sensory Impairment, Motor Paralysis, and Involuntary Movement

Yutaka Shimada

5.3.1 Overview of Disease

The origins of sensory impairment, motor paralysis, and involuntary movement are diverse. These symptoms of nerve and muscle diseases may be found in all parts of the body, including the central and peripheral nerves and muscles. Pathogenesis is also diverse, ranging from vascular disorders and degenerative, demyelinating, metabolic, and toxic diseases to trauma, tumors, and infection. These diseases are roughly classified into acute, subacute, and chronic phases, according to the period since onset, and may be progressive or recurrent.

5.3.2 Indications for Kampo Therapy

Since the effectiveness of Kampo therapy for sensory impairment and motor paralysis is determined by the primary disease, it is not possible to generalize about indications. When an effective Western medical therapeutic approach is available, however, this takes precedence. Kampo therapy may be considered when there is no treatment. Kampo therapy today is often used in the chronic phase.

Involuntary movement is classified into various types, and the causes of the disease may differ. In any case, Kampo therapy is chiefly applied to trembling and tics, which have a strong psychogenetic element. Muscle spasm is an extremely good target for Kampo therapy. Epilepsy is mainly treated with Western therapies.

5.3.3 Frequently Used Formulas (Table 5.8)

Sensory Impairment and Motor Paralysis

The causes of sensory impairment and motor paralysis are regarded as external pathogens, including wind, cold, dampness, and fire or heat. From the qi, blood[TM1], fluid[TM1] perspective, blood[TM1] deficiency and blood[TM1] stasis, qi deficiency and qi stagnation, and fluid[TM1] retention are important factors.

- **Keishikajutsubuto:** Widely used for numbness and paralysis in slight deficiency pattern patients with coldness. In this formula, *jutsu* with a fluid[TM1] regulating effect and *bushi* with a strongly warming effect are added to *keishito*.
- **Keishikaryojutsubuto**: Used in patients with slight deficiency pattern. In this formula, *bukuryo* with a fluid [TM1]regulating effect is added to *keishikajutsubuto*, which further enhances the effect on dampness, or fluid[TM1] retention.
- **Hachimijiogan**: Appropriate for slight deficiency pattern patients with numbness and weakness in the lower back and lower limbs in middle-aged and older patients. Especially indicated for elderly patients, who are also likely to have fatigue, malaise, urination disorder, and weakness of the lower abdominal region. *Hachimijiogan* is a typical kidney[TM1] deficiency formula, containing *keishi* and *bushi,* warming and heating herbs. This formula is used for people with coldness in the upper and lower limbs and can also be used in those with a burning sensation.
- **Goshajinkigan:** A formula consisting of *goshitsu* and *shazenshi* added to *hachimijiogan*. Used for relatively strong numbness and pain in slight deficiency pattern patients and *hachimijiogan* pattern patients with edema tendency.

---

22 Not available as a medical Kampo extract formulation.

23 Not available as medical Kampo extract formulation and OTC Kampo formulation.

Bushito: bushi 1.0, bukuryo・shakuyaku 4.0, jutsu 5.0, ninjin 3.0.

Table 5.8 Kampo formulas used for sensory impairment, motor paralysis, and involuntary movement, and their corresponding deficiency and excess patterns

<table>
<tr><th>Deficiency pattern</th><th>Slight deficiency pattern</th><th>Medium pattern</th><th>Slight excess pattern</th><th>Excess pattern</th></tr>
<tr><td></td><td>Keishikajutsubuto</td><td></td><td></td><td></td></tr>
<tr><td></td><td>Keishikaryojutsubuto</td><td></td><td></td><td></td></tr>
<tr><td></td><td>Hachimijiogan</td><td></td><td></td><td></td></tr>
<tr><td></td><td>Goshajinkigan</td><td></td><td></td><td></td></tr>
<tr><td></td><td>Rokumigan</td><td></td><td></td><td></td></tr>
<tr><td>Shimbuto</td><td></td><td></td><td></td><td></td></tr>
<tr><td></td><td>Ryokyojutsukanto</td><td></td><td></td><td></td></tr>
<tr><td></td><td></td><td colspan="2">Kakkonto</td><td></td></tr>
<tr><td></td><td></td><td>Goreisan</td><td></td><td></td></tr>
<tr><td></td><td>Tokishigyakukagoshuyushokyoto</td><td></td><td></td><td></td></tr>
<tr><td></td><td>Tokishakuyakusan</td><td></td><td></td><td></td></tr>
<tr><td></td><td></td><td colspan="2">Keishibukuryogan</td><td></td></tr>
<tr><td></td><td></td><td></td><td colspan="2">Tokakujokito</td></tr>
<tr><td></td><td></td><td>Sokeikakketsuto</td><td></td><td></td></tr>
<tr><td></td><td>Kamishoyosan</td><td></td><td></td><td></td></tr>
<tr><td></td><td>Hochuekkito</td><td></td><td></td><td></td></tr>
<tr><td>Juzentaihoto</td><td></td><td></td><td></td><td></td></tr>
<tr><td>Daibofuto</td><td></td><td></td><td></td><td></td></tr>
<tr><td></td><td colspan="2">Goshakusan</td><td></td><td></td></tr>
<tr><td></td><td colspan="2">Unkeito</td><td></td><td></td></tr>
<tr><td></td><td>Shokenchuto</td><td></td><td></td><td></td></tr>
<tr><td></td><td colspan="2">Sammotsuogonto</td><td></td><td></td></tr>
<tr><td></td><td></td><td>Shosaikoto</td><td></td><td></td></tr>
<tr><td></td><td></td><td></td><td colspan="2">Orengedokuto</td></tr>
<tr><td></td><td></td><td></td><td colspan="2">San'oshashinto</td></tr>
<tr><td></td><td></td><td>Shakuyakukanzoto</td><td></td><td></td></tr>
<tr><td></td><td></td><td></td><td>Yokukansan</td><td></td></tr>
<tr><td></td><td colspan="2">Saikokeishito</td><td></td><td></td></tr>
<tr><td></td><td></td><td>Chotosan</td><td></td><td></td></tr>
<tr><td></td><td>Keishikaryukotsuboreito</td><td></td><td></td><td></td></tr>
<tr><td></td><td></td><td></td><td>Saikokaryukotsuboreito</td><td></td></tr>
<tr><td></td><td>Kanbakutaisoto</td><td></td><td></td><td></td></tr>
</table>

- **Rokumigan:** A formula in which *keishi* and *bushi* are removed from *hachimijiogan*. Used for burning sensation in the upper and lower limbs in slight deficiency *hachimijiogan* pattern patients.
- **Shimbuto:** Used in deficiency pattern patients who have sensitivity to cold, gastrointestinal weakness, diarrhea tendency, and strong malaise, associated with motor paralysis and sensory impairment. This is formulas with processed aconite root.
- **Ryokyojutsukanto:** Appropriate for cold and weakness from the lower back to the lower limbs in slight deficiency pattern patients who have a tendency of frequent urination.

- **Kakkonto:** Used for abnormal skin sensation associated with common cold-like symptoms in medium to slight excess pattern patients.
- **Goreisan:** A typical fluid[TM1] retention formula used in medium pattern patients. Also used for pathologic conditions, including acute-phase neurological disorders in which localized edema may be assumed.
- **Tokishigyakukagoshuyushokyoto:** Effective for numbness and paralysis in slight deficiency pattern patients who have extreme coldness of the limbs.
- **Tokishakuyakusan:** Used for numbness and weakness in the limbs for slight deficiency pattern patients who have anemia and a tendency for edema. These patients also have blood[TM1] deficiency, blood[TM1] stasis, and fluid[TM1] retention.
- **Keishibukuryogan:** Used for medium to slight excess pattern patients who have hot flashes and facial redness, along with a tendency of blood[TM1] stasis, indicated by resistance and tenderness in the lower abdomen. These patients also have numbness in their limbs.
- **Tokakujokito:** Used for numbness of the limbs in slight excess to excess pattern patients who have constipation and a tendency of hot flashes with blood[TM1] stasis, indicated by lower abdominal cramps.
- **Sokeikakketsuto:** Appropriate for numbness and paralysis of the limbs in medium pattern patients who either have no or only slight coldness. Patients also have signs of blood[TM1] stasis, blood[TM1] deficiency, and fluid[TM1] retention.
- **Kamishoyosan:** Used for slight deficiency pattern patients who have psychoneurotic symptoms (such as anxiety and irritability) and diverse autonomic nervous symptoms (such as episodic sweating and sensation of heat) and complain of crawling, itchy, and ticklish sensations in the skin.
- **Hochuekkito:** Used for slight deficiency pattern patients who have motor paralysis, weakness in limbs, a tendency to fatigue, and no appetite. This is a typical qi deficiency formula.
- **Juzentaihoto:** Used for numbness, motor paralysis, and weakness of the limbs in deficiency pattern patients who are prone to fatigue and have no appetite. This is a representative formula for concomitant qi deficiency and blood[TM1] deficiency.
- **Daibofuto:** Used for motor paralysis, cramps, and numbness of the limbs in deficiency pattern patients who are sensitive to coldness. Patients also have signs of blood[TM1] deficiency, qi deficiency, and fluid[TM1] retention. This is formulas with processed aconite root.
- **Goshakusan:** Used for slight deficiency to medium pattern patients with a tendency of upper heat and lower cold, and numbness and paralysis affected by coldness or dampness.
- **Unkeito:** Used for burning sensation in the palms in slight deficiency to medium pattern patients with lip dryness, irregular menstruation, and pain in the lower abdomen.
- **Shokenchuto:** Used for burning sensation in the upper and lower limbs in slight deficiency pattern patients who are prone to fatigue and who also have abdominal weakness and strong abdominal muscle tension.
- **Sammotsuogonto:** Used for slight deficiency to medium pattern patients who complain of heat and burning sensation in the limbs.
- **Shosaikoto:** Used for heat and burning sensation in the limbs in medium pattern patients who have fullness and discomfort in the chest and hypochondrium.
- **Orengedokuto:** Used for sensory impairment such as numbness in the upper and lower limbs in slight excess to excess pattern patients who tend to have sensitivity to heat, hot flashes, facial flushing, and nervous imbalance.
- **San'oshashinto:** Used for slight excess to excess pattern patients with constipation who are irritable, cannot settle down, and complain of hot flashes, facial flushing, dizziness, and heavy-headedness as well as sensory impairment (such as numbness of the upper and lower limbs).

Involuntary Movement

Muscle spasm is regarded as a symptom of blood[TM1] deficiency, and formulas containing *shakuyaku* as the main ingredient, such as *shakuyakukanzoto,* are used. There is a close relation between the muscles and liver, and spasms seen in epilepsy and the like are considered to be induced by liver abnormality. Therefore, formulas of involving Bupleurum radix and *chotoko* are also used.

- **Shakuyakukanzoto:** Used for painful muscle spasms such as cramps in the leg [50–52]. Addition of *bushi* to *shakuyakukanzoto—shakuyakukanzobushito—*may be effective for patients with strong coldness and pain.
- **Yokukansan:** Used in slight excess pattern patients who have involuntary movement such as epilepsy, epilepsy-like spasms, childhood febrile convulsion, cramps and spasms in the eyelids, face, and limbs, as well as tremors and tics. Typical patients are oversensitive and short-tempered with a tendency toward irritability. *Yokukansankachimpihange* is effective for patients with gastrointestinal weakness and strongly palpable pulsation of the abdominal aorta (palpitation in the supra-umbilical region). Also effective for patients with intense muscle rigidity as seen in Parkinson's disease and Parkinsonian syndrome.
- **Saikokeishito:** Appropriate in slight deficiency to medium pattern patients with spasm and various involuntary movements observed in epilepsy. Typical patients have weak abdominal tone, fullness and discomfort in the

chest and hypochondrium, and palpitation in the supra-umbilical region.

- **Chotosan:** Can be expected to improve microcirculatory disorder because it contains *chotoko* that is effective for spasm [53]. Used for vascular parkinsonism in relatively older and medium pattern patients with slight tremor and rigidity.
- **Keishikaryukotsuboreito:** Used for spasms and tics aggravated by mental stress in slight deficiency pattern patients with weak abdominal tone and strong palpitation in the supra-umbilical region.
- **Saikokaryukotsuboreito:** Used for epileptic seizures and involuntary movement in slight excess pattern patients with psychoneurotic symptoms (including anxiety and irritation), normal or stronger abdominal tone, fullness and discomfort in the chest and hypochondrium, and palpitation in the supra-umbilical region.
- **Kanbakutaisoto:** A formula for hysteria attacks in slight deficiency pattern female patients. Used for similar involuntary movements, including spasms and tics.

5.4 Eczema, Urticaria, and Pruritus

Masaru Natsuaki

5.4.1 Overview of Disease

Eczema

Eczema, more precisely, is a general name for a group of diseases called "the eczema/dermatitis group." Clinically, it is associated with itchy sensations and emerges in various forms of exanthema, including erythema, papules, vesicles, pustules, erosion, crust, scale, and lichenification, and in various types of diseases, including contact dermatitis, seborrheic dermatitis, atopic dermatitis, nummular eczema, asteatotic dermatitis, stasis dermatitis, etc.

Urticaria

Urticaria (hives) is a transiently developing wheal or erythema caused by activation of dermal mast cells and is associated with severe itching. Individual exanthemas disappear within one to 24 h. The causes include food, pathogenic microbes, and physical irritation. In most chronic cases, the triggers are mental stress and fatigue.

Pruritus

Pruritus is a condition with no eruption associated with only an itchy sensation. However, it may be associated with eczematous lesions due to intense scratching. Senile pruritus is common due to aging-related impaired skin function but may reflect internal organ disease. Therefore, care must be taken to screen for conditions including diabetes, liver and kidney dysfunction, and malignancy in internal organs.

5.4.2 Indications for Kampo Therapy

The causes of the condition must be identified first in every case and be avoided or eliminated. In Western medicine, the basic treatments include the use of antihistamines for itching and topical steroids for inflammation control. External antifungal medications are appropriate for seborrheic dermatitis, and external tacrolimus or delgocitinib medications and dupilumab as a biological drug for atopic dermatitis.

In those cases in which the cause is not identified, however, Kampo therapy is indicated when standard treatment is not effective and the condition becomes chronic and intractable. The selection of formulas should not rely on deficiency or excess of physical strength but rather focus on therapy for improvement of symptoms (branch treatment) by assessment of the symptoms (exanthema) appearing on the skin as a "local pattern." Depending on the symptoms, two kinds of formulas are used concomitantly (combination of formulas). Thus, the individual patient's constitution is determined as a general pattern, and the constitution is improved (root treatment). Impaired autonomic nervous system and infection defense mechanism, regarded as qi deficiency, are treated with qi-tonifying formulas, whereas blood[TM1] tonifying formulas and cold-dispelling formulas are selected for blood[TM1] deficiency and cold constitutions. In cases where symptoms do not improve with Kampo medicines alone, combined use of antihistamines and topical steroids is preferable.

5.4.3 Frequently Used Formulas (Table 5.9)

The guideline for selecting therapeutic formulas with a focus on cutaneous symptoms classified by heat, fluid[TM1] retention, blood[TM1] deficiency, and blood stasis (not relying on deficiency or excess patterns) is shown in Table 1. Unfortunately, there is little high-level evidence for the effectiveness of each formula for the stated symptom, but these are experience-based selections of formulas with a long-time history in Kampo therapy.

Eczema

- **Byakkokaninjinto:** Often used for facial erythema in atopic dermatitis associated with hot sensation (flushing).
- **Orengedokuto:** Appropriate for patients having erythema with severe itching and heat sensation.
- **Jumihaidokuto:** Used for papules, pustules, etc. Also good for acne and folliculitis.
- **Eppikajutsuto:** Effective for exanthema with exudative tendency, associated with erythema and vesicles.
- **Shofusan:** Used for erythema, vesicles, exudate, crust, scale, and skin dryness.
- **Keishibukuryogan:** A typical blood[TM1] stasis resolving formula, used for shoulder stiffness, coldness in the limbs, and irregular menstruation. Particularly effective for

Table 5.9 Frequently used Kampo formulas for eczema, urticaria, and pruritus

Heat	Erythema, hot sensation in the face	Byakkokaninjinto
	Erythema, pruritus	Orengedokuto
	Papules, pustules	Jumihaidokuto
	Erythema, vesicles, exudate	Eppikajutsuto
	Wheals, constipation	Inchinkoto
Fluid[TM1] retention	Erythema, exudate, crust, scale	Shofusan
	Vesicles, edema, wheals	Inchingoreisan
Blood[TM1] deficiency	Skin dryness, pruritus	Tokiinshi
	Skin dryness, loss of vigor, coldness in the limbs	Juzentaihoto
Blood[TM1] stasis	Lichenification, pigmentation	Keishibukuryogan
	Lichenification, pigmentation, constipation	Tokakujokito

patients suffering from chronic exanthema with intense lichenification or pigmentation.

- **Tokakujokito:** Useful for patients with blood[TM1] stasis who have constipation, irregular menstruation, or mental anxiety.
- **Hochuekkito:** A typical qi-tonifying formula used to improve qi deficiency pattern. The long-term oral use for atopic dermatitis can effectively reduce the amount of topical steroid [54].
- **Juzentaihoto:** Used to improve both qi deficiency and blood[TM1] deficiency patterns, as well as loss of vigor, coldness in the limbs, and skin dryness.
- **Saikoseikanto:** Effective for chronic eczematous lesions in children who are prone to tonsillitis or lymphadenitis.
- **Ogikenchuto:** Used to improve constitution in nervous infants and children with repetitive infections.
- **Goreisan:** Used for patients who have local exudate with general thirst, reduced urine volume, and a tendency for edema.

Urticaria

- **Makyokansekito:** Used for alleviation of symptoms in acute urticaria.
- **Inchinkoto:** Effective for urticaria accompanied by constipation in patients with thirst and reduced urine volume.
- **Inchingoreisan:** Effective for urticaria with the tendency of severe edema in patients with thirst and reduced urine volume.
- **Maobushisaishinto:** First choice for cold urticaria.
- **Saikokaryukotsuboreito:** Appropriate for patients with qi stagnation pattern having insomnia and irritability.

Pruritus

- **Tokiinshi:** First choice for senile pruritus. Appropriate for patients who have slight skin dryness and pruritus with little inflammation findings (erythema or papules).
- **Goshajinkigan:** For elderly patients with a tendency to get cold in the lower body and with weakness in the lower abdominal region. Most appropriate for patients with lower limb numbness and itching associated with diabetes.
- **Orengedokuto:** Sometimes used successfully for pruritus with underlying disease such as renal failure.

6 Psychiatric Symptoms

6.1 Depressive State, Anxiety, and Insomnia

Hironobu Iguchi

6.1.1 Depressive State

Overview of Disease

According to the standardized diagnostic criteria (DSM-V [55] and ICD-11 [56]), a diagnosis of "depressive state" is made if the state associated with core symptoms—such as a depressed mood, a loss of interest or pleasure, decreased energy, proneness to fatigue, and decreased activity, as well as pessimism, loss of concentration and determination, anxiety and agitation, suicidal ideation, insomnia, and anorexia—lasts for at least 2 weeks, and if it hinders daily activities. A depressive state is commonly observed not only in so-called depression that primarily presents depressive state symptoms—major depressive disorder according to DSM-V, but also in psychiatric disorders, physical disorders, and drug use. In the latter cases, treatment for the primary disease is preferable.

DSM-V: Diagnostic and Statistical Manual of Mental Disorders 4th edition

ICD-11: International Statistical Classification of Diseases and Related Health Problems

Indications for Kampo Therapy

Among major depressive disorders, less severe conditions are considered good targets for Kampo therapy. These include mild conditions in which patients have no suicidal ideation and are able to endeavor partially to work and do housework and mild depressive states that do not meet the criteria for major depressive disorder (termed minor depressive disorder, for which the efficacy of general antidepressants has not been demonstrated). Once major depressive disorder reaches the intermediate or more severe stage, there is a particularly high risk of suicide. In this case, therapy should not consist of Kampo medicines alone. The combined use of antidepressants and Kampo medicines, however, is possible under the supervision of a psychiatrist. In cases where general antidepressant therapy is not effective, the situation may be improved by the additional administration of Kampo Formulas according to the pattern as those listed below.

Frequently Used Formulas (Table 5.10)

The pathologic conditions considered to be depressive states in Kampo medicine include those in which "internal causes" (sorrow, anxiety, pensiveness, anger, fear) arise with overwork and worry and in which qi stagnation and qi deficiency appear. In addition, patients can be presumed to have problems with heat/cold, fluid[TM1] retention, blood[TM1] stasis and blood[TM1] deficiency, as well as heart[TM1], liver[TM1], spleen[TM1] or kidney[TM1] issues. In Kampo therapy, these pathologic conditions are taken into consideration in deciding on the formulas suitable for the patient's pattern—this is the key to treatment.

- **Yokukansan**: Appropriate for patients with slight excess pattern who have a marked sense of agitation, including irritability and short temper, associated with eyelid spasms, trembling in the limbs (liver[TM1] agitation), and insomnia. If in addition, gastrointestinal symptoms are notable, the use of *yokukansankachimpihange* is recommended.
- **Kamikihito**: Effective for patients with slight deficiency or medium pattern who have marked loss of vigor, anxiety, heart palpitations, and insomnia. *Kihito* is an option if anxiety, agitation, and heat sensation are not prominent.
- **Hangekobokuto**: For patients with medium pattern who have symptoms of qi stagnation, such as obstructive discomfort in the throat and fullness in the chest, in association with anxiety, heart palpitations, dizziness, and insomnia. Also, patients tend to have abdominal splashing sounds and epigastric stuffiness. If gastroesophageal reflux disease is also present, *bukuryoingohangekobokuto* is indicated.
- **Kososan**: It is used for patients with slight deficiency pattern who tend to have depressive moods with headache and anorexia. This formula has a regulating effect on menstruation and is often used for women.
- **Saibokuto**: This formula is a mixture of *hangekobokuto* and *shosaikoto*. It's used for patients with a medium pattern who have symptoms of fullness and discomfort in the chest and hypochondrium in addition to the symptoms for which *hangekobokuto* is indicated. For example, it is thought to be effective in cases with asthma symptoms that are aggravated by stress and are accompanied by insomnia at night.
- **Kamishoyosan**: This formula is indicated for slight deficiency pattern patients with various physical complaints, including a tendency to fatigue, headache, and shoulder stiffness, as well as paroxysmal heat sensation in the upper body and sweating in association with anxiety, agitation, and insomnia. This formula is frequently used for patients with menopausal syndrome or premenstrual syndrome who also have blood[TM1] stasis.
- **Rikkunshito**: For patients with deficiency to slight deficiency pattern who have a feeling of enervation and postprandial bloating/fullness. If these symptoms are accompanied by fullness and discomfort in the chest and hypochondrium, *chikujountanto* is suggested. If general malaise is marked, *hochuekkito* is recommended.
- **Chotosan**: Effective for depressive states in medium pattern patients with a hypertensive tendency, particularly middle-aged or older. These patients also have chronic headaches (often worse in the morning), dizziness, and stiffness in the neck and shoulders.
- **Hachimijiogan**: Appropriate for middle-aged or older patients with slight deficiency pattern who have a tendency to fatigue, weakness, and pain in the lower body; numbness; coldness; and a tendency to edema; nocturia; and weakness of the lower abdominal region. *Rokumigan* is used for similar younger patients with no coldness.
- **Saikokaryukotsuboreito**: For patients with slight excess pattern who have anxiety, depression, insomnia, flightiness, irritability, and palpitation, with fullness and discomfort in the chest and hypochondrium. *Saikokeishikankyoto* should be used for patients with decreased physical strength, shortness of breath, coldness of the lower extremities, and night sweating.
- **Daisaikoto**: This formula is used for excess pattern patients with prominent fullness and discomfort in the chest and hypochondrium, and it also can be effective for depression and insomnia.
- **Nyoshinsan**: This formula is used for patients with medium to slight excess pattern, especially after childbirth or miscarriage, who are depressed and emotionally unstable. It can also be administered to patients with menopausal depression accompanied by dizziness, flushing, and heart palpitations.
- **Juzentaihoto**: This formula is used for deficiency pattern patients with a tendency to fatigue and malaise, as well as symptoms of blood[TM1] deficiency. It is used for people who are fatigued and weak from a variety of chronic diseases and can be used for depressive states as well.

6.1.2 Anxiety

1. **Overview of Disease**

In the DSM-V, generalized neurosis is classified as "anxiety disorders," such as generalized anxiety disorder, panic disorder, and social anxiety disorder, while psychosomatic anxiety symptoms are classified as "somatic symptoms."

2. **Indications for Kampo Therapy**

Kampo therapy may be tried for mild cases. "Somatic symptoms," in particular, is a condition in which complaints of pain, fatigue, digestive, and respiratory symptoms persist, which cannot be explained by organic abnormalities. This is a situation in which Kampo therapy should be tried as an alternative. Panic disorder, however, is a debilitating disease which presents with physical symptoms, and repeated attacks are often complicated by agoraphobia and depression. Therefore, if Kampo medicine has no effect, it is necessary to introduce evidence-based pharmacotherapy as soon as possible.

3. **Frequently Used Formulas (Table 5.10)**

Because anxiety is often observed together with depression, most formulas listed in the first section on depressive state can also be expected to be effective for anxiety. Qi counter flow and abnormalities of the heart[TM1] are assumed in cases of anxiety in Kampo medicine, and the following formulas can be considered as options. For physical symptoms, many other formulas not listed in Table 5.9 may be tried according to the Kampo medicine patterns.

- **Keishikaryukotsuboreito**: Effective for anxiety associated with flightiness and palpitation, similar to *saikokaryukotsuboreito*; for patients with slight deficiency pattern who have weaker physical strength, coldness in the lower limbs, and no fullness and discomfort in the chest and hypochondrium.
- **Orengedokuto**: Used for anxiety associated with agitation, irritability, and insomnia in patients with slight excess to excess pattern. Patients characteristically have a hypertensive tendency and facial redness. *San'oshashinto* is recommended for patients who also have constipation.
- **Shigyakusan**: Indicated for stomach and intestinal pain and/or discomfort in patients with medium to slight excess pattern. Patients may have fullness and discomfort in the chest and hypochondrium and abdominal muscle tension, accompanied by coldness of the extremities.
- **Hangeshashinto**: Used for patients with medium pattern with epigastric stuffiness and resistance and increased borborygmus, associated with eructation, stomatitis, nausea, loose stools, diarrhea, and other gastrointestinal symptoms.
- **Seishinrenshiin**: Effective for anxiety, insomnia, and depression in patients with slight deficiency pattern and gastrointestinal weakness who chronically complain of anxiety and proneness to fatigue along with residual urine sensation, pollakiuria, and miction pain. They also frequently have coldness in the lower limbs, but they have a red complexion.
- **Ryokeijutsukanto**: Effective for patients with slight deficiency pattern who have vertigo, heart palpitations, dizziness, anxiety, and a tendency to get cold.
- **Sansoninto**: Effective for patients with slight deficiency pattern who have tiredness, flushing, hot flashes, anxiety, restlessness, and difficulty sleeping well.

6.1.3 Insomnia

Overview of Disease: Indications for Kampo Therapy

The causes of insomnia are commonly divided into five categories: physical disorder (cardiac disease, respiratory disease, sleep apnea syndrome, etc.), physiologic insomnia (shift work, inappropriate sleep hygiene, etc.), psychological insomnia (stress, nervousness, and other personality traits, etc.), psychiatric disorder, and pharmacological insomnia (alcohol, caffeine, etc.). The top priorities are assessing the cause and appropriate medical interventions according to identified causes. After this, Kampo therapy is offered to those patients who have insomnia due to psychological causes or psychiatric or physical disorders. When benzodiazepines are not sufficiently effective, concurrent use of Kampo medicines could be helpful.

Frequently Used Formulas (Fig. 5.26)

Basically, sleep disturbance often has anxiety, depression, or related physical symptoms in the background. Therefore, improving depression, anxiety, or physical symptoms with the formulas listed in previous sections—A) Depressive State and B) Anxiety—can be expected to effectively treat insomnia. While Kampo medicines cannot be expected to have a direct hypnotic sedative action like benzodiazepines, continued oral administration two to three times a day will have good indirect effects for sleep disorders. However, since a mild sedation can be observed after oral administration of Kampo formulas [57], the nighttime and early morning doses may be taken before going to bed or upon awakening in the middle of the night or early in the morning. The following general categorization may be useful in selecting a formula: sleep-onset insomnia (mainly due to nervousness and anxiety), sound-sleep disorder (mainly due to anxiety and depression), and early morning awakening (mainly due to aging). Kampo Formulas that are expected to be particularly effective for insomnia are selected and pre-

Table 5.10 Frequently used Kampo formulas for depression and anxiety

Qi stagnation pattern	Kososan (slight deficiency pattern)	Cases with a tendency of depressed mood, and women with mild symptoms
	Hangekobokuto (medium pattern)	Uncomfortable feeling in the throat, nausea in addition to these symptoms, bukuryoingouhangekoubokuto is used for patients with gastroesophageal reflux disease
	Rikkunshito (slight deficiency pattern—deficiency pattern)	Abdominal bloating after eating, loss of appetite
Qi counter flow pattern	Ryokeijutsukanto (deficiency pattern)	Heart palpitations, dizziness, unsteadiness when standing up, easy to become cold
	Keishikaryukotsuboreito (slight deficiency pattern)	Anxiety, easily startled, easy to become cold
Psychological problems (anxiety, agitation)	Orengedokuto (slight excess pattern—excess pattern)	Anxiety, agitation, insomnia, heat pattern, tendency to hypertension
	Hangeshashinto (medium pattern)	Epigastric stuffiness and resistance, abdominal rumbling. Diarrhea, stomatitis
	Nyoshinsan (medium pattern—slight excess pattern)	Feeling of heat in the upper part of the body and cold in the lower part, dizziness, heart palpitations, emotional instability after childbirth
	Seishinrenshiin (slight deficiency pattern)	Psychoneurotic residual urine, complaints of frequent urination
	Chikujountanto (medium pattern)	Loss of appetite, restlessness, sleeplessness, cough, slightly warm tendency
Liver[TM1] problems (over-tension, irritability, depression)	Shigyakusan (medium pattern—slight excess pattern)	Fullness and discomfort in chest and hypochondrium, abdominal muscle tension, psychological gastrointestinal symptoms
	Saikokaryukotsuboreito (slight excess pattern)	Fullness and discomfort in chest and hypochondrium, anxiety, heart palpitations, easily startled
	Daisaikoto (excess pattern)	Fullness and discomfort in chest and hypochondrium, nausea, constipation
	Kamishoyosan (slight deficiency pattern)	Blood stasis pattern, easy fatigue, headache, stiff shoulders, tendency to feel cold and also have hot flashes
	Chotosan (slight deficiency pattern)	For post-middle age people, hypertension, headache worse in the morning, irascibility
	Yokukansan (slight excess pattern) Yokukansankachimpihange (slight deficiency pattern)	Irritability, eyelid spasms, gritting of teeth, face, or limb spasms if gastrointestinal symptoms are noticeable, use yokukansankachimpihange
Blood[TM1] deficiency pattern and qi deficiency pattern	Kamikihito (slight deficiency pattern—medium pattern) Kihito (slight deficiency pattern)	Loss of energy and appetite, anxiety, agitation, insomnia, amnesia, kihito is used when anxiety and agitation are low
	Sansoninto (slight deficiency pattern)	Mental and physical fatigue, feeling of body heat, anxiety, insomnia
	Hochuekkito (slight deficiency pattern)	Loss of appetite, sluggishness in the hands and feet, slight fever tendency
	Juzentaihoto (deficiency pattern)	Fatigue accompanied by blood[TM1] deficiency pattern, chronic symptoms
Kidney[TM1] deficiency	Hachimijiogan (slight deficiency pattern) Rokumigan (slight deficiency pattern)	For post-middle age patients, easy to fatigue, pain in lower half of the body, tendency to get cold; rokumigan is suitable for younger patients with no tendency of cold

sented in Table 5.1. For explanations of the formulas, please refer to previous sections on (A) Depressive State and (B) Anxiety.

6.2 Dementia and Abnormal Behavior

Eiichi Tahara

6.2.1 Overview of Disease

Dementia includes a range of diseases, primarily Alzheimer's disease, vascular dementia, and a mixture of these two. The core symptoms are memory disorder, disorientation, diminished thinking and calculation ability, and impaired judgment. Peripheral signs, otherwise termed behavioral and psychological symptoms of dementia (BPSD), are gaining attention. They include characteristic psychological symptoms (anxiety, excitement, depression, hallucinations, delusions, misperceptions, etc.) and behavioral disorders (wandering, untidiness, hyperactivity, sexually deviant behavior, etc.).

6.2.2 Indications for Kampo Therapy

Kampo medicines are used for dementia in general, but the best indication is BPSD. Spleen[TM1] and kidney[TM1] tonifying formulas such as *hachimijiogan* and *hochuekkito* improve

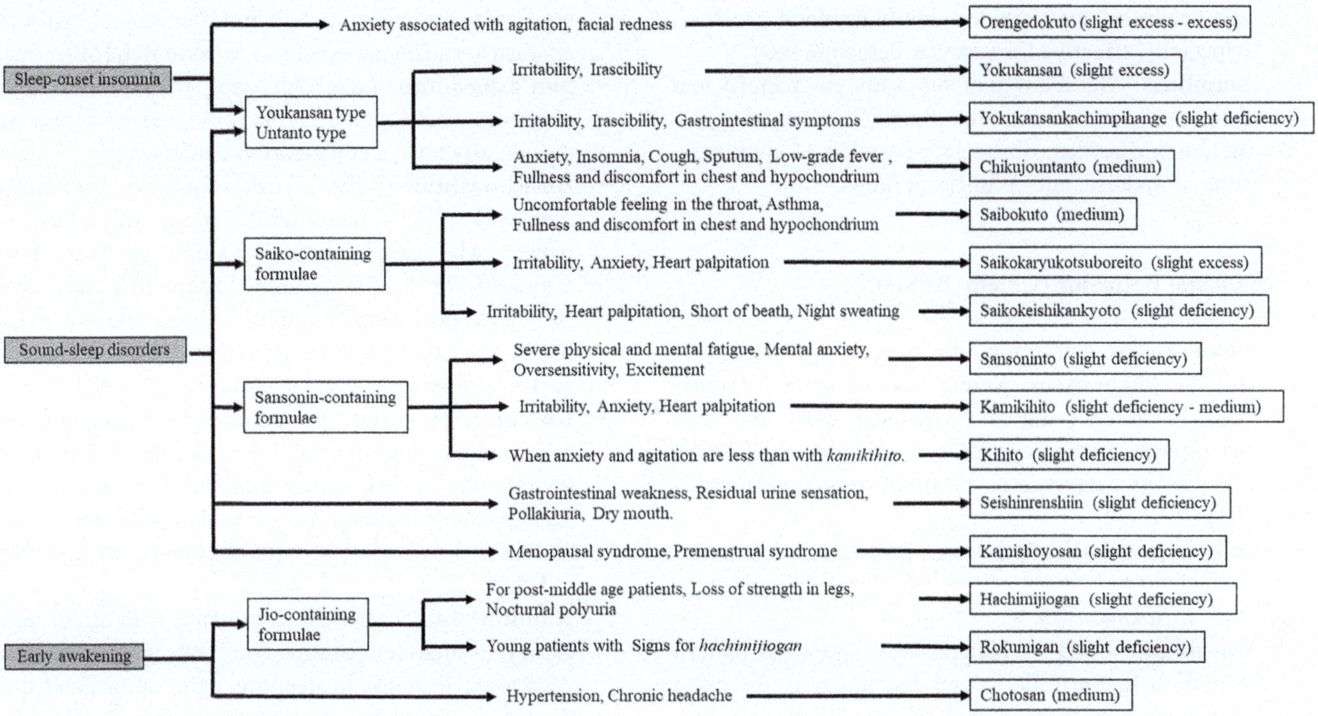

Fig. 5.26 Frequently used formulas for insomnia

qi deficiency and qi stagnation in those with depressive tendencies, mental anxiety, insomnia, impatience, etc. *Yokukansan* and *orengedokuto* are used for short temper and mental restlessness caused by liver[TM1] and heart[TM1] imbalance. Kampo formulas are extremely helpful because, unlike Western drug therapy, they don't cause central nervous system inhibition, aspiration pneumonia, or risk of falling.

6.2.3 Frequently Used Formulas

1. **Dementia**

- **Hachimijiogan**: A basic formula for yin pattern elderly patients with slight deficiency pattern. Effective for weakness, coldness, and numbness in the lower body; urinary disorder (such as nocturnal enuresis); weakness in the lower abdomen; mild tendency of edema; and coldness or heat with agitation in the limbs. This formula is sometimes taken concurrently or in combination with *ninjinto*. If coldness is marked, *bushi* is added [58].
- **Goshajinkigan**: Patients present a slightly more deficient pattern than those indicated for *hachimijiogan* and have a pronounced tendency of edema.
- **Hochuekkito**: One of the formulas containing *ninjin* and ogi (so-called *jingizai* in Japanese). Effective for patients with slight deficiency pattern. Used for general malaise, anorexia, low-grade fever, night sweating, visceral ptosis tendency, and lack of vitality in speech and eyes.
- **Rikkunshito**: Appropriate for patients with yin pattern and deficiency to slight deficiency pattern. They have impaired gastrointestinal function, anorexia, epigastric fullness, thick tongue fur, and splashing sounds in abdomen [59].
- **Shikunshito**: Used for patients with a more pronounced deficiency pattern than *rikkunshito*. They have general malaise, loss of appetite, poor complexion, and impaired gastrointestinal function. It is like *rikkunshito* but markedly effective in patients with qi deficiency, associated with a slight splashing sound and tongue fur.
- **Tokishakuyakusan**: Effective for patients with yin pattern and slight deficiency pattern. They have signs of blood[TM1] deficiency, static blood[TM1], and fluid[TM1] retention, associated with headache, dizziness, or edema. May be used in combination with *ninjinto* or *bushi*.
- **Keishibukuryogan**: Appropriate for patients with yang pattern and medium to slight excess pattern, who commonly have hot flashes with facial redness. Sometimes they have resistance and tenderness in the lower abdomen. Especially effective for patients suspected to have an underlying cerebrovascular disorder.
- **Chotosan**: Offered to patients with yang pattern and medium pattern. Generally used for shoulder stiffness

and headache due to underlying high blood pressure. Especially effective for vascular dementia [60].

- **Shimbuto:** Good for patients with yin pattern and deficiency pattern who have fluid[TM1] retention signs, including diarrhea, dizziness, sensation of shakiness, general malaise, and coldness in limbs.

2. **Abnormal Behavior (Chiefly BPSD)**

- **Yokukansan**: Appropriate for patients with yang pattern and slight excess pattern who are irritable, impatient, insomniac, and easily agitated. They may also have spasms in their eyelids, face, or limbs. Sometimes it is used by caregivers as a form of stress management [61].
- **Yokukansankachimpihange**: Effective for patients with slight deficiency pattern who have similar symptoms to *yokukansan.*
- **Daisaikoto**: Used for patients with an excess pattern who have severe fullness and discomfort in the chest and hypochondrium as well as constipation; sometimes associated with shoulder stiffness, heavy-headedness, dizziness, tinnitus, nausea, vomiting, depressive mood, nervous tension, and/or abdominal muscle tension.
- **Saikokaryukotsuboreito**: Effective for patients with a slight excess pattern who have relatively severe fullness and discomfort in the chest and hypochondrium, accompanied by anxiety, insomnia, and irritability. They may have strong pulsation in the abdominal aorta, heavy-headedness, headache, shoulder stiffness, or depressed mood.
- **Saikokeishikankyoto**: Appropriate for patients with slight deficiency pattern. Used for fatigue and malaise, palpitations, shortness of breath, or insomnia. They may suffer from upper heat and lower cold, sweating in the head, night sweating, thirst, lip dryness, nightmares, or slight fullness and discomfort in the chest and hypochondrium.
- **Kamishoyosan**: Used for patients with slight deficiency pattern, who have a tendency to fatigue, nervous anxiety, insomnia, irritability, or short temper. Associated with various symptoms including shoulder stiffness, headache, dizziness, burning sensation in the upper body, paroxysmal sweating, and skin formication. Proximate to *saikokeishikankyoto* but patients are differentiated by the tendency of fever and static blood[TM1].
- **Orengedokuto**: Appropriate for patients with yang pattern and slight excess to excess pattern who have hot flash tendency with facial redness, nervous anxiety, insomnia, and impatience. Often associated with epigastric stuffiness, epistaxis, or skin itch [62].
- **San'oshashinto**: Good for yang pattern and slight excess to excess pattern. Like *orengedokuto*, patients specifically have a constipation tendency.
- **Bushishashinto:**[24] This is *san'oshashinto* with *bushi.* Appropriate for patients with Yin pattern and excess pattern who have psychiatric symptoms like those indicated for *san'oshashinto*, except that they have somewhat poor facial complexion and coldness in the limbs. Patients may complain of stuffiness in the epigastric region when constipated.
- **Unseiin**: Appropriate for patients with yang pattern and medium pattern who have blood[TM1] deficiency (symptoms treated with *shimotsuto*) in addition to *orengedokuto* indications. They also have hot flashes and mental restlessness, with obviously dry and dark red skin.
- **Kamiuntanto:**[25] Offered to patients with slight deficiency to medium pattern, who have gastrointestinal weakness, difficulty in sleeping, palpitations, and startle easily. Effective against short temper, sense of urgency, and uneasiness.
- **Kamikihito**: Appropriate for patients with a slight deficiency pattern or medium pattern who have gastrointestinal weakness. They have a tendency of fatigue-induced bleeding and anemia, resulting in neurosis and amnesia. Sometimes associated with a tendency to have fever, irritability, impatience, or anxiety.
- **Shishishito:**[19] Effective for patients with deficiency pattern, who have precordial agony, insomnia, mental restlessness, and heat sensation in the chest. Some patients may complain of a downward pulling sensation on the shoulders, as though sinking, particularly in the morning. There are various *shishishito* variations for coexisting symptoms: *shishikankyoto*[18] for cold, *shishikanzoto*[18] for shallow breathing, *shishikobokuto*[18] for chest agitation with abdominal fullness, *shishishokyoshito*[18] for nausea, and so on.
- **Kihito**: Offered to patients with slight deficiency pattern who have gastrointestinal weakness. *Kihito* indications are similar to kamikihito indications, but *kihito* patients have no fever signs. Patients are likely to have

[24]Not available as a medical Kampo extract formulation or an OTC Kampo extract formulation.

Bushishashinto: daio 1.0, oren, ogon, bushi 0.5.
Shishikankyoto: sanshishi, kankyo 2.0.
Shishikanzoshito: sanshishi 3.0, koshi 5.0, kanzo 1.0.
Shishikobokuto: sanshishi 3.0, koboku 4.0, kijitsu 2.0.
Shishishokyoshito: sanshishi 3.0, koshi 4.0, shokyo 4.0.

[25]Not available as a medical Kampo extract formulation.

bleeding or anemia from overwork, causing neurosis and forgetfulness [63].

- **Kososan**: Appropriate for patients with deficiency pattern, associated with anorexia, gastrointestinal symptoms such as upper abdominal fullness, anxiety, insomnia, headache, and qi stagnation symptoms such as depressed mood.
- **Hangekobokuto**: Effective for patients with medium pattern, who have depressive tendencies. They complain of blocked throat sensation, sullen mood, insomnia, nervous anxiety, etc. Often used concomitantly with f formulas of involving Bupleurum radix.
- **Kanbakutaisoto**: Effective for patients with slight deficiency pattern, who have oversensitivity, general or local muscle rigidity/spasm, yawning and insomnia, pessimism, or fits of agitation.
- **Sansoninto:** Effective for patients with slight deficiency pattern, who have insomnia which is induced by severe physical and mental fatigue due to underlying anemia tendencies. This is sometimes associated with mental anxiety, oversensitivity, and overexcitement.
- **Keishikaryukotsuboreito:** Effective for patients with slight deficiency pattern, who complain of oversensitivity or mental anxiety. They may also have strong pulsation in the abdominal aorta, a tendency to fatigue, and night sweats. Also considered the formula for *saikokaryukotsuboreito* indications with different constitutions (deficiency pattern). May be effective for deviant sexual behavior in elderly people. In this case, pulsation in the abdominal aorta is not necessarily palpable [64].
- **Tokakujokito**: A typical blood[TM1] stasis resolving formula for slight excess to excess pattern patients who have hot flashes, headaches, dizziness, insomnia, agitation, and other symptoms in addition to constipation. Tenderness in the sigmoid colon region or resistance and sharp tenderness in the left iliac region is characteristic (lower abdominal cramp).

7 Whole Body

7.1 Fatigue and Malaise

Shinji Nishida

7.1.1 Overview of Disease

The origins of fatigue and malaise are very diverse. Acute diseases involve infection, dehydration, and electrolyte abnormalities. Chronic diseases involve organic pathologic changes, as seen in visceral diseases (affecting the kidneys and liver and the respiratory, endocrine, and cardiovascular systems) as well as blood disease, malignant tumors, collagen disease, chronic inflammatory disease, and neuromuscular disease. Chronic diseases also lead to mood disorders (such as depression) and psychiatric disorders (such as anxiety disorder). There are many pathological conditions (i.e., psychosomatic diseases), however, in which psychiatric and physical symptoms appear together and affect each other.

Recently a relevant concept of functional somatic syndrome (FSS) has been proposed. FSS is defined as "pathological conditions in which the existence of organic diseases cannot be explained in specific terms, despite thorough testing and examination." The chief symptoms include fatigue, pain (headache, joint pain, and muscle pain), palpitation, dizziness, and digestive symptoms. FSS includes irritable bowel syndrome, dysmenorrhea, fibromyalgia, jaw arthropathy, multiple chemical sensitivity, tension-type headache, and chronic fatigue syndrome. FSS is also associated with a high incidence of psychoneurotic symptoms such as depression and anxiety. Many sufferers have complex psychosocial backgrounds and find it difficult to build a satisfactory doctor-patient relationship. FSS must be treated as a psychosomatic disease in many patients.

Therefore, it is important for patients who complain of chronic fatigue and malaise not only to exclude organic disease but also to take a dual approach of addressing both psychological and physical aspects [65].

7.1.2 Indications for Kampo Therapy

Kampo therapy is appropriate for people suffering chronic fatigue or malaise if no organic disease has been found. This is the disease group that is equivalent to FSS. Among these, the typical disease is chronic fatigue syndrome. The recommended treatments include pharmacotherapy with vitamin C, melatonin, and antidepressants, as well as nondrug therapies such as cognitive behavior therapy. Tonic formulas such as *hochuekkito* and *juzentaihoto* are also considered effective.

In diseases that cause fatigue, there are not only the pathoconditions of qi deficiency and blood[TM1] deficiency that require tonic formulas, but often there are other conditions like qi stagnation and qi counter flow as well.

For actual differentiation of diseases, patients with depression or irritability as well as fatigue may generally be considered to have qi depression (*Kiutsu*). Those who complain of fatigue alone, rather than psychoneurotic symptoms, may mostly be considered to have qi deficiency. A point to note on differentiation is that qi stagnation often gets worse in the morning and at the start of the week, whereas qi deficiency commonly gets worse in the afternoon and at the end of the week.

Antidepressants, tranquilizers, and the like, as well as Kampo medicines, exhibit a certain efficacy in the treatment of qi stagnation. There are no therapeutic drugs in Western medicine for qi deficiency, which makes it a good target for Kampo therapy.

7.1.3 Frequently Used Formulas (Fig. 5.27)

Irritability or Depression-associated Fatigue and Malaise

- **Daisaikoto**: For patients with excess pattern and plump features. They appear to feel impatient but complain of their symptoms in a modest manner. Their complaints are mostly physical symptoms (malaise, shoulder stiffness, stomach pain, abdominal pain, constipation, etc.). Patients answer questions about psychoneurotic symptoms if asked, but relatively few patients regard psychoneurotic symptoms as their chief complaint. The abdominal pattern includes extreme fullness and discomfort in the chest and hypochondrium, epigastric stuffiness and resistance, and abdominal muscle tension.
- **Saikokaryukotsuboreito**: For patients with slight excess pattern who complain of depressed mood, impatience, and other psychoneurotic symptoms in addition to physical symptoms such as palpitations, lightheadedness, and headaches. In many cases, patients are suffering stress from unavoidable life situations, including workplace relations and care problems. The abdominal pattern includes marked fullness and discomfort in the chest and hypochondrium and pulsation of the abdominal aorta.
- **Saikokeishikankyoto**: For patients with slight deficiency pattern with abdominal pattern characterized by weak abdominal strength, tenderness directly below the sternal xiphoid process, and palpitation in the supra-umbilical region. Fullness and discomfort in the chest and hypochondrium are virtually imperceptible. Patients write in great detail about chief complaints, though extremely varied, on the history-taking questionnaire. In terms of character tendency, this formula is considered effective for patients who say, "I cheerfully look after guests when they visit but feel exhausted after they leave." Many patients like this are resistant to taking psychoactive drugs or cannot take such drugs because of lightheadedness after medication.
- **Kamikihito**: For patients with slight deficiency to medium pattern with poor complexion and intense depressive symptoms rather than impatience. Patients characteristically have sleep disorders (especially light sleep and profuse dreaming).

Fatigue and Malaise with Few Psychoneurotic Symptoms

- **Hochuekkito**: Used in slight deficiency pattern patients with symptoms such as drowsiness after meals, weak eyes, a heavy feeling in the limbs as though they will fall off, atony, low-grade fever (unidentified fever), and proneness to colds. Abdominal strength is medium or weaker. Effective for chronic fatigue syndrome in patients who have absolutely no psychoneurotic problems and for elderly patients with mild depression who experience malaise after taking antidepressants [66].
- **Rikkunshito**: Used for deficiency to slight deficiency pattern patients who complain of early satiety after meals. Abdominal strength is feeble, and a splashing sound is present. These findings are virtually equivalent to the postprandial distress syndrome of functional dyspepsia (FD).
- **Seishoekkito**: Used for slight deficiency pattern patients who have heat sensation, thirst, diarrhea, and weight loss in summer. Abdominal strength is medium to slightly weak.
- **Juzentaihoto**: Used for deficiency pattern patients with malaise who also have blurred vision, hair loss, and skin dryness. That is, qi deficiency in addition to blood[TM1] deficiency. Often effective as an adjunct therapy after malignant tumor surgery. Although *juzentaihoto* is used in patients with medium to weak abdominal strength, this does not apply in its use as an adjunct therapy for malignant tumors [67].
- **Ninjin'yoeito**: Used for slight patients deficiency pattern. Indications are similar to *juzentaihoto*, but the abdominal pattern often includes epigastric stuffiness and resistance. The constituent herbs suggest that this formula is more effective in patients with respiratory symptoms.
- **Tokishakuyakusan**: Used for slight deficiency pattern patients who have gastrointestinal weakness and blood[TM1] deficiency symptoms such as hypomenorrhea and hair loss, as well as fluid[TM1] retention such as edema. The abdominal pattern often includes splashing sounds and tender points indicative of blood[TM1] stasis.
- **Shimbuto**: Used for deficiency pattern patients who feel coldness, tend to have loose bowels, and have fluid[TM1] retention signs such as dizziness and edema. Abdominal strength is weak.

Fatigue and Malaise Largely Due to Constitution and Aging

- **Shokenchuto**: Used for slight deficiency pattern patients who are likely to suffer stress-related stomach trouble and cannot gain weight. This is used in irritable bowel syndrome cases. Abdominal examination shows strong muscle tension.
- **Ogikenchuto**: Used for deficiency pattern patients with excessive sweating and chronic inflammation of the skin. *Ogikenchuto* may be used for pressure sores not only for

Fig. 5.27 Frequently used Kampo formulas for fatigue and malaise

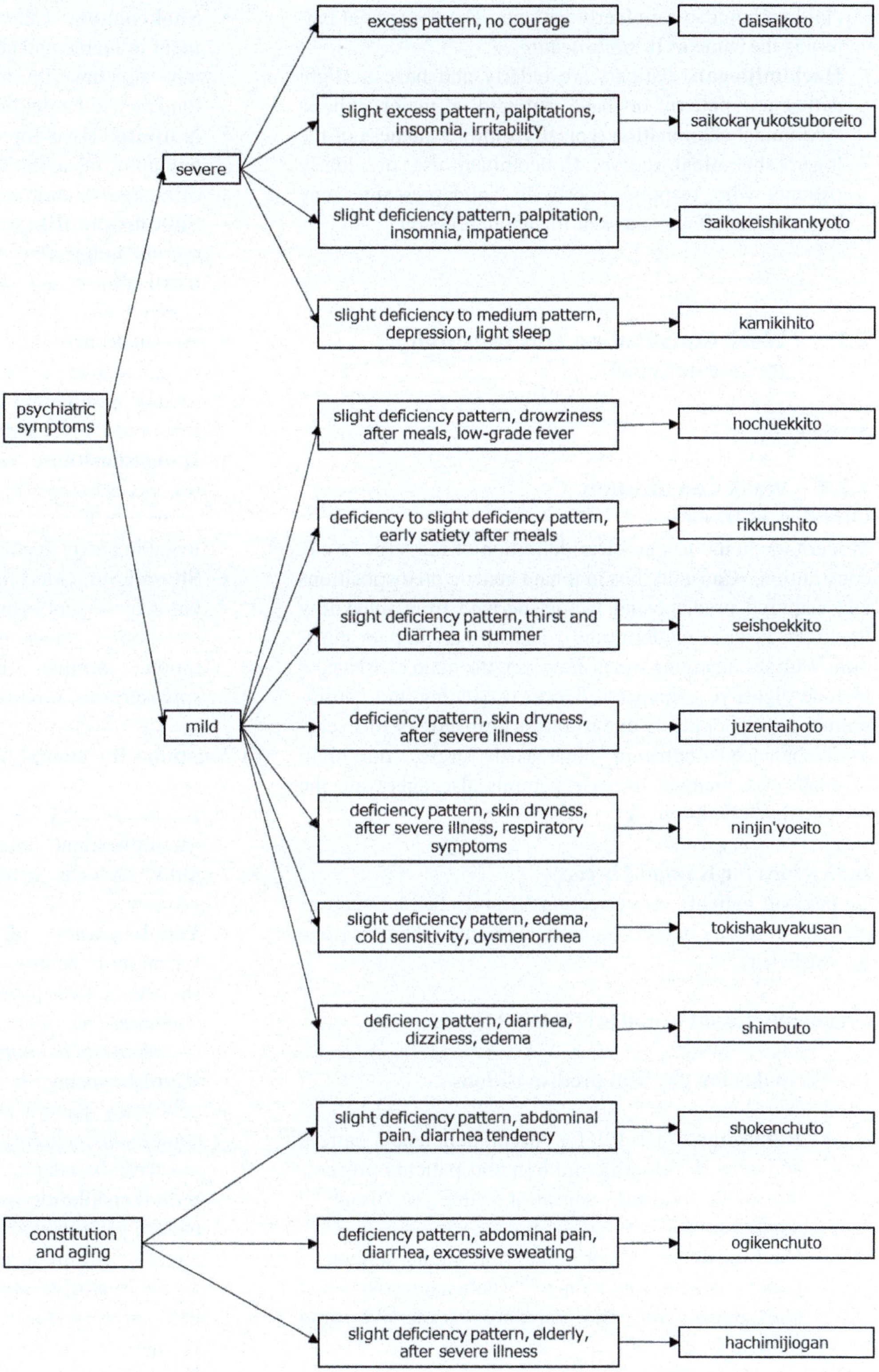

children but also for elderly patients. The abdominal pattern is the same as in *shokenchuto*.

- **Hachimijiogan**: Patients are elderly and have a slight deficiency pattern or have suffered a major illness. Abdominal examination typically shows weakness of the lower abdominal region. Concomitant use in elderly patients who respond poorly to antidepressants may improve the effectiveness of the antidepressant.

7.2 Weak Constitution and Sensitivity to Coldness [68]

Kenshu Lai

7.2.1 Weak Constitution

Overview of Disease

Modern medicine has no clear definition of the term "weak constitution." Causality lies in innate genetic predispositions and acquired predisposing factors derived from unhealthy lifestyles. Prior to modern times, causality lay in poor nutrition. With the changing times, however, the main causes now include digestive exhaustion due to overeating and cardiopulmonary hypokinesia due to physical inactivity or excessive/unbalanced nutrition. Increased stress, day-night reversal, and changed lifestyle patterns also aggravate the pathological conditions.

Indications for Kampo Therapy

Counseling patients on correcting lifestyle factors such as diet and everyday habits is important; Kampo therapy alone is insufficient.

Frequently Used Formulas (Table 5.11)

(a) **Formulas for physical predispositions**

- **Rokumigan**: Useful for slight deficiency pattern and slow-developing children and patients presenting with burning sensations due to fluid[TM1] depletion.
- **Hachimijiogan**: Appropriate for slight deficiency pattern patients with kidney[TM1] deficiency associated with aging and cold dampness (excessive fluid intake).
- **Shimbuto**: Used for deficiency pattern patients with symptoms caused by cold dampness (lightheadedness, diarrhea, etc.) or hypometabolism due to aging or chronic debilitating disease, in addition to gastrointestinal weakness.
- **Shokenchuto**: Effective for constitutional improvement in feeble and slight deficiency pattern. Patients, who also have lip dryness, nasal hemorrhage, and a tendency to be ticklish.
- **Ninjinto**: Used for deficiency pattern patients who complain of anorexia, hypersalivation, watery nasal discharge, or stomach pain when exposed to cold.
- **Shikunshito/Rikkunshito**: Good for anorexia or chronic indigestion. *Shikunshito* is for deficiency pattern patients, and *rikkunshito* is for the slight deficiency pattern patients.
- **Hochuekkito**: Used for slight deficiency pattern patients with constitutional atony (visceroptosis) chronic debilitating conditions with general malaise, low-grade fever, and night sweating.
- **Hangeshashinto**: Used for patients with medium (excess deficiency) pattern. Target signs include epigastric stuffiness, nausea/vomiting, and diarrhea with irritable bowel syndrome.
- **Shosaikoto**: Good for medium pattern. This formula has a biological response modification (BRM) function; long-term use is effective for improving constitution. Similar formulas include *saibokuto*, *saikokeishito*, *saikoseikanto*, and *keigairengyoto*.

(b) **Formulas for mental predispositions**

- **Kososan**: Used for deficiency pattern patients with gastrointestinal sickness and psychosomatic symptoms such as headache, dizziness, and allergic symptoms.
- **Yokukansan/Yokukansankachimpihange**: Used for infantile neurosis, tantrum, or irritability, and for short-tempered patients with slight excess pattern (*yokukansan*) or slight deficiency pattern (*yokukansankachimpihange*).
- **Kamishoyosan**: A typical formula used for slight deficiency pattern patients to alleviate a range of symptoms including irritability, headache, and climacteric disorders.
- **Saikokeishikankyoto**: Effective for slight deficiency pattern patients with head sweating, insomnia, and a tendency toward anxiety.
- **Hangebyakujutsutemmato**: Appropriate for slight deficiency pattern patients with headache and vertigo/dizziness.
- **Kanbakutaisoto**: Good for emotional lability and hysteria in slight deficiency pattern patients.
- **Ryokeijutsukanto**: Used for autonomic imbalance, cardiac neurosis, and anxiety tendency in slight deficiency pattern patients.

Table 5.11 Prescriptions for the weak constitution

Prescriptions for weak constitution		
Name	Deficiency and excess	Signs and symptoms
1. prescription mainly for physical symptoms		
Rokumigan	Slight deficiency	Slow-developing children and patients presenting with burning sensation due to fluid depletion
Hachimijiogan	Slight deficiency	Lower-region deficiency associated with aging and cold dampness (excessive fluid intake)
Shimbuto	Deficiency	Symptoms caused by cold dampness or hypometabolism due to aging or chronic debilitating disease
Shokenchuto	Slight deficiency	Feeble patients with lip dryness, nasal hemorrhage, and ticklishness tendencies
Ninjinto	Deficiency	Anorexia, hypersalivation, watery nasal discharge, or stomach pain when exposed to coldness
Shikunshito	Deficiency	Anorexia or chronic indigestion
Rikkunshito	Deficiency—slight deficiency	Anorexia or chronic indigestion (shikunshito + chimpi, hange)
Hochuekkito	Slight deficiency	Constitutional atony (viseroptosis), chronic debilitating conditions with general malaise, low-grade fever, nocturnal sweating, etc.
Hangeshashinto	Medium	Epigastric stuffiness, nausea, vomiting, and diarrhea with irritable bowel syndrome
Shosaikoto	Medium	Biological response modification (BRM) activity, effective for improvement of constitution with long-term use
2. prescription mainly for psychiatric symptoms		
Kososan	Deficiency	Gastrointestinal sickness, psychosomatic symptom such as headache, dizziness, and allergic symptoms
Yokukansan	Slight excess	Infantile neurosis, tantrum, or irritability, and in short-tempered patients
Yokukansankachimpihange	Slight deficiency	Same as yokukansan (with significant fluid retention in stomach)
Kamishoyosan	Slight deficiency	Irritability, headache, and climacteric disorders
Saikokeishikankyoto	Slight deficiency	Head sweating, insomnia, and anxiety tendency
Hangebyakujutsutemmato	Slight deficiency	Headache and vertigo/dizziness
Kanbakutaisoto	Slight deficiency	Emotional lability and hysteria
Ryokeijutsukanto	Slight deficiency	Autonomic imbalance, cardiac neurosis, and anxiety tendency
3. prescription for chronic fatigue		
(a) Formulas containing *ninjin* and *Ogi*		
Juzentaihoto	Deficiency	Pattern of both qi and blood deficiency, general malaise, and low-grade fever in patients with chronic debilitating conditions
Ninjin'yoeito	Slight deficiency	Pattern of both qi and blood[TM1] deficiency. Appropriate for Juzentaihoto pattern patients complaining of respiratory symptoms
Hochuekkito	Slight deficiency	Same as above
(b) Kenchuto group		
Shokenchuto	Slight deficiency	Same as above
Ogikenchuto	Deficiency	Chronic fatigue in patients with hypertonic constitution caused by qi deficiency
Kigikenchuto*	Deficiency	Pattern of both qi and blood[TM1] deficiency

*Not available as a medical Kampo extract formulation

(c) **Tonic formulas for chronic fatigue**

- **Formulas with *Ginseng and Astragalus root***
  - **Juzentaihoto**: A formula treating pattern of both qi and blood[TM1] deficiency by exerting immuno-enhancing/stimulating activity. Very useful for general malaise and low-grade fever in deficiency pattern patients with chronic debilitating conditions.
  - **Ninjin'yoeito**: Another formula for the pattern of both qi and blood[TM1] deficiency. Appropriate for *juzentaihoto* pattern patients complaining of respiratory symptoms. Physical strength shows a slight deficiency pattern.
  - **Hochuekkito**: Same as above.
- **Formulas in Kenchuto Group**
  - **Shokenchuto**: Same as above.
  - **Ogikenchuto**: This formula is *shokenchuto* with *ogi* added to tonify qi. Effective for chronic fatigue in deficiency pattern patients with hypertonic constitution caused by qi deficiency.
  - **Kigikenchuto**: This formula is *ogikenchuto* containing *toki* and is useful for deficiency pattern patients with both qi and blood[TM1] deficiency.

7.2.2 Sensitivity to Cold (Table 5.12)

Overview of Disease

The concept of "sensitivity to cold" does not exist in Western medicine. The temperature sensation of coldness is precisely a kind of subjective biological response to external stimuli, while objectively, there may be no coldness present at all. Conversely, the sufferer might not feel cold despite the

Table 5.12 Kampo frequently used formulas for sensitivity to cold

Formulas	Deficiency/excess	Indication for formulas
(a) Whole body type		
Shimbuto	Deficiency	As mentioned above
Hachimijiogan	Slight deficiency	As mentioned above
Ninjinto	Deficiency	As mentioned above
Shokenchuto	Slight deficiency	As mentioned above
Goshajinkigan	Slight deficiency	Edema who are indicated for *hachimijiogan*
Bushirichuto	Deficiency	*Ninjinto* pattern and intense interior cold
Keishininjinto	Slight deficiency	*Ninjinto* pattern with chronic headache
Ryokyojutsukanto	Slight deficiency	Low back and lower body coldness
Goshuyuto	Slight deficiency	Gastrointestinal weakness complains of headache, hiccup, vomiting, and shoulder stiffness
Daikenchuto	Slight deficiency—Deficiency	Cool abdomen and limbs with relatively strong abdominal pain with increased peristaltic movement, abdominal distension, or tympanites
Shigyakuto	Deficiency	Coldness of the limbs and lientery
Bukuryoshigyakuto	Deficiency	Shigyakuto pattern with dysphoria. Substituted by a combination of *ryokyojutsukanto*, *ninjinto*, and *bushi* powder extract formulations
(b) Upper heat and lower cold type		
Qi counter flow		
Keishikanzoto	Slight deficiency	Paroxysmal palpitation and chest distress
Keishikaryukotsuboreito	Slight deficiency	Hot flashes and more intense anxiety and qi abnormality than seen in *keishikanzoto* pattern
Qi counter flow and fluid[TM1] retention		
Ryokeimikanto	Slight deficiency	Blocked ear sensation and hot flashes associated with coldness in the limbs
Ryokeijutsukanto	Slight deficiency	See above
Qi counter flow and blood[TM1] stasis		
Tokakujokito	Slight excess—Excess	Hot flashes and constipation tendency, especially accompanied by psychoneurotic symptoms
Keishibukuryogan	Medium—Excess	To improve microcirculatory issues throughout the body
Unkeito	Slight deficiency—Medium	Lip dryness and heat agitation in the palms
Fluid[TM1] retention due to an unhealthy diet		
Goshakusan	Slight deficiency—Medium	Complain of lower abdominal or back pain, myalgia, and arthralgia following exposure to cold dampness Occasionally with lower cold upper heat
Orento	Medium	Complain of hot flashes and gastric pain due to tangled cold and heat condition
Choreito	Medium	Appropriate for hyperphagia/polydipsia with lower body coldness and heaviness, lower abdominal discomfort, cystitis-like symptoms, and tendency of diarrhea
Ryutanshakanto	Slight excess	Hyperphagia/polydipsia patients with lower body coldness and swelling, and leukorrhea/excessive menstrual bleeding
Daisaikoto	Excess	Lower cold upper heat, shoulder stiffness, abdominal pain/discomfort, and tendency of constipation
(c) Extremities type		
Blood[TM1] deficiency		
Shimotsuto	Slight deficiency	Chronic debilitating disease or a variety of serious illnesses related to immunity
Tokishakuyakusan	Slight deficiency	Heavy-headedness, swelling, and other fluid[TM1]retention symptoms
Tokishigyakukagoshuyushokyoto	Slight deficiency	Various painful diseases induced by cold, especially effective for chilblains and Raynaud's symptoms
Blood[TM1] stasis		
Keishibukuryogan	Medium—Excess	Same as above
Tokakujokito	Slight excess—Excess	Same as above
Others		
Byakkoto	Medium to slight	Body surface and limbs are cool despite interior heat
Byakkokaninjinto	excess	Byakkoto pattern with thirst

(continued)

Table 5.12 (continued)

Formulas	Deficiency/excess	Indication for formulas
(d) Psychosomatic correlation type		
Kamishoyosan	Slight deficiency	As mentioned above
Yokukansan	Slight deficiency	As mentioned above
Yokukansannkachimpihange	Slight deficiency	As mentioned above

objective presence of cold. Sensitivity to cold is generally more prevalent among women. The incidence among men as well as younger age groups, however, has increased remarkably in recent years.

Indications for Kampo Therapy

People whose energy production is low are prone to feeling cold, and also people whose gastrointestinal function is weak often feel coldness because energy is not properly supplemented or transported. Qi stagnation may intensify psychogenic senses of cold and chills. Furthermore, fluid[TM1] retention intensifies cold in the lower body, and blood[TM1] deficiency and blood[TM1] stasis cause coldness in the extremities.

Frequently Used Formulas

Patients should be counseled on lifestyle habits (appropriate exercise and redressing daily lifestyle factors, including food, clothing, and home).

(a) **Whole body type**

The whole body cools when physical energy is depleted or when energy supplementation and transportation are compromised.

- **Shimbuto**, **Hachimijiogan**, **Ninjinto**, **Shokenchuto** (mentioned above).
- **Goshajinkigan**: Useful for slight deficiency pattern patients with edema who are indicated for *hachimijiogan*.
- **Bushirichuto**: Effective for deficiency pattern patients with *ninjinto* pattern and intense interior cold.
- **Keishininjinto**: For slight deficiency pattern patients with *ninjinto* pattern with chronic headache.
- **Ryokyojutsukanto**: Used for slight deficiency pattern patients with low back and lower body coldness.
- **Goshuyuto**: Used for slight deficiency pattern patients with gastrointestinal weakness who complain of headache, hiccup, vomiting, and shoulder stiffness.
- **Daikenchuto**: Used for deficiency to slight deficiency pattern patients with cool abdomen and limbs who have relatively strong abdominal pain with increased peristaltic movement, abdominal distension, or tympanites.
- **Shigyakuto**:[26] Used for coldness of the limbs and lientery.
- **Bukuryoshigyakuto**:[20] For *shigyakuto* pattern patients with dysphoria. Can be substituted by a combination of *ryokyojutsukanto*, *ninjinto*, and *bushi* powder extract formulations.

(b) **Upper heat and lower cold type**

When the lower body is cool and there is insufficient Yang qi on the body surface, this can cause qi to rise, and a combination of *keishi* and *kanzo* is required to treat this. If fluid[TM1] retention is also present, *bukuryo* is added. If blood[TM1] stasis is present, blood[TM1] stasis resolving herbs are added. If the cause of the coldness is due to fluid[TM1] retention or food stasis from poor diet or neglect, however, this must be rectified.

- **Qi counter flow**
  - **Keishikanzoto**:[27] Effective for paroxysmal palpitation and chest distress.
  - **Keishikaryukotsuboreito**: Good for slight deficiency patients with hot flashes and more intense anxiety and qi abnormality than seen in the *keishikanzoto* pattern.
- **Qi counter flow** Qi counter flow **and fluid[TM1] retention**
  - **Ryokeimikanto**:[20] Used for blocked ear sensation and hot flashes associated with coldness in the limbs.
  - **Ryokeijutsukanto**: See above.
- **Qi counter flow** Qi counter flow **and blood[TM1] stasis**.
  - **Tokakujokito**: Used often for patients with slight excess to excess pattern with hot flashes and constipation tendency, especially when accompanied by psychoneurotic symptoms.
  - **Keishibukuryogan**: This formula improves microcirculatory issues throughout the body for medium to slight excess pattern patients.
  - **Unkeito**: Appropriate for slight deficiency to medium pattern patients with lip dryness and heat agitation in the palms.
- **Fluid[TM1] retention due to an unhealthy diet.**

[26] Not available as a medical Kampo extract formulation.

[27] Not available as medical Kampo extract formulation nor OTC Kampo extract formulation.

Keishikanzoto:keishi 4.0, kanzo 2.0.

Overeating causes stomach heat, and this makes qi rise (hot flash). When there is also phlegm-fluid retention from overdrinking, lower body coldness creates "lower cold, upper heat."

- **Goshakusan**: For slight to medium deficiency pattern patients who complain of lower abdominal pain, low back pain, myalgia, and arthralgia following exposure to cold dampness (air conditioning and cool drinks). Occasionally they also have lower cold upper heat.
- **Orento**: This formula is for medium pattern patients with signs similar to *hangeshashinto*. They also complain of hot flashes and gastric pain due to tangled cold and heat conditions.
- **Choreito**: Appropriate for hyperphagia/polydipsia patients with a medium pattern complaining of lower body coldness and heaviness, lower abdominal discomfort, cystitis-like symptoms, and a tendency to diarrhea.
- **Ryutanshakanto**: For hyperphagia/polydipsia patients with slight excess pattern, complaining of lower body coldness and swelling, and leukorrhea/excessive menstrual bleeding.
- **Daisaikoto**: Used for patients with excess pattern complaining of lower cold upper heat, shoulder stiffness, abdominal pain/discomfort, and a tendency toward constipation.

(c) **Extremities type**

Blood[TM1] deficiency and blood[TM1] stasis are the causes of vascular insufficiency in the extremities. The formulas containing *toki* should be selected for the treatment of blood[TM1] deficiency, and blood[TM1] stasis resolving formulas are used for blood[TM1] stasis.

- **Blood[TM1] deficiency**.
  - **Shimotsuto**: Used for slight deficiency pattern patients with chronic debilitating disease or a variety of serious illnesses suspected of being related to immunity.
  - **Tokishakuyakusan**: Appropriate for slight deficiency pattern patients with blood[TM1] deficiency, heavy-headedness, swelling, and other fluid[TM1] retention symptoms.
  - **Tokishigyakukagoshuyushokyoto**: Used for slight deficiency pattern patients with various painful diseases induced by cold, especially effective for chilblains and Raynaud's symptoms.
- **Blood[TM1] stasis**.
  - **Keishibukuryogan**, **Tokakujokito**: Same as above
- **Others.**
  - **Byakkoto[20]/Byakkokaninjinto**: For medium to slight excess pattern patients whose body surface and limbs are cool despite interior heat (reversal cold of extremities).

(d) **Psychosomatic correlation type**

- **Kamishoyosan, Yokukansan, Yokukansankachimpihange**: Same as above

7.3 Anemia and Bleeding Tendency

Takaaki Kosuge

7.3.1 Overview of Disease

Anemia

Anemia is defined as a condition of either absolute or relative reductions in erythrocyte count, hemoglobin level, and hematocrit value.

In Western medicine, the main causes of anemia are (1) insufficient materials for erythrocyte production (hypoferric anemia), (2) hematopoietic disorder (aplastic anemia, pure red cell aplasia, myelofibrosis, myelodysplastic syndrome, etc.), (3) impaired cell maturation (renal anemia, megaloblastic anemia, etc.), and (4) excessive erythrocyte destruction (hemolytic anemia, hypersplenism, hemoglobinopathy, etc.).

Bleeding Tendency

Bleeding diathesis (tendency) is an unusual susceptibility to bleeding in the skin or submucosal bleeding (1 and 2) or deep internal bleeding in joints, muscles, or organs (3 and 4) and includes the following: (1) skin or submucosal bleeding due to extravasation, as seen in allergic purpura, purpura simplex, and senile purpura; (2) temporary hemostasis (thrombocyte hemostasis) disorder, as seen in petechial hemorrhagic lesion and purpura, epistaxis and ulorrhagia, gastrointestinal hemorrhage, and hypermenorrhea; (3) secondary hemostasis (blood coagulation factor-mediated hemostasis) disorder; and (4) abnormally accelerated coagulation or fibrinolytic system.

7.3.2 Indications for Kampo Therapy

Anemia

International standard therapies exist for the various classes of anemia. Once a definitive diagnosis has been made, replacement of iron, vitamin B12, folate, and/or erythropoietin as well as blood transfusion should start immediately. Kampo is not the first choice therapy.

In Kampo medicine, however, anemia is considered to be a condition of blood deficiency. Kampo formulas may improve symptoms caused by blood characteristics, not just blood volume, as in (3) below.

1. Cases in which Western medicine is either ineffective or causes adverse effects
2. Cases that, under the international standard therapy, only require monitoring without treatment: mild aplastic anemia, myelodysplastic syndrome (especially low-risk group by International Prognostic Scoring System <IPSS>), and senile anemia [69]
3. Cases in which anemia symptoms continue despite blood values returning to normal

Bleeding Tendency
Western medical therapy is the first choice for (3) and (4) in section A-2 above, particularly for reasons of the severity of pathological conditions. Kampo medicines demonstrate effectiveness for (1) and (2).

There are therapeutic guidelines for (2) idiopathic thrombocytopenic purpura (ITP).

In Kampo medicine, these symptoms are regarded as blood circulation abnormalities caused by the failure of qi to control blood[TM1].

7.3.3 Frequently Used Formulas

Anemia (Table 5.13)

(a) **Blood[TM1] deficiency**

Patients experience lightheadedness and dizziness. The face becomes pale, and heart palpitations increase. Heaviness and numbness develop in the limbs. The skin loses color and dries out, head hair loss worsens, and anemia-like symptoms such as sleep disorders develop. The tongue becomes pale, and the pulse is thin.

- **Shimotsuto:** Generally used for slight deficiency pattern patients, but this is the primary formula for improving blood[TM1] deficiency. Widely used as a combined formula or an addition to other formulas.
- **Kyukikyogaito:** Used for bleeding associated with blood[TM1] deficiency in patients with slight deficiency pattern. Frequently effective for lower body bleeding such as atypical genital bleeding, hemorrhoidal bleeding, and hematuria.
- **Tokishakuyakusan:** For patients with a slight deficiency pattern who have a variety of symptoms from the combination of blood[TM1] deficiency and fluid[TM1] retention. It is used not only for anemia but also for gynecological disorder.

(b) **Pattern of both qi and blood[TM1] deficiency**

Qi deficiency and blood[TM1] deficiency are closely associated: many patients who have blood[TM1] deficiency symptoms also have qi deficiency symptoms. The tongue is pale, and the pulse is fine and vacuous.

- **Juzentaihoto:** *Shikunshito* and *shimotsuto* fortified with *keihi* and *ogi*. Most frequently used for the treatment of anemia. Effective for deficiency pattern patients with strong fatigue and malaise, general debility, night sweats, and coldness in hands and feet. There is abundant evidence of myeloid stem cell differentiation inducing effect of this formula in Western medical research.
- **Ninjin'yoeito:** Signs similar to *juzentaihoto* pattern, but for slight deficiency pattern; associated with coughing, sputum, shortness of breath, deficiency heat, and nervous imbalance.
- **Kihito:** For slight deficiency pattern patients with gastrointestinal and constitutional weakness who suffer bleeding or anemia because of overwork or nervous strain, who also present with psychiatric symptoms including amnesia, insomnia, enervation, and depressive tendency, in addition to strong blood[TM1] deficiency symptoms.
- **Kamikihito:** Useful for *kihito* pattern patients with slight deficiency to the medium pattern, suffering deficiency heat with hot flashes, burning sensation, chest tightness, irritability, and nervous excitement. Often used as the first choice for ITP, based on strong evidence in medical research.

(c) **Qi deficiency**

Patients present with weak, shallow breathing, have little vocal force, and speak in a whispering tone. They are easily startled and have facial pallor associated with intense limb or general malaise. Patients may also have anorexia, susceptibility to infection, and proneness to bleed. The tongue is pale and limp. Pulse is weak and soft and lacks vitality.

- **Shikunshito:** Typical formula for qi deficiency. For deficiency pattern patients who tend to have painful abdominal distension, epigastric discomfort, nausea, vomiting, diarrhea, and other symptoms of gastrointestinal weakness.
- **Rikkunshito:** Signs similar to *shikunshito* pattern, but patients have a deficiency to slight deficiency pattern. Beneficial for stronger gastrointestinal symptoms than those in *shikunshito* pattern patients, such as the sensation of epigastric blockage.
- **Hochuekkito:** Widely used in slight deficiency pattern patients with pronounced general malaise, constitutional weakness, and weak digestion. Patients may also com-

Table 5.13 Kampo frequently used formulas for anemia

Symptoms	Condition	Formulas	Deficiency/excess pattern	Features
Dizziness	Blood[TM1] deficiency	Shimotsuto	Slight deficiency	Primary prescription for improving blood deficiency
Pallor		Kyukikyogaito	Deficiency	Lower body bleeding such as atypical genital bleeding or hemorrhoidal bleeding
Palpitation		Tokishakuyakusan	Slight deficiency	Gynecological disorder
Limb malaise	Pattern of both qi and blood[TM1] deficiency	Juzentaihoto	Deficiency	Most frequently used for anemia treatment
Dry skin		Ninjin'yoeito	Slight deficiency	Coughing, sputum, shortness of breath, deficiency heat, nervous imbalance
Head hair loss		Kihito	Slight deficiency	Bleeding or anemia as a result of overwork or nervous strain
Sleep disorders		Kamikihito	Slight deficiency to medium	Kihito pattern patients suffering deficiency heat/the first choice for ITP
	Qi deficiency	Shikunshito	Deficiency	Typical prescription for qi deficiency
Pale tongue		Rikkunshito	Deficiency to slight deficiency	Stronger gastrointestinal symptoms than that of shikunshito pattern
Thin pulse		Hochuekkito	Slight deficiency	Notable general malaise, constitutional weakness/ sensation of visceroptosis
		Ninjinto	Deficiency	Sensitivity to cold stronger than that of rikkunshito pattern

plain of a sensation of visceroptosis or whole body ptosis, as well as taste disorder.

- **Ninjinto:** Appropriate for deficiency pattern patients with sensitivity to coldness as the chief symptom and also gastrointestinal weakness symptoms as seen in shikunshito- and rikkunshito-pattern patients

Bleeding Tendency

(a) **Excess heat**

Various symptoms associated with inflammation and congestion appear throughout the body in pathological conditions with excess heat in all the triple energizers. The most common manifestation in mucous membranes is bleeding, which comes under the broad definition of bleeding diathesis. This includes epistaxis from nasal mucous membranes, hemoptysis from bronchial mucous membranes, and hematemesis/melena from alimentary canal mucous membranes. Skin or submucosal bleeding in allergic purpura may also be included.

- **Orengedokuto:** A typical heat-clearing formula used in slight excess to excess pattern patients who are prone to hot flashes and irritability and complain of epigastric stuffiness and vexation with palpitations. The pharmacological actions of *oren* and *ogon* help clear heat, cool blood[TM1] and arrest hemorrhage.
- **San'oshashinto:** Among the formulas in shashinto group, *san'oshashinto* is the leading prescription for the excess pattern. Its purgative effect helps eliminate the excess heat in the triple energizers and arrest hemorrhage. Used for stronger excess patterns than that of *orengedokuto* patients, when patients have hot flashes, facial redness, nervous imbalance, and constipation tendency. Bleeding can effectively be stopped by using other *shashinto* formulas appropriate to the patient's pattern.

(b) **Spleen[TM1] deficiency**

In most patients with chronic bleeding tendency, spleen[TM1] deficiency causes poor production of qi and blood[TM1], disturbs blood circulation control, and leads to bleeding. In this sense, it is no exaggeration to say that the treatment of bleeding tendency is a matter of "tonifying the spleen[TM1]."

Qi-tonifying and qi and blood[TM1] tonifying formulas are frequently used.

See the previous section for details.

- **Kihito, Kamikihito**
- **Shikunshito, Rikkunshito, Hochuekkito**
- **Juzentaihoto, Ninjin'yoeito, Ninjinto**

- **Keihito:** Used when patients have stronger dyspepsia than *shikunshito* patients and remarkably watery or soft stool. Physical constitution is a slight deficiency pattern.

Other Pathologies and Formulas Related to Anemia and Bleeding Tendency

Blood[TM1] stasis and qi stagnation may also be causes of anemia-like symptoms, submucosal hemorrhage or hemorrhage in the skin (ecchymosis), or localized bleeding.

Blood[TM1] stasis resolving formulas and qi-regulating formulas may be useful.

- **Hangekobokuto, Kososan:** Qi-regulating formulas.
- **Kamishoyosan, Unkeito, Nyoshinsan, etc.:** Blood[TM1] stasis resolving formulas.

7.4 Metabolic Disease

Motoko Fukuzawa

7.4.1 Obesity

Overview of Disease

Obesity is a condition in which excessive adipose tissue is accumulated in the body. A person whose body mass index (BMI: body weight/body height as kg/m^2) is 25 or more is diagnosed as obese in Japan. A BMI of 25 or over associated with visceral fat accumulation or with concomitant presence of hypertension, dyslipidemia, and abnormal glucose tolerance is diagnosed as obesity requiring treatment. Metabolic syndrome (visceral fat obesity plus concomitant hypertension, dyslipidemia, and abnormal glucose tolerance) patients are susceptible to arteriosclerotic diseases such as ischemic heart disease and cerebral vascular disorder. In these patients, the treatment of obesity is very important.

Indications for Kampo Therapy

Drug therapy is offered for patients who do not respond to diet therapy and therapeutic exercise. The anorexiant mazindol is available in Western medicine, though its use is limited to patients with a BMI of 35 or more for a period of 3 months. Kampo medicines are not greatly effective in reducing weight but can be used for long periods regardless of the degree of obesity, bringing improvement of concomitant symptoms, quality of life (QOL), and weight loss outcomes. It was reported that *bofutsushosan* and *boiogito* have an anti-obesity effect enough to reduce visceral fat mass [70, 71].

Frequently Used Formulas (Fig. 5.28)

In Kampo medicine, the chief causes of obesity are "food disturbance" (the accumulation of food in the body that becomes pathological) and fluid[TM1] retention, which is frequently associated with static blood[TM1], qi counter flow, qi counter flow and qi stagnation. In patients with a solid build (regarded as excess pattern), food disturbance plays a role and is often accompanied by constipation. Obesity in patients with a flabby build (deficiency pattern) is often related to fluid[TM1] retention.

- **Bofutsushosan:** Patients have excess pattern with solid build, potbelly, hot flashes, edema, and constipation.
- **Daisaikoto:** Patients have excess pattern with solid build, shoulder stiffness, headache, and constipation tendency, in addition to fullness and discomfort in chest and hypochondrium.
- **Eppikajutsuto:** Used for excess pattern patients with swelling and pain in the joints (particularly the knees), edema, and reduced urine volume.
- **Tokakujokito:** Patients have slight excess to excess pattern with constipation, hot flashes, irritability, insomnia, and menstrual disorder, in addition to an abdominal pattern of lower abdominal cramps.
- **Saikokaryukotsuboreito:** Effective for slight excess pattern with hypersensitivity, palpitations, and insomnia, in addition to fullness and discomfort in chest and hypochondrium.
- **Yokukansan:** Used for slight excess pattern patients with irritability, intense agitation, and insomnia.
- **Keishibukuryogan:** Used for medium to slight excess pattern with hot flashes, facial redness, shoulder stiffness, headache, menstrual disorder, and signs of blood[TM1] stasis.
- **Hangekobokuto:** Effective for medium pattern patients with depression, anxiety, and insomnia.
- **Boiogito:** Patients have a slight deficiency pattern; patients with flabby builds, excessive sweating, edema, swelling, and pain in the knee joint.
- **Tokishakuyakusan:** Effective for slight deficiency pattern patients with coldness in hands and feet, dizziness, edema, and menstrual disorder.
- **Kamishoyosan:** Effective for a slight deficiency pattern patients with upper heat, lower cold, irritability, and insomnia.
- **Kumibinroto:** Useful for deficiency pattern patients with coldness in hands and feet, joint stiffness, lower limb fatigue, edema, and shortness of breath.

7.4.2 Diabetes Mellitus

Overview of Disease

Diabetes Mellitus (DM) is a disease that results from inadequate insulin secretion or inadequate insulin action (due to insulin resistance) and leads to hyperglycemia. DM is classified as type 1 or type 2.

Since complications such as retinopathy, nephropathy, and neuropathy reduce patients' QOL, preventing the onset and advance as well as controlling blood sugar are important treatment strategies. Diet therapy and therapeutic exercise are the basic treatments. Insulin treatment is used for type 1 diabetes. In type 2 diabetes, if glycemic improvement is inadequate, hypoglycemic drugs and insulin should be administered.

Indications for Kampo Therapy

Herbs such as *ninjin* and *jio*, and formulas such as *seishinrenshiin* and *hachimijiogan* reportedly have a hypoglycemic action. It is difficult, however, to clinically achieve sufficient

Pattern	Formula	Indications
Excess pattern	Bofutsushosan	excess pattern, solid build, potbelly, hot flashes, edema, constipation
	Daisaikoto	excess pattern, solid build, shoulder stiffness, headache, constipation tendency, fullness and discomfort in chest and hypochondrium
	Eppikajutsuto	excess pattern, swelling and pain in the joints (particularly the knees), edema, reduced urine volume
	Tokakujokito	slight excess to excess pattern, constipation, hot flashes, irritability, insomnia, menstruation disorder, resistance and marked tenderness in the left iliac region
	Saikokaryukotsuboreito	slight excess pattern, oversensitivity, palpitations, insomnia, fullness and discomfort in chest and hypochondrium
	Yokukansan	slight excess pattern, irritability, intense agitation, insomnia
Medium pattern	Keishibukuryogan	medium to slight excess pattern, hot flashes, facial redness, shoulder stiffness, headache, menstrual disorder, blood stasis
	Hangekobokuto	medium pattern, depression, anxiety, insomnia
Deficiency pattern	Boiogito	slight deficiency pattern, flabby build, excessive sweating, edema, swelling and pain in the knee joint
	Tokishakuyakusan	slight deficiency pattern, coldness in hands and feet, dizziness, edema, menstrual disorder
	Kamishoyosan	slight deficiency pattern, upper heat lower cold, irritability, insomnia
	Kumibinroto	deficiency pattern, coldness in hands and feet, joint stiffness, lower limb fatigue, edema, shortness of breath

Fig. 5.28 Frequently used formulas for obesity

hypoglycemic effect with Kampo therapy alone. Thus, Western medicinal treatment is preferred for blood sugar control. Kampo therapy is effective for the subjective symptoms and complications of diabetes.

Frequently Used Formulas (Fig. 5.29)

(a) **Hyperglycemia treatment**

Reportedly, herbs such as *ninjin, jio, sanyaku, bakumondo, gomishi*, and *sanshuyu*, as well as formulas such as *seishinrenshiin, goreisan, hachimijiogan, ninjinto, byakkokaninjinto, bakumondoto, chikuyosekkoto,*[28] *and zokumeito*[22] have a hypoglycemic effect. In addition, *bofutsushosan* and *goshajinkigan* have been shown to improve insulin resistance, while *bofutsushosan* and *boiogito* have been demonstrated to ameliorate blood sugar values through their anti-obesity action [72].

(b) **Treatment of subjective symptoms**

- **Daisaikoto:** Used for excess pattern obese patients with constipation and fullness and discomfort in the chest and hypochondrium.
- **Bofutsushosan:** Effective for excess pattern patients who have solid build with potbelly, hot flashes, and constipation.
- **Byakkokaninjinto:** Appropriate for medium to excess pattern patients with thirst, polydipsia, and polyuria.
- **Goreisan:** Used for medium pattern patients with thirst, reduced urine volume, edema, and dizziness.
- **Hachimijiogan:** Used for slight deficiency pattern patients with pollakiuria, nocturia, thirst, lower body cold and numbness, edema, and impotence.
- **Goshajinkigan:** Patients have a slight deficiency and *hachimijiogan* pattern with remarkable chills and lower limb edema.
- **Rokumigan:** Patients have a slight deficiency and *hachimijiogan* pattern without chills.
- **Seishinrenshiin:** Effective for sensitivity to cold in slight deficiency pattern patients with pollakiuria, gastrointestinal weakness, and oversensitivity.
- **Bakumondoinshi:**[29] Offered to deficiency pattern patients with thirst, polyuria, and dry skin.

(c) **Treatment of complications**

- **Diabetic neuropathy**
  - **Sokeikakketsuto:** Used for medium pattern patients with sensitivity to cold, lower body myalgia, arthralgia, and neuralgia (with more severe pain at night and dawn), in addition to blood[TM1] stasis.
  - **Hachimijiogan, Goshajinkigan:** Effective for slight deficiency pattern patients with lower body chills, numbness, pain, and impotence. *Goshajinkigan* has been reported to exert an aldose reductase inhibitory effect, a vasodilatory effect, and an analgesic effect.
  - **Keishikajutsubuto:** Used for slight deficiency pattern patients with sensitivity to coldness, low back

[28]Not available as a medical Kampo extract formulation.

[29]Not available as with Kampo extract formulation nor OTC Kampo formulation.

Bakumondoinshi: bakumondo 7.0, ninjin, karokon 2.0, chimo, kakkon 3.0, jio 4.0, bukuryo 6.0, gomishi, kanzo, chikuyo 1.0.

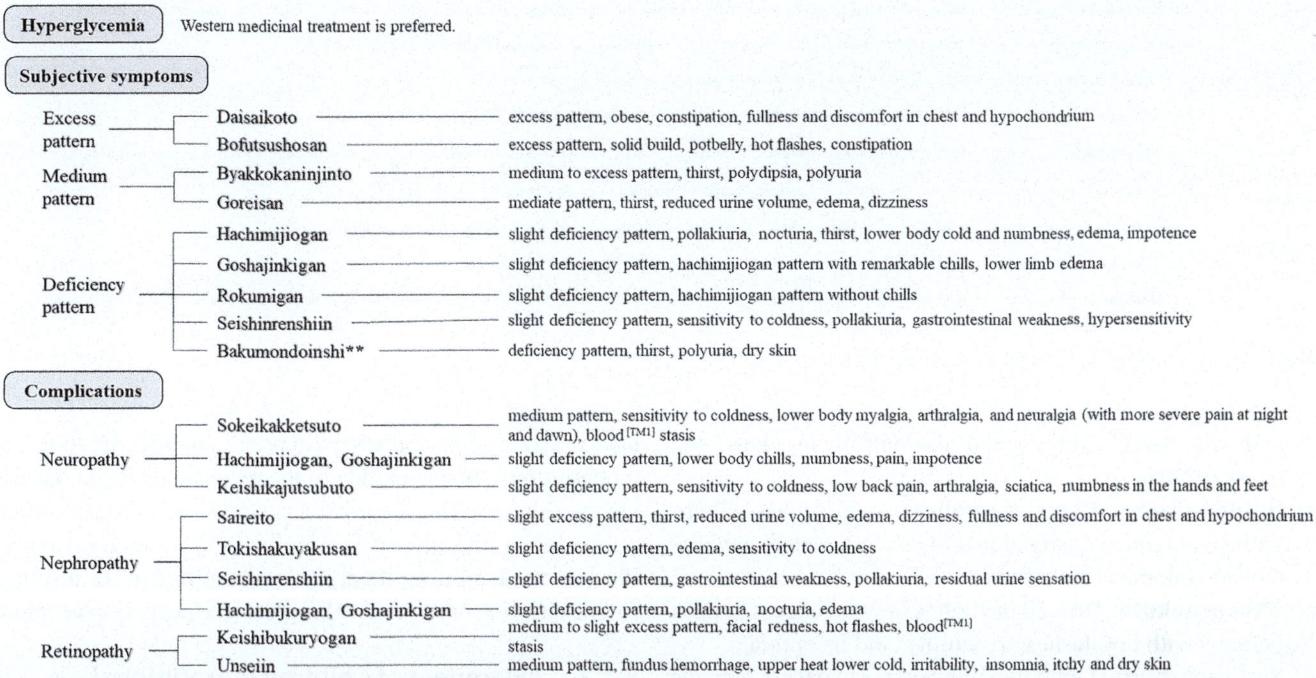

Fig. 5.29 Frequently used formulas for diabetes mellitus

pain, arthralgia, sciatica, and numbness in the hands and feet.

- **Diabetic nephropathy**
  - **Saireito:** Appropriate for medium pattern patients with thirst, reduced urine volume, edema, dizziness, and fullness and discomfort in the chest and hypochondrium. Reportedly, *saireito* may improve urinary albumin excretion.
  - **Tokishakuyakusan:** Effective for slight deficiency pattern patients with edema and sensitivity to cold.
  - **Seishinrenshiin:** Used for slight deficiency pattern patients who have gastrointestinal weakness and complain of pollakiuria and residual urine sensation.
  - **Hachimijiogan, Goshajinkigan:** Used for slight deficiency pattern patients with pollakiuria, nocturia, and edema.
- **Diabetic retinopathy**
  - **Keishibukuryogan:** Effective for medium to slight excess pattern patients with facial redness, hot flashes, and blood[TM1] stasis symptoms.
  - **Unseiin:** Used for fundus hemorrhage in patients who have the medium pattern with upper heat, lower cold, irritability, insomnia, and itchy, dry skin.

7.4.3 Dyslipidemia

Overview of Disease

Dyslipidemia is a lifestyle disease that occurs when dietary habits, lack of exercise, and other lifestyle imbalances combine with genetic factors. Hypercholesterolemia, LDL hypercholesterolemia, HDL hypocholesterolemia, and hypertriglyceridemia are major risk factors for arteriosclerosis and are treated to prevent arteriosclerotic diseases such as ischemic heart disease and cerebrovascular disorder.

Indications for Kampo Therapy

Several herbs and formulas have been demonstrated to improve blood lipid levels, but their effectiveness is not as great as Western drugs. Few Kampo medicines are helpful when aiming just to improve blood lipid levels. Instead, Kampo medicines are helpful when comprehensive treatment, including improvement of concomitant symptoms, is sought and when used for patients who cannot take Western medicines because of adverse reactions.

Frequently Used Formulas (Fig. 5.30)

Formulas with Bupleurum root and blood[TM1] stasis resolving formulas are frequently used.

- **Daisaikoto:** Appropriate for excess pattern patients with solid build, shoulder stiffness, and constipation tendency,

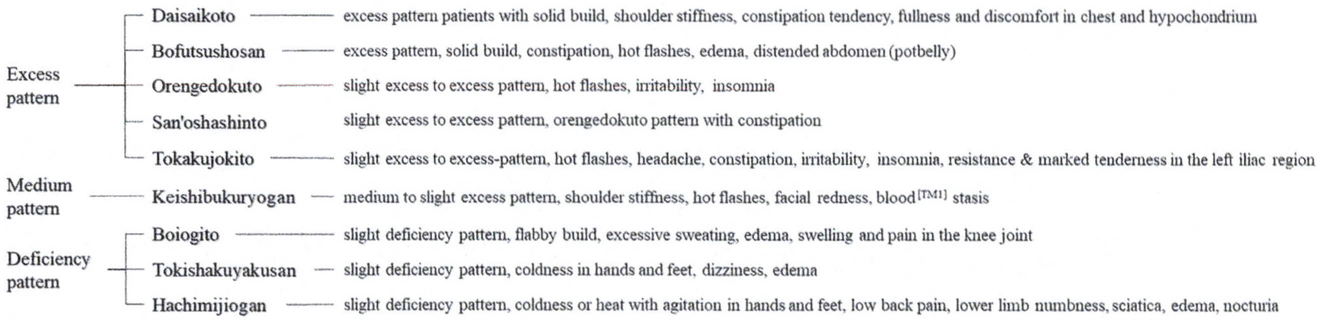

Fig. 5.30 Frequently used formulas for dyslipidemia

and who have fullness and discomfort in chest and hypochondrium.

- **Bofutsushosan:** Useful for patients with excess pattern with solid build, constipation, hot flashes, edema, and distended abdomen (potbelly).
- **Orengedokuto:** Offered in slight excess to excess pattern patients with hot flashes, irritability, and insomnia.
- **San'oshashinto:** Good for slight excess to excess patients with orengedokuto pattern with constipation.
- **Tokakujokito:** Appropriate for slight excess to excess pattern patients who have hot flashes, headaches, constipation, irritability, and insomnia, with lower abdominal cramps.
- **Keishibukuryogan:** Used for medium to slight excess pattern patients with shoulder stiffness, hot flashes, facial redness, and blood[TM1] stasis signs.
- **Boiogito:** Effective for patients with a slight deficiency pattern who have a flabby build, excessive sweating, edema, swelling, and pain in the knee joint.
- **Tokishakuyakusan:** Used for slight deficiency pattern patients with coldness in hands and feet, dizziness, and edema.
- **Hachimijiogan:** Effective for slight deficiency pattern patients with coldness or heat with agitation in hands and feet, associated with low back pain, lower limb numbness, sciatica, edema, and nocturia.

8 Others

8.1 Childhood Diseases

Hideaki Yamaguchi

8.1.1 Introduction

The Medical Service Act of Japan defines a child as a young person aged under 18. In modern pediatrics, however, a child is generally deemed a boy or girl up to junior high school age. Historically, Kampo treatment for children seems to have targeted acute and severe diseases, mainly infections. In modern times, however, due to the recent changes in our living environment and remarkable advances in Western pediatric medicine, the role of Kampo has shifted to areas where Western medical drug therapies are insufficient. In this article, descriptions are made taking these aspects into account.

8.1.2 Awareness of Children in Traditional Chinese Medicine

China has a long history of describing pediatric medicine. For example, *Xiǎoér Yào Zhèng Zhí Jué* (Keys to Pediatric Medicines and Patterns), the world's oldest existing systematic text on pediatrics, was written by Qián Yǐ in 1119 in the Southern Song Dynasty. This was followed by the publication of many pediatric textbooks. As such, historically formed awareness of children is summarized in Table 5.14 [73]. In China, these perceptions were summarized to characterize children as "being lively and active but immature and brittle." Furthermore, in describing excesses and deficiencies in their five zang organs, children were characterized by the phrase "*niyo sanbusoku*" (the liver[TM1] and heart[TM1] are vigorous, while the spleen[TM1], kidney[TM1], and lung[TM1] are weak). This may be reworded in modern fashion as follows: Children are susceptible to fevers that can cause convulsions and disturbance of consciousness (*shinjyoyuuyo*), are highly excitable and mentally unstable (*kanjyoyuyo*), are immature in digestive and respiratory functions and susceptible to hypofunctions (*haijyo, hijyobusoku*), and have is fragile vitality so they are susceptible to growth and developmental disorders (*jinjyobusoku*).

8.1.3 Features of Kampo Practices for Children

In pediatric medicine, Kampo practitioners should bear in mind that children are generally characterized by wide differences in disease structure among different ages because they are in the process of mental and physical development and growth. Accordingly, features of Kampo practices for pediatrics are compared with those for adults are shown in Table 5.15.

Table 5.14 Characteristics of children in traditional Chinese medicine (modified from Reference 73)

1. Lively and active, growing rapidly
2. The zang and fu organs are still functionally immature
3. In terms of pathology, likely to become diseased
4. Quick recovery because organs are intact

Table 5.15 Features of children compared with adults

1. There are many child-specific conditions and disorders
2. Simpler and easy to identify Kampo conditions
3. Good response to Kampo medicines, with quick manifestation of effects
4. Can be managed with a limited range of crude drugs and Kampo formulas
5. Side effects are less prevalent
6. Many cases require special effort to allow the child take the medication easily

8.1.4 Points to Note in Examinations of Children

Inspection

(a) **Overall observation**

During the examination, the child should be checked for monthly/yearly age-appropriate development and growth through greetings, responses to questions, calmness/restlessness, complexion, skin condition, etc.

(b) **Tongue examination**

Tongue changes are minor in children compared to adults. Whatever the age, the tongue's body is often colored light red with a thin white coating. It must be noted that when the child puts out his/her tongue under tension, the tip of the tongue tends to turn red. A geographic tongue is sometimes noted, and its extent often reflects the time course of the condition. Definitely, abnormal findings are only infrequently found in tongue examination, but Kampo practitioners should be vigilant of any such findings because they suggest severe mental or physical illness (refer to Chap. 3, Sect. 2.3).

Auscultation and Olfaction

The magnitude of voice reflects physical vigor, allowing assessment of qi deficiencies, including "innate qi"). In infants and young children, excess and deficiency patterns are sometimes determined by stool odor intensity.

Inquiry

In pediatric Kampo diagnosis, questioning is of paramount importance. In addition to the history of current illness, inquiries about heat/cold, sweating, thirst, appetite, urination and defecation, sleep, menstruation (prepuberty and older girls), and mental status provide important information for making a Kampo diagnosis. In addition, both aggravating and ameliorating factors for chief complaints are important. Generally, children are often more sensitive to heat, drink more, have a larger appetite, sleep better, and are more active than adults. In the growing phase of children, special attention should be paid to decreased digestive function and sleep disorders. Since the inquiry is mostly made with the child's family, particularly his/her mother, it should be taken into account that their account may be somewhat modified.

Palpation

(a) **Pulse examination**

In children, pathologic pulses are not highly defined and are difficult to identify. The classical literature says that pathologic pulses become identifiable at the age of three and older and that pulse examination should be checked mainly for floating/deep pulses, pulse rate, and pulse strength [74]. This is also helpful in the modern era. It should be noted, however, that children have variable pulse rates depending on age and tend to have rapid pulses due to the short distance from the heart to the wrists. Children tend to have rapid and wiry pulses due to their susceptibility to tension.

(b) **Abdominal examination**

In children, particularly infants and young children, abdominal patterns as found in adults are unlikely. The amount of abdominal strength, however, serves for reference purposes. Although schoolchildren and older may be examined in nearly the same manner as adults, typical abdominal patterns tend to be less likely to develop in younger children. Excessive ticklishness sometimes found in children is considered a findings that reflects their high tension and hypersensitivity.

Although the above examinations take longer than usual with children, the information obtained is essential to the diagnosis and treatment. This time is also important to enable the practitioner to build good relationships with patients and their families.

8.1.5 Diagnosis and Treatment 73) (Fig. 5.31)

As a general rule for diagnosis and treatment, information from inquiry and physical findings that have been collected from a Kampo viewpoint should be assessed to diagnose individual pediatric patients to choose the appropriate crude drugs and Kampo medications for each child. Understanding the pathophysiology in advance often contributes to choosing Kampo drugs. However, choosing a single formula for a single disease name should be avoided since it will lower treatment efficiency.

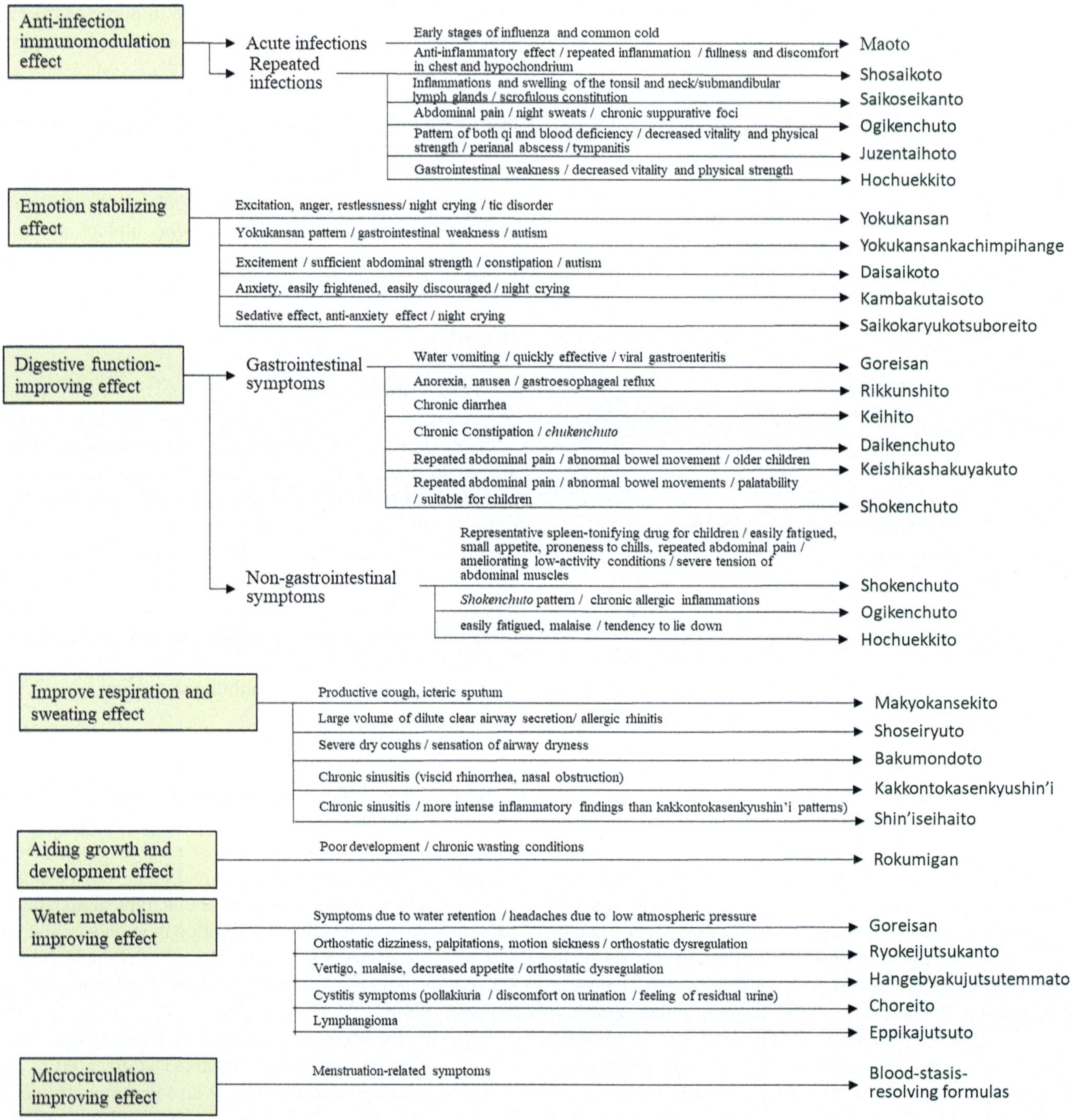

Fig. 5.31 Kampo medicines used frequently in children

With regard to Kampo medical diagnosis and treatment in children, little description appears in "*Shanghanlun*" or "*Jinguiyaolue*," with nearly no traditional rules of treatment. Historically, Kampo treatments of children became systematized to some extent by the late Edo period. After the Meiji period, pediatric Kampo treatments vanished from the center stage of medical practice for a time due to the policy on medical services of the Japanese government. After Kampo extracts were included in the National Health Insurance drug price list, however, this became useful in setting guidelines for pediatric medicine. Many extract formulas have been used in a wide variety of cases, and their utility has become recognized again in clinical settings. Modern pediatric Kampo medicine, however, seems to lack systematic conceptualization in its overall view. In this article, therefore, Kampo treatments are divided into seven approaches, bearing in mind the above-described characteristics of children, as well as water balance disorders and menstruation-related troubles. Kampo extracts suitable for pediatric use are described systematically with general remarks.

Regarding formula descriptions, deficiency, medium, and excess patterns in young children are not described, since they are often difficult to distinguish from each other in actual clinical settings because no specific definitions are available in pediatrics. However, sometimes this is not applicable to older children; refer to the relevant chapter for the choice of formulas for excesses and deficiency patterns.

Anti-infection Immunomodulation Effect

In children, fever-inducing acute infections and accompanying conditions are prevalent and are likely to change rapidly (*shinkanyuyo*). This is due mainly to the immaturity of biological functions (*hihaifusoku*).

(a) **Acute infections**

Historically, acute infections are considered to have been the most important issue in pediatric Kampo medicine. Classically, acute infections were considered to be manageable according to adult regimens for children 7 years or older or to be managed using pediatric doses for children younger than 7 years. In modern times, well-established preventive and therapeutic systems are available, so there is not a great need for practices with Kampo medications for acute infections in children. Hence, the description below focuses on *maoto*, on which there are relatively many clinical reports.

- **Maoto**: A representative formula for the early yang stage. It targets chills, anhidrosis, and floating tense pulses in the early stage of acute febrile diseases (which are difficult to distinguish in children). It's used for early stages of influenza and is also effective for children [74]. Pediatric use is acceptable in the absence of dehydration because disease-fighting reactions usually occur intensely in children. This formula should be discontinued when the fever has resolved.

(b) **Repeated infections**

For repeated infections such as tonsillitis, tympanitis, and perianal abscess, on the other hand, ameliorations are expected with a combination of *shosaikoto*, *saikoseikanto*, or the like that are based on Bupleurum root (*saiko*), which has an anti-inflammatory effect. Also, *ogikenchuto*, *juzentaihoto*, *hochuekkito*, or the like that are based on Astragalus root (*ogi*) or ginseng (*ninjin*), which are expected to improve immune functions, are used. These combinations can also be used for some diseases characterized by repeated autoinflammation.

- **Shosaikoto**: This is a formula for use in the late yang stage and can be used for a broad range of repetitive or chronic infections and inflammations with an expectation for a unique anti-inflammatory effect. Fullness and discomfort in the chest and hypochondrium are often noted in abdominal examination. This may be used in combination with *saikokeishito*, *saibokuto*, *saireito*, and other formulas, and find many opportunities for pediatric use.
- **Saikoseikanto**: Used in scrofulous children who repeatedly experience tonsillitis, cervical-submandibular lymphadenitis, and other diseases.
- **Ogikenchuto**: A combination formula of *shokenchuto* with Astragalus root (*ogi*), which is known as a highly effective drug for children, is expected to have a greater immune-potentiating effect than *shokenchuto* alone. Its use targets recurrent abdominal pain and night sweats. This formula can be used for skin lesions, chronic abscesses, etc.
- **Juzentaihoto**: Used for patterns of both qi and blood[TM1] deficiency with decreased immune function and chronic infections. Reportedly useful for chronic tympanitis [75] and perianal abscess [76].
- **Hochuekkito**: Used for dispirited children with gastrointestinal weakness. The general condition is not so bad as to require *juzentaihoto*.

Emotion-Stabilizing Effect

Among the wide variety of crude drugs, many have an emotion-stabilizing effect to various degrees. There are some formulas containing more than one such crude drug that are prepared with an expectation of emotion-stabilizing effects. In children, the body and mind are difficult to separate, and mental issues tend to become somatized. Even so, psychotropic drugs are difficult to use in children compared with adults. These Kampo medications can be said to be more suitable for use in children because they have not only emotion-stabilizing effects but also physical-function-improving effects (e.g., improving digestive function).

- **Yokukansan**: Having a sedative effect, this formula was used as an anticonvulsant in old times. Also useful for excitability, night crying, tic disorder, and autism spectrum disorder [77]. Although this formula is well known for use as the same medication for both mother and child, other formulas may be used in this way.
- **Yokukansankachimpihange**: A combination formula of *yokukansan* supplemented with Citrus unshiu peel (*chimpi*) and pinelliae tuber (*hange*) is more effective in

maintaining the digestive function and suitable for long-term treatment for autism spectrum disorder.

- **Daisaikoto**: Essentially, this formula is used for concurrent late and middle yang stage patterns. Having a sedative effect, this formula is particularly useful for excitation symptoms in autism spectrum disorder. This formula targets children with sufficient abdominal strength, fullness and discomfort in the chest and hypochondrium, and the tendency for constipation. Daisaikotokyodaio is used in the absence of constipation.
- **Kanbakutaisoto**: Having an anti-anxiety effect, this formula is used for children with discouraging conditions such as anxiety and a tendency to fright. Having a simple composition, this formula is sweet, palatable, and suitable for children. In Japan, this formula has been used as the first choice drug for night crying since the Edo period.
- **Saikokaryukotsuboreito**: This formula has sedative and anti-anxiety effects. Also useful for night crying. The rhubarb (*daio*)-free form is easy to use for children.

Digestive-Function-Improving Effect

Children are a growing entity, requiring much more energy in the form of qi than adults for development and growth. Because "acquired qi" is produced directly in the spleen[TM1] and stomach[TM1], it is of paramount importance to improve digestive function in children.

(a) **Treatments of direct gastrointestinal symptoms**

Basic gastrointestinal symptoms that can pose problems in clinical pediatrics include vomiting, diarrhea, constipation, and abdominal pain. These symptoms are caused by a broad range of pathologic conditions, whose differential diagnosis and treatment by Western medical approaches are, of course, important. However, many of the symptoms that are intractable using conventional methods are manageable with Kampo medications.

- **Goreisan**: This formula is quickly effective for vomiting in viral gastroenteritis, particularly water vomiting, a condition of "counterflow of water" where the patient vomits water soon after intake. This formula is administered little by little.
- **Rikkunshito**: Used for upper gastrointestinal dysfunction symptoms, such as anorexia, abdominal distention, and nausea. Useful for gastroesophageal reflux.
- **Keihito**: Used in cases of persistent diarrhea in the absence of a definite organic cause.
- **Daikenchuto**: Useful for constipation because it promotes intestinal peristalsis. This formula may be used in combination with *shokenchuto*, i.e., in the form of *chukenchuto*, to be more effective for chronic constipation.
- **Keishikashakuyakuto**: This formula is rich in peony root (*shakuyaku*) and has a spasmolytic effect. Suitable for older children with recurrent abdominal pain, constipation, etc. in conditions like hypersensitive bowel syndrome.
- **Shokenchuto**: This is a formula of *keishikashakuyakuto* supplemented with malt sugar (*koi*) to increase palatability and is suitable for children. This is the first choice drug for children with frequent abdominal pain, especially in conditions like hypersensitive bowel syndrome.

(b) **Treatment of gastrointestinal organs for non-gastrointestinal symptoms (qi-tonifying formula)**

In Kampo medicine, it is assumed that an impairment of digestive function (spleen[TM1] and stomach[TM1]) by a certain cause causes a secondary dysfunction in the entire body or in various parts of the body, which in turn can cause disease. Therefore, treatments that back up digestive function are meaningful for ameliorating chronic and/or recurrent symptoms and diseases that are not directly related to gastrointestinal organs. Formulas that ameliorate such functional impairments are known as "spleen[TM1]-tonifying formulas." This is also applicable to treatments of repeated infections.

- **Shokenchuto**: This is a representative spleen[TM1]-tonifying drug for children. It is effective in ameliorating low-activity conditions such as fatigability, small appetite, proneness to chillness, and repeated abdominal pain. This formula targets severe tension in abdominal muscles. This formula is sweet and palatable because it contains malt sugar (*koi*).
- **Ogikenchuto**: Comprising *shokenchuto* supplemented with Astragalus root (*ogi*), this formula can be used as a basic medicine for chronic allergic inflammations such as atopic dermatitis.
- **Hochuekkito**: Containing Astragalus root (*ogi*) and ginseng (*ninjin*), which have a qi-tonifying effect, and bupleurum root (*saiko*), which has an immunomodulatory effect, this formula is suitable for children. Used in cases of severe fatigue such as fatigability, malaise, tendency to lie down, and night sweats.

Improving Respiration and Sweating Effect

Children have immature respiratory function (lung insufficiency) and are therefore prone to coughing, which is likely to be prolonged. Some Kampo formulas have an affinity for the airway and can be used as antitussives for children. Any underlying disease, such as chronic sinusitis, as the cause of the coughing should be treated.

- **Makyokansekito**: This formula was used for bronchial asthma in old times and is used in cases of severe inflammation in the lower airway with productive cough and icteric sputum.
- **Shoseiryuto**: Used for fluid[TM1] retention with a large volume of dilute clear airway secretion in asthmatic bronchitis and allergic rhinitis. This formula becomes more effective for allergic rhinitis in older children when supplemented with a small amount of aconite root (*bushi*) powder.
- **Bakumondoto**: Used for the sensation of airway dryness and severe dry cough. This formula is effective for nocturnal cough when taken before bedtime. It's easily ingested and has a mild anti-anxiety effect.
- **Kakkontokasenkyushin'i**: This is the first choice drug for acute and chronic sinusitis, used in cases with nasal obstruction, rhinorrhea, or postnasal drip.
- **Shin'iseihaito**: Used in cases of more intense inflammations than those for which *kakkontokasenkyushin'i* is indicated. If purulent rhinorrhea is difficult to discharge, *hainosankyuto* is used in combination. This, however, can promote pus discharge and result in increased nocturnal cough.

Aiding Growth and Development Effect

Some crude drugs are used as kidney-tonifying formulas to aid in the growth of vital functions of children for conditions expected to mitigate aging. *Rokumigan* is a representative formula.

- **Rokumigan**: This is a kidney[TM1]-tonifying formula for children. This formula can be used in cases of development/growth retardation and considerable wasting due to chronic disease and seems to be more effective when used in combination with *shokenchuto* than alone.

Water-Metabolism-Improving Effect

Children are likely to experience dehydration, which can be managed using an appropriate infusion therapy. In modern times, treatment targets include headache, vertigo, dullness, malaise, nausea, and anorexia caused by a slight excess or imbalance of water.

- **Goreisan**: This is a representative formula used to improve water metabolism. It can be used for a wide variety of symptoms due to water retention, such as headache, vertigo, nausea, and edema. It's also useful in preventing migraines associated with low atmospheric pressure in children. Prophylactic use for periodic vomiting is possible in some cases.
- **Ryokeijutsukanto**: Can be used for orthostatic dizziness, palpitations, morning arousal disturbance, motion sickness, and other symptoms due to orthostatic dysregulation.
- **Hangebyakujutsutemmato**: Can be used in cases of vertigo, malaise, and decreased appetite due to marked orthostatic dysregulation.
- **Choreito**: Useful for acute cystitis with pollakiuria, discomfort in urination, etc. [78].
- **Eppikajutsuto**: Highly effective when used for lymphangioma in pediatric surgery [79].

Microcirculation-Improving Effect

In children, there are only a few conditions with static blood[TM1] as the main sign. However, blood[TM1]-stasis resolving formulas are useful in girls in the prepuberty stage and older with menstruation-related symptoms (refer to Sect. 4.3).

8.1.6 Doses and Medication Timing

Pediatric doses can be determined according to age (months/years) or body weight. The doses mentioned below were determined using the more convenient basis of age (Table 5.16).

Although the medication is usually taken orally before meals twice or thrice a day, it can be made more effective by flexibly making regimen changes, including on-demand administration and dosing time adjustments suitable for symptom onset and daily activity status.

8.1.7 Efforts to Increase the Ease of Administration

If the child has difficulty taking an extract formula, efforts should be made to increase the ease of use, such as dissolving it in hot water, mixing it with easy-to-swallow fluids such as cocoa or maltose, using it as a drug intake aid, and choosing a suitable dosage form.

Table 5.16 Pediatric doses; based on adult doses (relative to 1 for adults)

6 Months	1 Year	3 Years	7 Years	12 Years
1/5	1/4	1/3	1/2	2/3

8.1.8 Side Effects

Incidences of side effects as reported in adults are relatively low. However, children should be monitored carefully because they are not good at describing their symptoms. In children with lactose intolerance, the practitioner should be vigilant of diarrhea induced by lactose as an excipient for extract formulas.

Package inserts for extract formula bear the statement "Safety in children has not been established [insufficient clinical data]." Although this situation is not considered problematic, it should be borne in mind for caution's sake.

8.2 Treatment of the Elderly

Akito Hisanaga

8.2.1 Medical Services for the Elderly and Kampo

The World Health Organization (WHO) defines an "elderly person" as anyone 65 years and older. Japan is already a super-aging society. According to statistical data from the Ministry of Public Management, as of September 15, 2020, Japan's population of elderly persons accounts for 28.7% of the entire population. Even so, not all elderly persons experience substantial adverse health effects due to aging. Healthy elderly persons have recently been increasing due to supportive factors, such as improvements in nutrition by better food quality and supplies, technical developments, and advances in medical and healthcare services. Given this situation in Japan, the Japan Association of Gerontology and the Japan Geriatrics Society jointly proposed that it would be appropriate to define the elderly as being an age of 75 years or more, rather than 65 years or more.

Viewing their health qualitatively, elderly persons do not represent a uniform population at all but are instead highly diverse. In the past, medical services for elderly persons have been discussed on the basis of a general description of the medical characteristics of elderly persons with the assumption of progression of senescence. This standard view, however, is no longer suited to Japan's present status in which an increasing number of elderly persons maintain adequate physical strength and are relatively healthy even while under treatment for chronic diseases. In addition, the symptoms of elderly patients often manifest atypically, unlike those described in medical textbooks. Also, they often suffer from more than one chronic disease and multiple diseases increase the number of drugs taken, making drug interactions and adverse effects more likely to occur. Otherwise, the influence of environmental factors is likely to play a greater role. In view of these features, the methodology in Kampo medicine for comprehensive understanding and treatment of the patient's mental and physical conditions seems to be most suited for medical services for the elderly.

8.2.2 Senescence

The basic approach in Kampo medicine for the elderly is essentially the same as that for the young. The intention in Kampo medicine essentially is to provide individual care, whether or not the patient is elderly. Practitioners must avoid preconceptions like the patient has both a yin pattern and a deficiency pattern because he or she is an elderly person. As a basic rule, one must interpret the pathological condition of the patient one is facing, in a straightforward manner, using the four examinations. On the other hand, it is a fact that senescence is an unavoidable universal phenomenon, so a viewpoint on how to understand senescence is considered necessary as a general concept in Kampo theory. Therefore, how "senescence" is viewed in Kampo medicine, distinct from the modern viewpoint of "elderly persons" as represented in the title, is discussed below.

Conceptual Differences Between Western Medicine and Kampo Medicine.

There are some differences in conception and aims of treatment. The differences shown in Table 5.17 are recognized.

Aging and Kidney[TM1] Deficiency

The aging process is viewed as a diminishment of the kidney[TM1]. The kidney[TM1] in East Asian Medicine is a functional unit involving not only urogenital functions but also the bone, tooth, eye, ear, brain, and other tissues and organs. In Kampo medicine, nocturia is associated with renal hypofunction, and dysuria is associated with prostatic hypertrophy, decreased libido, osteoporosis, tooth loss, joint deformation, lumbago, decreased vision, hearing loss, and tinnitus as viewed as senescence phenomena. Also, symptoms such as shortness of breath and amnesia are interpreted as symptoms due to kidney[TM1] deficiency. In Kampo medicine, senescence is not viewed merely as breakdowns in an organism in the progression toward death, including chronic hypofunction associated with compromised metabolic turnover or irreversible changes due to age-related deterioration of organs. Kampo medicine is characterized by an effort to understand distortions in the biological activities of the body holistically with the viewpoint of disorders of the kidney[TM1] as a functional unit. In other words, Western medicine and Kampo medicine are in contrast because the former interprets aging from the viewpoint of death and the latter, from the viewpoint of life.

8.2.3 Therapeutic Strategies for Elderly Patients

Because elderly persons are inevitably subject to senescence, they must have some manifestations of kidney[TM1] deficiency, whether mild or severe. In elderly persons, not all physical disorders can be explained in terms of kidney[TM1] deficiency; disorders can occur due to causes other than kidney[TM1] deficiency. Even when the weakness of the lower

Table 5.17 Differences in view of senescence in Western medicine and Kampo medicine

	Western medicine	Kampo medicine
Conceptual philosophy	Interpretation from the viewpoint of "death" of life	Interpretation from the viewpoint of "living" as an organism
Interpretation of senescence	Viewed simply as a series of failures in an organism due to aging-related irreversible decline in physiological functions. This includes the inability to maintain homeostasis in a progression toward death. Morphological and functional breakdowns are diagnosed mainly on an organ basis	Viewed comprehensively from the standpoint of disorders in the functional unit known as kidney[TM1]. Thus, biological activities in the whole body become disrupted
Diagnosis	A diagnosis is made based on objective findings captured by means of inquiries and medical tests. The condition is diagnosed according to diagnostic criteria (uniform diagnosis)	Individual patterns are identified through the four examinations for Kampo diagnosis (personalized diagnosis).
Treatment goal	First priority is given to disease amelioration (including rehabilitation). If treatment is difficult, palliative care will be initiated	In addition to treatment to ameliorating the kidney[TM1] disorder and supporting disrupted functions. In addition, therapeutic approaches for functional units other than kidney[TM1] may be chosen

abdominal region is noted in abdominal examination (a sign of kidney[TM1] deficiency), if the kidney[TM1] deficiency suggested by a weak lower abdomen is not the primary aspect of the disease, the findings associated with kidney[TM1] deficiency should be regarded as having little significance. That is to say, kidney[TM1]-tonifying formulas should not be administered uniformly. One must avoid giving too much weight to only a portion of the findings. The patient's body and mind should be viewed as a whole to determine whether it is appropriate to make kidney[TM1] deficiency the target of treatment. When the condition is explainable in terms of spleen[TM1] deficiency, as a general rule, administration of kidney[TM1]-tonifying formulas is avoided, and priority is given to treating spleen[TM1] deficiency.

Case of Coexisting Kidney[TM1] Deficiency That Did Not Require Treatment

A 70-year-old man
[History of illness]

In the summer of 2 years ago, he underwent a distal gastrectomy for gastric cancer at the Department of Surgery of Hospital A. Around a year ago, symptoms such as abdominal discomfort, abdominal pain, anorexia, and heartburn developed. He was repeatedly admitted to and discharged from the hospital's Department of Surgery. However, extensive examination did not find gastrointestinal passage disorder, and it was determined that he was not indicated for re-surgery, so he was put on observation. At age 70, however, his symptoms got worse. They included abdominal pain, nausea, decreased appetite, loss of weight (7 kg lost in 2 weeks), and a sudden feeling of heat or cold (A). His fatigue intensified to the point of being unable to get up. He came to the hospital requesting Kampo treatment. At that time, he would become nauseous with the change of position or neck flexion. Thus, he was completely unable to get up from lying supine on the stretcher and could not even lift his head.

[General findings]

The patient was of average height and weight. His mind was clear. There were no neurological abnormalities. His face was pale. During the examination, the patient lay still and just moved his eyes. Although his voice was weak, his speech was intelligible.

[Kampo medicine findings].

Pulse findings: Between floating and sunken, medium strength, slightly large, tense.

Tongue findings: The tongue body is slightly swollen, dark red, and wet. The tongue surface geography looks like a mirror tongue, and glossy.

Abdominal findings: Extremely weak abdominal strength. Nauseous upon light compression in the upper abdomen and around the umbilicus. Bilateral fullness and discomfort in chest and hypochondrium. Pain with pressure on the right and below the umbilicus. The lower abdominal region was weak. A laparotomy scar was noted on the midline.

[Treatment & progress] The weakness in the lower abdominal region found in the abdominal examination suggested the kidney[TM1] deficiency. Nevertheless, taking into account that the chief complaints (A) were not associated with kidney[TM1] deficiency, and the marked fullness and discomfort in the chest and hypochondrium, a deficiency pattern of the late yang stage and a liver[TM1] disorder were diagnosed. After an extract of *saikokeishikankyoto* was administered three times a day for about 2 weeks, the patient's various symptoms were ameliorated. He was once more able to get out of bed and energetically engage in activity.

[NOTE] About Japan's health insurance system for generally healthy elderly persons

Kampo practitioners may sometimes be requested to administer Kampo treatments to prevent senescence or disease. Kampo medicine essentially treats patients on the basis of signs and symptoms. So even when no disease is identified by Western medicine, Kampo treatments based on symptoms are possible in the health insurance system. Treatments covered by health insurance cannot be provided with only the rationale of aging.

8.2.4 Special Considerations in Treating Elderly Persons with Progressed Senescence (Table 5.18)

Issues in the treatment of elderly persons and the significance of Kampo are shown below.

Key Points in Prescribing Kampo Medicines for the Elderly

Herbs that can cause side effects (refer to Chap. 4, Sect. 3.3.2).

(a) **Pseudoaldosteronism due to *kanzo***

Specifically, although *yokukansan* does not contain a large amount of *kanzo*, it can cause pseudoaldosteronism when used carelessly for long periods or in elderly persons over 85 years old [80]. Pseudoaldosteronism often results from prolonged administration of *shakuyakukanzoto* for cramps in the calf. An increase in the amount of *kanzo* from taking more than one Kampo extract preparation can raise the risk of side effects. There is a need to modify the regimen, such as once-a-day doses or taking only as needed.

Table 5.18 Characteristics of pathologies and diseases in the elderly

1.	A patient often has disease in more than one organ. (Significance of Kampo) One formula can be used to treat multiple conditions. This reduces medication consumption compared to Western medicine. (reduction of polypharmacy)
2.	Individual differences are great. (Significance of Kampo): Drugs are administered according to patterns (*sho*).
3.	Decreased defensive capacity of the body. (Significance of Kampo): A fair number of herbs have immune-stimulating effects.
4.	There are often cases that cannot be diagnosed due to a lack of objective findings, even though subjective symptoms are present. (Significance of Kampo): Conditions can be managed well as insipient diseases by treating the pattern (*sho*).
5.	More than treatments focused on visceral diseases to prolong life, there is a need for comprehensive holistic care in view of the quality of life (QOL). (Significance of Kampo): Excellent for alleviating symptoms (treatment by pattern) when radical treatment is difficult.
6.	Tendency of water, electrolyte, and metabolic abnormalities, so drug metabolism and drug responses differ from other adults. (Significance of Kampo): Effects are slow and the number of reports of side effects is fewer than with Western drugs. Caution should be exercised, however, for formulas containing certain herbs such as *kanzo* (glycyrrhiza).

(b) **Increased blood pressure and dysuria with the use of *mao* (Ephedra)**

Mao is an ephedrine-containing herb with sympathomimetic effects. Prolonged administration of *kakkonto* for stiff shoulders can cause hypertension. Dysuria can develop in cases with pre-existing prostatic hypertrophy. Large doses can cause symptoms like palpitations, so special caution should be exercised in patients with underlying heart disease. Reducing the amount of *MAO* and concomitant use of Western drugs with similar pharmacological effects (theophylline, sympathomimetic drugs) should be considered.

(c) **Gastromucosal disorders due to *jio* (*Rehmannia root*) and *senkyu* (*Cnidium Rhizome*)**

Special caution should be exercised with young adults and the elderly. Also, special caution is called for with the use of *hachimijiogan*, as it can cause gastric ulcerations. The dosing frequency should be reduced to once daily if there are any symptoms.

(d) **Others**

The side effects of *bushi* (aconite root), *ogon* (scutellaria root), and *sanshishi* (gardenia fruit) in the elderly are similar to those in youth and adults.

Polypharmacy of Kampo Extract Preparations (Refer to Chap. 1, Sect. 6.1.4).

The multiple uses of Kampo extract formulas carelessly to cope with multiple complaints can be raised as an issue. Kampo practitioners should always bear in mind that the standard practice is to use a single Kampo extract formula at one time. When encountering conditions that may benefit from multiple formulas, the practitioner should make a considered and manageable treatment plan by consulting the patient and deciding priorities in treatment.

8.2.5 Major Conditions and Frequently Used Formulas (Fig. 5.32)

Dementia

No Kampo formula has been shown to be more effective for the cardinal symptoms of dementia than any currently approved anti-dementia drugs in Japan.

Condition	Formula	Indication
Dementia	*Hachimijiogan*	Core symptoms of Alzheimer-type dementia [81]
Dementia	*Yokukansan*	Excitation and restlessness in Alzheimer-type dementia and Lewy body dementia[82-84]
Dementia	*Chotosan*	Apathies and sleep disorders associated with vascular dementia [85]
Dementia	*Tokishakuyakusan*	Sleep disorders and night delirium associated with Alzheimer-type dementia and vascular dementia [86]
Dementia	*Keishikaryukotsuboreito*	Sexual deviances [87]
Decreased appetite	*Rikkunshito*	Deficiency pattern to slight deficiency pattern / epigastric stuffiness and resistance and fluid[TM1] retention in stomach / non-PPI-responsive NERD [88]
Decreased appetite	*Hochuekkito*	Slight deficiency pattern / malaise, slight fever, muscle weakness
Decreased appetite	*Shokenchuto*	Slight deficiency pattern / abdominal muscle tension / for cases not indicated for ginseng
Constipation	*Daiokanzoto*	Medium pattern / abdominal distention with constipation
Constipation	*Jokito*	Severe abdominal distention with constipation / *daijokito, choijokito, tokakujokito* (see Constipation section)
Constipation	*Mashiningan*	Slight deficiency pattern to medium pattern / scybala / blood [TM1] deficiency
Constipation	*Bukuryoin* *Bukuryoingohangekobokuto*	Slight deficiency pattern / hypersensitive to rhubarb
Constipation	*Daikenchuto*	Deficiency pattern to slight deficiency pattern / abdominal distention with peristalsis agitation or intestinal gas / functional constipation as a stroke sequela [89]
Dysphagia	*Hangekobokuto*	Reportedly effective in ameliorating medium pattern / dysphagia [90]
Feeling cold	*Hachimijiogan*	Slight deficiency pattern / coldness in lumbar and lower limbs
Feeling cold	*Goshajinkigan*	Slight deficiency pattern / *hachimijiogan* pattern accompanied by numbness
Feeling cold	*Bushirichuto*	Deficiency pattern / decreased appetite, indigestion
Feeling cold	*Shimbuto*	Fluid [TM1] retention / chronic watery diarrhea, sensation of waivering, and dizziness in deficiency / yin pattern

Fig. 5.32 Major conditions and frequently used formulas for the elderly

- **Hachimijiogan**

Although a report is available on the effect of *hachimijiogan* on cardinal symptoms of Alzheimer-type dementia in deficiency [81], the duration of treatment was shorter at 8 weeks, with no evidence for prolonged effect equivalent to, or higher than, that of anti-dementia drugs (compared to clinical trial data for anti-dementia drugs.

- **Yokukansan**

Kampo medicines have been useful for behavioral and psychological symptoms of dementia (BPSD). With a deficiency pattern, *yokukansan* is effective for excitement and restlessness in Alzheimer-type dementia and Lewy body dementia, but its effect on depression is negligible [82–84].

- **Chotosan** [85]

Reportedly effective for apathy and sleep disorders associated with vascular dementia in deficiency pattern.

- **Tokishakuyakusan**

Reportedly effective for sleep disorders and night delirium associated with Alzheimer-type dementia and vascular dementia in deficiency pattern [86].

- **Keishikaryukotsuboreito**

Deficiency pattern: Reportedly effective for sexual deviance [87].

Decreased Appetite

In the case of markedly decreased appetite, efforts should first be made to prevent further weakness and restore normal physical function. Formulas such as *rikkunshito*, *hochuekkito*, and *shokenchuto* are administered for spleen[TM1] deficiency conditions that are both the causes and results of decreased appetite. All these formulas are used to target decreased abdominal strength.

- **Rikkunshito**

For deficiency to slight deficiency pattern patients with epigastric stuffiness and resistance as well as fluid[TM1] retention in the stomach. Reportedly effective in ameliorating stomach distention in elderly patients with conditions such as non-erosive reflux disease (NERD) refractory to proton pump inhibitors (PPI) and postprandial heartburns [88].

- **Hochuekkito**

For cases where a slight deficiency pattern is accompanied by malaise, slight fever, and muscle weakness.

- **Shokenchuto**

For slight deficiency pattern patients with abdominal muscle tension that is conspicuous or those who feel worse when taking *ninjin* (ginseng).

- **Others**

When the above formulas for suspected spleen[TM1] deficiency have no positive effect, suspect a secondary decrease in appetite. Consider the administration of formulas of involving Bupleurum radix, such as *yokukansan* or *yokukansankachimpihange*.

Constipation
It is a general rule in Kampo to use formulas with rhubarb for abdominal distention with feces (*jitsuman*) and to use formulas without *daio* for abdominal distention with gas (*kyoman*).

- **Daiokanzoto**

Widely used for abdominal distention in medium pattern.

- **Formulas in jokito group (daijokito, choijokito, tokakujokito)**

For excess pattern patients with severe abdominal distention who are not sufficiently responsive to *daiokanzoto* but have a good appetite, it is preferable that the condition be interpreted as gastrointestinal heat (*ikajitsu*), as mentioned in the definition for middle yang stage pattern. In these cases, use *choijokito* (medium pattern), *daijokito* (medium to slight excess pattern), or *tokakujokito* (slight excess pattern to excess pattern).

- **Mashiningan**

For slight deficiency to medium pattern patients with marked blood[TM1] deficiency signs, such as eliminating scybala.

- **Bukuryoin, Bukuryoingohangekobokuto**

In cases of slight deficiency pattern with hypersensitivity to rhubarb, *bukuryoin* or *bukuryoingohangekobokuto* should be considered.

- **Daikenchuto**

For deficiency to slight deficiency pattern patients with clearly unstable peristalsis or severe abdominal distention with intestinal gas. Often effective for compulsive constipation. This formula was reported to improve clinical scores for constipation and intestinal gas volume in patients with functional constipation from stroke sequelae when taken orally for 1 month in a randomized control trial (RCT) [89].

- **Others**

In cases of abdominal distention (gas bloating) in deficiency pattern patients who get poor results with *daikenchuto*, consider administration of *keishikashakuyakuto*, *shakuyakukanzoto*, or *shakuyakukanzobushito*. It is also important that the prescription of these formulas be combined with dietary instructions. This includes regular dietary habits and proper intake of water and dietary fibers.

Dysphagia
Mis-swallowing becomes more likely as pseudobulbar palsy occurs with the progression of cerebral infarction or cerebral degenerative disease.

- **Hangekobokuto**

For medium pattern, reportedly effective in ameliorating dysphagia regardless of the pattern [90]. However, since the progression of dysphagia cannot be prevented with this formula alone, other feasible measures, such as efforts for a better dietary regimen and swallowing training, should also be taken.

Feeling of Cold
If the patient has a severe feeling of cold due to decreased metabolism and disuse disorders associated with senescence, malaise and shortness of breath reduce activity and cause recumbency. This condition is interpreted as the "desire for sleep" condition precisely as given in the definition for the middle yin stage pattern. This is considered a good indication for formulas with processed aconite root, which has a metabolism-enhancing effect. Because the increase in muscle strength cannot be expected, however, physical rehabilitation should be started once the symptoms have been mitigated with Kampo medicines.

- **Hachimijiogan**

Indicted for slight deficiency pattern patients with coldness in lumbar and lower limbs.

- **Goshajinkigan**

Selected in cases of *hachimijiogan* pattern accompanied by numbness.

- **Bushirichuto**

For deficiency pattern patients with severe signs of decreased appetite and indigestion or associated malaise. It is desirable that preference be given to the treatment of spleen[TM1] deficiency, and that *bushirichuto* be administered, avoiding the use of kidney[TM1] tonifying formulas containing *jio*, such as *hachimijiogan* and *goshajinkigan*.

- **Shimbuto**

This formula is used for fluid retention in the yin pattern. Suitable for deficiency pattern patients with coldness and bad color in the limbs and who complain of chronic watery diarrhea, sensation of body motion, and dizziness. These patients have markedly decreased metabolism, often complaining of coldness in all parts of the body and severe general malaise to the extent of wanting to lie down and sleep.

8.2.6 Column

Ikuro WakayamaToshihiro Togo, and Takashi Seki

The Elderly and Acupuncture and Moxibustion

In Japan, the average life span in 2016 was 80.98 years for males and 87.14 years for females, and their differences from healthy life expectancy without the need for long-term care were approximately 9 and 12 years for males and females, respectively. The proportion of elderly persons living alone has been increasing yearly; statistics in 2015 showed that the proportion of the entire elderly population was 13.3% (1.92 million) and 21.1% (4.00 million) for males and females, respectively. Bearing in mind this situation of the Japanese elderly, it will be highly significant to maintain motor functions and manage and maintain a good eating status. Given this viewpoint, this article describes acupuncture/moxibustion treatment for spinal stenosis, dysphagia, and aspiration pneumonia, which markedly affect the quality of life (QOL) in the elderly.

Spinal Stenosis and Acupuncture/Moxibustion

Lower limb pain, including lumbago and knee pain, reduces activity in elders. Spinal stenosis is a disease characterized by severe lumbago, lower limb numbness, and intermittent claudication, in which the morbidity increases with age, and often, it is difficult to determine its surgical indication. Kasuya et al. conducted a comparative study of conservative treatments (acetaminophen treatment, exercise therapy, acupuncture/moxibustion) for lumbar spinal stenosis (LSS) in patients with fifth lumbar nerve root injury between the ages of 50 and 79. Acupuncture treatments were performed by applying electro-stimulation to the *Zusanli* (ST36) acupoint (peroneal nerve), Yanglingquan (GB34) acupoint (fibular head lateral deep peroneal nerve), and left and right Large Intestine Shu (BL25) acupoints (multifidus muscle). Results were evaluated using the Zurich claudication questionnaire (ZCQ), a specific QOL scoring system for lumbar spinal stenosis. They reported that acupuncture/moxibustion treatment was much more effective and more satisfactory than drug therapy and exercise therapy in terms of the ZCQ scale for "severity amelioration" and "physical function improvement."

Dysphagia, Aspiration Pneumonia, and Acupuncture/Moxibustion

Recently, it has been found in Japan that pneumonia ranks high as a cause of death. Statistics in 2019 showed that pneumonia was ranked fifth. More than 90% of relevant deaths occurred in elderly patients ≥65 years of age. In the elderly, the cause of pneumonia varies, but it involves high incidences of aspiration pneumonia due to mis-swallowing. This is caused mainly by reduced swallowing and cough reflex due to cerebrovascular disorder in the basal ganglion, as well as by pseudobulbar palsy associated with frontal lobe atrophy due to degenerative disease.

In the treatment of patients with dysphagia, oral drug therapy is often difficult. There is a need, therefore, to improve the swallowing reflex, not relying on oral administration. Seki et al. reported that swallowing reflex was improved by acupuncture treatment on the *Zusanli* (ST36) and *Taikei* (KI3) acupoints in patients with cerebrovascular disorder and a history of aspiration and that aspiration and pharyngeal retention decreased significantly on videofluorography. The swallowing reflex was also improved by electro-stimulation of these same acupoints using a skin surface electrode.

Points to Note in Japan's Health Insurance System for Generally Healthy Elderly Persons

Kampo practitioners may sometimes be requested to administer Kampo treatments to prevent senescence. Since Kampo medicine makes treatments essentially on a symptomatic basis, health insurance treatments with Kampo drugs are accepted just based on symptoms, even if no disease is identified by Western medicine. Medical services covered by health insurance cannot be provided with the only rationale of aging.

Japan's Mild Acupuncture/Moxibustion Stimulation and Elderly Treatment

Besides the aforementioned diseases, acupuncture/moxibustion treatment is applicable to chronic pain in the elderly. However, since strong acupuncture stimulation in the elderly can aggravate symptoms, it is important that efficacy be maximized with mild stimulation. In Japan, gentle acupuncture treatments are common, and generally, shallow insertions are performed with an insertion tube. These treatments are not inferior to those with deep insertions. It has been reported, for example, that in acupuncture treatment for osteoarthritis of the knee, shallow insertions were as effective against pain as deep insertions and were more effective in improving motor function.

8.3 Cancer

Yoshiharu Moto-o

8.3.1 Overview of Disease

Cancer occurs in various organs, with organ specificity. Its biological malignancy varies greatly according to histological type. Therefore, it is not possible to discuss cancer in various forms as a single entity. In Japan, one out of two people will have some form of cancer during their lifetime, and one out of three will die of it. Cancer has been the top cause of death since 1981. By organ, lung cancer is number one on the list of cancer mortality among Japanese, followed by stomach, colorectal, pancreas, and liver cancers in descending order (2018 List of Statistical Surveys conducted by Ministry of Health, Labor, and Welfare). There have been sharp increases in prostate cancer in men and breast cancer in women. Future countermeasures require urgent attention. The three major cancer therapies are surgery, radiation, and chemotherapy. Each patient requires the most appropriate multidisciplinary treatments, including immunotherapy and palliative care. Less invasive surgical procedures have been and continue to be devised one after another, and especially remarkable advances have been made in endoscopic surgery. In radiation therapy, complications decrease as the irradiation field is narrowed to a pinpoint. In chemotherapy, the development of new anticancer agents, molecular-targeted drugs, and immune checkpoint inhibitors is demonstrating survival advantages, particularly in colorectal, breast, and renal cell cancers. Now, chemotherapy can render unresectable cancers amenable to potentially curable resection. As a result, some patients are freed from cancer.

8.3.2 Indications for Kampo Therapy

While Chinese medicine does use herbs that are called "anticancer herbs," in Japan, it is virtually impossible to inhibit cancer growth with Kampo therapy alone within the framework of the health insurance system. Instead, Kampo medicines offer hope with the improvement of general conditions and indirect antitumor effects. Kampo can contribute to the following stages in the course of allopathic cancer management: treatment, follow-up, and palliative care. As stated above, Kampo is not used for direct antitumor effects in cancer treatment. Instead, the intention is to bring allopathic treatment to a successful conclusion with its chief goal of reducing or preventing the adverse effects of allopathic treatments. As detailed below, Kampo can be used for symptoms that Western medicine finds difficult to deal with, such as peripheral neuropathy, anorexia, general malaise, and delayed diarrhea. This suggests that administering Kampo medicines with follow-up care for chronic (inflammatory) disease, especially liver disease, can lead to chemoprevention of hepatocellular cancer. Kampo medicines can also be used in the follow-up after completion of postoperative adjuvant chemotherapy for all types of cancer. In palliative care, all kinds of Kampo medicines, especially prescriptions containing *bushi*, can be used to reduce adverse effects and overcome resistance, as well as to increase the efficacy of the opioids used for pain relief. The rich variety of Kampo formulas offers many choices for psychoneurotic, digestive, and respiratory symptoms, as well as pain management.

Signs and symptoms not described in "Frequently Used Formulas" will be summarized here.

For nausea and vomiting, there is no need to recommend Kampo medicines as the first choice. Instead, it is imperative to use 5-HT_3 and NK-1 receptor antagonists, dexamethasone, and others in accordance with the "Antiemetic Guidelines (2015)." However, in a randomized controlled trial (RCT), combined use of *rikkunshito* was reported to reduce nausea significantly following chemotherapy on day 14 and also alleviated vomiting and anorexia as well.

The liver injury here refers to hepatic damage resulting from the use of anticancer agents (drug-induced liver injury). Thus, essential treatment includes discontinuation of medication and liver-supporting therapy. Ursodeoxycholic acid (UDCA) is often used in liver-supporting therapy, but *inchinkoto* is one of the possible treatments for prolonged intrahepatic cholestasis. The level of evidence for its clinical effectiveness is not high, but there are detailed reports in basic experiments on the choleretic action mediated by the ingredient *genipin*.

Cancer patients and their families desire to enhance immune strength and prevent its deterioration. Many patients want to maintain or enhance their immunity while undergoing chemotherapy. This is also what attending physicians hope. There are, however, only a few high-quality reports demonstrating the actual clinical effectiveness of Kampo formulas in tumor immunity improvement. Among the formulas studied, *juzentaihoto* has been reported to suppress inflammation after hepatectomy and prevent the recurrence of hepatocellular carcinoma in RCTs. Also, it is reported to suppress inflammatory cytokine and reactive oxygen species production by Kupffer cells in a laboratory setting.

8.3.3 Frequently Used Formulas

Anorexia

- **Rikkunshito**: For patients with deficiency or slight deficiency pattern, the effectiveness of this prescription for anorexia following chemotherapy has been demonstrated in basic studies and clinical trials. It has also been found that *rikkunshito* reverses the blood acylghrelin decrease induced by chemotherapy (particularly cisplatin) and ghrelin receptor decrease in the hypothalamus.

Hematotoxicity

- **Kamikihito**: For patients with slight deficiency to medium pattern, the effectiveness of this formula has been demonstrated specifically for thrombocytopenia, though only in an observation study. The group treated with *kamikihito* showed milder thrombocytopenia and faster recovery than the untreated group.
- **Juzentaihoto**: Used for deficiency pattern patients with anemia and leukocytopenia, but only as an auxiliary role. Experimental studies have shown increases in spleen colony counts after irradiation, suggesting that *juzentaihoto* accelerates myeloid stem cell growth.

Stomatitis

- **Hangeshashinto**: Appropriate for patients with the medium pattern. Chemotherapy-induced stomatitis is considered to develop via the mechanism that oral mucosal cells with high cell turnover, induced by an anticancer agent, undergo apoptosis due to increases in reactive oxygen species, cytokines, and prostaglandins. It has been reported that *hangeshashinto* is effective for chemotherapy-induced stomatitis through the mechanisms involving the inhibition of prostaglandin E2 induction and the antibacterial action of the ingredient *oren*.

Bowel Movement Disturbance

- **Daikenchuto**: For patients with deficiency to slight deficiency pattern. This formula is used for the prevention of postoperative ileus and intestinal hypomotility. The efficacy of opioid-induced constipation is also promising.
- **Hangeshashinto**: This formula is effective for medium pattern patients with delayed diarrhea due to irinotecan hydrochloride (CPT-11). Dosing prior to CPT-11 is recommended as a prophylactic.

Peripheral Neuropathy

- **Goshajinkigan**: This formula has been used for slight deficiency pattern patients with peripheral neuropathy due to paclitaxel and oxaliplatin [91]. The chief symptom is numbness in the extremities. Chemotherapy must be discontinued before the onset of functional disorder. However, these two anticancer drugs differ in their mechanism of inducing peripheral neuropathy. Paclitaxel induces axonopathy, whereas oxaliplatin causes neuronopathy. Therefore, especially in cases treated with oxaliplatin, alternative Kampo formulas must be sought.

General Malaise and Cancer Cachexia

- **Hochuekkito**: Originally used for patients with slight deficiency pattern, but among the Kampo formulas available, this is most often administered to advanced and recurrent cancer patients with a complaint of general malaise as well as fatigue. While interleukin-6 (IL-6) is involved in cancer cachexia, the fact that *hochuekkito* has an IL-6 inhibiting activity is only mentioned in reports of invasive surgery and infection, and this does not appear in cancer-related reports. Further elucidation of the mechanisms of *hochuekkito* is expected, as activin receptor type IIB (ActRIIB) has recently been found to link with cancer cachexia [92].
- **Ninjin'yoeito**: Used for patients with slight deficiency pattern. The efficacy and mechanisms of *ninjin'yoeito* in cancer cachexia and sarcopenia have been elucidated, and this formula is recommended for elderly cancer patients.

References

1. Saylor D, Steiner TJ. The global burden of headache. Semin Neurol. 2018;38(2):182–90.
2. International Headache Society. The international classification of headache disorders, 3rd ed. Cephalalgia. 2018;38(1):1–211.
3. Harada Y, Yoshida K, Nojiri S, Kurihara Y, Kobayashi H, Arai H. Identification of chronic subdural hematoma types most responsive to Goreisan, Kampo medicine: a retrospective study. J Clin Neurosci. 2020;78:198–202.
4. Basura GJ, Adams ME, Monfared A, et al. Clinical practice guideline: Meniere's disease. Otolaryngol Head Neck Surg. 2020;162(2 suppl):S1–S55.
5. Bhattachayya N, Gubbels SP, Schwartz SR, et al. Clinical practice guideline, benign paroxysmal positional vertigo. Otolaryngol Head Neck Surg. 2017;156(3 suppl):S1–S47.
6. Tunkel DE, Bauer CA, Un GH, et al. Clinical practice guideline, tinnitus. Otolaryngol Head Neck Surg. 2014;151(2 suppl):S1–S40.
7. Japanese guideline for allergic rhinitis 2020 Allergology International 69, PP331-345 2020 Elsevier B.V.
8. Practical guideline for the management of allergic rhinitis in Japan p58 and p78, 2020 Life Science Tokyo.
9. Liu YF, Kim Y, Yoo T, et al. Burning mouth syndrome: a systematic review of treatments. Oral Dis. 2018 Apr;24(3):325–34.
10. Braud A, Boucher Y. Taste disorder's management: a systematic review. Clin Oral Investig. 2020;24(6):1889–908.
11. Taira K, Fujiwara K, Fukuhara T, et al. The effect of Hangeshashinto on oral mucositis caused by induction chemotherapy in patients with head and neck cancer. Yonago Acta Med. 2020;63(3):183–7.

12. Hottenbacher L, et al. Opinions on Kampo and reasons for using it--results from a cross-sectional survey in three Japanese clinics. BMC Complement Altern Med. 2013 May;16(13):108.
13. Takayama S, et al. A multi-center, randomized controlled trial by the integrative management in Japan for epidemic disease (IMJEDI study-RCT) on the use of Kampo medicine, kakkonto with sho-saikotokakikyosekko, in mild-to-moderate COVID-19 patients for symptomatic relief and prevention of severe stage: a structured summary of a study protocol for a randomized controlled trial. Trials. 2020;21(1):827.
14. Committee for the Japanese respiratory society. Second edition of Guidelines for management of cough. 2012.
15. Committee for the Japanese respiratory society. Guidelines for Appropriate Medication Use in Kampo Therapy. 2005.
16. Tatsumi K, et al. 2. Respiratory tract disease. In: Mizuno S, editor. Internal Kampo medicine. Kyoto: Medical Yukon; 2007. p. 121–84. Tatsumi K. Manual of Kampo therapy for respiratory diseases. Tokyo: Kyowa Kikaku. 2006.
17. Shinozuka N, Tatsumi K, Nakamura A, Terada J, Kuriyama T. The traditional herbal medicine Hochuekkito improves systemic inflammation in patients with chronic obstructive pulmonary disease. J Am Geriatr Soc. 2007;55(2):313–4.
18. Tatsumi K, Shinozuka N, Nakayama K, Sekiya N, Kuriyama T, Fukuchi Y. Hochuekkito improves systemic inflammation and nutritional status in elderly patients with chronic obstructive pulmonary disease. J Am Geriatr Soc. 2009;57(1):169–70. The Japanese Society of Allergology (supervised). Zensoku Yobo—Kanri Gaidorain (Asthma Prevention and Management Guidelines) 2015, Tokyo: Kyowakikaku Tsushin. Katsura H, et al. J Jpn Respir Soc. 38(3): 174–179, 2000
19. Ito T, et al. The effects of Hachimi – jio – Gan on chronic asthma (the second report). Kampo Med. 1996;47(3):443–9.
20. Shinozuka N, et al. The traditional herbal medicine Hochuekkito improves systemic inflammation in patients with chronic obstructive disease. J Am Geriatr Soc. 2007;55(2):313–4.
21. Yakubo S, et al. Clinical evaluation of Moku-boi-to (Mu-fang-yi-tang): a Japanese and Chinese traditional medicine for heart failure. J Trad Med. 2002;19:159–63.
22. Ezaki H, et al. Effects of Mokuboito， a Japanese Kampo medicine， on symptoms in patients hospitalized for acute decompensated heart failure – a prospective randomized pilot study. J Cardiol. 2019;74:412–7.
23. Katayose D, et al. The therapeutic application of Saiko-ka-ryukotsu-borei-to (Chai-Hu-Jia-Long-Gu-Du-Li-Tang) in the cardiological clinic. Kampo Med. 2001;52(1):25–38. (summary in English)
24. Tominaga K, et al. Kampo medicines for gastrointestinal tract disorders: a review of basic science and clinical evidence and their future application. J Gastroenterol. 2013;48:452–62.
25. Kubota T, et al. Gastrointestinal system. In: Introduction to KAMPO Japanese traditional medicine. Tokyo: Elsevier Japan K.K.; 2005. p. 118–21.
26. Textbook of Traditional Japanese Medicine, Part 1: Kampo. Health and Labour Sciences (Research Grant Research on the standardization of traditional Japanese medicine promoting integrated medicine). http://kampo-edu.med.u-tokai.ac.jp/textbook/pdf/Part1_Kampo_ Textbook_of_Traditional_Japanese_Medicine_en.pdf.
27. The Dictionary of Kampo Medicine (Basic terms). The Japan Society for Oriental Medicine, 2020, Tokyo.
28. Kainuma M, Sakai S,Sekiya N， et al.The effects of a herbal medicine (Mao-to) in patients with chronic hepatitis C after injection of IFN-beta. Phytomedicine 11(1): 5–10 2004.
29. Shimada Y, Fujimoto M, Nogami T, et al. Non-alcoholic fatty liver disease satisfactorily treated with traditional Japanese kampo medicine. Tradit Kampo Med. 2018;5(1):56–60.
30. Shoda J Matsuzaki Y Tanaka N， et al. The inhibitory effects of dai-chai-hu-tang (dai-saiko-to) extract on supersaturated bile formation in cholesterol gallstone disease. Am J Gastroenterol 91(4): 828–830 1996.
31. Nagasaka K, Fukuda H, Watanabe T. Report of four cases of chronic renal failure effectively treated with Astragi radix. Kampo Med. 2012;63:378–83.
32. Shoji T. Combined administration of shinbuto and boiogito prevents the progression of chronic kidney disease with minimal proteinuria in the long-term (part 2). Kampo Med. 2020;71:378–83.
33. Kamakami M. Experience of using Gosha-jinki-gan in patients with cerebrovascular disorders with frequent urination and urinary incontinence. J Trad Med. 1990;7:348–9.
34. Tokunaga S, Nakajima T, Yamaguchi K, et al. Clinical study of o Gosha-jinki-gan in patients with urination disorder. Department of Urology, Acta Urologica Japonica. 1992;54:1067–70.
35. Ikeuchi T, Ueno M. Clinical studies of chronic prostatitis and prostatitis-like syndrome (4)–(6). Acta Urologica Japonica. 1990;36:801–6. 37:1677–1682.1991; 39:321–325,1993
36. Sugaya Y, Nishizawa R, Noto H, et al. Effects of Chorei-to, Chorei-to-goshimotsu-to for urethra syndrome. Acta Urologica Japonica. 1992;38:731–5.
37. Ushiroyama T, Ikeda A, Sakai M, Hosotani T, Suzuki Y, Tsubokura S, Ueki M. Effects of *unkei-to*, an herbal medicine, on endocrine function and ovulation in women with high basal levels of luteinizing hormone secretion. J Reprod Med. 2001;46:451–6.
38. Ushiroyama T, Hosotani T, Yamashita Y, Yamashita H, Ueki M. Comparison of endocrinological effects of the traditional herbal medicines *Unkei-to* and *Touki-shakuyaku-san* in improving luteal phase defects in women of xu zheng, a deficient condition. Study of pulsatile secretion of gonadotropins. Herb Comp Med. 2002;3:53–61.
39. Ushiroyama T, Ikeda A, Sakuma K, Ueki M. Comparing the effects of estrogen and an herbal medicine on peripheral blood flow in post-menopausal women with hot flashes: hormone replacement therapy and *Guizhi-fuling-wan*, a Kampo medicine. Am J Chin Med. 2005;33:259–67.
40. Shigemi D, Hashimoto Y, Michihata N, Yasunaga H. Effect of Japanese herbal Kampo medicines on live birth rate in women with recurrent pregnancy loss. Int J Gynaecol Obstet. 2021;153(3):489–95.
41. Takakuwa K, Yasuda M, Hataya I, Sekizuka N, Tamura M, Arakawa M, Higashino M, Hasegawa I, Tanaka K. Treatment for patients with recurrent abortion with positive antiphospholipid antibodies using a traditional Chinese herbal medicine. J Perinat Med. 1996;24(5):489–94. https://doi.org/10.1515/jpme.1996.24.5.489.
42. Kano T, Shimizu M, Kanda T, Hijikata Y. Sairei-to therapy on alloimmune recurrent spontaneous abortions and autoimmune complicated recurrent spontaneous abortions. Am J Chin Med. 2010;38(4):705–12.
43. Yoichiro I. Regulatory mechanism for water metabolism of gorei-san through aquaporin. Sci Kampo Med. 2011;35(2):90–3.
44. Yasunaga H. Effect of Japanese herbal Kampo medicine Goreisan on reoperation rates after Burr-Hole surgery for chronic subdural hematoma: analysis of a national inpatient database. Evid Based Complement Alternat Med. 2015;2015:817616. https://doi.org/10.1155/2015/817616.
45. Yano Y, et al. Goreisan inhibits upregulation of aquaporin 4 and formation of cerebral edema in the rat model of juvenile hypoxic-ischemic encephalopathy. Evid Based Complement Alternat Med. 2017;2017:3209219. https://doi.org/10.1155/2017/3209219.
46. Matsuda A, et al. Therapeutic effect of Saireito (TJ-114) on autoimmune hepatitis-reduction of steroid dose and side effects. Shindan to chiryo (Diagnosis and treatment). 1993;81(4):911–5.
47. Kogure T. Recent clinical applications of Japanese oriental (Kampo) medicine for rheumatoid arthritis: search for Kampo responder. Altern Ther Health Med. 2013;19:50–2.

48. Kogure T, Harada N, Yamamoto K, et al. Positive effects of *Uyakujunkisan* therapy (Kampo medicine) for postherpetic neuralgia with concomitant pregabalin: two case reports with a literature review. Altern Ther Health Med. 2016;22:40–4.
49. Motoo Y, Tomita Y, Fujita H. Prophylactic efficacy of *ninjin-yoe-ito* for oxaliplatin-induced cumulative peripheral neuropathy in patients with colorectal cancer receiving postoperative adjuvant chemotherapy: a randomized, open-label, phase 2 trial (HOPE-2). Int J Clin Oncol. 2020;25:1123–9.
50. Kumada T, Kumada H, Yoshiba M, Nakano S, Suzuki H, Tango T. Effects of shakuyaku-kanzo-to (Tsumura TJ-68) on muscle cramps accompanying cirrhosis in a placebo-controlled double-blind parallel study. J Clin Ther Med. 1999;15(3):499–523. (in Japanese with English abstract)
51. Takao Y, Takaoka Y, Sugano A, et al. Shakuyaku-kanzo-to (Shao-Yao-Gan-Cao-Tang) as treatment of painful muscle cramps in patients with lumbar spinal stenosis and its minimum effective dose. Kobe J Med Sci. 2016;61(5):E132–7.
52. Ito Y, Murotani N, Ito K, et al. Effect of Shakuyaku-kanzo-to on muscle cramps in hemodialysis patients. J Jpn Soc Dial Ther. 2003;36(1):33–9.
53. Shimada Y. Effects of chotosan on cerebrovascular disorders. J Trad Med. 2012;29(4):157–68.
54. Kobayashi H, Ishii M, Takeuchi S, et al. Efficacy and safety of a traditional herbal medicine, Hochu-ekki-to in the long-term management of kikyo (delicate constitution) patients with atopic dermatitis- a 6-month, multicenter, double-blind, randomized, placebo-controlled study. Evid Based Complement Alternat Med. 2010;7:367–73.
55. NICE. Depression: the treatment and management of depression in adults (NICE clinical guideline 90). London: The National Institute for Health and Care Excellence; 2013.
56. Kleinstäuber M, Witthöft M, Steffanowski A, van Marwijk H, Hiller W, Lambert MJ. Pharmacological interventions for somatoform disorders in adults. Cochrane Database Syst Rev. 2014;2014:CD010628.
57. Shi M-M, Piao J-H, Xi-Lin X, Zhu L, Yang L, Lin F-L, Chen J, Jiang J-G. Chinese medicines with sedative–hypnotic effects and their active components. Sleep Med Rev. 2016;29:108–18.
58. Iwasaki K, Kobayashi S, Chimura Y, et al. A randomized, double-blind, placebo-controlled clinical trial of the Chinese herbal medicine "ba wei di huang wan" in the treatment of dementia. J Am Geriatr Soc. 2004;52(9):1518–21.
59. Utumi Y, Iseki E, Murayama N, et al. Effect of Rikkunshi-to on appetite loss found in elderly dementia patients: a preliminary study. Psychogeriatrics. 2011;11(1):34–9.
60. Imai H, Takeshima N, Oda H, et al. Choto-san versus placebo for patients with dementia: systematic review and meta-analysis. Psychogeriatrics. 2017;17(6):466–78.
61. Iwasaki K, Satoh-Nakagawa T, Maruyama M, et al. A randomized, observer-blind, controlled trial of the traditional Chinese medicine Yi-Gan San for improvement of behavioral and psychological symptoms and activities of daily living in dementia patients. J Clin Psychiatry. 2005;66(2):248–52.
62. Okamoto H, Chino A, Hirasaki Y, Ueda K, et al. Orengedoku-to augmentation in cases showing partial response to yokukan-san treatment: a case report and literature review of the evidence for use of these Kampo herbal formulae. Neuropsychiatr Dis Treat. 2013;9:151–5.
63. Watari H, Shimada Y, Matsui M, et al. Kihito, a traditional Japanese Kampo medicine, improves cognitive function in Alzheimer's disease patients. Evid Based Complement Alternat Med. 2019;2019 https://doi.org/10.1155/2019/4086749.
64. Niitsu T, Okamoto H, Iyo M. Behavioral and psychological symptoms of dementia in an Alzheimer's disease case successfully treated with natural medicine: association with gonadotropins. Psychogeriatrics. 2013;13(2):124–7. https://doi.org/10.1111/psyg.12010.
65. Henningsen P, Zipfel S, Herzog W. Management of functional somatic syndromes. Lancet. 2007;369(9565):946–55. https://doi.org/10.1016/S0140-6736(07)60159-7.
66. Wang XQ, Takahashi T, Zhu SJ, et al. Effect of Hochu-ekki-to (TJ-41), a Japanese herbal medicine, on daily activity in a murine model of chronic fatigue syndrome. Evid Based Complement Alternat Med. 2004;1(2):203–6. https://doi.org/10.1093/ecam/neh020.
67. Shin S, Park SJ, Hwang M. Effectiveness a herbal medicine (Sipjeondaebo-tang) on adults with chronic fatigue syndrome: a randomized, double-blind, placebo-controlled trial. Integr Med Res. 2021;10(2):100664. https://doi.org/10.1016/j.imr.2020.100664. Epub 2020 Sep 22
68. Weak constitution. Introduction to KAMPO – Japanese traditional medicine. The Japan Society for Oriental Medicine, 182–184, Elsevier, Japan, 2005.
69. Greenberg P, et al. Revised international prognostic scoring system for myelodysplastic syndromes. Blood. 2012;120(12):2454–65.
70. Hioki C, et al. Clin Exp Pharmacol Physiol. 2004;31:614–9.
71. Yamanaka J, et al. Evid Based Complement Alternat Med. 2013; https://doi.org/10.1155/2013/943075.
72. Yoshida M, et al. Effects of Boui-Ougi-to treatment on visceral fat obesity in patients with diabetes mellitus. Kampo Med. 1998;49(2):249–56. (summary in English)
73. Pediatrics. Introduction to KAMPO – Japanese traditional medicine. The Japan Society for Oriental Medicine, 172–175, Elsevier, Japan, 2005.
74. Kubo T, et al. Antipyretic effect of Mao-to, a Japanese herbal medicine, for treatment of type A influenza infection in children. Phytomedicine. 2007;14:96–101.
75. Ito M, et al. Randomized controlled trial of juzen-taiho-to in children with recurrent acute otitis media. Auris Nasus Larynx. 2017;44:390–7.
76. Sueyoshi R, et al. Combination therapy with traditional medicines for perianal abscess in children. Pediatr Int. 2019;61:1025–9.
77. Wake R, et al. Yokukansan for irritability with pervasive developmental disorder in children and adolescents. Psychopharmacology. 2013;23:329–36.
78. Kawashima N, et al. Choreito formula for BK virus-associated hemorrhagic cystitis after allogeneic hematopoietic stem cell transplantation. Biol Blood Marrow Transplant. 2015;21:319–25.
79. Ogawa K, et al. Effect of Japanese Kampo medicine, eppikajutsuto, in patients with lymphatic malformation: a retrospective observational study. Medicine (Baltimore). 2021;100(51):e28420.
80. Okahara K, Ishida Y, Hayashi Y, et al. Safety and efficacy evaluation of long term treatment with a traditional Japanese medicine, Yokukansan, on behavioral and psychological symptoms of dementia. Dement Jpn. 2012;26:196–205.
81. Iwasaki K, Kanbayashi S, Chimura Y, et al. A randomized, double-blind, placebo-controlled clinical trial of the Chinese herbal medicine "ba wei di huang wan" in the treatment of dementia. J Am Geriatr Soc. 2004;52:1518–21.
82. Iwasaki K, Satoh-Nakagawa T, Maruyama M, et al. A randomized, observer-blind, controlled trial of the traditional Chinese medicine Yi-gan san for improvement of behavioral and psychological symptoms and activities of daily living in dementia patients. J Clin Psychiatry. 2005;66:248–52.
83. Mizukami K, Asada T, Kinoshita T, et al. A randomized cross-over study of a traditional Japanese medicine (kampo), yokukansan, in the treatment of the behavioral and psychological symptoms of dementia. Int J Neuropsychopharmacol. 2009;12:191–9.
84. Mizukami K. Kampo therapy and behavioral and psychological symptoms of dementia. Tradit Kampo Med. 2014;1:11–8.

85. Terasawa K, Shimada Y, Kita T, et al. Choto-san in the treatment of vascular dementia: a double blind, placebo-controlled study. Phytomedicine. 1997;4:15–22.
86. Inanaga T, Dainoson K, Ninomiya Y, et al. Effects of Toki-Shakuyaku-San in patients with senile cognitive disorders. Prog Med. 1996;16:293–300.
87. Tahara E, Shintani T, Moriyama K, et al. Two elderly cases of deviant sexual behavior successfully treated with Keishi-ka-ryukotsu-borei-to. Kampo Med. 2003;54:957–61.
88. Sakata Y, Tominaga K, Kato M, et al. Clinical characteristics of elderly patients with proton pump inhibitor-refractory non-erosive reflux disease from the G-PRIDE study who responded to rikkunshito. BMC Gastroenterol. 2014;14:116. https://doi.org/10.1186/1471-230X-14-116.
89. Numata T, Takayama S, Tobita M, et al. Traditional Japanese medicine Daikenchuto improves functional constipation in poststroke patients. Evid Based Complement Alternat Med. 2014;2014:231–58.
90. Iwasaki K, Kato S, Monma Y, et al. A pilot study of banxia houpu tang, a traditional Chinese medicine, for reducing pneumonia risk in older adults with dementia. J Am Geriatr Soc. 2007;55:2035–40.
91. Kono T, Hata T, Morita S, et al. Goshajinkigan oxaliplatin neurotoxicity evaluation (GONE): a phase 2, multicenter, randomized, double-blind, placebo-controlled trial of goshajinkigan to prevent oxaliplatin-induced neuropathy. Cancer Chemother Pharmacol. 2013;72:1283–90. https://doi.org/10.1007/s00280-013-2306-7.
92. Zhou X, Jin Lin W, John L, et al. Reversal of cancer cachexia and muscle wasting by ActRIIB antagonism leads to prolonged survival. Cell. 2010;142:531–43.

Part II

Acupuncture and Moxibustion Treatment

6 General Theory of Acupuncture and Moxibustion

Ikuro Wakayama, Toshihiro Togo, Hitoshi Yamashita, and Yosuke Amano

1 Acupuncture and Moxibustion (Acu-Moxa)

Ikuro Wakayama

Japan, China, and Korea are the three main countries utilizing acupuncture and moxibustion (acu-moxa) as a treatment modality effective for many diseases. The licensure system in these countries, however, differs in terms of acu-moxa and herbal medicine. In China and Korea, acu-moxa is practiced by Chinese medical doctors and Korean medical doctors, and they also prescribe herbal medicine. In Japan, on the other hand, both Western medical doctors and acu-moxa practitioners (鍼灸師) can practice acupuncture and moxibustion, and Western medical doctors can prescribe Japanese herbal medicine (Kampo medicines, 漢方薬), while acu-moxa practitioners cannot. Acu-moxa practitioners practice acu-moxa, and Kampo doctors (Western medical doctors who specialize in Kampo medicine) practice Kampo. "Kampo" in a broad sense means traditional Japanese medicine, including Japanese herbal medicine and acu-moxa.

It is very important, therefore, that acu-moxa practitioners collaborate with Kampo doctors as well as other Western medical doctors. At present, however, most medical doctors (except Kampo doctors) do not have sufficient knowledge about acu-moxa. Conversely, acu-moxa practitioners are rather lacking the knowledge about what is practiced in Western medical hospitals.

Considering the future of the medical system in Japan, the combined use of acu-moxa with the modern Western medical treatment or with Kampo medicine treatment will greatly contribute to the betterment of patients. In some university hospitals and general hospitals in Japan, Kampo doctors and acu-moxa practitioners work together to provide treatment to their patients, but it will take some time for this system to spread throughout the country. Further development of medical doctor-acu-moxa practitioner collaboration will be needed.

1.1 Current Status of Acupuncture and Moxibustion in the World

Acu-moxa originated in ancient China and subsequently developed independently, mainly in Japan, China, and Korea in East Asia. It is now internationally recognized as one of the most useful non-pharmacological therapies.

In the 2000s, large-scale clinical trials were conducted mainly in Europe, and now many randomized controlled trials (RCTs) and systematic reviews (SRs) have been published in the Cochrane review. Thus, the clinical effect of acu-moxa has been extensively examined and incorporated into clinical practice guidelines (CPGs) for many diseases in many countries. However, acu-moxa has been a clinical treatment method very familiar to the people of Japan for a long time, and well accepted in their culture and daily living. Therefore, the idea that the clinical effects of acu-moxa have to be verified does not arise so much.

However, acu-moxa is regarded as a new physical therapy in Western countries, so clinical trials were needed to confirm the evidence of its efficacy.

According to a 2019 report by the World Federation of Acupuncture-Moxibustion Societies (WFAS), 101 countries

I. Wakayama
Kansai University of Health Sciences, Sennan-gun, Japan

T. Togo (✉)
Meiji University of Integrative Medicine, Nantan, Japan
e-mail: office@jsom.or.jp

H. Yamashita
Graduate School of Health Sciences, Morinomiya University of Medical Sciences, Osaka, Japan

Y. Amano
Nihon Isen, Tokyo, Japan

Kampo Medical Literature Editorial Committee, The Japan Society for Oriental Medicine (ed.), *Complete Japanese Traditional (Kampo) Medicine*, https://doi.org/10.1007/978-981-96-7143-4_6

around the world approved acu-moxa practice, 29 have legal systems for acu-moxa practice, and 18 cover acu-moxa practice with insurance [1]. The qualifications for acu-moxa vary from country to country. For example, in France, only medical doctors are allowed to practice acu-moxa, whereas in the United Kingdom, medical doctors, physiotherapists, nurses, and acu-moxa practitioners are allowed to practice [2]. (Actually, the practitioners in Western countries practice acupuncture, but very few of them practice moxibustion.) In the United States, acu-moxa can be practiced by medical doctors or by acu-moxa practitioners who hold a NCCAOM (National Certification Commission for Acupuncture and Oriental Medicine) license, or a qualification approved by the state of their residence [3]. In China and Korea, as mentioned above, medical doctors practice acu-moxa, but they have completed a different curriculum from Western medical doctors. That is, they are trained mainly in traditional medicine instead of Western medicine, which is to say traditional herbal medicine, acu-moxa, and tuina (massage).

Regarding licensure systems for acu-moxa practitioners, the NCCAOM in the United States is one of the most well-established ones. Nevertheless, no country except Japan has such a sophisticated and long history of education and licensure of acu-moxa; this is a major feature of Japanese acu-moxa.

At the General Assembly of the WHO in May 2019, ICD-11 (International Classification of Diseases, 11th Edition) was approved in which a chapter on traditional medicine was adopted for the first time in the history of ICD. Regarding acu-moxa, traditional medical diagnoses (patterns) as well as meridian patterns of the 12 main meridians and extra meridians were listed. In the future, therefore, using these patterns as a basis, the project of accumulating data on acu-moxa treatment needs to be started [4, 5].

2 Current Status of Acupuncture and Moxibustion in Japan

Ikuro Wakayama

2.1 Qualification, Education, and National Examination System for Acu-Moxa Practitioners in Japan

The licensure system for practicing acu-moxa in Japan is divided into two systems, one for acupuncturists (鍼師 orはり師) and the other for moxibustionists (灸師 or きゅう師). Most practitioners, however, have both licenses, and they are usually called acu-moxa practitioners (鍼灸師).

Acupuncture and moxibustion education in Japan includes three-year courses at vocational schools (81 schools) and four-year courses at universities (ten universities) as of August 2021. At any of these institutions, one who completes the course specified by the rules of the Ministry of Health, Labor and Welfare (MHLW) is eligible to take the national examination. In Japan, historically, visually impaired people have contributed to the development of acu-moxa. Therefore, acu-moxa education is also provided for the visually impaired at schools for the blind. These students take the same national examination as those with sight. (Of course, visual disability should not be a handicap, so the examination environment is arranged accordingly.) The national examination for acu-moxa is conducted once a year just as with other medical professions. In 2020, the numbers of examinees were 3853 for acupuncture and 3797 for moxibustion. The numbers of successful applicants was 2698 and 2740, and the pass rates were 72% and 72.2% for acupuncturists and moxibustionists, respectively.

2.2 Number of Acu-Moxa Practitioners in Japan

The number of acu-moxa practitioners in Japan is about 180,000 as of 2019, of which about 120,000 are engaged in clinical practice (end of 2018). It is less than half of the number of medical doctors that counts approximately 300,000. In addition, it is reported that only 4% of hospitals adopt acu-moxa for routine treatment9). Therefore, the most acu-moxa practitioners are practicing in private outpatient clinics.

2.3 Insurance Coverage for Acupuncture and Moxibustion

If certain requirements are met in acu-moxa treatments, national health insurance can be applied as "medical expenses". Regarding the payment of "medical expenses" for acu-moxa treatment, the national government notified prefectural governors in 1967, and in 2004, the following six diseases were eligible for insurance coverage when medical doctors agreed to the treatment of patients with acu-moxa. These are (1) neuralgia, (2) rheumatoid arthritis (this actually refers to diseases that cause swelling and pain in joints rather than rheumatoid arthritis per se), (3) low back pain, (4) frozen shoulder (scapulohumeral periarthritis), (5) cervicobrachial syndrome, and (6) cervical sprain sequelae (whiplash injury). In addition to the above, insurance can be applied to chronic painful diseases with consent from medical doctors. However, if a patient is currently being treated for the same diagnosis in a medical institution, acu-moxa treatment is not covered by health insurance.

2.4 Integrative Medicine and Acupuncture and Moxibustion: The Importance of Collaboration Between Medical Doctor and Acu-Moxa Practitioners

Integrative medicine is a therapy that combines modern Western medicine with complementary and alternative medicine and/or traditional medicine. There are various types of integrative medicine, but for acu-moxa, the combination of Western medicine and acu-moxa, or the combination of Kampo medicinal treatment and acu-moxa, is the most common form.

Collaboration between medical doctors/Kampo doctors and acu-moxa practitioners will be conducted either in the hospitals or in private outpatient acu-moxa clinics. In the latter cases, communication via medical letters is very important. In either case, however, a medical doctor should understand acu-moxa well, recognize it as one of the treatment options, and determine the indications, while the acu-moxa practitioner must understand the team approach to medical care, and must have the ability to communicate with medical doctors and other medical staff. The main purpose of this volume is to provide information about acu-moxa to medical doctors, and encourage collaboration with acu-moxa to make it possible to treat intractable conditions alongside Western medicine.

The Japan Society of Acupuncture and Moxibustion (JSAM) is currently developing a certified acu-moxa practitioner system to assure the public of the knowledge and skills of acu-moxa practitioners. Developing human resources who can collaborate with medical doctors is the most important aim of this system. Presently, there are not many hospitals in which acu-moxa practitioners work together with medical doctors or other medical staff as a team. Hospitals where acu-moxa practitioners are included in the medical team, however, have achieved many good results: (1) acu-moxa becomes a treatment option for symptoms that cannot be effectively treated with modern Western medicine: especially in palliative medicine, where acu-moxa has an important role in alleviating pain and improving QOL of patients, (2) medical doctors request acu-moxa treatment for diseases in which it has never been applied previously, (3) number of medical doctors who are not biased against traditional medicine has increased, (4) joint research between medical doctors and acu-moxa practitioners began, and (5) degree of patient satisfaction increased [6]. In addition, it is a good idea to treat the same patient by exchanging information between a medical doctor and an acu-moxa practitioner by way of medical referral letters. This kind of collaboration is not yet common in Japan, but its development in the future is expected.

2.5 Collaboration of Medical Doctors and Acu-Moxa Practitioners in Acupuncture and Moxibustion Research

Research on acu-moxa in Japan is progressing mainly at acu-moxa training institutions, especially in universities. When an acu-moxa practitioner conducted acu-moxa research in the past, he or she engaged in joint research in the laboratory of the faculty of medicine of a university to obtain a master's or a PhD degree. However, recently it has become possible to obtain these degrees in acu-moxa universities. Presently, most of the ten universities with acu-moxa departments offer a master's course, and more than half of them offer a PhD program, providing an opportunity to learn from and study alongside medical doctors or basic medicine researchers. Thus, most of the scientific research regarding acu-moxa published in 2020 in foreign journals written by Japanese researchers was conducted in acu-moxa universities.

3 Indications for Acupuncture and Moxibustion Treatment and Their Evidence

Ikuro Wakayama

3.1 Misunderstandings About Applicable Diseases for Acupuncture and Moxibustion

Regarding the indications for acu-moxa treatment, the WHO draft in 1996 and the National Institutes of Health (NIH) Consensus Development Statement in 1997 are well known in Japan. WHO held a meeting in Italy in 1996 and made a draft of the indications for acupuncture treatment. On the other hand, the United States established an Office of Alternative Medicine (OAM) in the National Institutes of Health (NIH) in 1992, and promoted clinical and basic research on complementary and alternative medicine. The NIH Consensus Development Statement in 1997 accelerated the trend toward acu-moxa research in the United States as well as in Europe. Presently, the National Center for Complementary and Integrative Health (NCCIH) is energetically continuing research and education in this field. Of course, this has also had a great influence on acu-moxa research in Japan.

None of the diseases listed as indications, however, have been developed based on sufficient evidence, and at present, only historical significance remains ~~13)14)~~. The WHO draft was just a draft, and therefore, the plenary session stated that "in the future, the indication of acupuncture must be decided based on RCT" [7].

In recent years, many RCTs of acupuncture, including those of the Cochrane review, and SRs analyzed based on these RCTs have been published, leading to the publication of many clinical practice guidelines (CPGs). Therefore, the evidence derived from these RCTs, SRs, and CPGs should be referred to for appropriate clinical decisions. In fact, positive results have been published regarding the efficacy of acupuncture for lower back pain and other pain conditions [8, 9].

Meanwhile, clinical research of acupuncture in Europe and in the United States cannot serve as good evidence for the practitioners and patients in Japan for the following reasons: (1) they mainly use Chinese acupuncture needles that are thicker than Japanese needles and also Chinese acupuncture techniques differ from Japanese; (2) the participants of these studies were Western people, whose race and lifestyle are quite different from Japanese; (3) they used very shallow (minimal acupuncture) or non-penetrating needles as sham/placebo intervention, which are regarded as real acupuncture in Japan; and (4) they concluded that acupuncture was not effective because the results with real acupuncture were not superior to their sham/placebo.

On the other hand, clinical trials of acu-moxa conducted in Japan also have problems because (1) most of them involved very small number of participants, (2) they could have publication bias [10], (3) they do not have a biostatistician on the research team in most clinical research. Therefore, it is necessary to wait for a large-scale and high-quality clinical trial of acu-moxa in Japan.It should be noted that very little of the above indications and research consider moxibustion. Both in Japan and abroad, the vast majority of research on acu-moxa is concerned with the effects of acupuncture, not moxibustion.

3.2 Toward Establishing Evidence for Acupuncture and Moxibustion in the Future

More than 80% of the pathological conditions treated by acu-moxa in Japan are musculoskeletal pain conditions [11]. However, acu-moxa is applied to many other conditions, such as fatigue, health promotion, eye strain, digestive system issues, tinnitus/hearing loss, urological symptoms, etc. Therefore, for pain conditions, it is important to accumulate more experience and evidence. Also, conversely, for diseases for which acu-moxa has not been fully utilized and evidence has not been established, acu-moxa should be more actively attempted.

In addition, evidence from Japan is needed instead of evidence from Europe and the United States. In other words, it is necessary to have the results of clinical research using Japanese-style acu-moxa treatment, and those in which Japanese people were recruited as participants for the study. Otherwise, the results of clinical research cannot be generalized to Japan. For that purpose, clinical trials in hospitals conducted by a team consisting of medical doctors, acu-moxa practitioners and other necessary members are needed. Unfortunately, however, such high-quality RCTs have yet to be reported, with a few exceptions. This is the challenge in conducting clinical trials of acu-moxa in Japan, so in addition to conducting RCTs, it would be advisable to build a patient registry system to accumulate individual experiences.

4 History of Acupuncture and Moxibustion in Japan

4.1 Ancient Times

Toshihiro Togo

The medical culture of the Chinese continent reached Japan through the Korean Peninsula between the fifth and sixth centuries. In this period, esteemed doctors were invited from the Korean Kingdoms Silla and Baekje, and there are records of request for gifts of medicinal substances. After the Sui Dynasty was established in 589, emissaries were sent from Japan to learn from the advanced culture and political system of China. This was the so-called Sui envoys. When the Tang Dynasty was established in 618, Japan sent Tang envoys, which led to the adoption of the political system (the Ritsuryo system of legal codes) and the medical system of the continent.

4.2 Middle Ages(Sixth to About Fourteenth Centuries)

Toshihiro Togo

4.2.1 Acupuncture and Moxibustion Under the Ritsuryo System

The Taiho Ritsuryo (Taiho Code), promulgated in 703, included medical laws that established rules for medical administration. Although the Ritsuryo code no longer exists, the details of the medical system of the time can be surmised from reproduced original sources.

In an imperial edict of 757, the text" *Koteidaikeitaiso* 黄帝内経太素 *Yellow Emperor's Inner Classic: Grand Basis*)" is included, and this text was used as a medical text for centuries. *Koteidaikeitaiso* is a commentary on the "*Koteidaikei*

黄帝内経 (*Yellow Emperor's Inner Classic*)," but it was lost in China in the Song Dynasty. In Japan, however, a Heian Period (794–1185) copy of the commentary was found in Ninnaji Temple (仁和寺), and this has become a precious resource for studying what the *Koteidaikei* was like before the Song revisions. (The above manuscript is a national treasure.)

4.2.2 The Compilation of Ishinpo (Tanba Yasuyori)

Tanba Yasuyori (912–995) compiled a comprehensive medical compendium entitled "*Ishimpo* 医心方 (*Prescriptions from the Heart of Medicine*)" consisting of 30 volumes from the over 200 Chinese medical texts that had been shipped to Japan up until his time. He presented this to Emperor Enyu in 984. *Ishimpo* includes quotations from Chinese documents along with the titles of the original texts, providing valuable material for researching the aspects of Chinese medical texts of that era. Although the *Ishimpo* does not include Tanba Ysuyori's own writings, the way he edited it suggests his thoughts on medicine. It has been pointed out that overall this text favors practical methods over medical theories.

An original copy of this text was preserved by the Nakarai family, who had received it as a gift from Emperor Ogimachi in 1573. It was purchased by the Ministry of Culture in 1982 and was designated as a national treasure 2 years later.

4.2.3 Acupuncture and Moxibustion in the Middle Age

The practice of acupuncture is considered to have declined in China during the Six Dynasties Period, and moxibustion became primary around the Tang Dynasty (seventh century). The following passage in the Chinese classic "*Gedaihiyoho* 外台秘要方 (*Arcane Essentials from the Imperial Library*)" (752) by Wang Tao illuminates this trend: "Acupuncture is very abstruse since ancient times, and isn't something people of this day can learn. Medical texts say that acupuncture can kill a person, but it cannot revive a person. If some reference is made (to acupuncture) here, there is risk that life will be harmed. Therefore, acupuncture classics will not be cited here, and only moxibustion texts will be referenced."

Thus, there was mention of the risks of acupuncture, but not much else. Even though the first medical policy in Japan included acupuncture under the Ritsuryo system, the actual practice of acupuncture was mostly limited to surgical applications. As for moxibustion, however, it is mentioned from time to time in the diaries of royalty, and it's apparent that it was popular. It should be noted, however, that the days and times as well as the location of the moxibustion application were strictly limited by the prohibitions in medical texts.

4.2.4 Medical Texts in the Kamakura and Nambokucho Periods (1337–1392)

When trade between Japan and Song began in the late twelfth century, many medical books printed using woodblock printing techniques began to reach Japan. This means that the results of the revision of medical books carried out during the Northern Song Dynasty in China were also transmitted to Japan. Buddhist monks played a major role in the transmission of medical texts in this era, and the practice of medicine also shifted from court physicians to monks. Representative Japanese medical texts in this period include Kajiwara Shozen's "***Ton-isho*** 頓医抄 (*Excerpts for Novice Doctors*)" (1303) and "*Man'ampo* 万安方 (*Prescriptions for Complete Safety*)" (1315) and Yurin's "*Fukudenho* 福田方 (*Prescriptions for Good Fortune*)" (1363). Both these authors were monks. The listing of acupuncture points in the "*Man'ampo* 万安方 (*Prescriptions for Complete Safety*)" is arranged by parts of the body rather than by the meridians, which was common among texts of the time. Also, most of the treatment protocols in this text were for moxibustion. Also, the "*Ton'isho* 頓医抄 (*Excerpts for Novice Doctors*)" and "*Man'ampo* 万安方 (*Prescriptions for Complete Safety*)" included figures of the organs and meridians from a Northern Song diagram "*Sonshinkanchuzu* 存真環中図 (*Illustration of Viscera and Meridians*)" (1113) in which Kajiwara's keen interest in anatomy is observed. Yurin's "*Fukudenho* 福田方 (*Prescriptions for Good Fortune*)" also has a section for the organs and the 12 meridians, but doesn't describe the meridians in any detail. The Japanese texts that followed mostly limited themselves to point location and did not go into detail about the meridians.

4.3 Late Feudal Period, Fourteenth to Nineteenth Centuries

Toshihiro Togo

4.3.1 Trade with Ming Dynasty China and Japanese Medicine

When the Yuan Dynasty came to an end in 1368, the subsequent Ming Dynasty forbade private trade and limited it to official tributary trade. Japan began paying tribute to the Ming Court in 1404 and sent trade missions 19 times until the mid-sixteenth century. Many monks traveled to China to study during this period, and the newest medical texts were brought back to Japan. Further, woodblock printing technology adopted in Japan made it possible to reproduce imported medical texts and promoted the circulation of commentaries that explained these texts in an easy-to-understand way for Japanese physicians, increasing access to medical knowledge.

4.3.2 Features of Acupuncture and Moxibustion in the Late Feudal Period

Monks replaced court physicians to become the main bearers of medicine in Japan after the Middle Ages, and the interpretation of Chinese medical texts began to reflect Buddhist views of the body. The relation between these Buddhist views of the body and acupuncture and moxibustion practice is a field requiring more research going forward. However, when one considers the development of traditional medicine in Japan after the Middle Ages, one must bear in mind that in some cases the medical theory was constructed based on the newest texts imported from China, and in other cases the practice was based on Buddhist views of the body.

In Japan in the Middle Ages, the abdomen containing the five Zang organs was considered important, and the presence of "worms" in the abdomen began to attract attention as the cause of disease. In the text "*Harikikigaki* 針聞書 (*Record of Oral Teachings on Acupuncture*)" by Ibaraki Genko (1568), 63 varieties of "worms" of unique shapes were illustrated as the cause of the Five Aggregations and Six Accumulations. Just as in the field of drug treatment, acupuncture and moxibustion took on the tradition of abdominal examination, and the abdomen became an important area for diagnosis. Thus, unique abdominal diagnosis systems were devised. The strike mallet needling method discussed below is an example where the abdomen as an area for diagnosis was converted into an area for treatment.

4.3.3 Formation of Different Styles

A wide variety of acupuncture and moxibustion styles developed in the late feudal period, and each style created its own names for points as well as needle techniques and transmitted these. Active research is currently underway concerning the characteristics of these styles and their inter-relationships.

4.3.4 Needle Techniques Developed in Japan: Strike Mallet Needling Method and Acupuncture Tube Inserting Method

Many needling techniques were developed in Japan, but here only the strike mallet needling method and the acupuncture tube inserting method will be discussed as representatives of Japanese innovations.

Strike Mallet Needling Method (*Dashin*)

In the strike mallet needling method or hammer needle technique, a needle is placed on a point and the head of the needle is hammered with a small mallet. This imparts some vibration to the body surface. This technique is thought to have been created by the monk Mubun and fully developed by Misono Isai (1557–1616).

As texts that outline the principles of this technique, there are "*Shindo Hiketsu Shu* 鍼道秘訣集 (*Compilation of Secrets of Acupuncture,* 1685)" and "*Ichugen'o* 意仲玄奥 (*Profound Knowledge of Isai's Abdominal Acupuncture, 1696*)". In this style, abdominal diagnosis was performed by palpating areas for the five Zang organs and six fu apportioned on the abdomen. After determining the location of the pathogenic qi, a needle was placed there and hit repeatedly with a mallet, and the needle was inserted this way. This was a holistic treatment using the abdomen as the site of diagnosis and treatment.

The Acupuncture Tube Inserting Method and the Sugiyama Shinden Style

The acupuncture tube, which is used in almost all countries today, was developed in Japan in the seventeenth century. After the death of the visually impaired acupuncturist Sugiyama Waichi (1610–1694), the legendary inventor of the acupuncture tube, his disciple Shimaura Wadaichi compiled the text "*Sugiyama Shindenryu* 杉山真伝流 (*Secrets of Sugiyama-style Acupuncture*)". This text not only described techniques using the acupuncture tube but included many manipulation techniques assuming subtle "exchanges of qi." A number of these techniques were listed in the modern text "*Shinkyu-no-Kagaku* 鍼灸の科学 (*The Science of Acupuncture: 1959*)" by Yanagiya Sorei (1906–1959) as "current needling techniques."

4.3.5 Achievement of Sugiyama: Acupuncture Training Centers

During the Genroku era in the early Edo Period (1688–1704), Sugiyama Waichi was elevated to the rank of top court acupuncturist for his successful treatment of the fifth Shogun Tokugawa Tsunayoshi (1646–1709), and he used his position to contribute to acupuncture education. In 1682, Sugiyama opened the world's first educational facility for the visually impaired, an acupuncture training center called the "Sugiyama-style Acupuncture Practice Center." By the era of his successor, Mishima Yasuichi, 45 acupuncture training facilities were established all over Japan. Until these training facilities were abolished by the Meiji Government in 1874, they served as education centers for the visually impaired in acupuncture and moxibustion.

4.3.6 Expounders of Medical Texts and Their Educational Activities

In the early Edo Period, there was a group of scholars known as expounders of medical texts, who specialized in explaining classical medical texts and promulgated medical theories. Even though most of these scholars didn't practice medicine, their analysis of Chinese medical texts was at a high level. After digesting the theory of Five Circuits and Six

Qi (a foundational theory at that time), these scholars illuminated fundamental issues regarding Chinese medical theory, including the organs and channel system.

4.3.7 Study of Acupuncture Points in the Late Feudal Period

Interest in the acupuncture points grew in Japan in the late feudal period, and many texts and commentaries were compiled. Particularly, the text "*Jushikeihakki*十四経発揮 (*Elucidation of Fourteen Meridians, 1341*)" written by Hua Shou (1304–1386) was used extensively as a resource for study and commentary.

4.3.8 Study of Early Classics in the Edo Period

Also, in the late feudal period in Japan, the earliest classics such as the "*Koteidaikei* 黄帝内経 (*Yellow Emperor's Inner Classic*)" and "*Nangyo* 難経 (*the Classic of Difficulties*" were reprinted or commentaries were published based on texts from the classics redaction in the Song Dynasty and were circulated widely.

In the late Edo Period (mid-seventeenth to mid-nineteenth centuries), physicians of the Taki and Esawa clans used comparative study of classics to pursue the "original form" of the oldest medical classics. Classics like "*Koteidaikeitaiso* ***黄帝内経太素*** (*Yellow Emperor's Inner Classic: Grand Basis*)" stored at the Ninnaji Temple in Kyoto or the original copy of "*Ishimpo* 医心方 (*Prescriptions from the Heart of Medicine*)" handed down in the Nakarai clan were earlier than the Song Dynasty redaction. When it became possible to view these texts that were unaltered and conveyed the original language of the Sui and Tang Dynasties, the members of the Edo Medical School worked to compile commentaries that included thorough textual analysis.

4.3.9 The Koho School and Eclectic School and Moxibustion

In the mid and late Edo Period, the Koho (classical way) school became prominent. This group was skeptical of the Yin and Yang and Five Phases theory, and valued testing ideas and real experience. Among these physicians, there were many who emphasized moxibustion therapy. For example, Goto Konzan (1659–1733) held that moxibustion, like balneotherapy, removed obstructions of Qi, and applied many cones of moxibustion in places along the spine that were depressed or tender. Kagawa Shu-an (1683–1755), the disciple of Goto, also emphasized palpation of the back and wrote about moxibustion targeting places on the skin surface that were protruding or depressed. Furthermore, the representative of the Eclectic School, Wada Tokaku (1744–1803), left some case studies of moxibustion therapy.

4.3.10 *Shiraku* Therapy in the Middle and Late Edo Period

Shiraku (pricking collaterals method), with the aim of eliminating stagnant blood from the body, is mentioned in the first chapter of the "*Koteidaikeireisu* 黄帝内経霊枢 (*Yellow Emperor's Inner Classic: Spiritual Pivot*). " The revival of *Shiraku* in the mid and late Edo Period (especially the latter half of the eighteenth century) was spearheaded by two great physicians of Kyoto. The first was Yamawaki Tomon (1736–1782), the second son of the famous Yamawaki Toyo, who belonged to the school combining Kampo and Dutch medicine. The other was Ogino Gengai (1737–1806), whose disciple Miwa Tosaku (1759–1818) recorded Ogino's teachings in "*Shirakubunkenroku* 刺絡聞見録 (*Memos on Shiraku (Pricking Collaterals)*)". In this text, the treatment methods of *Shiraku* for 104 conditions are listed. In modern times,

Kudo Kunimasa (1918–1989), who served as a military doctor in the Second World War, worked to promote *Shiraku* by publishing guidebooks on *Shiraku* therapy as well as reprinting the classic text "*Shirakubunkenroku* 刺絡聞見録 (*Memos on Shiraku (Pricking Collaterals)*) ".

4.3.11 The Inflow of Western Medical Knowledge (Anatomy) and Search for a New Concept of the Body

The eighth Shogun of the Edo Period, Tokugawa Yoshimune (in power 1716–1745), as part of his Kyoho Reforms, relaxed the restrictions on the import of Western books, and Dutch medical texts began to be introduced. This sparked an interest in real anatomy to replace the simplistic depictions in ancient Chinese texts. Dissections of cadavers of executed convicts became common from the 1750s onward because of the interest among physicians in the composition of the body, both by conventional physicians who practiced Kampo medicine and by those who practiced Dutch medicine. Based on these dissections, it became clear, when it came to the composition of the body, that the Western medical texts were more accurate than the Chinese texts based on Zang-fu and channel theories. Although this fact did not undermine the trust of physicians at the time in Chinese medicine as far as therapeutics, but without question, it provided grounds for criticizing Chinese medical theory.

Ishizaka Sotetsu (1770–1841) departed from the traditional Zang-fu and channel theories, and attempted to construct a new theory. As far as acupuncture technique goes, Ishizaka carried on the Sugiyama tradition, but he replaced key terms like Ying (nutritive) Qi, Wei (defensive) Qi, and Zong (pectoral) Qi with artery, vein, and nerve. Thus, he exchanged Western medical concepts for Chinese ones. This kind of adoption of Western medical concepts implies that a new theoretical model was being sought to replace Zang-fu and channel theories, even as traditional acupuncture techniques were retained as therapeutic methods.

4.4 Premodern (1868–1945)

Toshihiro Togo

4.4.1 New Medical Policy and Acupuncture and Moxibustion

The Tokugawa shogunate, which lasted 240 years, came to an end in 1868, and the Meiji government, which toppled the Tokugawa shogunate, soon after taking power, instituted a policy of making Western medicine the legitimate medicine of Japan. In 1874, Isei, the first modern medical policy in Japan, was promulgated. Under the policy, only those who had studied Western medicine were given a medical license, so in effect, those doctors who specialized in Kampo were prevented from practicing. Acupuncture and moxibustion, on the other hand, were allowed to continue under the policy, but it was limited to that performed under the supervision of Western-trained doctors. (This provision, however, was rescinded 1 year later.) Also, concerning the practice of acupuncture and moxibustion by the visually impaired, it was reported that there was no harm in this practice by the visually impaired, so this was allowed to go on.

4.4.2 The Transposing of Traditional Medicine with the Western Medical View

The "Revised Acupoints" Imposed by the Government

In the Meiji era, even in textbooks, acupuncture points (meridian points) were denoted as Koketsu, which meant "hole points," and mention of meridians was eliminated. Also, the descriptions for individual point locations and indications were changed to anatomical descriptions and Western disease names. Thus, the traditional medical view of the body, based on the Zang-fu and 12 meridians, was seldom referred to. This trend was solidified when, in 1913, the standardization of acupuncture points (commonly called the "revised acupuncture points") was initiated by the Ministry of Education. The Ministry of Education formed a committee of six experts from each field, including medical history, massage, and anatomy, and had them deliberate on the future of education concerning acupuncture points.

Scientific Approaches to Acupuncture and Moxibustion by Physicians

After the Meiji Restoration, much of the knowledge about acupuncture and moxibustion that had been handed down was transplanted with Western medical terms, and the ideological space surrounding acupuncture and moxibustion that had existed up until the late feudal period disappeared. Nevertheless, there were a few doctors and researchers who worked to validate acupuncture and moxibustion.

For example, Okubo Tekisai (1840–1911), in his text "*Shinchishinsho* 鍼治新書 (*New Text on Acupuncture Therapy*)" published in 1892, stated that needle stimulation affected the cardiac function by way of the sympathetic nerves. Thus, he raised the possibility that the autonomic nervous system was related to the therapeutic effects of acupuncture. Also, medical doctors like Miura Kin-nosuke, Goto Michio, and Toki-eda Kaoru, while taking a negative stance toward the theories in classical sources, sought scientific explanations for what kind of physiological changes occurred in the body with acupuncture and moxibustion and how this contributed to the healing of diseases. Below is a brief introduction to medical doctors in Japan before the Second World War who acknowledged the merits of acupuncture and moxibustion and contributed to its academic development.

Ishikawa Hidetsurumaru did not believe in Yin and Yang, Five Phases, or the meridian theory, but he had a keen interest in organ dysfunction and its relationship to reactions found on the body surface.

In 1947, when he was summoned to the Mie branch office of GHQ (General Headquarters), he explained the therapeutic effects of acupuncture in terms of Langley's dual control of the autonomic nervous system and impressed the American military doctor.

Hashida Kunihiko (1882–1945) was the second son of a Kampo physician belonging to the Asada school who became an assistant professor at the Tokyo Imperial University. He specialized in experimental physiology, especially electrophysiology, but on the other hand, he was very knowledgeable about Zen Buddhism. In particular, from Dogen's Zen text "*Shobogenzo* 正法眼蔵 (*Treasury of the True Dharma Eye*)", he extracted the concept of "Zenki (whole organism)," which was the idea that the body and its functions should be viewed as one organic whole. This concept is close to the "holism" of today, and Hashida decided to reconstruct medicine from this perspective. He viewed Kampo medicine, acupuncture, and moxibustion as modalities that supported his approach. When he assumed the position of Minister of Education in 1940, he planned to establish a medical institute specializing in traditional medicine, but this never came to pass.

Itakura Takeshi (1888–1958) was an internist in the hospital of the medical school associated with the Tokyo Imperial University. When the GHQ, the occupying authorities in Japan, issued a proclamation banning acupuncture and moxibustion in 1947, Itakura convinced Brigadier General

Crawford Sams to rescind this order by scientifically explaining the value and importance of acupuncture and moxibustion in Japan.

Hara Shimetaro (1882–1991), after graduating from medical school in Kyoto, started research at Kyushu University in 1924, and a year later, he began his research on the prophylactic effects of moxibustion therapy. Hara performed many experiments, but the most important experiment was the preventative effects of direct moxibustion against tuberculosis. The conclusion was that prophylactic and continuous moxibustion was effective in the treatment of tuberculosis. Hara himself applied moxibustion on his ST36 points and lived to well over 100. In recent years, MoxAfrica, an NGO based in England, has been conducting clinical trials and promoting moxibustion in Uganda in Africa as part of the self-care regimen for tuberculosis as a complication of AIDS. This work is based on the studies conducted by Hara.

4.4.3 Revival of Classical Acupuncture and Moxibustion in the Modern Era

The discussion around acupuncture and moxibustion from the late 1800s into the early 1900s was taken over by Western medical terminology and treatments remained in the realm of symptomatic relief. Around the 1920s, however, a movement began to reappraise the classical view of physiology and pathology and to apprehend the disease state of patients in a holistic manner. The two main actors in the revival of classical acupuncture and moxibustion were Sawada Ken (1878–1938) and Yanagiya Sorei (1906–1959).

Sawada and Taikyoku Therapy

Sawada Ken immigrated to the Korean Peninsula after learning the martial art Jujutsu, and he worked as a bone-setter. Sawada moved back to Tokyo in 1922 and opened an acupuncture and moxibustion clinic. In a period when the clinical practice of acupuncture and moxibustion had abandoned classical principles and only attempted to relieve symptoms, Sawada reappraised the significance of the five Zang organs (yin organs) and advocated the importance of an approach that addressed a broad variety of diseases by treating both the mind and body. This method was called Taikyoku (Taiji) Therapy and received a large following in pre-war Japan. The treatment was centered around moxibustion, and about 15 standard points (including GV12, CV12, TB4, Sawada's GB15, and KI3) received direct moxibustion along with points suited to each patient. Also, the importance of self-care was emphasized, and patients were expected to do regular moxibustion on themselves. In this sense, the Sawada style emphasized moxibustion as a means of life nurturing.

Yanagiya's Reappraisal of Classics and Creation of Meridian Therapy by His Students

The movement to revive Kampo medicine gained steam with the publication of texts like "*Kampoigakunoshinkenkyu* ***漢方医学新研究*** (*New Investigation of Kampo Medicine, 1926*)" by Nakayama Tadanao, "*Ikainotettsui* ***医界之鉄椎*** (*Iron Hammer to the Medical World, 1910*)" by Wada Keijuro, and "*Kokan'igaku*皇漢医学(*Traditional medicine originated in China and developed uniquely in Japan, 1927*)" by Yumoto Kyushin. In the fields of acupuncture and moxibustion, the revival of acupuncture based on the classics was undertaken after the 1930s, and Yanagiya Sorei (1906–1959) was at the center of this movement. Yanagiya aimed to rebuild the identity of acupuncture medicine by examining the theories and practical techniques described in classical texts. In addition to researching classical texts, he also worked hard to discover techniques transmitted from premodern times. He created a database of these methods and extracted those that were clinically effective.

Yanagiya had his students, Okabe Sodo (1907–1984), Inoue Keiri (1904–1967), and others, study the basic concepts in classical texts and had them report on their findings. Okabe and Inoue referenced the clinical approach of Yagishita Katsunosuke based on the tonifying and draining of the 12 meridians and combined this with the meridian and point selection principle in the "*Nangyo* 難経 (*Classic of Difficult Issues*)" to create a diagnosis and treatment system called Meridian Therapy after several years of trial and error. In Meridian Therapy, imbalances in meridians are considered to be at the background of every disease, and deficiency and excess in meridians are determined by Six Position Pulse Diagnosis at the radial artery. The essential points on the arms and legs are treated using the principles in Chapters 69 and 75 of the" *Nangyo* 難経 (*Classic of Difficult Issues*)", and then symptomatic treatment is provided for individual symptoms. The tonification and dispersion on essential points of the four limbs is called Root Treatment, and the treatment for the symptoms is called Tip Treatment.

Meridian Therapy is a diagnosis and treatment system created by clinicians who investigated methods in classical texts in Japan in the first half of the twentieth century. Because of its utility and the organizational power of Okaba, Ino-ue, and Takeyama Shin'ichiro (1900–1969), the influence of Meridian Therapy in postwar Japan grew to almost synonymous with traditional Japanese Acupuncture and Moxibustion. Concerning the conceptual details and techniques of this system, however, many variations have developed, and these are still being consolidated.

4.5 Modern Times (After 1945)

Toshihiro Togo

4.5.1 The "McArthur Storm" and Passing of Law No. 217

After World War Two ended in 1945, Japan came under the rule of the GHQ (General Headquarters of the Supreme Commander for the Allied Powers) until 1951. In September 1947, the GHQ recommended to the Medical System Council that acupuncture and moxibustion should be prohibited. Before this notice was issued, Ishikawa Hidetsurumaru had two times explained to the military doctor at GHQ's branch office in Mie about the safety and scientific basis of acupuncture and moxibustion. These explanations even included actual demonstrations. After the recommendation of prohibition was issued, Ishikawa visited the Ministry of Health and Welfare again and argued the scientific basis of acupuncture and moxibustion and their effectiveness. Within these professions, there was a strong resistance to this prohibition, both from sighted and from visually impaired practitioners, and a vigorous movement to repeal this prohibition started. After 3 months of this campaign, acupuncture and moxibustion gained a legal basis for continuation in the Diet in December 1947. Furthermore, not only sighted practitioners but those who were visually impaired were granted the same license.

4.5.2 Founding of Professional Associations (JAMA and JAMTA)

While the continued practice of acupuncture and moxibustion was secured, the recommendation of prohibition from the GHQ cited the lack of scientific evidence as one of the main reasons, so finding scientific evidence for the therapeutic effects of acupuncture and moxibustion became the urgent agenda for these professional associations. The Japan Society of Medical Acupuncture (JSMA) was founded in 1948, and the Japan Acupuncture and Moxibustion Society (JAMS) was founded in 1951. These two associations that worked after 1945 toward the aim of elucidating the scientific basis of acupuncture and moxibustion merged in 1980 to become the Japan Society of Acupuncture and Moxibustion (JSAM) to pursue their common goals.

4.5.3 Serizawa's Research on Acupuncture and Moxibustion and Contribution to Education

Serizawa Katsusuke (1915–1998) was one of the leaders among the visually impaired who protested the GHQ's prohibition of acupuncture and moxibustion, and he contributed greatly to the profession in postwar Japan in both research and education [12]. Serizawa wrote many textbooks as well as books to educate the public. He also worked to nurture those who came after him in scientific research. Further, with the awareness that an institution of higher learning for acupuncture and moxibustion was needed, he proposed the concept of an acupuncture and moxibustion junior college at the congress of the Japan Association of Massage & Acupuncture Teachers in 1972. This led to the foundation of the Meiji College of Acupuncture Medicine in 1978.

4.5.4 Founding of Institution of Higher Learning and Birth of Doctors of Acupuncture and Moxibustion

The Meiji College of Acupuncture Medicine mentioned above was upgraded to a four-year college in 1983, 5 years after its founding, and became the Meiji University of Oriental Medicine. In 1992 this university began to offer a predoctoral program, and in 1994, a post-doctoral program was added. The number of four-year colleges offering acupuncture and moxibustion degrees has increased since then, and there are 12 such colleges in Japan as of 2024.

4.5.5 Reports of Acupuncture Anesthesia and Progress of Related Research

In July 1971, preceding Nixon's visit to China, James Reston, a *New York Times* reporter who was staying in China, had surgery for appendicitis. He had post-surgical pain management with acupuncture, and he reported on this. This initiated a host of reports concerning acupuncture anesthesia, and there was a so-called acupuncture anesthesia boom. Acupuncture anesthesia received a great deal of attention as a revolutionary method that made it possible to perform open abdominal surgery with the patient alert. It gradually fell out of favor because there was an individual difference in the effect, and even though it did have an analgesic effect, it did not have the effect of relaxing muscles, which is indispensable for abdominal surgery. Also, with advances in anesthesiology, the merits of acupuncture anesthesia diminished. Thus, research shifted to the mechanism of pain reduction with acupuncture.

4.5.6 Ministry of Health and Welfare Scientific Research Department: Basic and Clinical Research on Acupuncture and Moxibustion (1975 Onward)

As acupuncture anesthesia attracted interest in the medical world in Japan as well as abroad, in 1975, under the direction of the Ministry of Health and Welfare of Japan, a research group focused on Oriental medicine was formed. In the collected works (Vol. 1) published in 1979, the following theory about the mechanism of pain reduction by acupuncture was proposed: "At the current time, our working theory on the mechanism of the analgesic effect of acupuncture is a type of negative feedback by the nociceptive system originating in polymodal receptors."

Many of the medical doctors who led this research group in 1978 and 1979 were also involved in the research sections of JSMA and JAMS. This contributed to the merger of these organizations into the Japan Society of Acupuncture and Moxibustion (JSAM), as well as the founding of the first college of acupuncture.

4.5.7 Return of China (PRC) to the International Community, Resumption of Japan–China Relations, and the Founding of WFAS

After the Cultural Revolution ended in 1976 and China's return to international society accelerated, academic societies and organizations of Traditional Chinese medicine began to be established within China. Academic exchanges with Japan also became frequent, and even with the Traditional Chinese medicine that was restructured during the Cultural Revolution started to become better known in Japan through medical journals such as "*Chuui Rinsho* 中医臨床 (*Clinical Journal of Traditional Chinese Medicine*)".

In this flow of events, Takagi Kentaro, the first president of the Japan Society of Acupuncture and Moxibustion, and Kurosu Yukio played key roles in the foundation of the World Federation of Acupuncture-moxibustion Societies (WFAS) in 1987.

4.5.8 International Standardization of Basic Acupuncture and Moxibustion Terminology at the WHO Western Pacific Regional Office (1989)

The necessity for the standardization of issues related to meridians and acupuncture points was recognized early in Japan. In 1973, an acupuncture point committee was formed with the participation of 11 associations related to acupuncture and moxibustion, and preparations were started for international standardization. Interest in acupuncture was growing, and in the beginning of the 1980s, the Western Pacific Region Office of the WHO formed a working group for standardizing acupuncture nomenclature. The final consensus was ratified at the WHO headquarters in Geneva in 1989 by the conference of a scientific group. In 1994, *the **Standard Acupuncture Nomenclature,*** **Part 2, Revised edition** was published. (The first edition was completed in 1984.)

4.5.9 Reprinting of Medical Classics and Preparing the Environment for Studies of Classical Literature (1980s)

The 1970s can be called a period of increased interest in the study of classics and the methodology of study in both acupuncture and moxibustion. In order to base clinical practice on classical texts, the collection of trustworthy original manuscripts and commentaries, and an accurate understanding of these texts became emphasized. Thus, many classical source materials were reprinted. Also, the full-scale reproduction and publication of rare texts began in the 1980s. With this, the majority of original texts about acupuncture and moxibustion that were transmitted or published in premodern times, as well as the subsequent studies of these texts, became available for review. Currently, many libraries with classical medical texts have an electronic archive for public viewing, and thus, an environment conducive to research has been created.

4.5.10 Trend of Research in Acupuncture and Moxibustion in Japan in the Last 30 Years (Since 1990)

Hitoshi Yamashita

Awareness of Importance of Clinical Trials

Viewed from the ratio of research papers published in Japan since the 1990s, the trend in acupuncture and moxibustion research in Japan has shifted from basic research and theories about therapeutic mechanisms using animals to clinical trials with human beings. At the background of this is the concept of Evidence-Based Medicine (EBM) that has become widespread in the medical world, and the awareness that clinical trials with a control group are necessary.

Clinical trials of acupuncture have been conducted in Japan in advance of the rest of the world in the 1960s by practicing acupuncturists, even though on a small scale. The first randomized controlled trial (RCT) for acupuncture in Japan was that published by Kinoshita Haruto in 1969 about the comparison of deep and shallow needling for sciatica.

In 1970, an article was featured in an acupuncture and moxibustion journal on the comparison of insertion into the carotid sinus and. Superficial insertion for hypotensive effect by Akio Debata.

What prompted clinical trials on acupuncture, especially RCTs, to be conducted again since the mid-1990s were the following factors that influenced acupuncture researchers at the time:

1. Criticism of the acupuncture profession from outside for claiming effectiveness without the evidence of clinical trials with controls.

2. Special international conferences on the methodology of clinical trials on acupuncture were convened several times in Japan, and the "Guidelines for Clinical Research on Acupuncture" were published by the WHO of the Western Pacific Region [13].

3. The annual discussion on the methodology of clinical trials on acupuncture, which young acupuncture researchers hold.

In the period between the 1970s and the 1990s, RCTs were published at a rate of about 10 per decade, but in the decade after 2000, 70 RCTs were published. This number further increased in the decade from 2010. While the scale remained small in most RCTs, the control shifted from a different acupuncture technique (comparing real acupuncture techniques to each other to see which was more effective) to sham needling. In other words, just like the RCTs conducted overseas, evidence was collected on whether or not the specific effect of acupuncture could be detected after eliminating the placebo effect and natural progress. Later, however, many researchers realized that, unlike the inactive placebos used in pharmacological experiments, sham needles elicited a physiological response. Therefore, in recent years, practical clinical trials on how the effects of acupuncture compare to standard treatments (drugs, plasters, etc.) have been reemphasized.

Many of the clinical trials on acupuncture were published in Japanese, but after 2000, many RCTs conducted in Japan were published in English in international professional journals. By 2020, about 30 studies were published internationally.

Collection and Evaluation of Clinical Evidence of Acupuncture

Clinical trials on acupuncture have become common in Japan as well as abroad. Following this trend, numerous RCTs of high quality have been reported in Germany, the US, Britain, and China since 2000 and 2010, respectively. However, the main RCTs included in the Cochrane review are those done abroad based on TCM-style acupuncture, which is different in many aspects from the diagnosis and level of stimulation in Japanese acupuncture.

Concerning the clinical practice guidelines in Japan, there has been an increase in documented recommendations for acupuncture treatment. Currently, in 2024, there is mention of evidence for acupuncture treatments and recommendations in 17 versions of clinical practice guidelines.

Other Trends in Acupuncture Research

Aside from clinical trials, since the 1990s, clinical research has been conducted to examine the possibilities for clinical applications of acupuncture from a new perspective. For example, the results of acupuncture have been analyzed by statistical studies of cases based on the characteristics of symptoms or the presence of physical findings. Also, single-case studies (N of one trial) are being done to assess effectiveness within one case. In terms of basic research, especially in the areas of neurophysiology, cardiovascular physiology, and molecular biology, research is ongoing with animals and normal human subjects.

Also, since 2000, in fields like medical sociology and educational methodology, the role of acupuncture and moxibustion is being examined from the perspectives of qualitative analysis, ethnography, and palliative care.

As far as international research exchanges are concerned, from 2006 to 2012, the Japan Society of Acupuncture and Moxibustion (JSAM) hosted three international acupuncture symposiums, and invited acupuncture researchers from abroad to discuss the situation of research in each country and exchange views.

The aforementioned World Federation of Acupuncture Societies held international symposiums in 1993 and 2016, at Kyoto and Tsukuba, respectively. In the 2016 symposium, especially, the many styles of Japanese acupuncture and moxibustion were introduced along with demonstrations and attracted the interest of overseas participants.

5 Therapeutic Effects of Acupuncture and Moxibustion

Toshihiro Togo

5.1 Mechanism of Receiving Acupuncture and Moxibustion Stimulation in Peripheral Regions: Polymodal Receptor Hypothesis

Acupuncture and moxibustion (AM) stimulation may evoke excitation of all receptors (low-threshold and high-threshold mechanoreceptors) on the surface of the skin, but the most responsive receptor to AM is a polymodal receptor. It is a kind of conceptual receptor identified by Burgess et al. in 1973 by electrophysiological experiments [14]. It responds to multiple modes of stimuli, such as mechanical, thermal, and chemical stimuli. Therefore, it is considered a candidate for a receptor for AM stimulation (mechanical/thermal). Regarding the relationship between AM stimulation and polymodal receptors, Takao Kumazawa (1932–2010) of Nagoya University proposed a hypothesis on the mechanism of acupuncture anesthesia in 1978. Among the various receptors on the skin, the reason why the polymodal receptor came to attention is that it responds to both mechanical stimuli by acupuncture and thermal stimuli by moxibustion [15]. Acupuncture stimulation evokes a sensation like deep pain called "*de qi* sensation." The sensation will be transmitted to the upper central nervous system, activate the endogenous analgesic system, and induce "acupuncture analgesia." It also affects the autonomic nervous system (such as blood pressure, respiratory rate, and heart rate). In addition, local inflammatory reactions known as "flare" or "wheal" observed on the skin after AM stimulation are also considered to be the result of the excitation of polymodal receptors. Polymodal receptors are composed of many receptors, such as mechanoreceptors, thermoreceptors, and chemoreceptors, that are expressed at free nerve endings, including opioid receptors, adenosine receptors, and cannabinoid receptors. Thermoreceptors include receptors that respond to stimuli with different temperatures, such as TRPV1, TRPV2, TRPV3, and TRPV4. Likely, ASIC2/3 and MRGRD are known as candidates of mechanoreceptors.

Diffuse noxious inhibitory controls (DNIC) is a phenomenon that suppresses the activity of wide dynamic range neurons involved in pain transmission in the dorsal horn of the spinal cord caused by noxious stimuli applied to tissues in various parts of the body. It is highly likely that polymodal receptors are also involved in the afferent pathway of DNIC.

Polymodal receptors evoke excitement even by mechanical stimuli that are not recognized as pain, such as scratching or rubbing the skin surface [16]. Actually, they respond to non-penetrating acupuncture stimuli or an intradermal needle. Therefore, polymodal receptors have many implications for the sham acupuncture setting in clinical trials of acupuncture.

In 2011, Denda showed that TRPV4 is expressed in keratinocytes of the skin [17], and further investigations about the relationship between AM stimulation and TRPV4 expression in keratinocytes are expected.

5.2 Mechanism of Acupuncture Analgesia

5.2.1 Endogenous Inhibitory System of Pain

In 1973, shortly after the press reports of acupuncture anesthesia, Han et al. reported from their experiments using rabbits that analgesic substances are released into the cerebrospinal fluid [18]. They showed that the analgesic effect was observed when the cerebrospinal fluid of a rabbit that received acupuncture stimuli was circulated into another rabbit. Eventually, it was clarified that endogenous opioids are involved in acupuncture analgesia by measuring the endorphin concentration in the cerebrospinal fluid after electroacupuncture stimulation.

In animal experiments on acupuncture analgesia, electroacupuncture is often used for equalizing the experimental conditions, but in subsequent studies, it was found that each opioid (endomorphine, β-endorphin, and dynorphin) acts differently depending on the stimulation frequency during electroacupuncture analgesia.

In 1982, Watkins and Mayer reported that the pain of conscious rats was relieved by electrical stimulation on the soles (footshock) [19]. They also found that stimulations on the forelimbs activate the endorphin neurons and induce opioid analgesia, but stimulations on the hind limbs activate inhibitory neurons of the brain stem. They named the latter phenomenon as non-opioid analgesia.

5.2.2 Descending Pain Inhibitory System

Many descending inhibitory nerves emerge from the brain stem, but the sites involved in analgesia include those from the periaqueductal gray matter (PAG) of the midbrain to the nucleus raphe magnus, and the nuclei gigantocellularis and its neighborhood. For the descending pain inhibitory systems, two systems, that is, the serotonin (5-HT) system and the noradrenaline system, are recognized. Serotonergic neurons that are scattered in the nucleus raphe magnus start from PAG and descend the dorsolateral funiculus of the spinal cord. Adrenergic neurons start from the locus coeruleus or nucleus subcaeruleus and descend the posterolateral funiculus of the spinal cord. Both neurons are engaged in analgesia in the posterior horn of the spinal cord.

5.2.3 Gate Control Theory

In addition to the mechanisms mentioned above, there is a gate control theory in which the pain signal caused by an excitation of the thin nerve fibers is suppressed in the dorsal horn of the spinal cord by an excitation of the thick myelinated nerve fibers (Aβ) of the peripheral nerves. This theory was proposed by Melzack and Wall in 1965 and has been the forerunner of analgesic research of AM that has been continued up to today. Although this theory was found to be inadequate by electrophysiological experiments, it explains the phenomenon very well, that a pain caused by injury is relieved by rubbing or pressing the surrounding skin. Therefore, interventions based on this theory, such as TENS (transcutaneous electrical nerve stimulation), in which electrodes are attached to the surface of the skin, are still used.

5.2.4 Peripheral Mechanism of Acupuncture Analgesia

In 2010, Goldman carried out an experiment in which animal models with inflammatory and neuropathic pain were successfully treated by acupuncture stimulation, and proposed that adenosine A1 receptors are involved in acupuncture analgesia. He hypothesized that adenosine triphosphate released from the tissue damaged by acupuncture stimulation is decomposed into adenosine by an action of an enzyme, bound to adenosine A1 receptors, which suppresses the firing of nociceptive neurons, leading to analgesia [20].

5.2.5 Analgesia and Visceral Function Adjustment by Acupuncture Stimulation, and Role of Oxytocin

Oxytocin, which works for uterine contraction, is known to be released by mother–child skinship or sexual behavior. Recent animal experiments, however, revealed that oxytocin and acupuncture analgesia are related. For example, it has been suggested that when ST-36 of a rat was stimulated by electroacupuncture at 10/20 Hz for 30 min, the effect of acupuncture analgesia was enhanced by intraventricular administration of oxytocin [21], and that oxytocin is involved in the regulation of visceral function by acupuncture stimulation [22].

5.3 Autonomic Nervous System Research and Acupuncture and Moxibustion [23]

Since the Meiji era in Japan, there have been many researchers who believe that the autonomic nervous system is involved in the curative mechanism of AM stimulation (Chap. 2). Among them, Tekisai Okubo (大久保適斎, 1839–1911), who studied Western medicine (Dutch medicine) before the Meiji Restoration and was the principal of Gunma Medical School, was the first person. In the book entitled *Shinchishinsho* 鍼治新書 (*New text on Acupuncture Therapy*) that he published in 1892, he explained that acupuncture stimulation will regulate visceral function when it acts on the sympathetic nerve [24]. Subsequently, Hidezurumaru Ishikawa (石川日出鶴丸, 1878–1947) of the physiology department of Kyoto Imperial University played an active role from the Taisho era to the Showa era, and led the research of viscero-cutaneous reflexes based on Langley's theory of autonomic nerve double innervation.

Later, research on the effects of AM stimulation on the autonomic nervous system was restarted by Akio Sato (1934–2006) of the Tokyo Metropolitan Institute of Gerontology. In the 1960s, he started the research of "somato-autonomic reflexes (reflexes whose afferent is a sensory nerve and efferent is an autonomic nerve)." The research was greatly progressed thereafter and is continuing to the present.

In the 1970s, Sato found that somatosensory stimuli in anesthetized animals cause reflexes that are specific to each organ. He published an article entitled *"Skin-Visceroautonomic Nerve Reflex"* in 1976, and showed that somatosensory stimulation affects heart rate, gastric motility, and urinary bladder activity based on the results of experiments conducted using anesthetized rats [25]. That is, stimulation on the skin (pinching pain using tweezers) reflexively increases or decreases the activity of the heart branch of the sympathetic nerve, resulting in an increase or decrease in heart rate. In addition, the stimulation of the abdominal skin reflexively increases the efferent discharge of the stomach, resulting in a decrease in gastric tonus, and the pain stimulation to the perineum suppresses the discharge of the pelvic nerve bladder branch, leading to the suppression of the micturition contraction of the bladder.

Sato then demonstrated that stimulation to the limbs evokes systemic reflexes and stimulation to the trunk evokes local reactions in anesthetized animals. In the 1990s, he also found that acupuncture stimulation induces visceral reflexes by activating nerves in the skin and muscles from the acupuncture stimulation experiments using anesthetized animals.

Based on the results of basic research conducted by Sato, various researchers examined systemic and segmental reactions caused by AM stimulation of limbs. Noguchi et al. examined the effect of electroacupuncture stimulation to the foot of an anesthetized rat, and found that acupuncture stimulation caused an increase in blood pressure, leading to an increase in blood flow in the skin and muscles. Similarly, Kobayashi et al. reported that manual acupuncture stimulation applied to the ST36-equivalent point of anesthetized rats increased or decreased the heart rate.

On the other hand, regarding the segmental reaction by AM stimulation, Sato and Yamaguchi used manual acupuncture and electroacupuncture stimulation, respectively, and found that both stimulations affected gastric motility [26, 27]. Tanaka et al. also found that moxibustion stimulation induced a change in duodenal motility [28]. They clarified that it was a segmental reflex because (1) the motility of the stomach and duodenum was suppressed by the stimulation of the somatosensory nerve of the trunk, and (2) it was not eliminated by the neck spinal cord amputation or decerebration.

Regarding the reaction of each organ to the somatosensory nerve stimuli of the trunk, Noguchi explained from a viewpoint of Oriental medicine that the functions of the transport point (兪穴) and alarm point (募穴) of the trunk are very similar to those of the visceral function of each segment.

5.4 Other Basic Research

5.4.1 Effect of Acupuncture and Moxibustion Stimulation on Oxidative Stress

In the living body, cytotoxic superoxide, reactive oxygen species (ROS) such as hydrogen peroxide, and free radicals are constantly generated, and a mechanism for removing them (antioxidant action) is also provided. A situation in which the production of free radicals exceeds the removal by antioxidants is called oxidative stress, and research on the removal of oxidative stress by AM stimulation is being conducted in Japan as well as in other countries. Some experiments used animals, and some used healthy adults. In animal experiments, (1) ischemia-reperfusion model [29], (2) Parkinson's disease model rat [30], and (3) essential hypertension model rat [31] were used. In experiments with healthy adults, the effect of acupuncture stimulation on oxidative stress induced by exercise load has been investigated [32].

5.4.2 fMRI Study Using Acupuncture and Moxibustion Stimulation

Although it has been recognized that the brain response during stimulation is very important to understanding the mechanism of action of AM, PET (positron emission tomography), which was developed in the 1980s, has been concerned about exposure to radioisotopes. But in the 1990s, almost non-invasive fMRI became widespread and was applied to research on AM, for example, that of mechanism of action, mechanism of *de qi* sensation, and assessment of placebo effect.

6 Meridians and Acupuncture Points

Yosuke Amano

6.1 Overview

Meridians and acupuncture points are employed as essential concepts for diagnosis and treatment in acupuncture and moxibustion. Meridians (also called channels) are pathways of Qi and Blood[TM1] which nourish and enable the body to function, and meridians consist of channels and collaterals. Acupuncture points (hereafter referred to as acupoints) are the main points that are on meridians among those reactive points where imbalances in the body are manifested, and also serve as treatment points (called Tsubo in Japan). These acupoints are engaged as reactive points, diagnostic points, and treatment points.

This chapter begins with the origins of meridians and acupoints from a historical perspective, then mentions the international standardization of acupoints, and finally details the theory of meridians and acupoints.

6.1.1 The Origins of Meridians and Acupoints

There is much that remains to be elucidated about the origins of the theory of meridians and acupoints. A portion of what is established from studies of the medical classics and, more recently, excavated writings will be introduced here.

It is believed that the meridians were organized by observation and views about the sections of the body (internal/external, surface/deep, front, side, and back), the circulatory system, the nervous system, the way stimulation was conducted in the body (needle sensation etc.), reaction phenomena of physical problems, and areas where therapeutic effects were obtained. Meridians were systematized using the "heaven, earth, and man theory" and the "Yin and Yang theory."

The acupoints were places where dysfunctions in the muscles and nerves often appeared and also served as treatment points. Also, they were places where dysfunctions in the Zang-fu often appeared and served as treatment points. Further, they were codified as effective sights for stimulation to treat specific symptoms, and by designating a name and location, these points became part of a shared tradition.

Later on, these were called acupoints, and those points that were located on a meridian came to be called meridian points. The concept of meridians and acupoints has not been uniform since the beginning, and it's apparent from excavated writings and various medical classics, including the "*Koteidaikei* 黄帝内経 (*Yellow Emperor's Inner Classic*)", that there were multiple views. Nevertheless, these concepts were organized between the Early Han and Late Han Dynasties.

In the tenth chapter of the **Vital Axis**, which was compiled in the Han Dynasty, 12 meridians are connected to the Zang-fu, and these meridians are interconnected, and it is said that Qi and Blood[TM1] circulated in them. This theory later gained collateral support to exert a strong influence in later ages, and the theory was organized and systematized including acupoints to become the mainstay of acupuncture and moxibustion therapy to this day.

6.1.2 International Standardization of Acupoints

The name, location, and affiliated meridian, as well as the primary indications, depend largely on the reaction of the body as described above. Thus, there is variation that results from accumulated clinical experience, and otherwise, in the process of historical transmission, the uniformity in its description is lost, and inevitably, differences have arisen. Given this historical background, the main texts that have been influential in some commonality in the description of acupoints are as follows: *K″oteimeido* (*kyo*) 黄帝明堂 (経) (*Yellow Emperor' s Bright Hall* (*abbreviated*))" (Han Dynasty), "*Shinkyukootsukyo* 鍼灸甲乙経 (*Systematic Classic of Acupuncture and Moxibustion*)" (Huang Fumi, 259), "*Koteidaikeimeido* 黄帝内経明堂 (*Yellow Emperor's Inner Classic: Bright Hall*)" (Yang Shangshan 655), and "*Dojinshuketsushinkyuzukyo* 銅人腧穴鍼灸図経 (*Illustrated Manual of Acupuncture Points of the Bronze Figure*)" (王惟一 Wang Weiyi, 1026). Nevertheless, in the transmission of classical medical texts and due to regional differences in treatment methods as well as the accumulation of clinical experiences, differences arose in countries of East Asia, primarily in the location of acupoints. After the modern era, when the institutional education of acupuncture and moxibustion became regulated, and as acupuncture and moxibustion began to gain international recognition, the project of standardizing acupoints also started in Japan, as well as abroad (see Chap. 6, Sect. 4).

In the case of Japan, ever since the Meiji Government officially adopted Western medicine (1874), regulations on acupuncture and moxibustion were also adopted, and an educational policy was also started. Given this trend, in 1913, the Ministry of Education commissioned a committee for the revision of acupoints. In 1918, this committee published the names and numbers of 120 revised acupoints. These revised acupoints were a reworking of acupoints based on a Western medical view, and located and classified points by body parts without regard to the concept of meridians. These were called "hole points" and were selected by eliminating those acupoints that were considered unimportant. Their locations were defined by anatomical terms and finger width measurements.

Much later, in 1965, the Japan Meridians and Acupuncture Points Committee was established with the aim of creating an international consensus about the meridians and acupoints. In the first World Congress of Acupuncture and Moxibustion that was held the same year, this committee proposed that the nomenclature for the meridians and acupoints be standardized. In 1973, the Japan Acupuncture Point Committee was established once more, involving 11 domestic organizations with the aim of standardizing the location of acupoints. Deliberations were thus made concerning the notation for acupoints and their locations. Internationally, WHO/WPR (World Health Organization/Western Pacific Region Office) took the lead in deliberations toward standardization, and by 1989 the English names and notations for the 12 regular meridians and eight extra meridians(extra meridians) and the acupoints of the 14 meridians (361 points) and their notations, as well as the extra points (48 points) and their names and notation were standardized. From 2003, the WHO/WPR initiated the international standardization of acupuncture point locations, and in Japan, the (Second) Acupuncture Point Committee was organized. After deliberations centering around Japan, China, and Korean delegates, the locations of 361 points were agreed upon. The details of this agreement were officially published in English in 2008 as *"WHO Standard Acupuncture Point Locations in the Western Pacific Region."* A year later, an official Japanese edition, *"WHO/WPRO hyojunkeiketsubui WHO/WPRO*標準経穴部位 *(WHO Standard Acupuncture Point Locations)"* was published. Following this, textbooks used in Japanese acupuncture and moxibustion schools were completely revised and the "New Edition: Introduction to Meridians and Acupoints" was published. The foundation for education and research in acupoints was established by this international standardization of acupoints, and it became a step toward sharing the medicine of acupuncture and moxibustion internationally.

6.2 The Theory of Meridians and Acupoints

Below is a summary of the theory of meridians and acupoints as applied in acupuncture and moxibustion. Refer to other texts for the exact course of the meridians and the location of points.

6.2.1 What are the Meridians?

Meridians (also called channels) are pathways of Qi and Blood[TM1], and they consist of channels, the primary pathway, and collaterals that branch off from these. There are 12 meridians and eight extra meridians (extra meridians), and 15 collateral vessels. Also, there are collateral vessels, tertiary vessels, and superficial collateral vessels. Further, there are meridian sinews and cutaneous regions in the skin and muscles associated with the meridians.

The body is nourished and functions with the Qi and Blood[TM1] that circulates in the meridians. Abnormalities in the meridians, that is, stagnation or excess or deficiency of Qi and Blood[TM1], cause dysfunctions in the body. Also, the meridians serve as pathways of invasion by pernicious influences.

These influences progress from the surface of the body to the interior (skin to tertiary vessels, to collateral vessels, to meridians, and finally to the Zang-fu) to attack the inside of the body.

Treatment consists of grasping the patho-condition, prognosticating, and providing treatment by detecting the reactions that appear in the meridians (cold/heat, depression, tenderness, avoidance of pressure, preference for pressure, hardness/softness, and dryness/moisture).

Meridians

Meridians are major pathways of Qi and Blood[TM1], and there are 12 meridians and eight extra meridians (extra meridians).

- Twelve Meridians (regular meridians, or 12 regular meridians)

The 12 meridians refer to those listed in the tenth chapter of the **Vital Axis**, and they are all linked to create a greater circulation to circulate Qi and Blood[TM1] through the body. These meridians are the foundation of the meridian theory, and are emphasized in diagnosis and treatment.

The Chinese character for meridian also has the meanings of manage, supervise, maintain, pass through, and record. The meridians manage the circulation of Qi and Blood[TM1] and flow through the whole body, and because they connect and unify the body, they are also called the meridian vessels, or regular meridians, or the 12 regular meridians.

The 12 regular meridians are divided into Yin meridians and Yang meridians, which are each divided into three. (**3 Yin meridians**: Taiyin, Shaoyin, and Jueyin. **3 Yang meridians**: Yangming, Taiyang, and Shaoyang.) The meridians flow in the upper and lower limbs, and they are also classified as the three Yin meridians of the arms, the three Yang meridians of the arms, the three Yin meridians of the legs, and the three Yang meridians of the legs.

Of all the flows of the 12 meridians through the whole body, flows on the outside of the body are called external paths, and flows inside the body are called internal paths. The external paths mainly supply the tissues (muscles, blood vessels, connective tissue, skin, and bone), while the internal paths mainly supply the Zang-fu.

The three Yin and three Yang meridians are in an external–internal relationship in terms of their paths. In other words, the Taiyin and Yangming, the Shaoyin and Taiyang, and the Jueyin and Shaoyang meridians are respectively in an external–internal relationship.

The 12 meridians are each closely connected to an organ (Zang or Fu), and also connect to an organ of the meridian with which it has an external–internal relationship. Yin meridians are associated with a Zang organ, and also connect to the Fu organ of its external–internal relationship. Yang meridians are associated with a Fu organ, and also connect to the Zang organ of its external–internal relationship. In addition, the aforementioned external–internal relationship of meridians also applies to the Yin and Yang organs of the Zang-fu, which are also in an external–internal relationship. Because of this relationship of associations and connections, the Zang-fu can be treated through the 12 meridians, and this contributes greatly to clinical results.

The 12 regular meridians begin at the middle burner and flow sequentially as ① arm Taiyin Lung[TM1] meridian→ ② arm Yangming Large Intestine[TM1] meridian→ ③ leg Yangming Stomach[TM1] meridian→ ④ leg Taiyin Spleen[TM1] meridian→ ⑤ hand Shaoyin Heart[TM1] meridian→ ⑥ hand Taiyang Small Intestine[TM1] meridian→ ⑦ leg Taiyang Bladder[TM1] meridian→ ⑧ leg Shaoyin Kidney[TM1] meridian→ ⑨ hand Jueyin Pericardium[TM1] meridian→ hand Shaoyang Triple Burner meridian→ leg Shaoyang Gallbladder[TM1] meridian→ leg Jueyin Liver[TM1] meridian.

Here it returns to the middle burner and connects back to ① arm Taiyin Lung[TM1] meridian to form a greater circulation.

The three Yin and three Yang meridians of the arms and the legs have a directionality. As a rule, the three Yin meridians of the arm flow from the chest to the arms and connect to the three Yang meridians of the arm. The three Yang meridians of the arm flow from the arms to the face and connect to the three Yin meridians of the leg. The three Yin meridians of the leg flow from the legs to the chest and connect to the three Yin meridians of the arm (Table 6.1). The general flow of the Yin meridians and Yang meridians is bottom to top for the Yin meridians and top to bottom for the Yang meridians when the arms are raised overhead (Table 6.1).

Table 6.1 Direction and connection of meridians

Meridians	Direction of flow	Connects to
Arm Three Yin	Chest to arms	Arm Three Yang
Arm Three Yang	Arms to face	Leg Three Yang
Leg Three Yang	Head to legs	Leg Three Yin
Leg Three Yin	Legs to chest	Arm Three Yin

Eight Extra Meridians (Extra Meridians) (奇経八脈)

The extraordinary meridians intensify the connections between the 12 regular meridians and regulate the circulation of Qi and Blood[TM1]. They are the Du, Ren, Chong, Dai, Yangqiao, Yinqiao, Yangwei, and Yinwei meridians. These are collectively called the eight extra meridians (extra meridians).

The eight extra meridians (extra meridians) do not have an association or connection to the Zang-fu. Since they have a different characteristic from the 12 meridians, they are called extraordinary meridians in contrast to the regular meridians.

Among the eight extra meridians, the Du (Governor) and Ren (Conception) meridians flow on the center line of the body, and are used frequently in clinical practice; the combination of the Du and Ren meridians with the 12 meridians are called the "14 meridians."

Collaterals

The collaterals are branches of meridians, and together with the meridians connect the whole body to form a system of circulating Qi and Blood[TM1]. The bigger collaterals are called great collaterals or divergent collaterals, while the smaller ones are called collateral vessels (narrow sense), tertiary vessels, and superficial collateral vessels.

- 15 collateral vessels

They are also called the 15 great collaterals, or the 15 divergent collaterals. These 15 include the great collateral of the Spleen[TM1], which separates from the Zang-fu, in addition to collaterals for the 12 meridians and the Ren and Du meridians. The site where these collaterals branch off is called a collateral connecting point.

The collateral vessel of the Ren meridian separates from the inferior aspect of the xyphoid process and disperses into the abdomen. The collateral vessel of the Du meridian separates from the bottom of the coccyx and travels up either side of the spine. The great collateral of the Spleen[TM1], after branching off from the Spleen[TM1], emerges on the side of the chest and distributes over the thorax and costal regions.

- Collateral vessels (narrow sense), tertiary vessels, and superficial collateral vessels.

The branches that separate from the 15 collateral vessels are called collateral vessels (in the narrow sense). Those branches that divide off these collateral vessels (narrow sense) are called tertiary vessels. Those which distribute close to the surface of the body are called superficial collateral vessels.

12 Meridian Sinews • 12 Cutaneous Regions

The meridian sinews are groups of muscles and joints that are organized in terms of which meridians nourish them with Qi and Blood[TM1]. In the 13th chapter of the Vital Axis (on meridian sinews), the location and distribution of the meridian sinews are organized by the three Yin and three Yang meridians of the arms and legs, and these are described along with symptoms from invasion of external pathogenic factors, such as pain and cramping.

Cutaneous regions are skin areas supplied by the collateral vessels that branch off from the meridians that have been classified systematically. They are also called the 12 cutaneous regions. Also, in the 56th (cutaneous regions) chapter of "*Somon* 素問 (*Basic Questions*)", there is a description of the cutaneous regions of the three Yin and three Yang meridians, and these are also called the six cutaneous regions.

6.2.2 What are Acupoints?

Acupoints, or so-called Tsubo, are acupuncture points. Acupoints appear as a reaction to dysfunctions in the body, and further, these are places where therapeutic effects tend to be obtained with treatment. These effects can occur at the acupoint, or adjacent to it, or distal to it, or even in the whole body. Acupuncture points are classified into acupoints, extra points, and Ahshi points.

Classification of Acupoints

Among all points, acupoints are those on the 14 meridians (12 meridians plus Du and Ren meridians), and their names and locations are established. In contrast to extra points, they are also called "proper points." With the leadership of the WHO, the names and locations of points associated with the meridians (361 in total) have been standardized, and this is applied to the education and research of acupuncture and moxibustion in Japan and around the world.

Extra points have established names, locations, and indications, and tend to show clear physical reactions and effects. These points, however, are not on the 14 meridians or are not associated with them. So, they are not directly linked to the meridian system, but have been recognized and applied as points that show special reactions or effects. Also, among the extra points, those that have been recognized since 1901 are called new points.

Ouch points don't have a specific name or location like acupoints and extra points, but appear as reactions depending on the patho-condition. They are points that can serve as treatment points, and are sometimes called "reactive points."

Method for Determining Location of Acupoints

Among methods of locating acupoints, there is the location of points by anatomical landmarks, that by bone standard, and that by finger measurement. The bone standard is a method by which each skeletal frame is used as the standard, regardless of height or differences in weight, to measure the length and width of the body. Finger measurement means using the width of the patient's fingers as a standard to determine point location, and it's used as an expedient to the bone standard. In actual practice, these methods are used as the basis to find palpable reactions, which are then used as the treatment location.

Essential Points

Among the acupoints, those deemed to have clinically important effects are collectively called essential points. These include the five essential points, five transport points (five phase points), four command points, eight meeting points, confluence point of eight vessels, crossing points, and lower sea points. Among these categories, the five essential points, five transport points (five phase points) will be discussed below.

- Five essential points

These are the important acupoints that are often used clinically. The source points, cleft points, connecting points, transport points, and alarm points are collectively called the five essential points.

Source points are where these source qi of the Zang-fu collects, and they are used as reactive points and diagnostic points, as well as treatment points for the Zang-fu. They are located close to the wrists and ankles, and there are two for every meridian, one on each side.

There are cleft points for each of the 12 meridians as well as for the Yangqiao, Yinqiao, Yangwei, and Yinwei meridians. They are located on the forearms or the calves, and are used as reactive points and diagnostic points as well as treatment points for acute symptoms.

The connecting points are where these collaterals branch off from their associated meridians, as mentioned above, and there are 15. The connecting points of the 12 meridians connect the meridians in an external–internal relationship. Thus, connecting points tend to show reactions from the opposite meridian in this relationship, and treating this point influences both meridians in the external–internal relationship. When imbalances in a meridian become chronic, it often spreads to the meridian in an external–internal relationship, so connecting points are used as reactive points and diagnostic points as well as treatment points for chronic diseases.

There are 12 transport points and 12 alarm points each corresponding to one of the 6 Zang and 6 Fu. These points reflect the condition of the Zang-fu and are used as diagnostic points and treatment points for the Zang-fu. The alarm points are located on the chest and abdomen, and the transport points are located on the back. To distinguish these transport points from the five transport points associated with the five phases, they are also called the back transport points.

- Five transport points (five phase points)

The 5 transport points are 5 points on the 12 meridians among those points at or distal to the elbow and knee joints. From the fingertip (or toe-tip) proximal, they are called the Well point, Brook.

Point, Stream point, River point, and Sea point. These names refer to the flow of water, and they refer to the size and depth of flow of the meridians at these points. Each of the five transport points has a five-phase characteristic, and they are also known as five phase points. They are used for tonification and dispersion treatments, applying the creative cycle and controlling cycle of the five phases. Also, each of the five transport points has indications that are clinically useful.

Addendum: diagram of 12 meridians and eight extra meridians (extra meridians).

Often as diagrams of the 12 meridians or eight extra meridians (extra meridians), one sees points on the surface of the human body, and these points are connected by lines. This is an abstraction of one aspect of the abovementioned concept of meridians. It is important to recognize this fact if one intends to fully utilize all the aspects of the meridian theory in clinical practice.

6.3 Meridian Symptomologies and ICD-11

Various things appear as abnormalities in the meridians, including invasion of external pathogens, dysfunctions in the Zang-fu, and abnormal conditions in the Qi and Blood[TM1]. These changes are captured through palpation, observation, and questioning, and can be regulated through acupuncture and moxibustion. This is the characteristic of acupuncture and moxibustion therapy. Abnormalities in the meridians manifest as various reactions, symptoms, and diseases, but the meridian symptomologies are a compilation of such symptoms associated with meridians. The primary source of meridian symptomologies includes the symptomology of the 12 meridians found in the tenth chapter of the Vital Axis, and the symptomology of the eight extra meridians (extra meridians) in the 29th chapter of the Classic of Difficulties.

In the World Public Health General Congress held in May of 2019, the International Disease Categories 11th edition (ICD-11) was officially adopted. In module I (traditional medicine pathologies) in the 26th chapter of this document, a section on Meridian and Collateral Patterns was included, and this included Main Meridian Patterns and Extra Meridian Patterns. With this, it has become possible to collect statistical data in relation to meridian symptomologies, and there is hope for the future application of this standard.

References

1. Ishizaki N, Tsuru H, Saito M, et al. Academic exchange at WFAS Turkey 2019 and review of RCTs conducted in China. J Jpn Soc Acupunct Moxibust. 2020;70(1):75–91.
2. Kincaid C. In Britain acupuncture is gaining in popularity every year. J Jpn Soc Acupunct Moxibust. 2018;68(4):347–52.
3. Hillairet A, Kobayashi A. Becoming an acupuncturist in the US. J Jpn Soc Acupunct Moxibust. 2018;68(3):208–14.
4. Saito M, Murase T, Watsuji T. Trial survey on clinical use of acupuncture and moxibustion of meridian and collateral patterns in international classification of diseases 11th revision. J Jpn Soc Acupunct Moxibust. 2018;68(4):300–4.
5. Watsuji T. "East Asian traditional medicine" and "meridian and collateral patterns" in the international classification of disease, 11th revision. J Jpn Soc Acupunct Moxibust. 2018;68(4):329–36.
6. Wakayama I, Katai S, Furuya Y, et al. Acupuncture and Moxibustion in hospitals- how have general hospitals changed after introducing acupuncture and Moxibustion in routine care? Kampo Med. 2021;72(1):72–88.
7. Takasawa N. Report on 2007 annual conference of the Society for Acupuncture Research. The status and future of acupuncture research: 10 years post NIH consensus conference (Baltimore MD, USA). J Jpn Soc Acupunct Moxibust. 2008;58(1):87–92.
8. Qaseem A, Wilt TJ, McLean RM, Forciea MA. Clinical guidelines committee of the acu-moxaerican College of Physicians. Noninvasive treatments for acute, subacute, and chronic low back pain: a clinical practice guideline from the acu-moxaerican College of Physicians. Ann Intern Med. 2017;166(7):514–30.
9. National Institute for Health and Care Excellence. Chronic pain (primary and secondary) in over 16s: assessment of all chronic pain and management of chronic primary pain. NICE guidance [NG193] published: 07 April 2021. https://www.nice.org.uk/guidance/ng193NICEguidelineweb. Accessed on Jan 2021.
10. Shikura T, Wakayama I, Kawasaki K. Publication bias of abstracts of clinical trials presented at the 2006-2010 annual meeting of the Japan Society of Acupuncture and Moxibustion: implications and suggestions for the future clinical research in Japan. J Jpn Soc Acupunct Moxibust. 2018;68(1):21–31.
11. Ishizaki N, Yano T, Kawakita K. Public status and prevalence of acupuncture in Japan. eCAM. 2010;7(4):493–500.
12. Matsui S. Distinguished achievement of the visually handicapped in the medical history of the acupuncture and moxibustion. J Jpn Soc Acupunct Moxibust. 2006;56(4):596–604.
13. WHO Regional Office for the Western Pacific. Guidelines for clinical research on acupuncture. WHO Regional Publications Western Pacific Series No. 15 1995.
14. Burgess PR, Peral ER. Cutaneous mechanoreceptors and nociceptors. In: Iggo A, editor. Handbook of sensory physiology, vol. 2. Berlin: Springer; 1973. p. 29–78.
15. Mizumura K. On the polymodal receptor with characteristics suitable for a receptor that transmits acupuncture/moxibustion stimuli. Kampo Med. 2011;62(2):196–205.
16. Kawakita K, Gotou K. Role of polymodal receptors in the acupuncture-mediated endogenous pain inhibitory system. In: Kumazawa T, et al., editors. The polymodal receptor-a gate way to pathological pain, vol. 113. Elsevier; 1996. p. 507–23.
17. Denda M, Tsutsumi M. Roles of transient receptor potential proteins (TRPs) in epidermal keratinocytes. Adv Exp Med Biol. 2011;704:847–60.
18. Research group of Acupuncture Anesthesia. The role of some neurotransmitters of brain in finger acupuncture analgesia. Sci Sinica. 1973;117:112–30.

19. Watkins LR, Mayer DJ. Organization of endogeneous opiate and non-opiate pain control systems. Science. 1982;216:1185–92.
20. Goldman N, Chen M, Fujita T, et al. Adenosine A1 receptors mediate local anti-nociceptive effects of acupuncture. Nat Neuroscie. 2010;13:883–8.
21. Yang J, et al. Effect of oxytocin on acupuncture analgesia in the rat. Neuropeptides. 2007;41(5):285–92.
22. Yoshimoto S, Babygirijia R, Dobner A, Ludwig K. Anti-stress effects of transcutaneous electrical stimulation (TENS) on colonic motility in rats. Dig Dis Sci. 2012;57(5):213–1221.
23. Sato Y, Uchida S, Noguchi E, et al. Memorial symposium in honour of professor Akio Sato. J Jpn Soc Acupunct Moxibust. 2010;60(4):672–92.
24. Noguchi E, Ohsawa H. Autonomic nervous system. Textbook of Traditional Japanese Medicine Part2: Acupuncture and Moxibustion. Research on the Standardization of traditional Japanese medicine promoting integrated medicine. Health and Labour Sciences Research Grant, Ministry of Health, Labour and Welfare of Japan. pp 53–79, 2013.
25. Sato A, Sato Y, Torigata Y. Cutaneo-visceral reflexes. Shinkei Kenkyu no Shinpo. 1976;20(2):210–7.
26. Sato A, Sato Y, Suzuki A, Uchida S. Neural mechanisms of the reflex inhibition and excitation of gastric motility elicited by acupuncture-like stimulation in anesthetized rats. NeurosciRes. 1993;18:53–62.
27. Yamaguchi S, Okada K, Ohsawa H, et al. Effect of electro-acupuncture stimulation on gastric motility in anesthetized rats. J Jpn Soc Neurovegitative Res. 1996;33(1):39–45.
28. Tanaka H, Noguchi E, Kobayashi S, et al. The effect of moxibustion on duodenal motility in anesthetized rats. J Jpn Soc Acupunct Moxibust. 2002;52(4):427–34.
29. Chen Y, Zhou J, Li J, et al. Electroacupuncture pretreatment prevents cognitive impairment induced by limb ischemia-reperfusion via inhibition of microglial activation and attenuation of oxidative stress in rats. Brain Res. 2012;1432:36–45.
30. Yu YP, Ju WP, Li ZG, et al. Acupuncture inhibits oxidative stress and rotational behavior in 6-hydroxydopamic lesioned rat. Brain Res. 2010;1336:58–65.
31. Lai X, Wang J, Nabar NR, et al. Proteomic response to acupuncture treatment in spontaneously hypertensive rats. PLoS One. 2012;7(9):e44216.
32. Fujimoto H, Hayashi T, Sakai T, et al. Effect of electroacupuncture on the change in glutathione concentration in the blood by ergometer exercise. J Jpn Soc Balneol Climatol Phys Med. 2013;76(2):105–16.

Acupuncture and Moxibustion Treatment and Safety

7

Toshihiro Togo and Masanori Takashi

1 Acupuncture and Moxibustion Treatment: Varieties of Basic Techniques

Toshihiro Togo

1.1 Overview: Features of Diagnostic and Treatment Techniques of Japanese Acupuncture and Moxibustion

In 2011, a joint statement was adopted by the Japan Society of Acupuncture and Moxibustion and the Traditional Japanese Acupuncture and Moxibustion Society titled "Tokyo Declaration concerning Japanese Acupuncture and Moxibustion: To contribute to improved medical care in the twenty-first century in Japan as well as the world." In this statement, the features of acupuncture and moxibustion (hereafter acu-moxa) practiced in Japan were explained as follows:

"On the clinical side of acu-moxa in Japan, thin needles are employed and inserted shallowly, and otherwise it includes non-insertion skin stimulation techniques. Many acupuncturists use subtle needling techniques that are minimally invasive to the patient, and have received the support of their citizens. The appraisal of these needling techniques has been increasing in the world.

In the patient examination, palpation is emphasized, and even when determining the acupoint or site of treatment, most all practitioners employ the method of palpating the body surface to confirm the reaction of the patient. Also, there is an understanding of the need for individualized treatment with consideration to individual differences."

T. Togo (✉)
Meiji University of Integrative Medicine, Nantan, Japan
e-mail: office@jsom.or.jp

M. Takashi
Acupuncture & Moxibustion NAS Clinic, Chigasaki, Japan

In this statement, ① thinness of needles used, ② light and subtle stimulation, and ③emphasis on palpation in the examination were raised. Actually, there are cases where thick needles are used, and needle techniques that elicit a strong needle sensation (*de qi* sensation) are practiced, so a diverse range of styles are practiced in Japan. Nevertheless, the "Sugiyama style" created in premodern Japan has a large variety of skin stimulation techniques employing the acupuncture tube, so it's apparent that subtle stimulation has been preferred in Japan. Also, in the field known as *Shonishin* (pediatric acupuncture), which grew in prominence in the Kansai region, tools based on non-insertion were developed. Furthermore, even three-edge needles (for bloodletting) have been used without insertion to apply light and subtle skin stimulation.

As far as the emphasis on palpation is concerned, there is a tradition of abdominal palpation and diagnosis in Japan since the middle age. In the field of acu-moxa, especially with the increase in visually impaired practitioners early on, it is presumed that various findings on the skin (protrusions, depressions, dampness, nodules, etc.) came to be considered important. Also, since these findings on the skin and stimulation on these sites came to be emphasized, it came to the attention of physiologists after the Meiji Era (1863), and this led to physiological research on the somatovisceral reflex in Japan in the early twentieth century.

1.2 Varieties and Standards of Needles

The first chapter of the *Koteidaikeireisu* 黄帝内経霊枢 *(Yellow Emperor's Inner Classic: Spiritual Pivot)* lists 9 types of needles that are now called "the ancient nine needles." This was not simply a classification of needles but an expression of the acupuncture treatment system of the time, which included the field of surgery. As for the shape of these needles, there is no description in the *Koteidaikeireisu* in terms of a figure. The figure in the *Ruikyo* 類経 *(Classified*

Kampo Medical Literature Editorial Committee, The Japan Society for Oriental Medicine (ed.), *Complete Japanese Traditional (Kampo) Medicine*, https://doi.org/10.1007/978-981-96-7143-4_7

Classic) (by Zhang Jingyue: 1563–1640) was copied multiple times in premodern Japan, and needles were made based on this. In modern Japan, except for the stiletto needle that is specialized for cutting like a scalpel that is outside the scope of practice for an acupuncturist, many of the other "nine needles" are applied in modern practices with various innovations. In this chapter, needles will be roughly divided into ① needles that are inserted and ② needles that are not inserted.

1.2.1 Needles That Are Inserted (Filiform Needle, Intradermal Needle, and Thumbtack Needle)

Filiform Needle

The needle that is used most in practice today is the filiform needle, and this consists of the needle body that is inserted under the skin and the needle handle that the practitioner holds. In Japan, filiform needles made of silver and gold have been produced since premodern times, and many different shapes were also devised including different tips such as the pine needle tip, tapered tip, willow leaf tip, and slanted tip. As mentioned in Chap. 6, Sect. 4.3.4, the acupuncture tube was invented in Japan in the Edo period (1611–1863) and its use became widespread. Stainless steel needles were developed in the 1960s, and in the 1980s, disposable needles with plastic tubes (single-use filiform needles) were marketed and became popular. Disposable needles rapidly spread throughout Japan and the world. Needles produced in Japan are between 15 and 150 mm in length, and 0.1 and 0.34 mm in diameter. Also, disposable needles under **Act on Securing Quality, Efficacy and Safety of Products Including Pharmaceuticals and Medical Devices** are classified as medical devices (class II) and in 2005 were established under Japan Industrial Standards as "JIS T9301: single use filiform needles." (Since ISO standard of "ISO17218: Sterile acupuncture needle for single use" was established in 2016, a revised JIS standard has been issued.)

Intradermal Needle

The intradermal needle consists of a very short needle body and a needle head. The purpose of this needle is to provide prolonged mechanical stimulation by fixing the protruding needle head in place with tape. This needle was devised by Akabane Kobei (1895–1983), who made his work public in his text *"Hinaishinho 皮内鍼法 (Intradermal Needling Method)"* (1952, Ido-no-Nippon Co.). The needle is between 0.16 and 0.2 mm in diameter, and the length is about 5 mm. The practitioner uses a pair of tweezers to insert the needle into the desired acupoint and then fixes it with a piece of tape. Along with the next item, the thumbtack needle, there is an international standard for these needles (IS 18746: Sterile intradermal needle for single use).

Thumbtack Needle

The needle consists of a short needle 1–3 mm in length and tape or adhesive material about 1.5 cm in diameter. Just as with the intradermal needle, the aim is to insert and fix in place in acupoints to provide prolonged mechanical stimulation (Fig. 7.1).

1.2.2 Needle-Like Tools That Are Not Inserted

The Tokyo Declaration concerning Japanese Acupuncture and Moxibustion of 2011 mentions "subtle needling techniques that are minimally invasive to the patient," as one of the features of acupuncture in Japan. The subtle stimulation mentioned here includes needle techniques including that using the filiform needle, but many kinds of tools that allow mechanical stimulation to be applied on the body surface were developed in Japan. These tools are used for "needle techniques that don't involve insertion (contact needling method)." Among the tools that are not meant to be inserted, there are those that are variations on the classical needles like the Teishin and the Enshin. Further, there are those that have been invented or developed in Japan in the modern age. Especially when treatments for children (*Shonishin* or pediatric acupuncture) became popular around the Kansai region in the first half of the twentieth century, many tools that were not meant for insertion were invented. These are now used not only for children and infants, but widely for sensitive patients in general (Table 7.1 and Fig. 7.2).

1.3 Needle Techniques

Many schools of acupuncture emerged in premodern Japan (see Sect. 4.3 in Chap. 6), and a variety of needle techniques were created, but after the Meiji period, very few carried on the tradition and their details became obscure. There are over 100 needle techniques listed in the text ***Sugiyama Shinden***

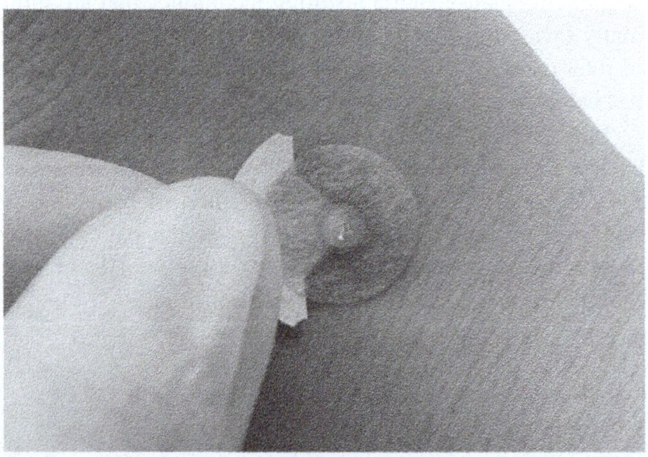

Fig. 7.1 Thumbtack needle. (Provided by SEIRIN Corporation)

Style, but the actual method and clinical applications of these are still being researched. In this section, the representative needle techniques will be listed based on the text ***Science of Acupuncture & Moxibustion: Techniques Volume*** (1959), and techniques will be divided into the categories of ① those that involve insertion beneath the skin, and ② "contact needling method" that does not involve insertion beneath the skin.

1.3.1 Acupuncture Techniques Involving Insertion

Basic techniques using filiform needles are listed (17 needle techniques) as follows (for intradermal needle and thumbtack needle, refer to the previous section):

- Simple insertion: After reaching the desired depth, the needle is withdrawn right away without adding any technique.

Table 7.1 Tools not meant for insertion, their shape, name, and primary use

Shape	Name(incl. Product name)	Primary use
With smooth surface	Plectrum type/blade type/ Choki-shin/Zan-shin/triangle needle	Friction pressure
With protrusion on main part	Broom needle/scraping needle/ pine needle type	Scratching
With thick needle body and round tip	Teishin(with spring without spring)/Enshin	Pressure friction
Rolling disk	Roller needle	Friction scratching
Collection of short needles	Cluster needle/Baika-shin/ seven star needle	Tapping

- Sparrow pecking: Adding in and out movements after inserting the needle.
- Intermittent: After inserting to a certain depth, lifting the needle and then inserting back to depth, and repeating this several times.
- Dripping: ① inserting one third of the way and pausing at each level and ② same as above but sparrow pecking is added at each level.
- Flicking: After reaching a certain depth, the handle or body of needle is flicked back and forth with the inserting hand.
- Retained needle: Leaving the needle in place for a while after inserting the needle in an acupoint.
- Twisting: Twisting the needle during insertion or withdrawal.
- Rotating: ① The needle is rotated in one direction with insertion and then rotated in the other direction with withdrawal. ② After reaching a certain depth, the needle is rotated in one direction.
- Mixed technique: Combining many techniques mentioned here in one insertion.
- Additional stimulation: Using the acupuncture tube or fingers to add stimulation to the skin around inserted needle.
- Index finger strike: After reaching a certain depth, placing the acupuncture tube over the needle and striking with the index finger.
- Following breath: The practitioner follows the patient's breathing to insert with exhale and pause insertion with inhale, and repeats this until reaching desired depth.
- Internal regulation: After needle reaches depth, the handle of the needle is held in the supporting hand and struck with the acupuncture tube held in the inserting hand.

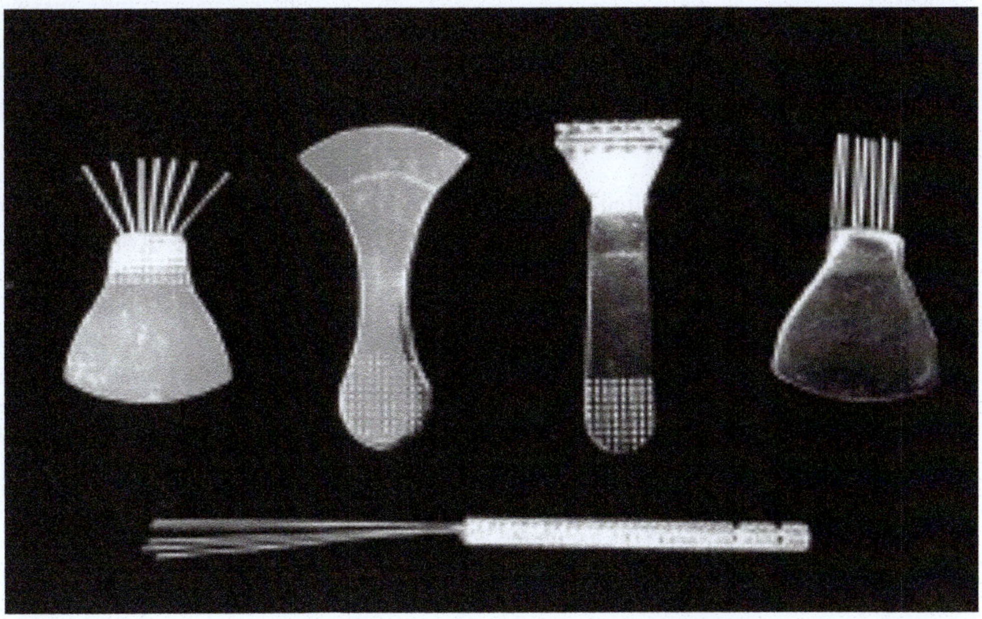

Fig. 7.2 Tools not meant for insertion. Top row from left: pine needle type, blade type, scraping needle, and pine needle type. Bottom row: broom needle

- Minute striking: Needle is placed on skin with acupuncture tube, and the head of the needle is hit lightly repeatedly. When needle starts to go in, it is lifted out again and striking is continued.
- Tube dispersion: The tube is placed on the point without a needle, and the top of the tube is struck repeatedly with the index finger.
- Needle-tip manipulation: With needle tip inserted just beneath the skin, the body of the needle is held in both hands and the skin is moved back and forth in various directions.
- Needle redirection: Withdrawing a needle most of the way after going to depth, the angle of the needle is changed and then it is reinserted.

1.3.2 Non-insertion Acupuncture Techniques(Contact Needling Method)

The contact needling method, which does not involve insertion beneath the skin and aims to stimulate the skin surface, is used for the purpose of addressing issues on the skin surface and regulating the autonomic nervous system. In addition, it is used for patients sensitive to acupuncture and children. The contact needling method is divided into five basic techniques based on the approach to the skin, but there are subtle variations in technique depending on the desired outcome:

- Touching: The tip of the needle or tool is brought into contact with acupuncture points or the body surface.
- Tapping: Tapping (striking) the skin surface with a needle or tool. (The strike mallet needling method/ tap mallet needling method is classified separately.)
- Friction: A needle or tool is used to friction the skin surface.
- Pressure: A needle or tool is used to add pression on acupuncture points or specific areas of the body surface.
- Scratching: A needle or tool is used to scratch the skin surface.

In actual practice, most often several techniques are selected from among the above basic techniques and serially combined (e.g., tapping and friction, or friction and pressure are combined).

1.3.3 Dashin (Strike Mallet Needling Method/ Tap Mallet Needling Method)

In Dashin, or the strike mallet needling method/tap mallet needling method, a needle is held on an acupuncture point and hammered on the top with a special hammer to apply vibration to the body surface. This technique was developed in premodern Japan, and even though it was listed in the text ***Science of Acupuncture & Moxibustion: Techniques Volume*** (1959), very few practiced it. Later on, however, a modern Dashin technique "without insertion" was developed based on ***Compilation of the Secrets of Acupuncture*** (1685), the original classic on Dashin.

1.3.4 Pricking Collateral Method (Shiraku)

In this needling technique, small amounts of bleeding are caused at Jing Well Points, small collateral vessels/thread-like collateral vessels, or areas with congestion (hemostasis) with the aim of activating a healing response. Aside from filiform needles, one of the 9 classical needles, the spear-like needle (three-edge needle), is used. This treatment of expelling blood that has become stagnant in the body is mentioned in the Chinese classic, *Kouteidaikei* 黄帝内経 *(Yellow Emperor's Inner Classic)*, and it was very popular in the Edo period (1611–1863). In modern times, in the "regulation concerning the practice of acupuncture and moxibustion" issued by Ministry of the Interior in 1911, there was an article that forbade pricking collateral method (*Shiraku*) in acupuncture. (This article was deleted in the regulations after 1945.) In the 1950s, Kudo Kunimasa (1918–1989), who was originally a military doctor, began publishing texts about pricking collateral method (*Shiraku*). Along with this, he worked to promote this technique through activities such as republication in 1985 of a late Edo period text, *Shiraku* Observation Record. Currently, the Japan Association of *Shiraku* Acupuncture is promoting this technique through seminars and a certification system along with compiling a manual that considers safety.

1.3.5 Low-Frequency Electroacupuncture Therapy

Low-frequency electroacupuncture therapy has been clinically applied primarily for pain reduction since the 1970s, after "acupuncture anesthesia" became publicized. Since that time, however, neurological and neurochemical studies on animals and healthy human subjects have been conducted, and it has been found that it has a variety of effects aside from pain reduction (improved circulation, immune modulation, autonomic regulation, and relaxation). Thus, it has come to be used not only for pain conditions but also for a wide variety of ailments. Its clinical application dramatically increased especially since the 1990s, when the techniques of low-frequency electroacupuncture therapy were improved, and needle insertion and direct electrostimulation of pathological tissues (such as muscles, nerves, subcutaneous connective tissue, and ligaments) became the practice.

The five categories in which low-frequency electroacupuncture therapy can be applied clinically are ① muscle pulse, ② nerve pulse, ③ subcutaneous pulse, ④ intervertebral pulse, and ⑤ reactive point pulse (Tsukuba University system). The aim, object, and method involved in these applications are shown in Table 7.2.

Table 7.2 Categories of low-frequency electroacupuncture therapy in Tsukuba University

	Name	Aim	Object	Method
1	Muscle pulse	To improve circulation in muscle, alleviate muscle hardness and shortening	Skeletal muscles	Low-frequency electrostimulation between 1 and 10 Hz that causes twitching. Depending on situation, intermittent simulation of about 30 Hz is used. Continuous high-frequency electrostimulation can cause pain, so sometimes the amount of current cannot be raised to produce adequate twitching
2	Nerve pulse	To normalize threshold of somatic nerves	Nerves	The frequency of electrostimulation is normally 1 Hz. Sometimes, higher frequency is effective, but it can produce strong muscle contractions and pain when a motor branch is stimulated. So, start with low frequency at a level that causes twitching and work up to a higher frequency. Insert needle adjacent to the target nerve and add current to selectively stimulate never fibers. The verification of whether the intended nerve has been stimulated is obtained by observing twitching in the muscles controlled by that nerve
3	Subcutaneous pulse	To alleviate pathology of subcutaneous connective tissues	Subcutaneous connective tissue	The standard frequency is 30–50 Hz. This stimulation is applied with horizontal needling just under the skin, so higher frequency is used. Be careful, however, because this can cause tetanus if the horizontal needle contacts a skeletal muscle. Use 30 Hz for itching in skin in the active stage of AD, urticaria, eczema, and RA and dialysis patients. Use 1 Hz in the remission stage of RA
4	Intervertebral pulse	To alleviate pathology of soft tissues in intervertebral joints and foramina (except nerves)	Intervertebral joints	Location of insertion is the same as for nerve pulse to treat cervical and lumbar vertebrae. After confirming radiating pain with insertion, stimulate with 1 Hz, and after confirming that the nerve pulse is initiated, gradually lift the needle to a depth where the nerve pulse disappears. Confirm that there is a deep knocking sensation. The standard frequency is 1 Hz. The needle penetrates the erector spinae muscles with insertion around the intervertebral joins, and high frequency sometimes leads to pain, so start with low frequency
5	Reactive point pulse	Autonomic nervous system regulation	Reactive points	Among the conditions/symptoms that can be alleviated are essential hypertension, degree and frequency of repeated tonsillitis, and dyspnea from bronchial asthma

Compiled based on references [3 and 4]

1.3.6 Domestic and International Standards for Low-Frequency Electroacupuncture Devices

As for international standards for low-frequency electric stimulation devices, there is IEC 60601-2-10:1987 "Medical electrical equipment. Part 2: Particular requirements for the safety of nerve and muscle stimulators." Also, based on this there is a domestic standard, "Medical electrical equipment—Section 2-10: individual requirements regarding the safety of nerve and muscle stimulators, JIS T 0601-2-10: 2005."

Concerning low-frequency electroacupuncture devices, however, even though there was an attempt to draft standards for them during the revision of pharmaceutical laws in 2005, it was not adopted. After that, with a focus on the issue of certain metals dissolving when acupuncture needles are used for an electrode, an attempt was made to establish standards to ensure safety. In 2011, the Japan Society of Acupuncture and Moxibustion issued "A report concerning the standards to secure safety of low frequency electroacupuncture devices." Based on this report, the Ministry of Health, Labor and Welfare has issued certification standards that limit the maximum current per session to 1C or less. The ISO standard for the device, after a long discussion at TC249, was published in 2022 as ISO 24571 Traditional Chinese medicine—general requirements for the basic safety and essential performance of electroacupuncture stimulators.

1.4 Moxa and Its Classifications

Until the Middle Ages, acupuncture was primarily concerned with surgery, and its complete adoption did not happen until the Kamakura or Muromachi periods (approx. 1200–1600). In contrast to this, ever since Chinese medicine first arrived in Japan, moxibustion has been widely practiced in Japan throughout its history. Even after the modern era when Western medicine became mainstream in Japan, moxibustion has been used not only in specialized clinics, but also at home for health preservation, as well as provided in places like temples for the purpose of prevention.

Because of the historical precedent of being used widely by the public, moxa material used for moxibustion is still classified among miscellaneous items, and there is no standard or acceptable certification standard as a medical device. Nevertheless, high-quality moxa material is produced by moxa producers in Japan that boast a long history, and different quality moxa is produced according to application. Also, in recent years smokeless moxa with reduced amounts of smoke, as well as electromoxibustion that uses electricity as

Table 7.3 Classification of grades of moxa (The raw material for the moxa in Japan is primarily the leaves of *Artemisia princeps Pamp*)

Grade	Use	Details
High grade	Direct moxibustion	This is just the extraction of the hairs (trichomes) on the back of mugwort leaves and is divided into 3–4 grades according to level of refinement. A stone grinder is used in the manufacturing process, and the end product is gold-colored and shiny. The more the fibers are short and round and even, the higher the quality. Moxa with longer fibers or black specs is of a lower quality. The higher the quality, the easier it is to form into rice-grain-sized cones, and the combustion temperature is lower so it can be applied without causing burns
Medium grade	*Kyutoshin* (warm needling)	This contains not only trichomes on the back of mugwort leaves but also powdered remnants of the mugwort leaves itself. Therefore, its color is a little greener or brownish compared to moxa for direct moxibustion. Because the combustion temperature is high, it is suitable for applying radiant heat to the skin surface by burning a ball of moxa on the head of a needle. It is divided into 3 to 4 grades according to level of refinement, and the higher quality material has fewer leaf remnants so it forms a better ball on the needle and it doesn't fall apart after burning
Low grade	Indirect moxibustion	The content of processing remnants is higher than *Kyutoshin* (warm needling) moxa material. The color is also darker brown or green. Further, since the combustion temperature is higher, it is suited for moxa stick, placing in a box or on top of insulating material like a piece of ginger or garlic. It is divided into 2 or 3 grades according to level of refinement

a heat source, has been developed. The classification of grades of moxa is shown in Table 7.3. Also, ISO issued in 2015 ISO 18666 moxibustion device regarding international standards for the devices used in moxibustion therapy.

1.5 Moxibustion Methods

Moxibustion methods can roughly be divided into "direct moxibustion" and "indirect moxibustion." The moxa cone is placed directly on the skin in the former, and an insulating material like ginger or garlic or a piece of cardboard is placed between the skin and the moxa cone in the latter, to provide indirect heat stimulation. Further, in direct moxibustion there is the distinction of "scarring moxibustion" and "non-scarring moxibustion," depending on whether a burn is created on the skin. The types of moxibustion methods and the grades of moxa used are shown in Table 7.4.

Table 7.4 Moxibustion methods and corresponding grades of moxa

Moxibustion methods			Grade of moxa
Direct moxibustion	Scarring moxibustion	Tonetsu-kyu (heat-penetrating moxibustion)	High grade
		Shoyaku-kyu (cautery moxibustion)	High grade
		Dano-kyu (suppurative moxibustion)	High and medium grade
	Non-scarring moxibustion	Chinetsu-kyu (non-scarring direct moxibustion)	High, medium, and low grade
Indirect moxibustion	Non-scarring moxibustion	Insulated moxibustion (ginger, garlic, salt, miso, etc.)	Medium and low grade
		Moxa products with cardboard base	Medium and low grade
	Non-scarring moxibustion	Warming moxibustion and electromoxibustion devices	-------
	Non-scarring moxibustion	Moxa stick moxibustion	Medium and low grade
Kyutoshin (warm needling)			Medium and low grade

1.5.1 Heat-Penetrating Moxibustion

This method employs high-grade moxa with little remnants for point moxibustion. A string of moxa material rolled into rice-grain-sized, half-rice-grain-sized, or string-like cones is placed directly on acupuncture points and burned to provide heat stimulation. This is a type of scarring moxibustion. The size and shape of the moxa cones depend on the application. Currently, it is common to use cone-shaped cones, but in texts like *"Gaikyutsusetsu* 艾灸通説 *(Prevailing Ideas on Moxa and Moxibustion)"* (1809) by Goto Chin-an, there is mention of a method of spindle-shaped cones with a smaller area at the base. Also, there is a method where, in order to reduce the amount of heat felt by the patient, the cone is extinguished before it burns completely. This is the so-called 70% moxibustion method which is non-scarring.

1.5.2 Suppurative Moxibustion/Pustulating Moxibustion (Dano-Kyu)

In this method, a moxa cone with the size of the end of the thumb or bigger is burned on the skin all the way. A special cream is applied on the burn which becomes infected, and the aim is to cause release of pus for several weeks. This is a variety of scarring moxibustion. It has been practiced in temples and clinics with a family moxibustion tradition with the aim of increasing resistance and preventing disease.

1.5.3 Cautery Moxibustion (Shoshaku-Kyu)

Moxa cones are burned repeatedly on warts and corns with the aim of burning off these growths.

1.5.4 Non-scarring Direct Moxibustion (Chinetsu-Kyu)

Cone-shaped moxa about 1 cm in diameter at the base and roughly the size of the end of the index finger is placed directly on the skin of the patient and burned. As soon as the patient feels heat, the moxa cone is removed. This is a type of non-scarring moxibustion. Ino-ue Keiri, one of the founders of meridian therapy devised this method and reported it in the general meeting of the Japan Meridian Therapy Association in 1951.

1.5.5 Moxa Stick Moxibustion (Bo-Kyu)

In this method, moxa material is wrapped in Japanese paper, etc., and formed it into sticks. The practitioner lights one end and holds the stick with the hand to provide radiant heat to treatment areas. Another application is to place something like a loquat leaf on the skin and place cloth or thick paper over this and press the burning end of the stick to heat the skin. Sometimes, just a towel is placed over the skin and the stick is pressed on over this. When radiant heat is being provided, the temperature is adjusted by changing the distance from the skin. There are devices designed to hold a stick in place over the body to provide continuous heat (Fig. 7.3).

1.5.6 Insulated Moxibustion (Kakubutsu-Kyu)

This is a general term for a method of placing material between the moxa cone and the skin. Insulating material such as a thinly sliced piece of garlic or ginger, or some salt or miso is placed between the skin and the moxa cone. This is a type of non-scarring moxibustion.

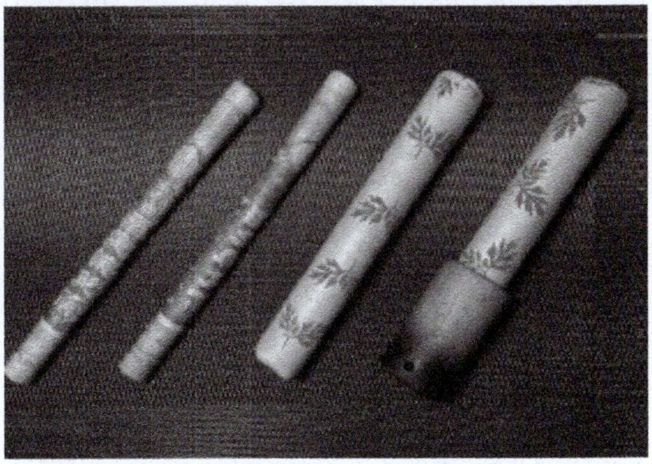

Fig. 7.3 Moxa stick: thin (left) moxa stick for holding over the body, thick (right) moxa stick for pressing into fabric, etc

1.5.7 Stick-on Moxa with Pedestal (Daiza-Kyu)

Stick-on moxa with pedestal is a method using commercially produced moxibustion products with a cardboard base with moxa rolled in paper above it. A fixed amount of moxa is in a small cylinder on the top, and it's designed with a hole so that there is space between the skin and the moxa. The base has adhesive so it stays on the skin. The top moxa is lit, and it burns down to provide indirect heat on a point. In recent years, there are smokeless stick-on moxa products made with charcoaled moxa, as well as those with special scents on the market (Fig. 7.4).

1.5.8 Electromoxibustion Devices

These are devices that use electricity as the heat source instead of moxa, since there are restrictions to the use of smoke-producing moxibustion in facilities like hospitals and nursing homes. In these facilities, electromoxibustion devices can be used. There are devices that target a small point and those that can stimulate a large area at once. There are a large variety of materials used for the contact surface with the skin including ceramics. The advantages of electric moxibustion devices, in addition to not producing smoke, are the temperature can be set so there is a low risk of burns. Further, these devices are portable, and they can be used in any environment including outdoors since no fire is used. Also, those devices designed to make a sound when a certain temperature is reached can be used by visually impaired people (Fig. 7.5).

1.5.9 Warm Needling (*Kyutoshin*)

A round ball of moxa or a precut cylindrical piece of moxa is placed on the head of a needle that is retained in a point. The moxa is lit and burned so the mechanical stimulation of the needle and the radiant heat stimulation from the head of the needle on the surrounding skin is combined. The heat that is conducted into the skin through the body of the needle is minimal. Since moxa is burned on the head of the needle, the needle handle must be stainless steel. The moxa material used is medium grade specially made for warm needling.

2 Acupuncture Using Various Approaches

2.1 Ryodoraku Therapy

Masanori Takashi

2.1.1 Introduction

Ryodoraku therapy, which was invented for acupuncture and moxibustion by Yoshino Nakatani in the 1950s, is a system of diagnosis and therapy for the regulation of the autonomic nervous system. The basis of Ryodoraku therapy is that

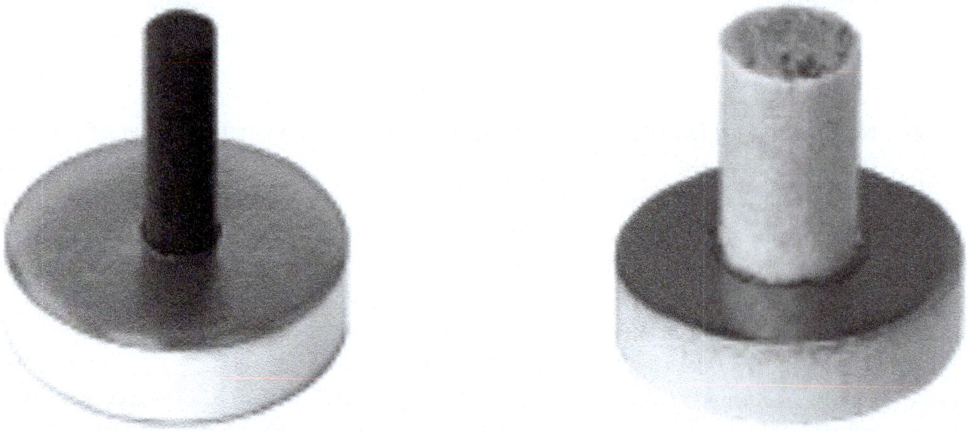

Fig. 7.4 Stick-on moxa with pedestal. (Provided by SENEFA Corporation)

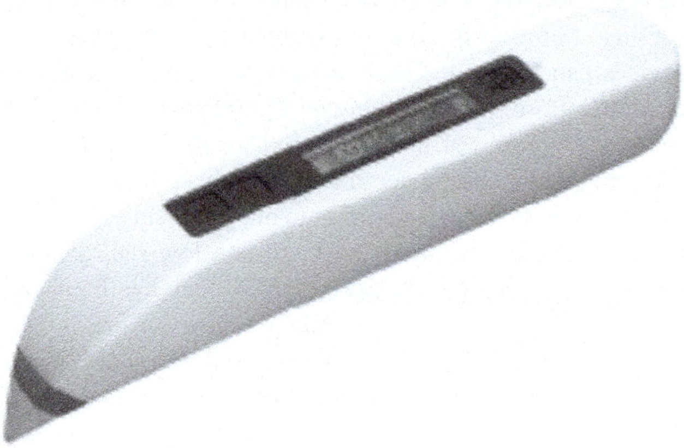

Fig. 7.5 Electromoxibustion device. (Provided by SEIRIN Corporation)

Ryodoten (electroconductive points), where there is low resistance in the skin to electrical current, connect to form lines named Ryodoraku (electroconductive lines). These are similar to the 12 meridians of acupuncture and moxibustion. Ryodoraku therapy regulates the function of sympathetic and parasympathetic nerves associated with imbalances in the 12 Ryodoraku to alleviate dysfunction and disease. This therapy is named Ryodoraku Autonomic Nerve Regulation Therapy.

2.1.2 Diagnostic Procedure

① The Neurometer is the instrument that has been developed to detect Ryodoten, where there is low resistance to electrical current in the skin. This instrument has two electrodes to measure the balance of the 12 Ryodoraku. The electrical resistance values were measured on the skin surface of the primary points of the meridian with a direct current of 21 Volts. These findings are recorded on a chart and are evaluated to decide treatment.

② The point of lowest resistance to electrical current is sought with a direct current reduced from 21 V to 12 V. These points are called Reactive Ryodoten. It is considered that Reactive Ryodoten are reflexes appearing on the skin surface from abnormal functioning and pathophysiological phenomenon of internal organs. These points are used for the focal treatment.

2.1.3 Ryodoten, Ryodoraku and Point, Meridian

Ryodoraku is lines and points based on the physiology and pathology of meridians determined from the standpoints of electrophysiology and the autonomic nerves.

The fluctuation of Ryodoraku and meridians is revealed by measurement of electrical resistance of skin. Thereby, the fluctuation and balance of the autonomic nerve system are checked indirectly.

2.1.4 Excitation Points

H13: LU9, H21: PC9, H31: HT9, H43: SI3, H51: TE3, H611: LI11.

F12: SP2, F29: LR8, F37: KI7, F41: BL67, F52: GB43, F65: ST41.

2.1.5 Inhibition Points

H18: LU5, H23: PC7, H33: HT7, H48: SI8, H510: TE10, H62: LI2.

F15: SP5, F22: LR2, F31: KI1, F43: BL65, F57: GB38, F61: ST45.

The Name of 12 Ryodoraku

Ryodoraku on the upper extremities are named [H] and numbered, and those on the lower extremities are named [F] and numbered.

2.1.6 Method of Treatment

The method of treatment is the adjustment of Ryodoraku and the adjustment of Active Ryodoten. The adjustment of Ryodoraku is applied to chronic diseases and addresses the deviations in physiological limits of Ryodoraku, individually. The focal care of Active Ryodoten is applied to specific complaints by probing electrical resistance of skin in local area.

2.1.7 Limits of Physiology

The values obtained by the Neurometer are inconsistent for healthy people and vary with age, lifestyle, and seasons. These variations are within permissible range of health and are called the limits of physiology. The limit of physiology is 1.4 cm based on measured data. Values over the physiological limit are called "agitation," and the values below the physiological limit are called "restraint." If the measured values at 12 volts are under 10 and the limits of physiology are a single line, the Neurometer measurements must be taken at 21 volts.

2.1.8 Abnormal Ryodoraku

The values over and under the limit of physiology are considered abnormal Ryodoraku. Excitation points are stimulated for cases of restraint, and inhibition points are stimulated for cases of agitation. The method of treatment is weak stimulation to excitation points and strong stimulation to inhibition points.

Please refer to the text for more details.

2.2 Trigger Point Acupuncture Therapy

Masanori Takashi

2.2.1 Outline

It is thought that trigger points create hard nodules in muscle tissue, strain tendons, and compromise blood circulation, causing a deficiency in oxygen and nutrition for metabolism, as well as accumulation of metabolic products. It has also been found that trigger points are a sensitive reflection of stress and a cause of pain in soft tissue.

Definition

Trigger points are the hard nodules in soft tissue of the human body, including the fascia, periosteum, tendons, and skin. Further, trigger points are responsive to mechanical stimulus and can cause various symptoms in other areas.

Feature

Trigger points are a complex soft tissue pathology caused by motor, sensory, and autonomic nerves. Therefore, they can't be grasped completely. It is significant that trigger points are hard nodules in the soft tissue which causes pain with stimulation. The features of trigger points in the fascia include hard nodules, tenderness with pressure, referred pain, decline of muscle strength, restriction of movement, autonomic reflex, focal simple contractive reflex, and escape reflex from stimulation.

The Cause of Trigger Points

Trigger points can be caused by weakness of contraction, imbalance of pressure within muscles, surface wound, excessive eccentric contraction, eccentric contraction of fatigued muscles, and excessive isotonic contraction.

Pathophysiology of Trigger Points

The precise details of mechanisms causing trigger points are not clear, but it's explained by the hypothesis of integration and motor point dysfunction. The assumption is that trigger points are formed and propagated not just by physical damage to muscles, but also by agitation of sympathetic nerves from mental stress. Therefore, clinically it is important to seek the cause of trigger point formation from different angles, including the social background of patients.

Classification of Trigger Points

Trigger point can be palpated as hard nodules in muscles. The hard nodules of trigger points vary in size from rice to thumb size. Trigger points are classified by the location of formation. The hard nodules formed in the center of the muscle fibers are called "central trigger points." The hard nodules that form at the attachment of muscles are called "adherent trigger points." Trigger points are also classified by the degree of seriousness. They are "actual trigger points" and "potential trigger points." Actual trigger points have spontaneous focal and referred pain, and potential trigger points have no focal and referred pain without stimulus.

Diagnosis

There are four prerequisites needed for the diagnosis of trigger points:

- The palpation of hard nodules in muscle
- The existence of severe tenderness in hard nodules
- The reproduction of tenderness with stimulation
- The restriction in range of motion with pain

Method of Detection

The flat examination is used for the detection of trigger points. In this examination, the skin over the trigger point is drawn to one side and the tip of finger is rolled across the muscle fiber to confirm pain. The "jump sign" will often occur as a response to escape from pain.

The Referred Pain of Trigger Points

The symptom of trigger points is focal pain (tenderness and spontaneous pain) and referred pain. Pain in an area distant from the origin is called referred pain. Referred pain is a phenomenon that is difficult to understand because of various patterns, according to the degree of seriousness.

Often in clinic, practitioners overlook trigger points that are the cause of the pain, by focusing on the site of the referred pain. The area where a trigger point first causes referred pain is called the first zone of referred pain. Subsequently, the area of pain from a more serious trigger point is called the second zone of referred pain.

Please refer to other text for more detail.

2.3 YNSA (Yamamoto New Scalp Acupuncture)

Masanori Takashi

2.3.1 Outline

YNSA is a scalp acupuncture system devised by the anesthesiologist Yamamoto Toshikatu, who made it public at the general assembly of Japan Ryodoraku Congress in 1973. There were other scalp acupuncture methods devised in China in the latter half of the 1960s, but these are different from this system. YNSA is an independent system of diagnosis and treatment for scalp acupuncture based on Yamamoto's clinical experience. The basic points from Point A to Point E in the frontal region were made public in 1973. Thereafter, the basic points from Point F to Point I were gradually added on to the other points. These points are shown in Table 7.5 in detail.

Applicable diseases include not only cerebral nerve disease, but also neck pain, lumbago, shoulder pain, headache, neurologic conditions (vertigo, tinnitus, and insomnia), complaints of general malaise (menopausal disorders, etc.). YNSA has high renown in the world, and was adapted in the health insurance system in Germany and Italy and is used for treatment by many doctors. The YNSA Association promulgates the YNSA method in Japan, and the method will be developed in the future.

2.3.2 Diagnosis and Treatment in YNSA

The meridians and points based on the acupuncture classics are not used on the YNSA system. YNSA uses a unique diagnostic method and treatment points based on Yamamoto's clinical experience. In the beginning, Doctor Yamamoto based his Ryodoraku therapy. Nevertheless, he emphasized palpating tenderness and hard nodules. Also, he developed unique methods of diagnosis and sites of treatment. In the early stage of YNSA development, the target of palpation was the abdomen and standard points. Yamamoto discovered

Table 7.5 Basic point

	Point A	Point B	Point C
Location	On the head, directly above BL 2, on the anterior hairline	About 1 cm lateral to point A on both sides	65 degrees to the top of the nose, crossing the hairline, on both sides
Region	Head, cervical vertebrae, shoulder	Cervical vertebrae, shoulder, shoulder joint	Scapula joint Shoulder joint Arm
	Point D	Point E	Point F
Location	Extension from end of eyebrow crossing hairline in temporal muscle on both sides	1 cm above midpoint of eyebrow, at a 15 degree to the top of the nose; 15 cm in length	Mastoid process
Region	Lumbar vertebra	Thoracic vertebra	Ischium
`	Point G	Point H	Point I
Location	Under mastoid process on both sides	Just above point B	1 cm diagonally posterior to point C
Region	Knee	Leg	Leg (whole)

that the reactive points of some diseases exist on the neck (sternocleidomastoid muscle, trapezius muscle, omohyoid muscle) at the secondary stage, and these reactive points were incorporated into the neck examination.

More recently, palpation of LI4 and the upper arms was added, and thus, the examination system of YNSA was achieved. The palpation of both LI4 is done first, and the side of treatment is decided. Next, upper arm palpation is performed to locate reactive points (corresponding to the lumbar, thoracic, and cervical vertebra, brain stem, cerebellum, and cerebrum). Then, the indicated zones on the scalp are treated. If this treatment has no effect, then the neck and abdomen are palpated and treatment is provided based on these findings according to the disease and symptoms.

Please refer to other text for more detail.

2.4 M-Test

Masanori Takashi

2.4.1 Introduction

The M-Test is a method of diagnosis and treatment based on meridians and points associated with pain, which was created by Mukaino Yoshito M.D. Mukaino treated athletes over a long time and discovered that the pains caused or aggravated by the body movement are on the lines of meridians. Thus, the postures that cause or aggravate the pain confirm the meridians and points for treatment. M-Test is also useful for judging the effect right after treatment.

The meridians and points for treatment can be decided quickly and precisely with the M-Test. It is also useful as a measure of treatment outcome. Also, it is possible to monitor the pathological condition that changes continuously. Mukaino has applied this method for diseases other than musculoskeletal injury.

Features

The pathological condition of patients with various symptoms that arise with movement of body and limbs can be understood based on the theory of meridians and points. Activities of daily living and lifestyle can be surmised, and explanation and guidance for self-care can be provided to patients. Thus, motivation for treatment is increased and this contributes to shortening the course of treatment and prevention.

Diagnosis and Therapy

- Diagnosis
  ① There are 30 basic movements to identify the abnormal meridians. They consist of anterior stretch, posterior stretch, and lateral-medial stretch of the limbs and body. The basic movements are classified into three blocks for upper limbs and three blocks for lower limbs, for a total six blocks (Table 7.6).
  ② The movements/stretches in the six blocks correspond to two meridians each.
  ③ The stretches related to the occurrence or exacerbation of symptoms are noted and scored with numerical rating scale (NRS). The two meridians with the highest score become the target for treatment.

Treatment

① The two meridians with the highest score are targeted for treatment.
② The main points for treatment are four points based on five-phases theory and proximal tight point on the meridians.

Table 7.6 Classification of M-Test blocks and meridians for treatment

		Meridians
A block	The upper anterior limbs	Lung[TM1] and large intestine[TM1]
B block	The upper posterior limbs	Heart[TM1] and small intestine[TM1]
C block	The upper lateral limbs	Pericardium[TM1] and Sanjiao[TM1]
D block	The lower anterior limbs	Spleen[TM1] and stomach[TM1]
E block	The lower posterior limbs	Kidney[TM1] and bladder[TM1]
F block	The lower lateral limbs	Liver[TM1] and gall bladder[TM1]

③ The four points associated with two meridians are pressed lightly with a finger as the movement causing pain is repeated, and the points that are most effective for the pain are determined. The effective points are then stimulated with needles. The movement causing pain is repeated to check the effect.
④ The same manner of the examination (movement) and stimulation is repeated on a proximal tight point. A short needle is effective for stimulation. A thumbtack needle or bandage with a short needle or tape that has about 400 microspikes protruding per 1 cm^2 is used for treatment. There is no any stress for patients because the stimulation is minimal and effective.
⑤ When treatment of the meridians in the block with the highest score is effective, symptoms associated with other blocks will also improve. Every block influences every other based on the five-phases theory.
⑥ If the treatment is not effective, Yin-Yang crossover point combinations and the flow chart of M-Test are used (Fig. 7.6).

The basic 24 points of 6 blocks (Fig. 7.7).
Lung[TM1] meridian (LU5, LU9), large intestine[TM1] meridian (LI2, LI11),
Heart[TM1] meridian (HT7, HT9), small intestine[TM1] meridian (SI3, SI8), pericardium[TM1] meridian (PC7, PC9), triple energizer meridian (TE3, TE10), spleen[TM1] meridian (SP2, SP5), stomach[TM1] meridian (ST41, ST45), kidney[TM1] meridian (KI1, KI7), bladder meridian (BL65, BL67), liver meridian (LV2, LV8), and gallbladder[TM1] meridian (GB38, GB43).

Please refer to other text for more detail.

2.5 Meridian Therapy

Toshihiro Togo
Meridian therapy devised during and after the Second World War in Japan is a system of diagnosis and therapy based on Chinese medical classics. Meridian therapy was devised by the students of Yanagiya Sorei who, from the 1930s, promoted the revival of acupuncture based on Chinese classics. These students were Okabe Sodo, Inoue Keiri, and Takeyama Shinichiro.

The main principle of meridian therapy is that disorders of the mind and body are caused by deficiency and excess of the 12 meridians. The deficiency or excess of the 12 meridians is judged by symptoms and six-position pulse diagnosis. The five-phases points of the upper and lower limbs are used to tonify deficiency and drain excess (*Honchiho*: root treatment). Afterward, this symptomatic treatment is provided for

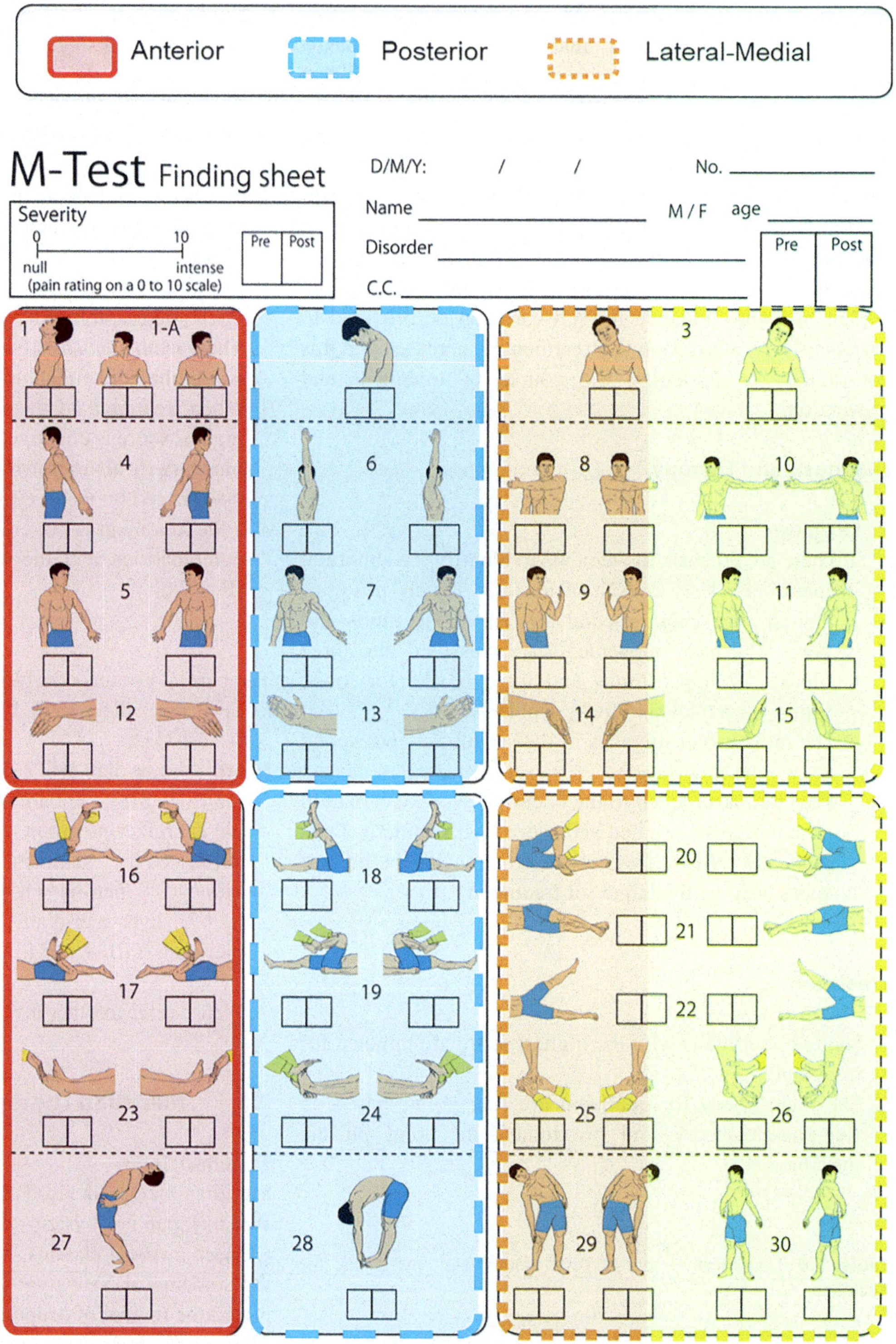

Fig. 7.6 M-Test finding sheet. (*Illustrated M-Test* Supervised by Mukaino Yoshito, Ishiyaku Publishers, Inc., 2012)

the symptoms (*Hyochiho*: branch treatment). The deficiency of meridians judged by diagnosis is called "Sho" based on the diagnosis by Koho (herbal) School. Acupuncture is performed in *Honchiho*, and moxibustion is performed in *Hyochiho*. In this way, meridian therapy is different from Taiji therapy, which regulates the balance of five organs with moxibustion pulse.

Meridian therapy has a premise that yin deficiency or *Zokyo* (deficiency in Zang organ) is the underlying cause of disease. *Zokyo* starts with deficiency in one of four yin meridians (lung[TM1], spleen[TM1], liver[TM1], and kidney[TM1]). This can be determined by pulse diagnosis. For these four yin meridians, deficiency can be tonified and excess can be drained. This treatment is based on Chapters 69 and 75 of the

Fig. 7.7 M-Test 24 Points. (*Illustrated M-Test* Supervised by Mukaino Yoshito, Ishiyaku Publishers, Inc., 2012)

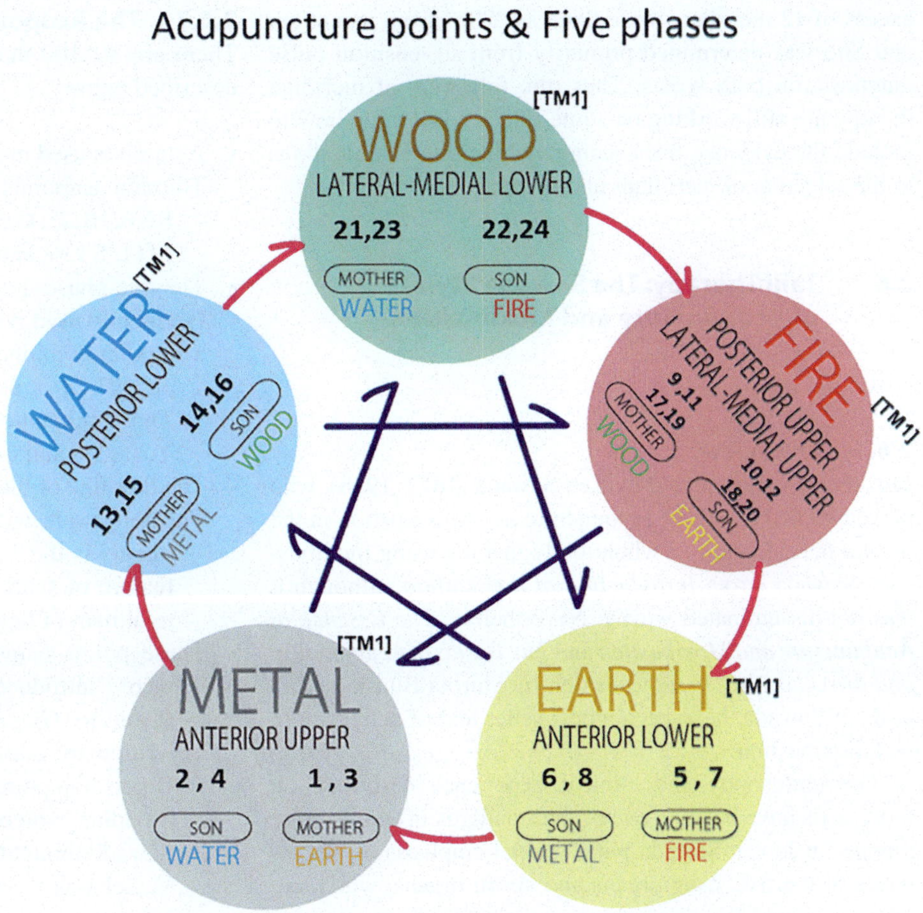

面(Phase)		陰(Yin M.)	陽(Yang M.)
Anterior	**Upper (metal)**	1. LU9 2. LU5	3. LI11 4. LI 2
	Lower (earth)	5. SP2 6. SP5	7. ST41 8. ST45
Posterior	**Upper (fire)**	9. HT9 10. HT7	11. SI3 12. SI8
	Lower (water)	13. KI7 14. KI1	15. BL67 16. BL65
Lateral-Medial	**Upper (fire)**	17. PC9 18. PC7	19. TE3 20. TE10
	Lower (wood)	21. LR8 22. LR2	23. GB43 24. GB38

Nanjing. Chapter 69 of the *Nanjing* explains the principle that the mother points must be used to tonify deficiency and that child points must be used to drain excess. This principle is used in *Honchiho* (root treatment) of meridian therapy to select the meridians and points for treatment.

For example, in cases judged to be deficiency of lung[TM1] meridian by pulse diagnosis, LU8 of the same meridian and SP5 of the mother meridian are selected along with LU9 of the same meridian and SP3 of the mother meridian are being selected for treatment, and these points are tonified.

Meridian therapy originated over 70 years ago. Since then, the followers of Okabe, Inoue et al. have developed various methods of diagnosis, selection of meridians and points, and ways of needle insertion. The deficiency and excess of 12 meridians were fixed as "Sho" from inception, and Sho was determined primarily from six-position pulse diagnosis on both wrists. Thus, the followers of meridian therapy are still working on some issues concerning how to include the evidence from seeing and hearing examinations in the selection of meridians and points.

2.6 Taiji Therapy: The Sawada Style of Acupuncture and Moxibustion

Toshihiro Togo

2.6.1 Overview

This therapy was created by Ken Sawada (1877–1938), who played on active part of acupuncture and moxibustion in the Showa period, and is a whole-body therapy using moxibustion. Sawada wrote *Introduction of the Sanjiao*, although it was not disseminated widely. Nevertheless, *The Essence of Acupuncture and Moxibustion* and *The Basics of Acupuncture and Moxibustion Therapy*, written by Shirota Bunshi, a disciple of Sawada, have been a best seller text of acupuncture and moxibustion.

The philosophy and clinical experience described on those texts have become one of the standards in acupuncture therapy in Japan. Sawada put a special emphasis on imbalances of the five Zang organs and six fu organs, which are diagnosed from the signs and symptoms of patients. Sawada did not put emphasis on the diagnosis of diseases based on Western medicine. He treated patients with moxibustion using acupoints based on his own theory of pathology. Below is an outline of the Taiji therapy described in *The Basics of Acupuncture and Moxibustion Therapy* (7th edition).

2.6.2 Theory

When Sawada studied Judo, when he was just starting out in massage therapy, he treated patient by stimulating acupoints with heated stones. He found that this was effective and decided to treat mainly with moxibustion. At first, Sawada referred to the text *Wakan Sansai Zue* (和漢三才図会 *Japanese-Chinese Encyclopedia*) to find the acupoints; later, he studied the classics *Shisi Jing Fahui (*十四経発揮 *Elaboration of the 14 Meridians)* and *Nangyo Tekkan (*難経鉄艦 *Iron Ship of the Classic of Difficulties*). Thus, Sawada devised a unique theory of moxibustion therapy. He emphasized in the text he wrote himself that the Sanjiao was important as the root of the fundamental power of body temperature. Sawada thought that moxibustion was beneficial for the energy of Sanjiao and for the general wellbeing of body. The classification of the Sanjiao (three burners) in Taiji therapy is that the upper burner is lung[TM1] and heart[TM1], the middle burner is spleen[TM1] and stomach[TM1], and the lower burner is kidney[TM1] and bladder[TM1].

2.6.3 The Acupoints Used for Therapy

There are 80–100 major acupoints used in Taiji therapy as described below:

- Acupoints used most frequently
  Thirteen acupoints were used frequently: left SJ4, RN12, RN6, BL23, GB25, BL32, BL20, BL18, BL17, DU12, LI11, ST36, and KI13.
- The five-phases points of each meridian

– Frequently used point combinations
  The point combination of left SJ4, RN12, BL20, BL18, and BL23 is used with BL22 and DU20 frequently. The combination of SJ4, RN12, and DU20 is named Yokankai and used frequently.

– The first line of bladder[TM1] meridian of Foot Taiyang
  The points selected frequently for moxibustion were used mainly in the Sawada style. Shirota referred to another feature of school of the Sawada style, which was the treatment of first line of bladder[TM1] meridian.
  These points named Huato Jiaji Xue 「華佗挟脊穴」 were introduced in *Shinkyusetsuyaku* 鍼灸説約 *(Concise Guide to Acupuncture and Moxibustion)* written by Ishizaka Sotetsu. Sawada recognized the Huato Jiaji points as the first branch of the bladder[TM1] meridian which is 1.5 cm lateral to the Du Vessel. Sawada thought that the line 1.5 cm lateral to the Du Vessel was the first line of the bladder[TM1] meridian. When he detected tenderness on points on these lines, he presumed the presence of heat in the organ associated with the tender points. Sawada treated this heat with acupuncture. These tender points on the first bladder[TM1] meridian lines are said to be found 1.5 cm above the corresponding organ points on the second bladder[TM1] meridian lines. Shirota emphasized that the first bladder[TM1] meridian lines were not described in the classics, and were discovered by Sawada, and were not taught by predecessors. Shirota claimed that acupuncture on points of the first bladder[TM1] meridian lines had wide applications.

3 Safety of Acupuncture and Moxibustion

Toshihiro Togo

This chapter details the minimum knowledge necessary for safety when engaging in acupuncture and moxibustion treatment. Regarding safety in the field of acupuncture and moxibustion, **Acu-moxa Safety Strategy Guidelines**, 2020 edition (from Ishiyaku Publishing; hereunder referred to simply as "Guidelines") has been published by the Safety

Committee of the Japan Society of Acupuncture and Moxibustion. Further, the website of the above Society offers the Japanese and English version of this document [1]. Also, the Japan Traditional Medicine Text: acupuncture and moxibustion edition includes detailed explanation based on safety research in and outside of Japan. The information in this chapter follows the information in the Guidelines and the above text, but please refer to the above resources and website for more details and the latest information.

3.1 Introduction

3.1.1 About Medical Accidents and Harmful Incidents with Acupuncture and Moxibustion

A medical accident is defined as "Personal injury that occurs in the site of medical treatment through the entire process of medical care regardless of the presence or lack of excesses or negligence on the part of medical providers." Accidents include both physical injury and psychological injury, and the victim includes not only the patient but the medical provider as well.

Medical accidents are exam and treatment records of incidents of harm that have been retroactively investigated by a third party. The event about which information is collected is called an "adverse event," and these are classified into the following four cases based on the cause-and-effect relationship:

① Side effect (harmful reaction): unintentionally occurring physical reaction.
② Negligence: an event arising from the negligence of the practitioner or the facility, lack of knowledge, or intentional act.
③ Unavoidable accident: natural disasters, etc.
④ Event with no cause-and-effect relationship with the treatment or the practitioner.

3.1.2 Study on the Frequency of Occurrence of Adverse Events

Until the first half of the 1990s, reports on adverse events with acupuncture and moxibustion were often featured in medical journals as case studies after the incident. These reports were weak in terms of accurately conveying the frequency of adverse events. After the mid-1990s, however, proactive studies on adverse events began independently in Japan [2], England [3], and Germany [4].

It has been determined that serious adverse events occur very infrequently in standard acupuncture treatments.

3.2 Side-Effects, Negligence, and Adverse Events with Acupuncture and Moxibustion

3.2.1 About Side-Effects (Adverse Events) with Acupuncture and Moxibustion

There is no way of avoiding a certain number of incidents during or after treatment. Undesirable reactions of the body are called side-effects (harmful reactions). The side-effects of acupuncture and moxibustion can be divided into systemic and local effects as follows:

① Systemic side-effects: strong fatigue or lassitude, excessive drowsiness, feeling unwell, etc.
② Local side-effects: pain with insertion, minute bleeding, itchiness in needled area, pain in area needled after treatment, etc.

Among the systemic side-effects, fatigue or lassitude after treatment tends to occur after the first treatment. As for drowsiness and lassitude, these pose a risk for those who drive or have to do work that requires concentration after the treatment. Therefore, patients must be informed before the treatment so they can be careful. The local side-effects such as bleeding and subcutaneous hemorrhaging occur most often with electroacupuncture therapy [5].

3.2.2 Malpractice and Incidents with Acupuncture and Moxibustion

Medical malpractice is defined as "One type of medical accident in which medical workers in the course of carrying out their duties go against the standards of medical practice and cause harm to patients." On the other hand, those things do not cause personal or financial loss to the patients, but unintentional occurrences that the alarm or alert practitioners are called incidents. In acupuncture and moxibustion, these are ① forgetting to remove a needle, ② causing a burn or a blister, ③ pneumothorax, ④ needle breaking. These are reported as being adverse events with the highest likelihood of malpractice.

3.2.3 Main Adverse Events in Acupuncture and Moxibustion and Their Prevention

Adverse events connected to acupuncture include (1) infectious diseases, (2) organ damage (including pneumothorax and puncture of blood vessels), (3) nerve damage, (4) skin diseases, (5) broken needle and needles left in place. In the **Acu-moxa Safety Strategy Guidelines,** the following items are listed as preventative measures for adverse events:

① Treatment of immunocompromised patients (diabetics, long-term steroid users): The appropriateness of treatment should be determined in each case.

② Insertion into joint cavities: This should not be done, from the perspective of preventing infection.
③ Treatment in areas with artificial parts (artificial joints, artificial vessels, pacemakers, etc.): From the perspective of preventing infection, direct insertion into the area should be avoided, and treatment of surrounding area should proceed with caution.
④ Insertion into upper back and thoracic area: This must be done very carefully in order to prevent pneumothorax.
⑤ Heart damage (cardiac tamponade, etc.): From the perspective of prevention, deep insertion in the anterior chest should be avoided. Also, one must be careful about a sternal hiatus at CV-17.
⑥ Treatment in area with large blood vessels: Deep needling and rough techniques must be avoided due to risk of blood vessel damage.
⑦ Treatment of patients with bleeding tendency (hemophilia, etc.): Be thorough about clean needle technique because they have a higher risk of bleeding and infection than normal patients.
⑧ Treatment in area with large nerves: Avoid deep needling and rough techniques.
⑨ Treatment on posterior cervical area: Due to the risk of injury to the central nervous system (brain and spine), caution is required with deep needling and rough techniques.

Also, the **Acu-moxa Safety Strategy Guidelines** respectively defines "broken needle, needles left in place, and foreign objects left in the body" as "needle remaining in body unintentionally, broken needle body remaining in body, and objects in body other than normal cells." It then goes on to list precautions as follows:

① Needles that remain in the body can cause chronic pain, or could move through the body to injure internal organs, nerves, or blood vessels, so attention must be paid to avoid leaving broken needle parts in the body.
② Needle embedding treatment, where needles are left in the body permanently, must not be practiced.
③ To avoid broken needles, single-use needles are recommended. When needles made for reuse are used, they must be inspected at their body and handle and the attachment before used to be sure they are sound.
④ If the needle handle breaks off and the needle becomes difficult to remove, the patient must be informed of this. Also, they should be referred to a medical facility to consult whether the needle needs to be removed.
⑤ Embedded needles can cause chronic pain, so when giving treatment it is desirable to inquire about history of embedded needle treatments especially with elderly patients.

As for adverse events related to moxibustion, there are reports about burns and cancerous changes at the site of moxibustion. As for the cancerous changes, they are the result of self-treatment, and they occurred through applying huge cones of moxa over many years (something that is rarely these days). This must be considered in another category from adverse events from moxibustion by licensed practitioners:

① There is a risk of infection, ulceration, or symptom exacerbation with moxibustion on areas with inflammation, infection, open wound, or circulatory impairment. Therefore, avoid treating such areas.
② Inquire about diseases that could cause sensory impairment (pain or heat sensation). Be very careful when treating local areas with sensory impairment.
③ Immunocompromised patients (diabetics, long-term steroid users) are at a higher risk of infection or ulceration compared to normal patients. Therefore, avoid excessive stimulation and reconsider suitability of treatment when the disease state doesn't improve.
④ When an unintended burn is caused, quickly rinse the area with cold water when the burn is mild (first degree). When the burn is medium (second degree) or more and there is a greater risk of infection, refer the patient to a dermatologist.
⑤ Excessive heat stimulation on the same point over a long period can become a cause of adverse events, so be careful to avoid this.

3.2.4 Prevention of Adverse Events Associated with Low-Frequency Electroacupuncture

Perform electroacupuncture only after first confirming that there are no contraindications. In the **Acu-moxa Safety Strategy Guidelines,** the following precautionary items are listed for practicing low-frequency electroacupuncture.

- **Precautions concerning the needles used for electroacupuncture**
  ① The needles used must be able to withstand corrosion due to electrolysis (electrolytic corrosion), which can cause needle breakage, as well as external forces of muscle contractions during treatment. Also, in view of

preventing adverse events such as needle breakage, they should be sterilized single-use stainless steel needles, and a thickness of more than 0.20 mm is advised. Further, needle lengths of over 30 smm are strongly advised.

② Silver needles should not be used because electrolysis tends to occur.

- **Precautions concerning the machines used for electroacupuncture**

① Use machines that are approved as devices for low-frequency electroacupuncture.

② Check the electroacupuncture device and its cords before starting treatment and perform periodic maintenance.

③ Don't use direct current pulsing which tends to cause electrolytic corrosion.

Also, as contraindications for electroacupuncture the following are listed: (①) Performing electroacupuncture on patients with medical implants such as pacemakers or defibrillators. (②) Simultaneous application of medical devices (such as electrocardiograms) and electroacupuncture.

3.3 Contraindications for Acupuncture and Moxibustion

In view of ensuring safety, the sites where acupuncture and moxibustion are contraindicated are listed in the **Acu-moxa Safety Strategy Guidelines,** as shown in Table 7.7.

Table 7.7 Sites contraindicated for acupuncture and moxibustion. Treatment is contraindicated on sites in which there is a risk of damaging organs or vital systems, and sites with potential for exacerbating symptoms

Intervention	Contraindicated sites or procedures
Acupuncture	Anterior fontanel of infants, posterior fontanel, external genitalia, nipples, navel, eyeballs, infected area, site of acute inflammation, large blood vessels, internal organs, central nervous system, site of malignant tumors
Moxibustion	Face, external genitalia, nipples, navel, site of infection, malignant tumors or acute inflammation, direct (scarring) moxibustion on area with skin disease

Special caution must be exercised when treating areas close to the abovementioned places (complied from Acu-moxa Safety Strategy Guidelines, 2020, Ver. 1.1.1)

References

1. JSAM. Safety Guidelines for Japanese Acupuncture and Moxibustion Practice 2020 Ver.1.1 by The Japan Society for Acupuncture and Moxibustion (JSAM) https://safety.jsam.jp/_src/37/safety_guidelines_of_jsam_eng_20210607.pdf
2. Yamashita H, Tsukayama H, Tanno Y, et al. Adverse events related to acupuncture. JAMA. 1998;280:1563–4.
3. MacPherson H, Thomas K, Walters S, et al. The York acupuncture safety study: prospective survey of 34000 treatments by traditional acupuncturists. BMJ. 2001;323:486–7.
4. Witt CM, Daniel P, Brinkhaus B, et al. Safety of acupuncture: results of a prospective observational study with 229,230 patients and introduction of a medical information and consent form. Frosch Komplementmed. 2009;16:91–7.
5. Yamashita H, Tsukayama H, Sugishita C. Local adverse reactions commonly seen in Japanese-style medical acupuncture practice. Clin Acupunc Orient Med. 2001;2:132–7.

Part III

Commentary of Kampo Formulas and Lists of Crude Drugs

Commentary of Kampo Formulas

8

Takao Namiki

安中散

Anchusan (ACS) ān zhōng sǎn
Manifestation

1. Symptoms

   - Epigastric pain: Either acute or chronic, but convulsive pain
   - Heartburn, belching
   - Stomach distention, anorexia
   - Nausea, vomiting
   - Cold feeling in the abdomen(cold stomach[TM1] and spleen[TM1])
   - Menstrual pain

2. Signs
   (i) Inspection: The complexion is often bad, and the body is often thin.
   (ii) Tongue examination: The tongue body is unremarkable, and tongue coating is often thin and white.
   (iii) Pulse examination: Often weak.
   (iv) Abdominal examination:
   Abdominal strength: Soft or slightly soft (1/5-2/5)
   Abdominal manifestations
   Abdominal pulsation (usual)
   Splashing sound: (often)
   Epigastric stuffiness and resistance (often)
   Subjective epigastric stuffiness (sometimes)
   Feeling of fullness in epigastric region (sometimes)
3. Indications
   Indicated for the following symptoms in patients with medium or deficiency pattern whose abdominal muscles tend to lack tone and who have stomachache or abdominal pain. Also, sometimes accompanied by heartburn, belching, anorexia, nausea, etc.: neurotic gastritis, chronic gastritis, and gastrointestinal weakness.

T. Namiki (✉)
International University of Health and Welfare Narita Hospital, Narita, Japan

Kampo Medical Literature Editorial Committee, Narita, Japan
e-mail: office@jsom.or.jp

胃苓湯

Ireito (IRT) wèi líng tāng
Manifestation

1. Symptoms

   - Diarrhea: Often watery. Diarrhea from summer to autumn is a good indication.
   - Vomiting.
   - Dry mouth, decreased urine volume.
   - Anorexia.
   - Postprandial stomach rumbling, abdominal pain.

2. Signs
   (i) Inspection: The face and limbs may be edematous.
   (ii) Tongue examination: In acute cases, the tongue is unremarkable. In chroniccases, tongue coating is often sticky and thick.
   (iii) Pulse examination: In cases with fever, the pulse is often floating and rapid.
   (iv) Abdominal examination:
   Abdominal strength: Moderate (3/5)
   Abdominal manifestations
   Splashing sound (usual)
   Distention (usual)
   Epigastric stuffiness (often)
   Borborygmus after a meal (sometimes)
3. Indications
   Indicated for the following symptoms in patients with medium pattern who have watery diarrhea and vomiting accompanied by thirst and decreased urine volume: food poisoning, heat stroke, cold abdomen, acute gastroenteritis, and abdominal pain.

Kampo Medical Literature Editorial Committee, The Japan Society for Oriental Medicine (ed.), *Complete Japanese Traditional (Kampo) Medicine*, https://doi.org/10.1007/978-981-96-7143-4_8

茵陳蒿湯

Inchinkoto (ICKT) Yīn chén hāo tāng
Manifestation

1. Symptoms

- Discomfort in epigastric region and chest: abdomen, especially fullness in upper abdomen. There is indescribable discomfort from the epigastrium to the inside of the chest. The patient is feeling a blockage in their chest and complains of nausea.
- Thirst, decreased urine volume: drinks a lot of water, but less urine than expected.
- Rash: Urticaria, eczema, dermatitis, etc. Often accompanied by pruritus.
- Constipation.

2. Signs
   (i) Inspection: Jaundice may be seen.
   (ii) Tongue examination: The tongue body may be red, and the tongue coating may be yellow.
   (iii) Pulse examination: Rapid.
   (iv) Abdominal examination:
   Abdominal strength: Slightly strong—strong (4/5–⑤/5)
   Abdominal manifestations
   Mild distension in upper abdomen (usual)
   Subjective epigastric fullness (usual)
   Epigastric stuffiness and resistance (sometimes)
3. Indications
   Indicated for the following symptoms in patients with medium and excess pattern who have thirst, decreased urine volume, and constipation: jaundice, hepatic cirrhosis, nephrosis, urticaria, and stomatitis.

茵陳五苓散

Inchingoreisan(IGRS) Yīn chén wǔ líng sǎn
Manifestation
This formula is a combination of goreisan and inchinkoto

1. Symptoms

- Thirst, decreased urine volume: Thirst, drinks a lot of water, but less urine than expected
- Jaundice
- Urticaria
- Edema, ascites
- Vomiting, anorexia
- Headache, dizziness/vertigo

2. Signs
   (i) Inspection: The face and limbs may be edematous.
   (ii) Tongue examination: The tongue body is unremarkable, and the tongue coating is slightly yellow.
   (iii) Pulse examination: Sometimes slippery pulse.
   (iv) Abdominal examination:
   Abdominal strength: * Slightly soft (2/5)
   Abdominal manifestations
   occasional splashing sound (usual)
   Feeling of fullness (sometimes)
   Epigastric stuffiness (sometimes)
3. Indications
   Indicated for the following symptoms in patients with medium or excess pattern who have thirst and decreased urine volume: vomiting, urticaria, hangover, and edema.

温経湯

Unkeito (UKT) Wēn jīng tāng
Manifestation

1. Symptoms

- Vexing heat in the palms and soles. The feeling of warmth in the palms is important; it is also used for eczema and dermatitis in the same area.
- Dry lips.
- Irregular menstruation/dysmenorrhea: May complain of abnormal menstrual flow.
- Cold sensitivity, chilblains.
- Lower abdominal pain due to cold.
- Infertility.

Signs
   (i) Inspection: Dry lips, redness of palms, and dry skin are often seen.
   (ii) Tongue examination: Tongue body is often pale and may have ecchymosis. Tongue coating is unremarkable.
   (iii) Pulse examination: There may be deep pulse.
   (iv) Abdominal examination:
   Abdominal strength: Soft to slightly soft (1/5 to 2/5)
   Abdominal manifestations
   Distention in lower abdomen (often)
   Occasional tenderness in lower abdomen (often)
   Cold lower abdomen (sometimes)
2. Indications
   Indicated for the following symptoms in patients with medium or deficiency pattern who have heat in the limbs and dry lips: irregular menstruation, dysmenorrhea, leukorrhea, climacteric disturbance, insomnia, neurosis,

eczema, cold feeling in the lower limbs and waist, and chilblain and dry skin (eczema and dermatitis in hand).

温清飲

Unseiin (USI) Wēn qīng yǐn
Manifestation

1. Symptoms

- Dryness and itching of the skin: The skin color is dark brown or tan. Characterized by brown skin. This is especially common in chronic dry skin diseases. It is usually not suitable for moist skin.
- Redness, hot, dry rash: Chronic rash that has become lichen-like. The itching is strong.
- Hotflash, bleeding tendency: Patient may have uterine bleeding, hemoptysis, melena, nosebleeds, etc.
- Irregular menstruation, dysmenorrhea
- Allergic constitution

2. Signs
   (i) Inspection: Often complexion is sallow.
   (ii) Tongue examination: The Tongue body may be reddish or red on the tip of the tongue.
   (iii) Pulse examination: May have rapid pulse.
   (iv) Abdominal examination:
   Abdominal strength: Moderate (3/5)
   Abdominal manifestations
   Abdominal muscle tension (usual)
   Fullness and discomfort in chest and hypochondrium (usual)
   Epigastric stuffiness and resistance (often)
   Occasional tenderness in lower abdomen (often)
3. Indications
   Indicated for the following symptoms in patients with medium pattern who have dry skin, bad skin color, and hot flushes: menstrual irregularity, dysmenorrhea, automatic imbalance syndrome unique to women resembling climacteric disturbance, neurosis, eczema, and dermatitis.

越碑加朮湯

Eppikajutsuto (EPTJ) Yuè bì jiā shù tāng
Manifestation

1. Symptoms

- Edema: The skin is tight but not swollen.
- Sweating tendency.
- Thirst, decreased urine volume: Edema and sweating deplete fluids, which causes reduced urine volume.
- Edema: Especially on the face.
- Skin heat and eczema: Especially seen on the face and the head.
- Joint pain and edema: Present in limb joints.

2. Signs
   (i) Inspection: The face may be edematous.
   (ii) Tongue examination: The tongue body is unremarkable, and tongue coating may be white.
   (iii) Pulse examination: Deep and rapid in some cases.
   (iv) Abdominal examination: Nothing notable.
   Moderately to slightly hard abdomen (3/5-4/5)
3. Indications
   Indicated for the following symptoms in patients with medium or excess pattern who have edema, thirst, diaphoresis, and sometimes decreased urinary volume: edema, swelling and pain of joint, arthritis, eczema/dermatitis, nocturnal enuresis, and itching or pain of eye.

黄耆建中湯

Ogikenchuto (OKT) Huáng qí jiàn zhōng tāng
Manifestation

1. Symptoms

- Patient presents a more deficient pattern than shokenchuto: In addition to symptoms for shokenchuto pattern, such as fatigue and abdominal pain, this patient presents a weak tendency, such as night sweats, thinness, and shortness of breath.
- Frail child, nocturnal enuresis.
- Eczema, dermatitis: Chronic rash such as atopic dermatitis in patients with Xiaojianzhong pattern.
- Granulation tissue growth disorder: Wound is difficult to heal, such as anal fistula and intractable ulcer.

2. Signs
   (i) Inspection: The complexion is pale, and the patient often looks tired.
   (ii) Tongue examination: The tongue is pale, and white moss may be seen.
   (iii) Pulse examination: Often deep or weak.
   (iv) Abdominal examination Abdominal strength: Soft to slightly soft (1/5-2/5).
   Abdominal manifestations
   Abdominal muscle tension (usual)
   Occasional abdominal pain (often)
3. Indications
   Indicated for the following symptoms in patients with deficiency pattern who are easily fatigued: delicate constitution, weakness during convalescence, night sweating, exanthema and dermatitis, erosive skin, abdominal pain, and coldness.

黄芩湯

Ogonto (OT) Huáng qín tāng
Manifestation

1. Symptoms

- Abdominal pain: Often complains of pain in the umbilical region and paraumbilical region. It can be used not only for diarrhea due to acute enteritis and dyspepsia but also for inflammation such as appendicitis and uterine adnexitis, as well as abdominal pain.
- Fever: Chills are observed, but sweating is not often observed.
- Diarrhea (with tenesmus): A person who feels sick to the stomach and has one bowel movement after another. The stool is not watery but muddy or mucous-like.
- Nausea and vomiting.
- Bitter taste in mouth.
- Dryness in mouth.

2. Signs
   (i) Inspection: Dehydration may cause a decrease in skin luster.
   (ii) Tongue examination: The quality of the tongue is unremarkable, and tongue coating may be white.
   (iii) Pulse examination: It may be deep or slow.
   (iv) Abdominal examination:
   Moderate abdominal strength (3/5)
   Abdominal manifestations
   Epigastric stuffiness and resistance (usual)
   Abdominal muscle tension (often)
   Tenesmus (sometimes)
3. Indications
   Indicated for the following symptoms in patients with medium pattern who have abdominal pain, epigastric fullness, sometimes with chills and fever: Diarrhea, gastroenteritis.

黄連解毒湯

Orengedokuto (OGT) Huáng lián jiě dú tāng
Manifestation

1. Symptoms

- Heat sensation: Symptoms such as dry mouth, dry skin, rash, and flushing of the face are observed. It can be used in the acute phase of febrile disease or a chronic excess heat pattern. Symptoms associated with inflammation and hyperemia due to the fever of the whole body are indicated. Unexpected symptoms such as numbness, chilliness, and mucosal inflammation may appear when administered to those with a cold and deficiency pattern.
- Bleeding: Bleeding symptoms such as hematemesis, hemoptysis, epistaxis, hematuria, and melena are exhibited due to inflammation and hyperemia.
- Psychiatric symptoms: irritability, insomnia, and anxiety. Insomnia is characterized by sleep onset disorders and cases where frustration prevents sleep.

2. Signs
   (i) Inspection: Face is often red (qi counter flow) due to inflammation and hyperemia.
   (ii) Tongue examination: The Tongue body is red, and the tongue coating may be yellow.
   (iii) Pulse examination: It tends to be deep and is often excess and rapid.
   (iv) Abdominal examination:
   Abdominal strength: Moderate to full (3/5-5/5)
   Abdominal manifestations
   Fullness and discomfort in chest and hypochondrium (usual)
3. Indications
   Indicated for the following symptoms in patients with medium or excess pattern who have a ruddy face, a touch of hot flushes, and a tendency toward irritability: nose bleeding, hypertension, insomnia, neurosis, gastritis, alcoholic hangover, miscellaneous symptoms related to menstruation, dizziness, palpitation, climacteric disturbance, eczema/dermatitis, itching of skin, and stomatitis.

黄連湯

Orento (ORT) Huáng lián tāng
Manifestation

1. Symptoms

- Abdominal pain: Mainly epigastric pain.
- Stagnation and/or feeling pressure in the epigastric region and anorexia: Burning sensation and discomfort from the chest to the upper abdomen due to acute gastritis and reflux esophagitis.
- Nausea and vomiting: Nausea, vomiting, and stomach discomfort due to a hangover.
- Diarrhea: Defecation abnormalities and viral enteritis associated with fever; often not accompanied by tenesmus.
- Stomatitis, angular cheilitis, bad breath: Especially recurrent stomatitis.

- Others: Concomitant symptoms include hot flashes, cold feet, headache, and fever.

2. Signs
   (i) Inspection: Flushing of the face is often seen.
   (ii) Tongue examination: Apical redness may be observed in the tongue body.
   Tongue coating is often moist and smooth; moss is white or white-yellow and thicker at the root of the tongue.
   (iii) Pulse examination: It is often wiry. Sometimes it is soft.
   (iv) Abdominal examination:
   Abdominal strength: Moderate to slightly strong (3/5–4/5)
   Abdominal manifestations
   Occasional abdominal pain in the epigastric region (usual)
   Epigastric stuffiness and resistance (usual)
   Chest anguish (often)
   Cold epigastrium when touched (sometimes)
3. Indications
   Indicated for the following symptoms in patients with medium pattern who have heavy obstructive feeling and/or oppressive feeling in stomach, anorexia, and sometimes nausea and vomiting: epigastralgia, acute gastritis, hangover, and stomatitis.

乙字湯

Otsujito (OJT) Yǐ zì tāng
Manifestation

1. Symptoms

- Hemorrhoids: Used in general for hemorrhoids such as anal fissure, anal prolapse of the anus, and hemorrhoidal prolapse in patients with constipation. However, for hemorrhoids that are caused mainly by blood[TM1] stasis rather than constipation, priority is given to blood[TM1] stasis resolving formulas such as keishibukuryogan. Consider other prescriptions for patients without constipation but who have marked flaccid anal prolapse or severe hemorrhoidal prolapse or marked bleeding.
- Itching and pain in the genital area: It can also be used for itching and pain in the vagina, perineum, and anus.

2. Signs
   (i) Inspection: Signs of blood[TM1] deficiency and blood[TM1] stasis, such as dry skin and chloasma, may be observed.
   (ii) Tongue examination: The tongue body is unremarkable, and there may be a dry white tongue coating.
   (iii) Pulse examination: Often excess.
   (iv) Abdominal examination:
   Abdominal strength: Moderate or higher (3/5–5/5)
   Abdominal manifestations
   Paraumbilical tenderness and resistance (usual)
   Fullness and discomfort in chest and hypochondrium (often)
3. Indications
   Indicated for the following symptoms in patients with medium or excess pattern who have constipation with hard stools: hemorrhoids (wart hemorrhoids) and anal fissures, constipation, and mild anal prolapse.

葛根湯

Kakkonto (KT) Gé gēn tāng
Manifestation

1. Symptoms

- General symptoms of the common cold in the initial stage: Headache, fever, and chills without spontaneous sweating.
- Diarrhea: A febrile illness at the initial stage accompanied by diarrhea, or diarrhea from a common cold in the initial stage.
- Stiff shoulders, neck pain, back pain: Stiffness and pain along the spinal column (Bladder[TM1] Meridien).
- Headache: Associated with tension headache and sinusitis.
- Others: Not only upper respiratory tract inflammation but also other inflammatory diseases such as mastitis, otitis media, conjunctivitis and keratitis, tonsillitis, rhinitis, periodontitis, insufficient breast milk production, nocturnal enuresis, and erosion around children's nose pillar and mouth.

2. Signs
   (i) Inspection: Nothing remarkable
   (ii) Tongue examination: Nothing remarkable
   (iii) Pulse examination: Floating, tight, and excess
   (iv) Abdominal examination: No specific abdominal manifestations
   Acute state: Abdominal strength: Not remarkable
   Chronic: Moderate or higher (3/5–5/5)
   Occasional tenderness beside the umbilicus (umbilical pain)
3. Indications
   Indicated for the following symptoms in patients with medium and excess pattern: The initial stage of the com-

mon cold (without spontaneous sweating), rhinitis, headache, shoulder stiffness, muscle pain, and pain in the arm and shoulder (Fig. 8.1).

葛根加朮附湯

Kakkonkajutsubuto (KTJB) Gé gēn jiā shù fù tāng
Manifestation

1. Symptoms

   In addition to the symptoms of kakkonto, there are the following indications. All patients tend not to sweat and have stiffness in the back of the neck, and the symptoms are exacerbated by cold and high humidity.

   - Swelling and pain: Acute/chronic swelling and pain of muscles and joints. Neuralgia, such as trigeminal neuralgia.
   - Rash: Acute or chronic urticaria, herpes zoster, etc.

2. Signs
   (i) Inspection: Unremarkable
   (ii) Tongue examination: Unremarkable
   (iii) Pulse examination: Unremarkable
   (iv) Abdominal examination: No literature
   Abdominal strength: Unremarkable
3. Indications

   Indicated for the following symptoms in patients with medium or excess pattern: swelling and pain of joint(s), neuralgia, muscle pain, rheumatic arthritis, shoulder stiffness, headache, and the initial stage of skin disease such as urticaria.

葛根湯加川芎辛夷

kakkontokasenkyushin'i (KTSS) Gé gēn tang jiā chuān xiōng xīn yí
Manifestation

1. Symptoms

   - Nasal congestion, runny nose, post-nasal discharge, acute/chronic rhinitis, sinusitis. Since it contains Magnolia kobus and Cnidium mofficinale, which have a heating effect, it may not be suitable for people with significant heat signs such as yellow purulent nasal discharge.

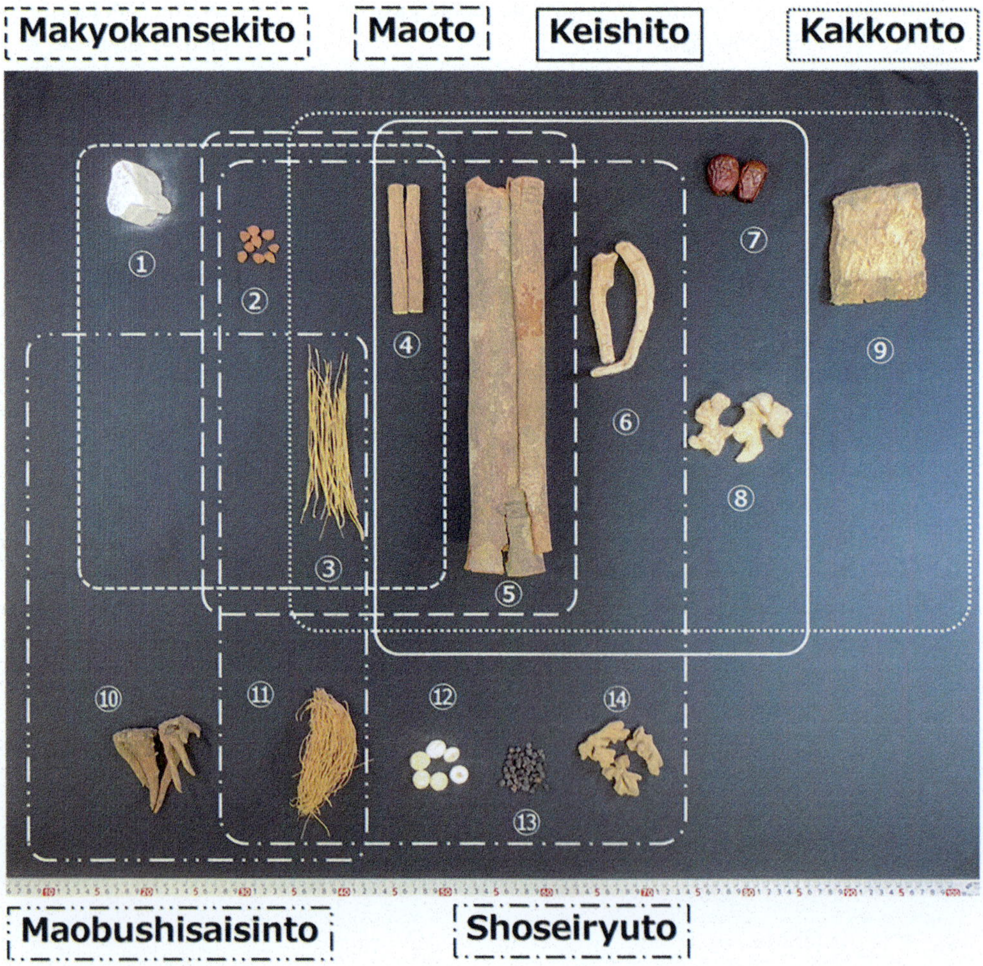

Fig. 8.1 Formulas in Keishito and Maoto groupsDuring the early yang stage pattern period, a formula containing ⑤ Cinnamon Bark and ③ Ephedra Herb (exterior releasing formulas) is used to induce sweating. If the patients have strong heat patterns, use ① Gypsum, which has a heat-clearing effect. If the patients have strong cold patterns and the disease has progressed to the middle yin stage pattern, use Processed Aconite Root, which has a warming effect, ② Apricot Kernel, ④ Glycyrrhiza, ⑥ Peony Root, ⑦ Jujube, ⑧ Ginger, ⑨ Pueraria Root, Asiasarum Root, Pinellia Tuber, Schisandra Fruit, Processed Ginger

- Headache, heavy head, and neck stiffness: Same as Kakkonto, it is used when there is an exterior pattern including chills, headache, and neck stiffness.
- Others: It is also used for various inflammation, pain, and hotness in the face and head, such as chronic otitis media, chronic tonsillitis, trigeminal neuralgia, and toothache.

2. Signs
   (i) Inspection: Unremarkable.
   (ii) Tongue examination: The tongue body is sometimes red, and the tongue coating is thin white moss.
   (iii) Pulse examination: Often float and tight.
   (iv) Abdominal examination:
   No special abdominal manifestation is reported.
   Moderate abdominal strength or higher (3/5-5/5).
3. Indications
   Indicated for the following symptoms with medium or excess pattern: nasal obstruction, empyema, and chronic rhinitis.

加味逍遙散

Kamishoyosan (KSS) Jiā wèi xiāo yáo sàn
Manifestation

1. Symptoms

- Symptoms of autonomic imbalance or menopause: general malaise, stiff shoulders, hot flashes and chillness, headache, various physical pains, insomnia, anxiety, anger, etc. It is often used for middle-aged women, but it can be used for men and women of all ages with a neurotic tendency.
- Symptoms of blood[TM1] stasis: Symptoms that occur with the menstrual cycle, such as menstruation disorders, irregular menstruation, premenstrual syndrome, neurosis, and depressive symptoms.
- Cold sensitivity.
- Constipation: Not severe.

2. Signs
   (i) Inspection: It is often used for women who are relatively thin and tend to give a nervous impression.
   (ii) Tongue examination: The tongue body may show red spots, and tongue coating is unremarkable.
   (iii) Pulse examination: Often deep and deficient and sometimes wiry.
   (iv) Abdominal examination: Abdominal strength: Soft to slightly soft (1/5 to 2/5).
   Abdominal manifestations
   Fullness and discomfort in chest and hypochondrium (usual)
   Infra-umbilical tenderness (sometimes)
   Abdominal pulsation (sometimes)
3. Indications
   Indicated for the following symptoms in persons with medium or deficiency pattern who are apt to have hot flashes, stiff shoulders, easy fatigue, and neuropsychiatric symptoms such as anxiety and irritability, and occasional constipation.
   Cold sensitivity, weak constitution, irregular menstruation, dysmenorrhea, menopausal disturbance, miscellaneous symptoms related to menstruation, and insomnia.

甘草湯

Kanzoto (KZT) Gān cǎo tāng
Manifestation

1. Symptoms

- Objective inflammatory findings such as redness and edema are not strong, but they are indicated when the symptoms are severe, sudden, and imminent.
- Sore throat
- Stomach pain
- Toothache
- Urination pain
- Hemorrhoids, pain associated with anal prolapse
- Spastic cough

2. Signs
   (i) Inspection: Unremarkable
   (ii) Tongue examination: Unremarkable
   (iii) Pulse examination: Unremarkable
   (iv) Abdominal examination:
   Abdominal strength (3/5)
   Abdominal manifestations
   Occasional abdominal muscle tension (usual)
3. Indication
   Indicated for the following symptoms in patients with any pattern: severe cough, sore throat, stomatitis, and hoarseness. External medicine: hemorrhoid and anal pain

甘麦大棗湯

Kambakutaisoto (KTT) Gān mài dà zǎo tāng
Manifestation

1. Symptoms

- Mental excitement: Emotions change quickly due to passionate and excitable nature. Patients can become uncontrollable. Sometimes patients make noises as if mad.
- Emotional incontinence: Sadness for no reason and quick to tears.
- Insomnia.

- Decreased responsiveness to stimulus: Response to external stimuli is sluggish.
- Yawning: Frequent.
- Gastrointestinal weakness.
- Child's tantrums and night crying.

2. Signs
   (i) Inspection: There may be a state of mental excitement, such as crying loudly. In addition, yawning may occur frequently.
   (ii) Tongue examination: Unremarkable
   (iii) Pulse examination: Sometimes rapid.
   (iv) Abdominal examination:
   Abdominal strength: Soft to slightly soft (1/5 to 2/5)
   Abdominal manifestations
   Abdominal muscle tension (usual)
3. Indications
   Indicated for the following symptoms in patients with medium or deficiency pattern: tendency of nervousness, startling easily, occasional yawning and insomnia, night crying, and convulsions in children.

桔梗湯

Kikyoto (KYT) Jié gěng tāng
Manifestation

1. Symptoms

- Throat pain: There is not much fever. It can be used as a mouthwash for throat pain.
- Dry throat: Throat is dry, but patients don't want to drink much water.
- Coughing.
- Purulent and viscous sputum.

2. Signs
   (i) Inspection: Unremarkable.
   (ii) Tongue examination: Unremarkable.
   (iii) Pulse examination: There may be a rapid pulse during fever.
   (iv) Abdominal examination:
   No specific abdominal manifestation reported
   Abdominal strength: Moderate (3/5)
3. Indications
   Indicated for the following symptoms with any pattern involving painful, swollen throat and occasional coughing: tonsillitis and peritonsillitis.

帰脾湯

Kihito (KIT) Guī pí tāng
Manifestation

1. Symptoms

- Amnesia
- Palpitations, insomnia, depressed mood, mental anxiety
- Anemia
- Night sweating

2. Signs
   (i) Inspection: The face may be pale.
   (ii) Tongue examination: The tongue body is pink, and the tongue coating may be moist white moss.
   (iii) Pulse examination: Often deficient.
   (iv) Abdominal examination:
   Abdominal strength: Soft to slightly soft (1/5 to 2/5)
   No specific abdominal manifestation reported.
3. Indications
   Indicated for the following symptoms in patients with medium or deficiency pattern with general malaise and mental fatigue and pale complexion: Anemia, insomnia, neurosis, and anxiety.

加味帰脾湯

Kamikihito (KKT) Jiā wèi guī pí tāng
Manifestation

1. Symptoms
   (There are the following symptoms in addition to symptoms of kihito.) Amnesia, palpitations, insomnia, depressed mood, mental anxiety, anemia, and night sweats.

- Irritability, frustration
- A feeling of heat

2. Signs
   (i) Inspection: The face may be pale.
   (ii) Tongue examination: The tongue body is normal pink, and the tongue coating may have moist white moss.
   (iii) Pulse examination: Often deficient.
   (iv) Abdominal examination:
   Abdominal strength: Soft to slightly soft (1/5 to 2/5)
   Abdominal manifestations
   Occasional abdominal pulsations (sometimes supra-umbilical or infra-umbilical pulsations) (often)
   Fullness and discomfort in chest and hypochondrium (sometimes)
3. Indications
   Indicated for the following symptoms in patients with medium or deficiency pattern with general malaise and mental fatigue, pale complexion, and sometimes feverish: Anemia, insomnia, anxiety, and neurosis.

芎帰膠艾湯

Kyukikyogaito (KKGT) Qiōng guī jiāo ài tāng
Manifestation

1. Symptoms

- Subcutaneous bleeding
- Hemorrhoid bleeding, genital bleeding
- Left lower abdominal pain

2. Signs
   (i) Inspection: The face is pale, bruising is often formed, and the skin is often dry.
   (ii) Tongue examination: The tongue body is unremarkable. Tongue coating may be moist or non-mossy.
   (iii) Pulse examination: There are cases of deep and deficiency.
   (iv) Abdominal examination:
   Abdominal strength: Soft to slightly soft (1/5–2/5)
   Abdominal manifestations
   Abdominal muscle tension (often)
   Tenderness (sometimes)
3. Indications
   Indicated for the following symptoms in patients with medium or deficiency pattern with cold sensitivity, bleeding tendency, but without gastrointestinal disorders: Hemorrhoidal bleeding, anemia, menstrual disorders, menorrhagia, uterine irregular bleeding, and subcutaneous bleeding.

芎帰調血飲

Kyukichoketsuin (KCI) Qiōng guī diào xuè tāng
Manifestation

1. Symptoms

- Various symptoms in postpartum: Anemia, lochia, weakness, dizziness, tinnitus, etc.
- Postpartum fever
- Irregular menstruation, menstrual pain

2. Signs
   (i) Inspection: The complexion may be dark and dull.
   (ii) Tongue examination: The tongue body is a normal pink color and may be accompanied by ecchymosis, which is a sign of blood stasis. Tongue coating is unremarkable.
   (iii) Pulse examination: It may be weak and thin.
   (iv) Abdominal examination:
   There is little literature.
   【reference】
   Abdominal strength: slightly soft 1/5–2/5. It may be very soft, like cotton.
3. Indications
   Indicated for the following symptoms in patients with medium or deficiency pattern: During postpartum, it can be used regardless of physical strength: Irregular menstruation, neurosis, or weakness in postpartum

九味檳榔湯

Kumibinroto (KBRT) Jiǔ wèi tuǒ láng tāng
Manifestation

1. Symptoms

- Cold feeling of limbs, cold feeling of the whole body.
- General malaise: Often accompanied by shortness of breath.
- Edema: Strong malaise in the lower limbs, often accompanied by edema.
- Strong sensation of joint rigidity: A strong sense of rigidity may be experienced in the joints of the neck, hips, and limbs.
- Paresthesia of limbs.

2. Signs
   (i) Inspection: Edema is found on the face and eyelids. The tip of the nose appears shiny due to the edema of the face.
   (ii) Tongue examination: The tongue body is unremarkable, and tongue coating often has thin white moss.
   (iii) Pulse examination: Fast pulse (quick rise and fast disappearance), often rapid.
   (iv) Abdominal examination:
   Abdominal strength: Unremarkable
   Abdominal manifestations
   Epigastric stuffiness (often)
   A feeling of fullness in the epigastrium (often)
3. Indications
   Indicated for the following symptoms in patients with medium or excess pattern who have general malaise, especially marked malaise in lower limbs: fatigue, menopause, palpitations, shortness of breath, edema, neurosis, gastroenteritis, and swelling in joints.

荊芥連翹湯

Keigairengyoto (KRT) Jīng jiè lián qiáo tāng
Manifestation

1. Symptoms

- Weak constitution: It is used to improve frail constitution and tendency to catch colds, as well as delicate constitution in adolescence with tendency to catch colds; also for otitis media and sinusitis after suffering from colds since childhood.

- Ear pain: Acute/chronic otitis media and acute mastoiditis (add sentai: cicada shell).
- Mankeishi: Vitex rotundifolia fruit, otitis externa.
- Nose pain: Acute/chronic maxillary sinus suppuration (add shin'I, Magnolia salicifolia), hypertrophic rhinitis.
- Others: Tonsillitis, nasal bleeding (add Cimicifuga rhizome and mountain cortex), acne, pulmonary tuberculosis, baldness, etc.

2. Signs
   (i) Inspection: Skin is dark and glossy. Sweating is seen on the palms and soles. Sometimes patients may be slim and have a thin neck.
   (ii) Tongue examination: The tongue body may look pale white, as with the shimotsuto pattern, or red, as with the orenren-gedokuto pattern. Tongue coating is often yellow-white.
   (iii) Pulse examination: Often tight.
   (iv) Abdominal examination:
   Abdominal strength: Moderate to slightly hard (3/5–4/5)
   Abdominal manifestations
   tension in the entire rectus abdominis muscle (usual)
3. Indications
   Indicated for the following symptoms in patients with medium or excess pattern who have dark skin, who tend to have greasy sweating seen on the palms and soles, and have tension in the abdominal wall: empyema, chronic rhinitis(sinusitis, chronic tonsillitis, and acne).

桂枝加黄耆湯

Keishikaogito (KSTO) Guì zhī jiā huáng shī tāng
Manifestation

1. Symptoms

- Common cold: In case of night sweats with keishito pattern
- Hyperhidrosis
- Cutaneous pruritus: Often reddish. May be accompanied by blisters and exudates.

2. Signs
   (i) Inspection: Reddish rash and moist skin may occur.
   (ii) Tongue examination: The tongue body is normal pink, and the tongue coating is moist and maybe non-moss or slightly white coating.
   (iii) Pulse examination: May be floating and weak.
   (iv) Abdominal examination:
   There is little literature.
   Abdominal strength: Unremarkable.
3. Indications
   Indicated for the following symptoms in patients with deficiency pattern: Night sweating, heat rash, eczema, and dermatitis.

桂枝加葛根湯

Keishikakakkonto (KSTK) Guì zhī jiā gé gēn tāng
Manifestation

1. Symptoms

- Early stage of common cold: A person with naturally weak immunity complains of chills, fever, headache, spontaneous sweating, and stiff shoulders in the early stage of the common cold.
- Rear neck stiffness: Chronic posterior neck stiffness.

2. Signs
   (i) Inspection: Almost the same as keishito. Glind's eyes may be weak.
   (ii) Tongue examination: Unremarkable
   (iii) Pulse examination: Floating, rapid, weak, and not tight.
   (iv) Abdominal examination:
   There is little literature.
   Abdominal strength: Unremarkable.
3. Indications
   Indicated for the following symptoms in patients with medium or deficiency pattern who sweat and have shoulder stiffness or headache: Early yang stage of a common cold.

桂枝加厚朴杏仁湯

Keishikakobokukyoninto (KSTKK) Guì zhī jiā hòu pǔ xìn grén tāng
Manifestation

1. Symptoms

- Cough: May be severe. Nocturnal coughing (sounds like a dog barking). Acute upper respiratory tract inflammation in patients with bronchial asthma, asthmatic bronchitis in children, etc.
- Bronchial asthma: Patients with bronchial asthma who feel tired and get worse when using formulas with ephedra herb.
- Chest fullness, wheezing.
- Abdominal distention, abdominal pain.

2. Signs
   (i) Inspection
   (ii) Tongue examination: Unremarkable

(iii) Pulse examination: Floating, slightly weak. Sometimes deep and tight during abdominal pain
(iv) Abdominal examination:
There is little literature.
Abdominal strength: Unremarkable.

3. Indication
Indicated for the following symptoms in patients with deficiency pattern: Cough, bronchitis, and bronchial asthma.

桂枝加芍薬湯

Keishikashakuyakuto (KSTS) Guì zhī jiā sháo yào tāng
Manifestation

1. Symptoms

- Diarrhea or constipation: Diarrhea is often accompanied by tenesmus. Keishi-ka-shakuyaku-daio-to is used in the case of heavy tenesmus. Rhubarb is added when the smell of flatulence or stools is strong.
- In addition, in the situation that diarrhea and constipation appear alternately, or that there is only abdominal pain and not having good stools when using laxatives, it is very useful. It is because taking a large amount of rhubarb may cause abdominal pain or swelling.
- Abdominal distension/fullness
- Abdominal pain: The natural constitution is that the intestines are weak, and it is often easy to feel a cold sensation.

2. Signs
(i) Inspection: Unremarkable.
(ii) Tongue examination: The tongue body is unremarkable, and tongue coating may be moist.
(iii) Pulse examination: Sometimes floating and weak.
(iv) Abdominal examination:
Abdominal strength: Soft to slightly soft (1/5 to 2/5)
Abdominal manifestations
Distension (usual)
Abdominal muscle tension (usual)
Abdominal pain (often)

3. Indications
Indicated for the following symptoms in patients with medium or deficiency pattern who have abdominal distension: tenesmus, abdominal pain, diarrhea, and constipation.

桂枝加芍薬大黄湯

Keishikashakuyakudaioto (KSTSD) Guì zhī jiā sháo yào dà huáng tāng
Manifestation

1. Symptoms

- Diarrhea or constipation: Diarrhea is often accompanied by tenesmus. This drug is used in cases of heavy tenesmus. Rhubarb is added when the smell of flatulence or stools is strong.
- In addition, it is very useful in situations where diarrhea and constipation appear alternately, or there is only abdominal pain without good bowel movements when using laxatives. This is because taking a large amount of rhubarb may cause abdominal pain or swelling.
- Abdominal distension/fullness.
- Abdominal pain: Constitutions with weak intestines and a tendency to feel a cold sensation.

2. Signs
(i) Inspection: Unremarkable
(ii) Tongue examination: The tongue body is unremarkable, and the tongue coating may be slightly dry and sometimes with no moss.
(iii) Pulse examination: Sometimes floating and weak.
(iv) Abdominal examination:
Slightly soft to moderate abdominal strength (2/5–3/5)
Abdominal manifestations
Distension (usual)
Abdominal muscle tension (usual)
Abdominal pain (often)
Tenesmus (sometimes)

3. Indications
Indicated for the following symptoms in patients with medium and deficiency pattern who have abdominal distension, abdominal pain, and constipation: Constipation and tenesmus.

桂枝加朮附湯

Keishikajutsubuto (KSTJB) Guì zhī jiā shù fù tāng
Manifestation

1. Symptoms

- Neuralgia/arthralgia: The pain is relieved by warming in a bath. The pain gets worse in the cold. The affected area is cold to the touch.
- Easy to sweat.
- Common cold.
- Tendency to catch a cold.
- Nervous tendency: Sensitive to pain.
- Flushing.
- Palpitations
- Weak gastrointestinal tract: Ephedra causes gastrointestinal symptoms.

2. Signs
   (i) Inspection: Physically poor nutrition, slimming, fair skin, easy to sweat, and moist skin.
   (ii) Tongue examination: Unremarkable.
   (iii) Pulse examination: It may be floating and weak.
   (iv) Abdominal examination:
   Abdominal strength: Soft to slightly soft (1/5 to 2/5)
   Abdominal manifestations
   Splashing sound (sometimes)
   Abdominal muscle tension (sometimes)
   Abdominal pulsations above umbilicus (sometimes)
3. Indications
   Indicated for the following symptoms in patients with deficiency pattern with sweating, cold limbs, stiff limbs, and occasional low urine output: arthralgia, neuralgia.

桂枝加苓朮附湯

Keishikaryoujutsubuto (KSTRJ) Guì zhī jiā líng shù fù tāng
Manifestation

1. Symptoms

- Neuralgia/arthralgia: The pain is relieved by warming in a bath. The pain gets gets worse in cold. The affected area is cold to the touch.
- Tendency to sweat.
- Cold.
- Tendency to catch a cold.
- Nervous tendency: Sensitive to pain.
- Flushing.
- Palpitations.
- Weak gastrointestinal tract: Ephedra causes gastrointestinal symptoms.

2. Signs
   (i) Inspection: poor nutrition, slimming, fair skin, easy to sweat, and moist skin.
   (ii) Tongue examination: Unremarkable
   (iii) Pulse examination: May be floating and weak.
   (iv) Abdominal examination: There is little literature.
   Abdominal strength: Unremarkable
3. Indications
   Indicated for the following symptoms in patients with deficiency pattern who have cold limbs and stiff limbs, low urine output, occasional palpitation, dizziness, and muscle cramps: arthralgia and neuralgia.

桂枝加竜骨牡蛎湯

Keishikaryukotsuboreito (KSTRB) Guì zhī jiā long gǔ mǔlì tāng

1. Symptoms

- Hair loss.
- Decreased libido, nocturnal emission.
- Flushing.
- Copious dandruff.
- Dizziness.
- Weak constitution: excitability and easy to fatigue.
- Insomnia: frequent dreams; patients can't sleep well due to unpleasant dreams.
- Easy to be surprised: palpitations, neurosis with palpitation as a subjective symptom.
- Enuresis, nocturnal emission.

2. Signs
   (i) Inspection: The body is not very sturdy. Some patients appear pale and lacking in energy.
   (ii) Tongue examination: The tongue body is unremarkable; the tongue coating may be moist.
   (iii) Pulse examination: Wide and large, but sometimes weak.
   (iv) Abdominal examination:
   Abdominal strength: Soft to slightly soft (1/5 to 2/5)
   Abdominal manifestations
   Occasional abdominal pulsations above umbilicus (usual)
   Muscle tension in lower abdomen (usual)
3. Indications
   Indicated for the following symptoms in patients with medium and deficiency pattern who are easily tired, nervous, and excitable: neurasthenia, insomnia, nocturnal crying in children, nocturnal enuresis, eye strain, and neurosis.

桂枝芍薬知母湯

Keishishakuyakuchimoto (KSCT) Guì zhī sháo yào zhī mǔ tāng
Manifestation

1. Symptoms

- Joint pain.
- Joint deformity: It is often used for thin patients with rheumatoid arthritis who are weakened, but it can also be used when patients who have no thinning of the lower limbs or no joint swelling are obese.
- Emaciation.
- Dizziness.

2. Signs
   (i) Inspection: Often accompanied by thinness and swelling in the knee joint. Dryness of skin may be observed.

(ii) Tongue examination: The tongue body is dry or slightly moist, and tongue coating may be lacking.
(iii) Pulse examination: May be floating, rapid, and slightly strong.
(iv) Abdominal examination:
There is little literature.
Abdominal strength: Unremarkable.

3. Indications
Indicated for the following symptoms in patients with deficiency pattern who have dry skin or chronic swelling of limbs or joints with pain: swelling: swelling and pain in joints, arthritis, and neuralgia.

桂枝湯

Keishito (KST) Guì zhī tāng
Manifestation
When used for chronic diseases, it is prescribed to patients with weak constitutions with floating and weak pulses.

1. Symptoms

- Aversion to cold, aversion to wind, fever; it is associated with the early stage of the common cold.
- When used for chronic diseases, it does not have to be accompanied by chills, a bad cold, or fever.
- Headache: It is caused by qi counter flow and may be accompanied by a rash.
- Perspiration: The target sign for use is sweat oozing out, but it can also be used in patients without sweat.
- Body pain.

2. Signs
(i) Inspection: Often has a weak body shape.
(ii) Tongue examination: tongue body is pink, and the tongue coating may be absent or slightly white.
(iii) Pulse examination: Often floating and weak.
(iv) Abdominal examination:
Abdominal strength
Acute: Unremarkable
Chronic: Soft to slightly soft (1/5 to 2/5)
Abdominal manifestation:
Occasional mild abdominal muscle tension (often)

3. Indications
Indicated for symptoms in patients with deficiency pattern with perspiration and common cold during the initial phase (Fig. 8.1).

桂枝人参湯

Keishininjinto (KNT) Guì zhī rén shēn tāng
Manifestation

1. Symptoms

- Headache: Headache and chronic headache associated with cold-like symptoms
- Fever, chills: Easy to merge at the time of cold
- Diarrhea: Watery diarrhea in the acute phase when exposed to cold
- Abdominal pain: Sometimes accompanied by severe abdominal pain
- Gastrointestinal weakness
- Feeling of fatigue in limbs
- Cold feet

2. Signs
(i) Inspection: Often the body appears weak.
(ii) Tongue examination: The tongue body is unremarkable, and tongue coating may be moist.
(iii) Pulse examination: Floating and weak, floating and loose, or weak.
(iv) Abdominal examination:
Abdominal strength: Soft to slightly soft (1/5 to 2/5)
Abdominal manifestations
Epigastric stuffiness and resistance (usual)
Abdominal pulsations (sometimes)

3. Indications
Indicated for the following symptoms in patients with deficiency pattern of digestive system and sometimes with fever and chills: Headache, palpitation, chronic gastroenteritis, gastrointestinal weakness, diarrhea, common cold, digestive symptoms (Fig. 8.2).

桂枝茯苓丸

Keishibukuryogan (KBG) Guì zhī fú líng wán
Manifestation

1. Symptoms

- Flushing: Red face
- Headache: Tension headache
- Stiff shoulders
- Dizziness
- Irregular menstruation, dysmenorrhea, infertility, uterine fibroids
- Cold feet

2. Signs
(i) Inspection: Often has a reddish face and a solid physique. The skin may be dark and rough.
(ii) Tongue examination: The tongue body is dark red or red tongue, and there may be distension of capillaries. Tongue coating is unremarkable.

(iii) Pulse examination: Pulse may be tense, deep, and slow.
(iv) Abdominal examination:
Abdominal strength: Slightly moderate (3/5 to 4/5)
Abdominal manifestations
Tenderness both in the paraumbilical region and lower abdomen

3. Indications
Indicated for the following symptoms in patients with excess pattern who have lower abdominal pain, shoulder stiffness, a dull headache, and a feeling of a hot head with cold feet: menstrual irregularity, dysmenorrhea, menstrual pain, climacteric disturbance, shoulder stiffness, dizziness, dull headache, bruise, frostbite, age spots, eczema, dermatitis, and acne (Fig. 8.2).

桂枝茯苓丸料加薏苡仁

Keishibukuroganryokayokuinin (KBGY) Guì zhī fú líng wán liào jiā yìyǐ rén
Manifestation

1. Symptoms

- Flushing: Red face
- Headache: Tension headache
- Stiff shoulders
- Dizziness
- Irregular menstruation, dysmenorrhea, infertility, uterine fibroids
- Cold feet
- Acne, age spots, rough hands

2. Signs
(i) Inspection: Often has a reddish face and a solid physique. The skin may be dark and rough.
(ii) Tongue examination: The tongue body is dark red or red tongue, and there may be distension of capillaries. Tongue coating is unremarkable.
(iii) Pulse examination: Pulse may be tense, sunken, and slow.
(iv) Abdominal examination:
Abdominal strength: Moderate or higher (3/5 to 4/5)
Abdominal manifestations

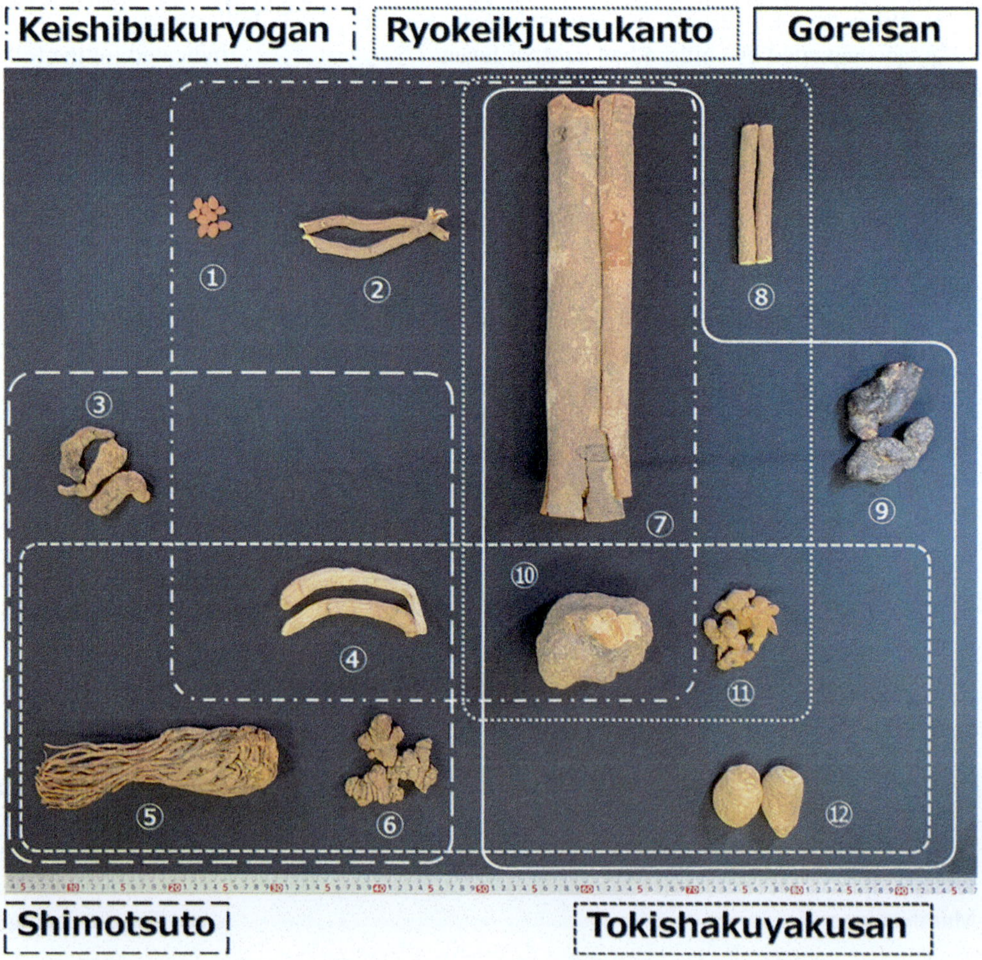

Fig. 8.2 Formulas related to blood[TM1] and fluid[TM1]There are formulas containing ③ Rehmannia Root, ⑤ Japanese Angelica Root, ④ Peony Root, etc. to improve blood[TM1] deficiency (blood[TM1] tonifying formulas), The formulas containing ⑥ Cnidium Rhizome, ① Peach Kernel, ② Moutan Bark, etc. eliminate blood[TM1] stagnation (blood[TM1] stasis resolving formula), and the formula containing Poria Sclerotium, Alisma Tuber, and ⑨ Polyporus Sclerotium eliminate fluid[TM1] retention (fluid[TM]-regulating formula). ⑦ Cinnamon Bark, ⑧ Glycyrrhiza, Atractylodes Rhizome

Tenderness both in the paraumbilical region and lower abdomen (usual)

3. Indications

Indicated for the following symptoms in patients with excess pattern who have lower abdominal pain, shoulder stiffness, a dull headache, and a feeling of hot flushes with cold feet: acne, age spots, rough skin on limbs (eczema and dermatitis on hands and feet), menstrual irregularity, and climacteric disturbance.

啓脾湯

Keihito (KHT) Qǐ pí tāng
Manifestation

1. Symptoms

- Anorexia
- General malaise
- Diarrhea: Chronic diarrhea without tenesmus (frequent defecation and occasionally awareness of heat sensation of the anus after tenesmus). Often diarrheal stool with a lot of foam that is discharged together with gas. Frequency is not so high at one to three times a day.
- Abdominal pain: Abdominal pain is usually mild but present.
- Vomiting: Occasionally accompanies other symptoms.
- Thirsty: May be accompanied by burning feelings in limbs, etc.

2. Signs
   (i) Inspection: Patients may be thin and have a pale complexion.
   (ii) Tongue examination: The tongue body is pale red, moist, and swollen. The tongue coating may be white and wet.
   (iii) Pulse examination: It may be deep and/or weak.
   (iv) Abdominal examination:
   Abdominal strength: Soft to slightly soft (1/5 to 2/5)
   Abdominal manifestations
   Mild abdominal pain (sometimes)
   Epigastric stuffiness and resistance (sometimes)

3. Indications

Indicated for the following symptoms in patients with deficiency pattern who are thin and tend to have diarrhea: weak digestive system, chronic gastroenteritis, dyspepsia, and diarrhea.

桂麻各半湯

Keimakakuhanto (KMK) Guì má gè bàn tāng
Manifestation

This is for an intermediate pattern between keishito and maoto and is used when coughing is protracted due to a prolonged cold.

1. Symptoms

- Headache: It is associated with the common cold, accompanied by neck stiffness.
- Chills: Chills accompany fever.
- Fever: Waves of heat often come repeatedly, but a feeling of heat is the main symptom.
- Sore throat.
- Cough: Prolonged coughing.
- Itching of the skin: Itching in skin with almost a rash.

2. Signs
   (i) Inspection: May have a reddish face.
   (ii) Tongue examination: The tongue body tends to be slightly dry, and tongue coating may be absent.
   (iii) Pulse examination: Often floating.
   (iv) Abdominal examination:
   There is little literature.
   Abdominal strength: Unremarkable.

3. Indications

Indicated for the following symptoms in patients with medium or slight deficiency pattern: colds, coughs, and itching.

香蘇散

Kososan (KOSS) Xiāng sū sǎn
Manifestation

1. Symptoms

- Cold: Elderly patients or when cold symptoms persist.
- Chronic headache, dull headache, feeling of wearing a hat: Often associated with depression.
- Chills: Often mild.
- Anxiety.
- Insomnia.
- Depression.
- Hysteria.
- Anorexia: There is a feeling of obstruction in the epigastric region.
- Abdominal pain: Accompanying a cold.
- Menstrual pain, irregular menstruation.

2. Signs
   (i) Inspection: Often nervous and appears unwell.
   (ii) Tongue examination: Sometimes a slightly white coating.
   (iii) Pulse examination: Deep and weak. In the case of cold symptoms, it is often floating and weak.

(iv) Abdominal examination:
Abdominal strength: Soft to slightly soft (1/5 to 2/5)
Abdominal manifestations
Epigastric stuffiness (usual)
Epigastric stuffiness and resistance (often)

3. Indications

Indicated for the following symptoms in nervous patients with a weak gastrointestinal tract in the early stage of a common cold or climacteric disturbance.

五積散

Goshakusan (GSS) Wǔ jī sǎn
Manifestation

1. Symptoms

- Abdominal pain: Chills and pain in the stomach
- Cold lower body: The upper body heats up and the lower body gets cold.
- Low back pain: Muscles feel tense from the low back to the thighs.
- Neuralgia: Sciatica and various neuralgias.
- Menstrual pain: Lower abdominal pain.
- Headache: Accompanied by flushing.

2. Signs

(i) Inspection: Sometimes pale complexion
(ii) Tongue examination: The tongue body may be between dry and wet, and the tongue coating may be wet and white.
(iii) Pulse examination: Sometimes floating and wiry or deep and slow.
(iv) Abdominal examination:
Abdominal strength: Soft to slightly soft (1/5 to 2/5)
Abdominal manifestations
Epigastric stuffiness and resistance (often)
Lower abdominal pain (sometimes)

3. Indications

Indicated for the following symptoms in patients with medium or slight deficiency pattern with cold body: Gastroenteritis, low back pain, neuralgia, arthralgia, myalgia, headache, climacteric disturbance, and common cold.

牛車腎気丸

Goshajinkigan (GJG) Niú chē shèn qì wán
Manifestation

1 Symptoms

In addition to the pattern of hachimijiyogan, it is used when edema and numbness are remarkable.

- Edema: It is used for swelling of limbs. It is also used for nephritis, nephrotic syndrome, and lymphedema.
- Numbness and pain: Used for peripheral neuropathy due to diabetes and anticancer drugs and numbness and pain of limbs (especially lower limbs) caused by spinal disorders.
- Cold: Cold limbs (especially legs).
- Dysuria, pollakiuria: Difficulty urinating; paradoxically, polyuria and pollakiuria may occur.
- Low back pain.

2 Signs

(i) Inspection: The limbs may be edematous.
(ii) Tongue examination: The tongue body may be moist, and the tongue coating may be white.
(iii) Pulse examination: Sometimes deep and deficient.
(iv) Abdominal examination:
Abdominal strength: Unremarkable
Abdominal manifestations
Weakness of the lower abdominal region (usual)
Abdominal muscle tension (lower abdomen)

3 Indications

Indicated for the following symptoms in patients with medium or deficiency excess pattern with a tendency of fatigue and feeling cold in the limbs, decrease in urine, edema, and occasional dry mouth: Leg pain, low back pain, numbness, blurred vision in old patients, pruritus, dysuria, frequent urination, edema, and symptoms accompanying hypertension (stiff shoulders, headache, and tinnitus).

呉茱萸湯

Goshuyuto (GSY) Wú zhū yú tāng
Manifestation

1. Symptoms

- Nausea and vomiting: Vomiting of saliva or gastric juices rather than food. Often associated with headaches
- Headache: Often used for severe headaches such as migraine
- ·Stiff shoulders
- Cold limbs
- Hiccups: Used for people who have a cold stomach
- Menstrual pain

2. Signs

(i) Inspection: Often has cold limbs.
(ii) Tongue examination: The tongue body is unremarkable, and the tongue coating may be white.
(iii) Pulse examination: sometimes deep or slow.

(iv) Abdominal examination:
Abdominal strength: Soft to slightly soft (1/5 to 2/5)
Abdominal manifestations
Splashing sound (often)
Feeling of fullness in epigastrium (often)
Epigastric stuffiness and resistance (often)
Agony (sometimes)

3. Indications

Indicated for the following symptoms in patients with medium or slight deficiency pattern who tended to have cold limbs, shoulder stiffness, and occasionally abdominal distention: headache and headaches associated with nausea, vomiting, and hiccups.

五淋散

Gorinsan (GS) Wǔ lín sǎn
Manifestation

1 Symptoms

- Frequent urination
- Pain with urination
- Feeling of residual urine
- Urinary turbidity: cloudy urine, hematuria, and pyuria
- Use Ryutanshakanto for those with excess pattern
- Use Seishinrensin'in for those who have poor heat generation and are prone to have septic cystitis with fatigue

2 Signs
(i) Inspection: Unremarkable
(ii) Tongue examination: The tongue body may be reddish, and the tongue coating may be slightly yellow.
(iii) Pulse examination: Deep and rapid.
(iv) Abdominal examination:
There is little literature.
【reference】
Abdominal strength: Medium (2.3/5).

3 Indications

Indicated for the following symptoms in patients with medium pattern: frequent urination, pain in urination, feeling of residual urine, and urinary turbidity.

五苓散

Goreisan (GRS) Wǔ líng sǎn
Manifestation

1 Symptoms

- Thirst, decreased urine volume: Feeling of heat, thirst, and desire to drink, but urine output is low in relation to the fluid intake.
- Edema
- Tendency to sweat
- Headache: It is suitable for both migraine and tension-type headaches. Headaches may have a tendency to get worse the day before rain.
- Counterflow of water-like vomiting: "Counterflow of water[TM1]" is a condition in which one wants to drink but immediately vomits. The nausea is not severe.
- Watery diarrhea
- It can be used even if all the symptoms are not present. Migraine does not have to be associated with dry mouth or decreased urine volume.

2 Signs
(i) Inspection: The face and limbs may often be edematous.
(ii) Tongue examination: The tongue body may have tooth marks, and tongue coating may be white.
(iii) Pulse examination: Floating and rapid.
(iv) Abdominal examination: Moderate abdominal strength (3/5)
Abdominal manifestations
Splashing sound (usual)
Epigastric stuffiness (often)
Abdominal pulsations (sometimes)

3 Indications

Indicated for the following symptoms in all patients regardless of their pattern who have oral dryness, decreased urine volume, dizziness, nausea, vomiting, stomachache, headache, and edema: watery diarrhea, acute gastrointestinal pain (do not use for gastrointestinal pain with tenesmus), heatstroke, headache, and hangover.

柴陥湯

Saikanto (SAK) Chái xiàn tāng
Manifestation

1 Symptoms

- Palpitations with chest pain.
- Discomfort from the epigastric region to the hypochondrium (fullness and discomfort in chest and hypochondrium)
- Anorexia

2 Signs
(i) Inspection: Unremarkable.
(ii) Tongue examination: The tongue body is unremarkable, and the tongue coating may be white or yellow.
(iii) Pulse examination: Wiry or slippery and rapid.
(iv) Abdominal examination:
Abdominal strength: Moderate (3/5)
Abdominal manifestations
Fullness and discomfort in chest and hypochondrium (usual)

Epigastric stuffiness and resistance (usual)
Chest pain (sometimes)
Chest oppression (sometimes)

3 Indications

Indicated for the following symptoms in patients with medium or slightly excess pattern who have occasional pain from the side of the abdomen to the epigastrium, bitterness in the mouth with anorexia, white tongue coating, strong coughing, difficulty in expectorating sputum, and occasional chest pain: coughing, chest pain, and bronchitis.

柴胡加竜骨牡蛎湯

Saikokaryukotsuboreito (SRB) Chái hú jiā long gǔ mǔlì tāng
Manifestation
The target of prescriptions containing dragon bones or oysters is thoraco-abdominal pulsations.

1. Symptoms

- Pulsations in the thoraco-abdominal region are the target for formulas containing dragon bones and oysters.
- Psychoneurological symptoms: irritability, anxiety, nervousness, agitation, insomnia, nightmares, confusion, etc.
- Palpitations/pulsations in the chest and abdomen
- Discomfort from the epigastric region to the hypochondrium (fullness and discomfort in chest and hypochondrium).
- Headache, heavy head, stiff shoulders
- Constipation: Some extracts contain rhubarb, and some do not. Use of these depends on the presence or absence of constipation.

* Symptoms are often exacerbated by stress.

2. Signs
   (i) Inspection: May be restless
   (ii) Tongue examination: Unremarkable
   (iii) Pulse examination: sometimes excess and tense.
   (iv) Abdominal examination: Abdominal strength: Moderate to slightly hard (3/5 to 4/5):
   Abdominal manifestations
   Abdominal pulsations, especially above the navel (usual)
   Fullness and discomfort in chest and hypochondrium (usual)
   Epigastric stuffiness and resistance (sometimes)
3. Indications

Indicated for the following symptoms in patients with medium or slightly excess patterns who have palpitations, insomnia, and constipation: Symptoms accompanying hypertension (palpitation, anxiety, and insomnia), neurosis, climacteric disorder, childhood nocturnal crying, and constipation.

柴胡桂枝乾姜湯

Saikokeishikankyoto (SAKK) Chái hú guì zhī gān jiāng tāng
Manifestation
Nausea, vomiting, and 胸脇苦満hypochondriac discomfort and distension

1. Symptoms

It is the most deficiency-prescription among the formulas involving Bupleuri radix. It is indicated for the same symptoms as saikokaryukotsuboreito but is used for those who are more deficient than saikokaryukotsuboreito. Symptoms are often exacerbated by stress.

- Psychoneurological symptoms: Nervousness, insomnia.
- Mild dissatisfaction from the epigastric region to the hypochondrium (fullness and discomfort in chest and hypochondrium).
- Sweating: Head sweating, night sweats.
- Alternating chills and fever: Fever and chills appear alternately.
- Hot flash: feel cold, but have a hot flash.
- Dry mouth.
- Palpitations in chest and abdomen, short of breath.

2. Signs
   (i) Inspection: In many cases, the complexion is not good.
   (ii) Tongue examination: Unremarkable.
   (iii) Pulse examination: Unremarkable.
   (iv) Abdominal examination:
   Abdominal strength: Soft to slightly soft (1/5 to 2/5)
   Abdominal manifestations
   Mild fullness and discomfort in chest and hypochondrium (usual)
   Abdominal pulsation (supra-umbilical) (usual)
   Epigastric stuffiness and resistance (sometimes)
3. Indications

Indicated for the following symptoms in patients with medium or slight deficiency pattern with oversensitivity to cold, slight anemia, nervousness, palpitation, shortness of breath, sometimes night sweat, head sweat, and thirst: climacteric disturbance, insomnia, neurosis, palpitation, shortness of breath, symptoms of late-stage common cold, and bronchitis.

柴胡桂枝湯

Saikokeishito (SAKT) Chái hú guì zhī tāng
Manifestation
It includes both the symptoms of the keishito pattern (fever, chills, sweating, headache) and the shosaikoto pattern

1. Symptoms

- Mild fever
- Coldness
- Headache
- Sweating
- Nausea and vomiting
- Stomachache
- Fullness and discomfort from the epigastric region to hypochondrium (fullness and discomfort in the chest and the hypochondrium).

2. Signs
 (i) Inspection: Unremarkable
 (ii) Tongue examination: Unremarkable
 (iii) Pulse examination: Often floating, wiry, and weak
 (iv) Abdominal examination:
  Abdominal strength: Slightly soft to moderate (2/5 to 3/5)
  Abdominal manifestations
  Abdominal muscle tension (usual)
  Epigastric stuffiness (often)
  Fullness and discomfort in chest and hypochondrium (often)
  Abdominal pain (upper abdomen) (often)
  Obstructive sensation in epigastrium
3. Indications
 Indicated for the following symptoms in patients with medium or slight deficiency pattern often accompanied by abdominal pain, occasional mild fever, rigors, headache, and nausea: gastroenteritis, middle and late stages of the common cold (Fig. 8.3).

柴胡清肝湯

Saikoseikanto (SSET) Chái hú qīng fèi tāng
Manifestation

1. Symptoms

- Swelling and sublingual swelling, pain: Chronic and recurrent lymphadenitis and tonsillitis (so-called adenopathy). Often used for children
- Insomnia, crying at night: Nervousness and irritability

2. Signs
 (i) Inspection: The skin may be dark.
 (ii) Tongue examination: Unremarkable.
 (iii) Pulse examination: Unremarkable.
 (iv) Abdominal examination:
  Abdominal strength: Slightly soft to moderate (2/5 to 3/5)
  Abdominal manifestations
  Bilateral rectus abdominis muscle tension (usual)
  Fullness and discomfort in chest and hypochondrium (usual)
  Abnormal hypersensitivity (ticklishness) of the abdominal wall (sometimes)
3. Indications
 Indicated for the following symptoms in patients with medium patterns who tend to be irritable: neurosis, chronic tonsillitis, and eczema. Also for improving the constitution of children.

柴朴湯

Saibokuto (SBT) Chái pǔ tāng
Manifestation

1. Symptoms
 It includes both the symptoms of Shosaikoto (such as hypochondrium discomfort) and Hangekobokuto (such as laryngopharyngeal hypersensitivity).

- Subjective symptoms
- Psychiatric symptoms: Anxiety, depression
- Foreign body sensation and obstruction in the throat and esophagus (feeling of pharyngeal obstruction)
- Wheezing, coughing
- Palpitations, dizziness
- Anorexia, nausea
- Mild discomfort from the epigastric region to the hypochondrium (fullness and discomfort in chest and hypochondrium).

2. Signs
 (i) Inspection: Unremarkable.
 (ii) Tongue examination: The tongue body is pink, and the tongue coating is often thin white moss.
 (iii) Pulse examination: Wiry, often a little rapid.
 (iv) Abdominal examination:
  Abdominal strength: Moderate (3/5)
  Abdominal manifestations
  Fullness and discomfort in chest and hypochondrium (usual)
  Epigastric stuffiness and resistance (often)
  Feeling of fullness in epigastrium (sometimes)

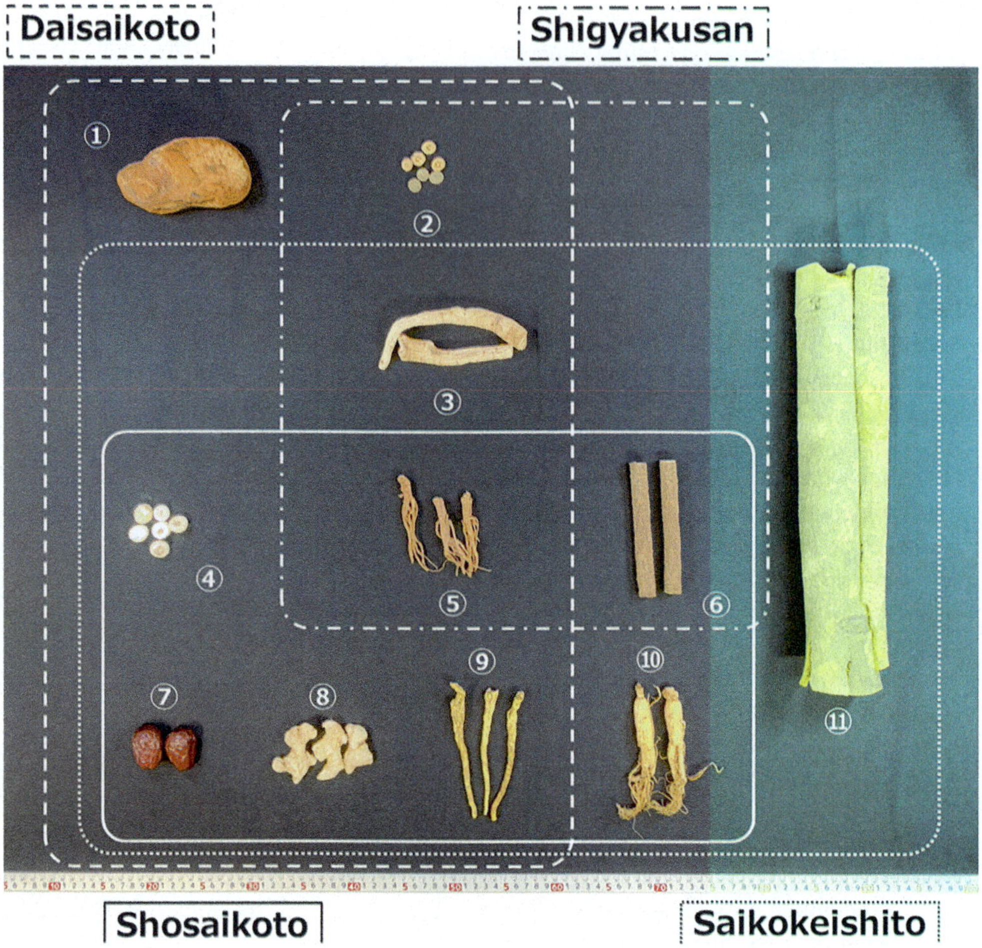

Fig. 8.3 Formulas containing Bupleurum RootDuring the late yang stage pattern, harmonizing formulas containing ⑤ Bupleurum root, and ⑨ Scutellaria root are used to harmonize pathogenic qi that has invaded half-exterior and half-interior in the body. Bupleurum Root is also prescribed in the formulas to eliminate qi stagnation① Rhubarb, ② Immature Orange, ③ Peony Root, ④ Pinellia Tuber, ⑥ Glycyrrhiza, ⑦ Jujube, ⑧ Ginger, Ginseng, Cinnamon Bark

3. Indications

   Indicated for the following symptoms in patients with medium pattern who have depressed feelings, a feeling of a foreign body in the throat and esophagus, a tendency to catch cold, and sometimes have palpitations, dizziness, nausea, etc.: Infantile asthma, bronchial asthma, bronchitis, coughing, anxiety neurosis, and weak constitution.

柴苓湯

Saireito (SRT) Chái líng tāng

Manifestation

It includes both the symptoms of shosaikoto (hypochondriac discomfort and distension, etc.) and goreisan (dry mouth, decreased urine, swelling, etc.).

1. Symptoms

   - Thirst
   - Reduced urine
   - Swelling feeling
   - Nausea and vomiting
   - Anorexia
   - Diarrhea
   - Stomachache
   - Dizziness
   - Mild fever
   - Mild discomfort from the epigastric region to the hypochondrium (fullness and discomfort in chest and hypochondrium).

2. Signs

   (i) Inspection: Unremarkable.

   (ii) Tongue examination: The tongue body is often pink, and the tongue is often covered with thin white moss.

   (iii) Pulse examination: Wiry, slightly floating, often rapid.

   (iv) Abdominal examination: Moderate abdominal strength (3/5)

   Abdominal manifestations

   Fullness and discomfort in chest and hypochondrium (usual)

   Occasional splashing sound (often)

   Epigastric stuffiness and resistance (sometimes)

   Abdominal muscle tension (sometimes)

Abdominal pain (sometimes)

3. Indications

Indicated for following symptoms in patients with medium pattern who have thirst, oliguria sometimes accompanied by anorexia and edema: watery diarrhea, acute gastroenteritis, sunstroke, and edema.

三黄瀉心湯

san'oshashinto (SOST) Sān huáng xiè xīn tāng
Manifestation

1. Symptoms

- Psychoneurological symptoms: Irritability, anxiety, insomnia, mood instability.
- Noboru, stiff shoulders, heavy tinnitus.
- Bleeding: Epistaxis (throat), hematemesis, melena, hemoptysis, hemoptysis, cerebral bleeding, hemoptysis, uterine bleeding, etc. When one is surprised or anxious when bleeding, one's mood can be calmed and bleeding stopped.
- Constipation.

2. Signs
   (i) Inspection: The face is often flushed.
   (ii) Tongue examination: The tongue body is often crimson. Tongue coating may be dry, white, or yellow.
   (iii) Pulse examination: Often large or buoyant.
   (iv) Abdominal examination:
   Abdominal strength: Moderate to slightly hard (3/5 to 4/5)
   Abdominal manifestations
   Epigastric stuffiness and resistance (usual)
3. Indications

Indicated for the following symptoms in patients with medium or excess pattern who have a slight feeling of flushing and have facial flushes, mental instability, epigastric stuffiness, and a tendency to be constipated: symptoms associated with hypertension (flushing, shoulder stiffness, tinnitus, dull headache, insomnia, and anxiety), nose bleeding, hemorrhoidal bleeding, constipation, and climacteric disturbance.

酸棗仁湯

Sansoninto (SSNT) Suān zǎo rén tāng
Manifestation
It is widely used for insomnia even if all the symptoms indicated for the condition are not present, but those who are presumed to have a deficiency pattern.

1. Symptoms

- Drowsiness
- Lethargy
- Many dreams
- Psychoneurological symptoms: Anxiety, neurasthenia, irritability, and easy to be startled
- Night sweats

2. Signs
   (i) Inspection: The face may be pale.
   (ii) Tongue examination: The tongue body is unremarkable, the tongue is moist, and often there is no coating.
   (iii) Pulse examination: Often deep, or deep and narrow, or deep and deficient, or deficient and rapid.
   (iv) Abdominal examination:
   Abdominal strength: Soft to slightly soft (1/5 to 2/5)
   Abdominal manifestations
   Fullness and discomfort in the chest (often)
3. Indications

Indicated for the following symptoms in patients with medium or slight deficiency pattern who suffer from physical and mental fatigue and weakness, anxiety, and inability to sleep well: insomnia and neurosis.

三物黄芩湯

Sammotsuogonto (SOT) Sān wù huáng qín tāng
Manifestation

1. Symptoms

- Hot limbs (oppressively hot): It makes you want to get your feet out of the futon (not limited to puerperal fever).
- Redness, heat, dryness, and pustules of palms and foot kicks.
- Anxiety.
- Insomnia.
- Palpitations.
- Thirst or dry mouth.
- Headache: May be present.

2. Signs
   (i) Inspection: The lips may be dry.
   (ii) Tongue examination: The tongue body is unremarkable, and the tongue coating may be white and slightly dry.
   (iii) Pulse examination: Unremarkable.

(iv) Abdominal examination:
No specific abdominal manifestations are reported.
Abdominal strength: Slightly soft (2/5)
3. Indications
Indicated for the following symptoms in patients with medium or slight deficiency pattern who have hot flushes in the limbs: Eczema, dermatitis, rough hands and feet (eczema/dermatitis on the hands and feet) and insomnia.

滋陰降火湯

Jiinkokato (JKT) Zī yīn jiàng huǒ tāng
Manifestation

1. Symptoms

- Cough: Dry and intermittent; tendency to cough especially at night when warmed with a heater or quilt. Not violent enough to vomit. Mostly subacute and chronic.
- Sputum: No sputum, or sputum that is viscous and stringy.
- Dry skin.
- Xerostomia: A feeling of dryness in the oral cavity and throat.
- Mild fever.

2. Signs
(i) Inspection: Often lean. The skin may be dry and dark. The mouth may be dry.
(ii) Tongue examination: The tongue body is unremarkable, and the tongue coating is often dry and slightly white.
(iii) Pulse examination: Rapid and may be weak.
(iv) Abdominal examination:
No specific abdominal manifestations are reported.
Abdominal strength: Slightly soft (2/5).
3. Indications
Indicated for the following symptoms in patients with deficiency pattern who have dry mouth and throat, cough up sticky sputum, have dry and dark skin, and are often constipated: bronchitis and cough.

滋陰至宝湯

Jiinshihoto (JST) Zī yīn zhì bǎo tāng
Manifestation

1. Symptoms

- Cough: Chronic and relatively severe.
- Sputum: Often viscous and difficult to expectorate.
- Mild fever.
- Dry mouth, dry throat.
- Night sweats: Elderly people may have night sweats and insomnia.
- Malaise.
- Anorexia.
- Hot palms and limbs.

2. Signs
(i) Inspection: Often thin.
(ii) Tongue examination: The tongue body is often crimson. Tongue coating is absent or slightly white and dry.
(iii) Pulse examination: Often thready and rapid, or wiry and thready.
(iv) Abdominal examination:
Abdominal strength: Slightly soft to moderate (2/5 to 3/5)
Abdominal manifestations
Mild hypochondriac discomfort and distension (often)
3. Indications
Indicated for the following symptoms in patients with deficiency pattern: chronic coughing and bronchitis.

紫雲膏

Shiunko (SK) Zǐ yún gāo
Manifestation

1. Symptoms

- Dry skin, rough skin, pain: Trauma, burns. Not suitable for moist skin with many exudates, but not limited to use on dry skin
- Pain associated with hemorrhoids and anal lacerations

2. Signs
(i) Inspection: Unremarkable
(ii) Tongue examination: Unremarkable
(iii) Pulse examination: Unremarkable
(iv) Abdominal examination:
No literature.
3. Indications
Indicated for skin cracks, chapped skin, chilblains, clavus (corn), prickly heat (heat rash), skin erosion, trauma, burns, pain associated with hemorrhoids, anal lacerations, and eczema/dermatitis.

四逆散

Shigyakusan (SGS) Sì nì sǎn
Manifestation

1. Symptoms

- Discomfort from the epigastric region to the hypochondrium (fullness and discomfort in chest and hypochondrium).
- Stomachache.

- Diarrhea: Diarrhea of Yang pattern, which has a strong odor and makes the anus feel hot after defecation (tenesmus), or abdominal pain without bowel movement. Often "diarrhea with a griping pain."
- Psychoneurological symptoms: Anxiety, depression, insomnia, etc.
- Cold limbs.
- Cough.
- Palpitations.

2. Signs
   (i) Inspection: Often has a whitish face. The expression may be dark.
   (ii) Tongue examination: The tongue body is unremarkable, tongue coating is white, and it is often slightly dry.
   (iii) Pulse examination: Often tight and wiry.
   (iv) Abdominal examination:
   Abdominal strength: Moderate (3/5)
   Abdominal manifestations
   Abdominal muscle tension (usual)
   Fullness and discomfort in chest and hypochondrium (usual)
   Epigastric stuffiness and resistance (often)
   Abdominal pain (sometimes)
3. Indications
   Indicated for the following symptoms in patients with medium or excess pattern who have discomfort from the epigastric region to the hypochondrium, often accompanying anxiety and insomnia: gastritis, abdominal pain, and neurosis (Fig. 8.3).

四君子湯

Shikunshito (SKST) Sì jūn zǐ tāng
Manifestation

1. Symptoms

- Anorexia: One can eat, but one doesn't have an appetite.
- Stomach discomfort and bloating: Bloating tends to occur especially after eating, and drowsiness is likely.
- Nausea and vomiting.
- Abdominal sounds.
- Diarrhea: Lots of loose stools and almost no abdominal pain.
- General malaise, limb malaise.
- Easy to catch a cold.

2. Signs
   (i) Inspection: Often thin and a pale complexion. Anemic and often dullness in eyes
   (ii) Tongue examination: The tongue body is unremarkable, and tongue coating is often absent or a moist, slightly white coating.
   (iii) Pulse examination: Often deep, thread, and weak
   (iv) Abdominal examination:
   Abdominal strength: Soft to slightly soft (1/5 to 2/5)
   Abdominal manifestations
   Splashing sound (usual)
   Borborygmus (often)
   Epigastric stuffiness (sometimes)
   Feeling of fullness in epigastrium (sometimes)
3. Indications
   Indicated for the following symptoms in patients with deficiency pattern who are thin and easily fatigued and have bad complexion and anorexia: Weak digestive system, chronic gastritis, heaviness in stomach, vomiting, and diarrhea.

梔子柏皮湯

Shishihakuhito (SSHK) Zhī zi bǎi pí tāng
Manifestation

1. Symptoms
   - Jaundice: There may or may not feel heat and there is no nausea, vomiting, abdominal distention, or lateral chest discomfort, but there is an annoying feeling (heart trouble) in the chest. Sometimes there is itching, redness, or melanin deposits (discoloration) in skin. Jaundice is milder than Kyosatsukoto pattern.
2. Signs
   (i) Inspection: Jaundice may be visible.
   (ii) Tongue examination: Unremarkable
   (iii) Pulse examination: Unremarkable
   (iv) Abdominal examination:
   There is little literature.
   [Reference] Abdominal strength: Unremarkable
   Typically no fullness (negative findings)
3. Indications
   Indicated for the following symptoms in patients with medium pattern who sometimes feel heat and itching: Itchy skin and bloodshot eyes.

七物降下湯

Shichimotsukokato (SCMKT) Qī wù xiáng xià tāng
Manifestation

1. Symptoms

- Stomach, stiff shoulders, dull headache, dizziness: Symptoms associated with hypertension
- Tinnitus

- Easy fatigue
- Coldness

2. Signs
   (i) Inspection: Often thin build and anemic. The skin is often dry.
   (ii) Tongue examination: The tongue body is pale pink, and the tongue coating is often absent.
   (iii) Pulse examination: Often deep, thread, and unsmooth.
   (iv) Abdominal examination:
   There is little literature.
   【reference】
   Moderate or less abdominal strength (1/5 to 3 5).
3. Indications
   Indicated for the following symptoms in patients with medium or deficiency pattern who have a bad complexion, are easily fatigued, and do not have digestive disturbance: symptoms associated with hypertension (hot flashes, stiff shoulders, dull headache, and dizziness).

四物湯

Shimotsuto (SMT) Sì wù tāng
Manifestation

1. Symptoms

- Dry skin diseases, spots
- Cold sensitivity, cold limbs, chilblains
- Menstrual disorders: Dysmenorrhea, irregular menstruation, menorrhagia, etc.
- Infertility, pre- and postnatal fatigue.
- Insomnia
- Menstruation-related symptoms: Psychoneurological and physical symptoms such as anxiety and irritability that appear with changes in female hormones such as menstruation, pregnancy, childbirth, postpartum, and menopause.

2. Signs
   (i) Inspection: Moderate to slightly weak. Anemic complexion, dry skin, and dry mucous membranes.
   (ii) Tongue examination: Tongue body is pink and often dry, and the tongue coating is scanty.
   (iii) Pulse examination: Often tight and irregular or deep and weak.
   (iv) Abdominal examination: Abdominal strength: Soft to slightly soft (1/5 to 2/5)
   Abdominal manifestations
   Pulsations in supra-umbilical region (usual)
3. Indications
   Indicated for the following symptoms in patients with deficient constitution who have cold sensitivity, dry skin, and a bad complexion without gastrointestinal disorder: irregular menstruation, dysmenorrhea, climacteric disturbance, menstruation-related symptoms, hypersensitivity to cold, chilblains, spots, anemia, and recovery from fatigue in pre/postpartum (Fig. 8.2).

炙甘草湯

Shakanzoto (SKZT) Zhì gān cǎo tāng
Manifestation

1. Symptoms

- Palpitations, shortness of breath: There may be no irregular pulse. There is a slight tendency toward neurosis and hypochondriasis.
- Unpleasant burning sensation in limbs (oppressively hot).
- Dry mouth.
- Skin dryness.
- Stool is hard and there is a tendency of constipation.
- Fatigue.

2. Signs
   (i) Inspection: The nutritional status may be slightly compromised; the skin may be dry.
   (ii) Tongue examination: Unremarkable.
   (iii) Pulse examination: May be irregular.
   (iv) Abdominal examination:
   Abdominal strength: Soft to slightly soft (1/5 to 2/5)
   Abdominal pulsations (usual)
3. Indications
   Indicated for the following symptoms in patients with deficiency pattern who are easily fatigued and who sometimes feel heat in the limbs: palpitation, shortness of breath, and irregular pulse.

芍薬甘草湯

Shakuyakukanzoto (SKT) Sháo yào gān cǎo tāng
Manifestation

1. Symptoms

- Skeletal muscle spasms and pain: Severe muscle spasms of limbs, abdomen, lower back, etc.
- Smooth muscle spasms and pain: Gastrointestinal tract, gallbladder, bronchi, urinary tract. It can also manifest as menstrual pain, hiccups, etc.
- Children's night crying, infant's vomiting.

2. Signs
   (i) Inspection: Unremarkable
   (ii) Tongue examination: Unremarkable
   (iii) Pulse examination: Sometimes tight due to pain
   (iv) Abdominal examination:
   Moderate abdominal strength: Any strength is appropriate.
   Abdominal manifestations.
   Abdominal muscle tension (often).
3. Indications
   Indicated for the following symptoms in patients without regard to physical strength who have a pain accompanied by sudden muscle spasm: cramps, muscle spasms, abdominal pain, and lumbago.

芍薬甘草附子湯

Shakuyakukanzobushito (SKB) Sháo yào gān cǎo fùzǐ tāng
Manifestation

1. Symptoms
   For those who have chills and cold sensations in addition to the pattern of shakuyakukanzo-to

   - Skeletal muscle spasms and pain: Severe muscle spasms of limbs, abdomen, lower back, etc.
   - Smooth muscle spasms and pain: Gastrointestinal tract, gallbladder, bronchi, and urinary tract pain caused by smooth muscle spasms. It also applies to menstrual pain, hiccups, etc.

2. Signs
   (i) Inspection: Unremarkable
   (ii) Tongue examination: Unremarkable
   (iii) Pulse examination: It may be tight due to pain.
   (iv) Abdominal examination:

   - There is little literature.
   - [Reference].
   - Moderate or less abdominal strength (1/5 to 3/5).
   - Abdominal manifestations.
   - Abdominal muscle tension.

3. Indications
   Indicated for the following symptoms in patients with medium or slight deficiency pattern who have cold sensation: cramps, muscle spasms, abdominal pain, lumbago, and neuralgia.

十全大補湯

Juzentaihoto (JTT) Shí quán dà bǔ tāng
Manifestation

1. Symptoms

   - Fatigue: Used to improve general condition, but especially to improve physical strength associated with malignant tumors and collagen disease constitutions. It's not used, however, for the active phase of disease or those with high fever.
   - Anorexia: Nevertheless, use with caution for those with extremely weak gastrointestinal tract from vomiting, diarrhea, etc., as it may cause gastrointestinal disorders.
   - Cold limbs.
   - Night sweats.

2. Signs
   (i) Inspection: Thin type, often with poor complexion and dry skin. May be accompanied by erosion of skin and mucous membranes.
   (ii) Tongue examination: The tongue body tends to be dry and may have tooth marks. Tongue coating may be slightly white coating.
   (iii) Pulse examination: Often deep and deficient.
   (iv) Abdominal examination:
   No specific abdominal manifestations are reported.
   Abdominal strength: Soft to slightly soft (1/5 to 2/5).
3. Indications
   Indicated the following symptoms in patients with weakness and deficiency pattern: loss of physical strength after a disease or operation, fatigue, anorexia, night sweats, cold limbs, and anemia.
   Precautions for use
   Pay attention to pseudoaldosteronism and myopathy as serious side effects.

十味敗毒湯

Jumihaidokuto (JHT) Shí wèi bài dú tāng
Manifestation

1. Symptoms
   - Rash: Inflammatory reactions such as redness and swelling, heat sensation, pain, and itching are often obvious. Use within a few days of onset in cases of carbuncle and furuncle.
2. Signs
   (i) Inspection: Abnormalities such as skin suppuration and eczema are often found. Often no dryness is seen.
   (ii) Tongue examination: The tongue body may be pink, and tongue coating may be dry and white.
   (iii) Pulse examination: sometimes floating and excess, or floating and tight.

(iv) Abdominal examination:
Moderate abdominal strength: Moderate or stronger (3/5 to 5/5)
Abdominal manifestations
Fullness and discomfort in chest and hypochondrium (usual)
Epigastric stuffiness and resistance (sometimes)

3. Indications

Indicated for the following symptoms in patients with medium pattern who have skin disease with reddening that is sometimes suppurative: symptoms in the early stage of suppurative dermatosis or acute dermatosis, urticaria, acute eczema, and tinea pedis.

潤腸湯

Junchoto (JCT) Rùn cháng tāng
Manifestation

1. Symptoms
   - Habitual constipation: It is a drug supplying fluid[TM1] and is used for flaccid constipation and spasmodic habitual constipation caused by lack of mucus in the large intestine. Also recommended for use when other drugs are not effective. Side effects and habituation are unlikely to occur even after long-term continuous use.
2. Signs
   (i) Inspection: Skin may be dry.
   (ii) Tongue examination: The tongue body is crimson and dry, and often there is little tongue coating.
   (iii) Pulse examination: sometimes rapid.
   (iv) Abdominal examination:
   No specific abdominal manifestations are reported.
   Slightly soft abdomen (1/5 to 2/5)
   Abdominal manifestations
   Tactile stool mass (often)
3. Indications

Indicated for the following symptoms in patients with medium or slight deficiency pattern who sometimes have dry skin: constipation.

小建中湯

Shokenchuto (SHKT) Xiǎo jiàn zhōng tāng
Manifestation

1. Symptoms
   - Easy fatigue/frail constitution: Also applied to improve the constitution of frail children, spinal caries, arthritis, hair loss, gastritis, hepatitis, bronchial asthma, stuttering, etc.
   - Stomach ache
   - Palpitations
   - Hot limbs
   - Cold sensitivity
   - Frequent urination, polyuria
   - Dry mouth
   - Nocturnal emission
2. Signs
   (i) Inspection: Frequently pale complexion.
   (ii) Tongue examination: Tongue body is normal to pink. Tongue coating is slightly white coating.
   (iii) Pulse examination: Generally tight, sometimes weak and wiry, but sometimes floating and weak with fever. It is not constant.
   (iv) Abdominal examination:
   Abdominal strength: Soft to slightly soft (1/5 to 2/5)
   Abdominal manifestations
   Abdominal muscle tension (usual)
   Abdominal pain (often)
   Supra-umbilical pulsations ("Shinju palpitation")
3. Indications

Indicated for the following symptoms in patients with deficiency pattern who are easily fatigued, with abdominal pain, poor complexion, sometimes accompanied by palpitation, hot flushes of the limbs, coldness, night sweating, nasal bleeding, pollakiuria, or polyuria: Delicate constitution in childhood, fatigue and malaise, nervousness, chronic gastroenteritis, nocturnal enuresis in children, and night crying.

小柴胡湯

Shosaikoto (SSK) Xiǎo chái hú tāng
Manifestation

1. Symptoms
   - Alternating chills and fever: A fever which is generated when chills stop, and then chills occur again. This is a fever type of late Yang stage.
   - Digestive symptoms: Mouth is bitter/sticky. Anorexia, nausea/vomiting, and a feeling of pressure and discomfort from the epigastic region to the hypochondrium.
   - Also discomfort in chest, dry throat, palpitations, dry mouth, abdominal pain, palpitations in epicardium, urinary inconvenience, mild fever, cough, stiff neck, and vexing heat in the palms and soles.
2. Signs
   (i) Inspection: Unremarkable.
   (ii) Tongue examination: The tongue body is strongly reddish, and the tongue coating is often dry and white or whitish yellow.
   (iii) Pulse examination: Often wiry.

(iv) Abdominal examination:
Abdominal strength: Moderate (3/5)
Abdominal manifestations
Fullness and discomfort in chest and hypochondrium (usual)
Epigastric stuffiness and resistance (often)
Abdominal muscle tension (sometimes)

3. Indications
Indicated for the following symptoms in patients with medium pattern who sometimes feel bilateral fullness and discomfort from abdomen to epigastrium, anorexia, bitterness in mouth, and have white moss on tongue: anorexia, nausea, gastritis, stomachache, chronic gastrointestinal disorder, fatigue, and symptoms accompanying the late stage of a cold.

小柴胡湯加桔梗石膏

Shosaikotokakikyosekko (SSKKS) Xiǎo chái hú jiā jié gěng shí gāo
Manifestation

1. Symptoms

- Alternating chills and fever: A fever which is generated when chills stop, and then chills occur again. This is a fever type of late Yang stage.
- Digestive symptoms: Mouth is bitter/sticky. Anorexia, nausea/vomiting, and feeling of pressure and discomfort from the epigastric region to the hypochondrium.
- Also discomfort in chest, dry throat, palpitations, dry mouth, abdominal pain, palpitations in epicardium, urinary inconvenience, mild fever, cough, stiff neck, and heat in limbs.
- The Sho-saiko-to kakikyo-gypsum pattern often exhibits stronger thirst and inflammation of the tonsils and throat (exhaustion, pus, etc.).

2. Signs
(i) Inspection: Unremarkable.
(ii) Tongue examination: The tongue body is strongly reddish, and the tongue coating is often dry and white or whitish yellow.
(iii) Pulse examination: Often wiry.
(iv) Abdominal examination:
Abdominal strength: Moderate (3/5)
Abdominal manifestations
Fullness and discomfort in chest and hypochondrium (usual)
Epigastric stuffiness and resistance (often)
Abdominal muscle tension (sometimes)

3. Indications
Indicated for the following symptoms in patients with excess pattern who sometimes feel bilateral fullness and discomfort from abdomen to epigastrium, anorexia, bitterness in the mouth, and have white moss on the tongue as well as a painful swollen throat: sore throat, tonsillitis, and peritonsillitis.

小青竜湯

Shoseiryuto (SST) Xiǎo qīng lóng tāng
Manifestation

1. Symptoms

- Fever
- Cough: Often accompanied by thin and copious saliva-like expectoration and wheezing
- Watery nasal discharge
- Edema
- Reduced urine volume

2. Signs
(i) Inspection: Unremarkable.
(ii) Tongue examination: The tongue body is unremarkable, and the tongue coating may be moist and white.
(iii) Pulse examination: Often floating and weak or floating, weak, and rapid.
(iv) Abdominal examination: Soft to slightly soft (1/5 to 2/5):
Abdominal manifestations
Splashing sound (usual)
Muscle tension in upper abdomen (sometimes)

3. Indications
Indicated for the following symptoms in patients with medium or slight deficiency pattern, who have cough and nasal discharge accompanied by watery sputum: Bronchitis, bronchial asthma, rhinitis, allergic rhinitis, edema, cold, and pollinosis (Fig. 8.1).

小半夏加茯苓湯

Shohangekabukuryoto (SHB) Xiǎo bàn xià jiā fú líng tāng
Manifestation

1. Symptoms

- Nausea and vomiting: Consider Goreisan in cases with severe dry mouth.
- Dizziness
- Motion sickness
- Palpitations
- Reduced urine volume

2. Signs
(i) Inspection: Unremarkable

(ii) Tongue examination: The tongue body is unremarkable. Tongue coating is moist and may be thick and white.
(iii) Pulse examination: It may be deep and weak.
(iv) Abdominal examination:
Abdominal strength: Soft to slightly soft (1/5 to 2/5)
Abdominal manifestations
Splashing sound (usual)
Epigastric stuffiness and resistance (sometimes)

3. Indications

Indicated for the following symptoms in patients of any pattern who have nausea and sometimes vomiting: Hyperemesis gravidarum (morning sickness) and vomiting, nausea, and gastritis.

消風散

Shofusan (SFS) Xiāo fēng sǎn
Manifestation

1. Symptoms
   - Eczema: Stubborn eczema with redness and swelling, a lot of exudate and moistening, forming crust, complaints of severe pruritus, and dry mouth. Symptoms often worsen in summer.
2. Signs

(i) Inspection: Unremarkable.
(ii) Tongue examination: The tongue body is crimson, and tongue coating is often slightly yellow.
(iii) Pulse examination: Floating and strong.
(iv) Abdominal examination:
No specific abdominal manifestations are reported.
Moderate abdominal strength: Moderate or higher (3/5 to 5/5).

3. Indications

Indicated for the following symptoms in patients with medium or excess pattern who have a skin disease with severe itching and exudation, and who sometimes feel heat in the affected parts: eczema, dermatitis, urticaria, athlete's foot, and heat rash.

升麻葛根湯

Shomakakkonto (SMKT) Shēng má gé gēn tāng
Manifestation

1. Symptoms

- Headache
- Fever
- Muscle pain
- Joint pain
- Rash

2. Signs

(i) Inspection: May present in anguish. A rash may be observed.
(ii) Tongue examination: Tongue body is crimson. Tongue coating is moist and sometimes light white.
(iii) Pulse examination: Sometimes floating and rapid.
(iv) Abdominal examination:
There is little literature.
【reference】.
Moderate abdominal strength: (3/5)

3. Indications

Indicated for the following symptoms in patients with medium pattern who have headache, fever, chills, etc: common cold during the initial phase, eczema, and dermatitis.

四苓湯

Shireito (SHRT) Sì líng tāng
Manifestation

1. Symptoms

- Epigastric stuffiness
- Feeling of heaviness in body
- Indigestion
- Diarrhea

2. Signs

(i) Inspection: The face may lack expression.
(ii) Tongue examination: The tongue body is unremarkable; tongue coating may be white or greasy white.
(iii) Pulse examination: May be slippery.
(iv) Abdominal examination:
No literature

3. Indications

Indicated for the following symptoms in patients with any pattern of thirst, decreased urine output despite water intake, nausea, vomiting, abdominal pain, edema, etc.: illness caused by the summerheat, acute gastroenteritis, and edema.

辛夷清肺湯

shin'iseihaito (SSHT) Xīn yí qīng fèi tāng
Manifestation

1. Symptoms

- Purulent nasal discharge: Colored and viscous nasal discharge. When the amount is large, post-nasal drip occurs, causing discomfort in the pharynx and wheezing.

- Nasal congestion: When inflammation worsens, pain, heat sensation, and decrease or loss of smell occur. Mouth breathing causes dry mouth.

2. Signs
   (i) Inspection: Mild swelling of the face and redness of the forehead and cheeks may be observed.
   (ii) Tongue examination: Tongue body is crimson; tongue coating is dry and white to yellow.
   (iii) Pulse examination: Sometimes floating, surging, thin, and rapid.
   (iv) Abdominal examination:
   No specific abdominal manifestations reported
   Abdominal strength: Moderate (3/5)
3. Indications
   Indicated for the following symptoms in patients with medium or excess pattern who have thick nasal discharge, occasional heat sensation: nasal obstruction, chronic rhinitis, and empyema.

参蘇飲

Jinsoin (JSI) Cān sū yǐn
Manifestation

1. Symptoms

- It is used at the beginning of a cold or when it is a little prolonged.
- Fever.
- Headache.
- Sputum: Often purulent.
- Epigastric stuffiness.
- Anorexia.
- Nausea and vomiting.
- Depression.

2. Signs
   (i) Inspection: A depressed facial expression may be observed. The face may be mildly flushed.
   (ii) Tongue examination: Tongue body tends to be unremarkable; tongue coating may be greasy white.
   (iii) Pulse examination: Sometimes floating and weak or floating and soft.
   (iv) Abdominal examination:
   Slightly soft to moderate abdominal strength (2/5 to 3/5)
   Abdominal manifestations
   Feeling of fullness in epigastrium (often)
   Epigastric stuffiness and resistance (often)
3. Indications
   Indicated for the following symptoms in patients with deficiency pattern who have gastrointestinal weakness: common cold and cough.

神秘湯

Shimpito (SPT) Shén mì tāng
Manifestation

1. Symptoms uptight

- Cough, wheezing, shortness of breath: Although there is little sputum, coughing is relatively severe and tends to be prolonged. It is also used to treat asthma attacks as well as prevent attacks.
- Depressive mood or anxiety: Often there are neuropsychiatric symptoms such as depression and anxiety. Disposition may be nervous, and there is a tendency to get tense.
- Rhinitis symptoms: Effective for nasal congestion. Amount of nasal discharge is not very great.
- Feeling of fullness and discomfort in chest: There is often a feeling of heat associated with coughing and wheezing. In addition, one may notice a discomfort like something is stuck in the chest.
- Epigastric stuffiness and oppression in the right flank region.

2. Signs
   (i) Inspection: The complexion is often poor, but the face may be reddish. Tendency of depression, anxiety, and nervousness.
   (ii) Tongue examination: Tongue body is pink, without swelling or tooth marks. Tongue coating is often dry and white.
   (iii) Pulse examination: Floating; often wiry.
   (iv) Abdominal examination:
   Abdominal strength: Slightly soft to moderate (2/5 to 3/5)
   Abdominal manifestations
   mild hypochondriac discomfort and distension (usual)
   Epigastric stuffiness (sometimes)
3. Indications
   Indicated for the following symptoms in patients with medium or slightly excess pattern who have coughing, wheezing, shortness of breath, but little sputum: infantile asthma, bronchial asthma, and bronchitis.

真武湯

Shimbuto (SIT) Zhēn wǔ tāng
Manifestation

1. Symptoms

- Diarrhea: Much watery diarrhea without tenesmus. Tendency of diarrhea at dawn.

- Abdominal pain: Tends to get worse by cold stimulation, but it is often mild.
- General malaise: Frequent complaint of strong general malaise and wanting to lie down and sleep. Fatigue may occur after defecation.
- Cold limbs: Limbs are cold and color is poor.
- Dizziness: Floating dizziness; complaint that fixed objects move like "crossing in front of me."
- Feeling of physical agitation: Complaint of physical agitation "as if one were on a ship" or "as if one were walking on a cloud."
- Skewed feeling: Patient intends to walk straight but goes diagonally.
- Palpitations: Palpitations and shortness of breath may be accompanied by anxiety.
- Motor neuralgia and sensory neuralgia may be observed.
- Reduced urine volume, enuresis.
- Fever: Occasionally observed.
- This can be widely used even if all the indicated symptoms do not appear. Cold and fluid[TM1] poisoning are targeted.

2. Signs
   (i) Inspection: The complexion looks bad. The patient's voice is often weak. The body is thin, and the face is often edematous.
   (ii) Tongue examination: The tongue body is pink or reddish pink and swollen with teeth marks. Tongue coating may be moist and white.
   (iii) Pulse examination: Often, deep, small, and deficient, or floating and deficient.
   (iv) Abdominal examination:
   Abdominal strength: Soft to slightly soft (1/5 to 2/5)
   Abdominal manifestations
   Pulsations in epigastrium (usual)
   Splashing sound (often)
   Abdominal muscle tension (sometimes)
3. Indications
   Indicated for the following symptoms in patients with deficiency pattern who have cold sensations, general fatigue, occasional diarrhea, abdominal pain, and dizziness: diarrhea, acute and chronic gastroenteritis, gastrointestinal weakness, dizziness, palpitation, common cold, edema, eczema/dermatitis、 and skin itching.

清上防風湯

Seijobofuto (SJBT) Qīng shàng fang fēng tāng
Manifestation

1. Symptoms

- Red face: Complexion is red, oily, and prone to hyperemia.
- Hot flash: There is a feeling of redness on the face and a feeling of a heavy head, while the feet are cold.
- Eczema, dermatitis: Hyperemic and intense redness is observed. Acne that is large, reddish, and has pus at the tip. Acne is likely to occur not only on the face but also on the precordium and back.
- Eye redness.
- No sweating: There is little tendency to sweat, and the skin other than the face tends to be dry.
- Reduced urine volume.
- Constipation: Often tends to be constipated.

2. Signs
   (i) Inspection: Flushing, hot flashes, and an oily face may be observed. Redness may be observed in the bulbar conjunctiva. Acne and dermatitis are often found on the face due to the tendency to rash.
   (ii) Tongue examination: The tongue body is red to bright red, and the tongue coating is often yellow and moderately moist.
   (iii) Pulse examination: Often a floating, rapid, and strong.
   (iv) Abdominal examination:
   There is little literature.
   (reference)
   Abdominal strength: Moderate (3/5).
3. Indications
   Indicated for the following symptoms in patients with medium or excess pattern who have a reddish face, occasional hot flashes: acne, facial/head eczema/dermatitis, rosacea.

清暑益気湯

Seishoekkito (SET) Qīng shǔ yì qì tāng
Manifestation

1. Symptoms

- Chest pain: Complaints of mild chest pain
- Cough/wheezing: May be effective for patients with mild dry chronic cough and bronchial asthma
- Throat discomfort, dry throat

2. Signs
   (i) Inspection: Often has a bad complexion, tends to sweat, sluggishness, and lack of vigor.
   (ii) Tongue examination: The tongue body is crimson to bright crimson. Tongue coating is often dry and yellow. Tongue coating may also be mirror tongue with little moss.
   (iii) Pulse examination: Often floating and deficient or deep and deficient.

(iv) Abdominal examination:
Abdominal strength: Soft to slightly soft (1/5 to 2/5)
Abdominal manifestations
Epigastric stuffiness (sometimes)
Discomfort and restlessness in chest (sometimes)

3. Indications
Indicated for the following symptoms in patients with tendency to fatigue, anorexia, and occasional thirst: heat stroke, anorexia/diarrhea due to heat, emaciation in summer, general malaise, and physical decline /anorexia due to chronic disease.

清心蓮子飲

Seishinrenshiin (SRI) Qīng xīn lián zǐ yǐn
Manifestation

1. Symptoms

- Difficulty urinating, pain when urinating
- Residual urination/frequent urination: Relatively chronic cystitis, urethritis, and psychogenic nonspecific urinary complaints.
- Cloudy urine: May be purulent, bloody, or mixed with urine sand. It tends to recur with fatigue and often takes a chronic course.
- Leucorrhea: Sometimes has the appearance of milk.
- spermatorrhea/dry mouth
- Depressed state
- General malaise
- Insomnia
- Gastrointestinal weakness/anorexia

2. Signs
(i) Inspection: Often appears frail and nervous.
(ii) Tongue examination: The tongue body is crimson; tongue coating is dry to medium moisture, and seldom white.
(iii) Pulse examination: Often deep, slightly weak, thin and rapid or deep, thin and without strength.
(iv) Abdominal examination:
Abdominal strength: Soft to slightly soft (1/5 to 2/5)
Abdominal manifestations
Epigastric stuffiness and resistance (often)

3. Indications
Indicated for the following symptoms in patients with medium or deficiency pattern who have gastrointestinal weakness, general malaise, dry mouth or dry tongue, and difficulty urinating: residual urine, pollakiuria, micturition pain, cloudy urine, difficulty urinating, and leucorrhea.

清肺湯

Seihaito (SHT) Qīng fèi tāng
Manifestation

1. Symptoms

- Cough: Violent coughing accompanied by sputum; coughing does not stop until exhaustion of sputum.
- Sputum: Often a large amount of thick, viscous, and purulent sputum.
- Hoarseness
- Sore throat

2. Signs
(i) Inspection: Prolonged severe coughing and thick sputum may drain physical strength.
(ii) Tongue examination: The tongue body may be crimson. Tongue coating may be slightly moist or dry and slightly white.
(iii) Pulse examination: Often wiry, slightly weak or thin, and rapid.
(iv) Abdominal examination:
There is little literature.
【reference】
Abdominal strength: Slightly soft to moderate (2/5 to 3/5).

3. Indications
Indicated for the following symptoms in patients with medium or slight deficiency pattern with continuous coughing with copious sputum that is hard to expectorate: Coughing accompanied by copious sputum, bronchitis.

川芎茶調散

Senkyuchachosan (SCCS) Chuān xiōng chá diào sǎn
Manifestation

1. Symptoms

- Headache: General headache. Early stage of cold syndrome, sinusitis, headache associated with menstrual cycle, tension-type headache, migraine, chronic headache, etc.
- Nasal congestion
- Nasal discharge
- Fever
- Sputum
- Joint pain in limbs
- Muscle pain

2. Signs
   (i) Inspection: Unremarkable.
   (ii) Tongue examination: The tongue body is unremarkable, and tongue coating may be slightly white coating.
   (iii) Pulse examination: Often floating.
   (iv) Abdominal examination:
   No specific abdominal manifestations reported
   Abdominal strength: Unremarkable
3. Indications
   Indicated for the following symptoms in patients of any pattern who have a headache: common cold, miscellaneous symptoms associated with menstruation, and headaches.

疎経活血湯

Sokeikakketsuto (SOKT) Shū jīng huó xiě tāng
Manifestation

1. Symptoms

- Joint pain.
- Neuralgia.
- Muscle pain.
- Low back pain.
- The nature of this pain is a stinging pain that runs all over the body, and it may be accompanied by numbness. It may be exacerbated by coldness and consumption of alcohol.

2. Signs
   (i) Inspection: Mild edema and congestion may be seen in the lower limbs.
   (ii) Tongue examination: The tongue body is often, pink and tongue coating is absent or slightly white.
   (iii) Pulse examination: Often slightly weak to deep and thin.
   (iv) Abdominal examination:
   Abdominal strength: Slightly soft to moderate (2/5 to 3/5)
   Abdominal manifestations
   Tenderness in lower abdomen (often)
3. Indications
   Indicated for the following symptoms in patients with medium pattern who have pain and sometimes neuralgia: joint pain, neuralgia, low back pain, and myalgia.

大黄甘草湯

Daiokanzoto (DKZT) Dà huáng gān cǎo tāng
Manifestation

1. Symptoms

- Constipation
- Vomiting: Those who vomit when eating because their gastrointestinal tract is blocked by chronic constipation

2. Signs
   (i) Inspection: Unremarkable
   (ii) Tongue examination: Unremarkable
   (iii) Pulse examination: Sometimes deep
   (iv) Abdominal examination:
   No specific abdominal manifestations reported.
   Abdominal strength: Around moderate (3/5)
   Abdominal manifestations
   Mild distention of abdomen (often)
3. Indications
   Indicated for the following symptoms in patients of any pattern: Constipation, various symptoms associated with constipation, such as a dull headache, hot flashes, eczema, dermatitis, pimples (acne), anorexia (loss of appetite), abdominal distension, abnormal intestinal fermentation, and hemorrhoids.

大黄牡丹皮湯

Daiobotanpito (DBT) Dà huáng mǔ dān pí tāng
Manifestation

1. Symptoms

- Lower abdominal pain: For acute abdominal inflammation such as appendicitis, it is used when the general condition is good and abscess formation is not remarkable even in early/mild cases or advanced cases.
- Abdominal distension
- Constipation tendency

2. Signs
   (i) Inspection: Unremarkable.
   (ii) Tongue examination: The tongue body is unremarkable. Tongue coating may be slightly yellow.
   (iii) Pulse examination: Deep, tense, or slow.
   (iv) Abdominal examination:
   Abdominal strength: Moderate to full (4/5 to 5/5)
   Abdominal manifestations
   Tenderness in the ileocecal region (usual)
   Lower abdominal resistance and fullness (sometimes)
3. Indications
   Indicated for the following symptoms in patients with medium or excess pattern who have lower abdominal

pain and who are likely to have constipation: menstrual irregularity, dysmenorrhea, menstrual pain, constipation, and hemorrhoids.

大建中湯

Daikenchuto (DKT) Dà jiàn zhōng tāng
Manifestation

1. Symptoms

- Abdominal pain: Paroxysmal colic-like abdominal pain that may come from gas accumulation or cold
- Increased intestinal peristalsis (stomach rumble)
- Fullness of abdomen
- Vomiting: Accompanied by ileus
- Cold: May feel cold in their limbs and abdomen

2. Signs
   (i) Inspection: Intestinal peristalsis may be observed.
   (ii) Tongue examination: Unremarkable
   (iii) Pulse examination: Deep, weak, and slow
   (iv) Abdominal examination:
   (i) No specific abdominal manifestations reported.
   (ii) Abdominal strength: Soft to slightly soft (1/5 to 2/5)
   (iii) Abdominal manifestations
   (iv) Unstable peristalsis (usual)
   Abdominal distention (usual)
   Coldness in the abdomen (often)
   Abdominal pain (often)
3. Indications
   Indicated for the following symptoms in patients with deficiency pattern who have pain due to cold in abdomen: lower abdominal pain and abdominal distention.

大柴胡湯

Daisaikoto (DST) Dà chái hú tāng
Manifestation

1. Symptoms

- Unpleasant fullness, oppression, and tension on the sides of the chest (fullness and discomfort in chest and hypochondrium)
- Constipation tendency
- Stiff shoulder
- Tendency to sweat, sensitivity to heat
- Depressive tendency
- Nausea, vomiting, anorexia
- Shortness of breath

2. Signs
   (i) Inspection: Physique is solid and may be obese or muscular.
   (ii) Tongue examination: The tongue body is unremarkable; the tongue coating is slightly dry and greasy white or yellow.
   (iii) Pulse examination: Deep and excess.
   (iv) Abdominal examination:
   Abdominal strength: Slightly hard to full (4/5 to 5/5)
   Abdominal manifestations
   Strong epigastric stuffiness and resistance (usual)
   Fullness and discomfort in chest and hypochondrium (usual)
   Abdominal muscle tension (often)
3. Indications
   Indicated for the following symptoms in patients with excess pattern who have a tendency to constipation accompanied by fullness and discomfort from lateral abdomen to epigastrium: gastritis, constipation, shoulder stiffness/headache/constipation associated with hypertension and obesity, neurosis, and obesity (Fig. 8.3).

大柴胡湯去大黄

Daisaikotokyodaio (DSTKD) Dà chái hú tāng qù dà huáng
Manifestation

1. Symptoms

- Unpleasant fullness, oppression, and tension on the sides of the chest (fullness and discomfort in chest and hypochondrium)
- Stiff shoulders
- Tendency to sweat, sensitivity to heat
- Depressive tendency
- Nausea, vomiting, anorexia
- Shortness of breath

2. Signs
   (i) Inspection: Physique is solid; may be obese or muscular.
   (ii) Tongue examination: The tongue body is unremarkable; the tongue coating is slightly dry and thick white or yellow.
   (iii) Pulse examination: Sunken and excess.
   (iv) Abdominal examination:
   There is little literature.
   【reference】
   Abdominal strength: Slightly hard to full (4/5 to 5/5)
   Abdominal manifestations
   Epigastric stuffiness and resistance (usual)
   Fullness and discomfort in chest and hypochondrium (usual)

3. Indications

   Indicated for the following symptoms in patients with medium or excess pattern who have fullness and discomfort from lateral abdomen to epigastrium: gastritis, stiffness/headache/constipation associated with hypertension and obesity, and neurosis.

大承気湯

Daijokito (DJT) Dà chéng qì tāng
Manifestation

1. Symptoms

   - Abdominal distension: There is a feeling of fullness around umbilicus. Do not use for those with weak pulse or rapid pulse and those with ascites or abdominal distention (due to gas), even if there is this sign.
   - Constipation: The stool is tightly constricted.
   - Thirst
   - Intermittent fever: Fever that occurs in the middle yang stage, which spreads throughout the body at a fixed time like the rising tide. There are no chills.
   - Psychiatric symptoms: anxiety, insomnia, agitation, etc.
   - Diarrhea: Accompanied by abdominal tenesmus
   - spontaneous urination

2. Signs
   (i) Inspection: The abdomen is often distended. Sometimes consciousness is not clear with incoherent speech.
   (ii) Tongue examination: The tongue body is unremarkable. Tongue coating is dry, and sometimes it is a black coating.
   (iii) Pulse examination: Often strong, sometimes deep and slow.
   (iv) Abdominal examination:
   No specific abdominal manifestations reported.
   Abdominal strength: Slightly strong to strong (4/5 to 5/5)
   Abdominal manifestations
   Abdominal distention (rigid fullness in abdomen) (usual)
3. Indications

   Indicated for the following symptoms in patients with medium or excess pattern who have constipation associated with fullness of abdomen: acute and chronic constipation, neurosis, hypertension, headache, pneumonia, encephalitis, mania, and depression.

大防風湯

Daibofuto (DBFT) Dà fang fēng tāng
Manifestation

1. Symptoms

   - Joint swelling, pain, and deformity: The muscles around the joint are atrophied, and swelling and deformity in joints are conspicuous.
   - Difficulty in flexing and extending joints: Ankylosis and contracture cause joints to become stiff.
   - Muscle weakness.
   - Difficulty walking.
   - Paralysis of limbs.
   - Staggering.
   - Unsteadiness
   - Hypersensitivity to cold.

2. Signs
   (i) Inspection: Malnourished, anemic, pale complexion, and often thin. Joints may be deformed, and muscles may be atrophied.
   (ii) Tongue examination: The tongue body is pink and atrophied; the tongue coating may be absent.
   (iii) Pulse examination: Often deep, weak, and thready.
   (iv) Abdominal examination:
   There is little literature.
   【reference】
   Abdominal strength: Soft to slightly soft (1/5 to 2/5)
3. Indications

   Indicated for the following symptoms in patients with deficiency pattern who are exhausted, weakened, and tend to be anemic: chronic arthritis, arthralgia, and neuralgia.

竹茹温胆湯

Chikujountanto (CUT) Zhú rú wēn dǎn tāng
Manifestation

1. Symptoms

   - Cough, sputum: Prolonged cough accompanied by sputum
   - Mild fever: Mild fever that is difficult to cure
   - Insomnia, anxiety: Always nervous and anxious and cannot sleep
   - Chest clogging: Sensation like heat in the chest
   - Easy to startle: Easily startled by noise

- Mild palpitations
- Amnesia
- Tendency to be irritable

2. Signs
   (i) Inspection: The face may be flushed due to fever. One may be ecstatic and dreamy or may talk deliriously. Tendency to be surprised and frightened.
   (ii) Tongue examination: The tongue body is unremarkable, and the tongue coating is often white. Yellow coating may be found in the center of tongue.
   (iii) Pulse examination: The pulse is slippery and often deficient.
   (iv) Abdominal examination:
   Abdominal strength: Slightly soft (2/5)
   Abdominal manifestations
   Mild fullness and discomfort in chest and hypochondrium (usual)
   Splashing sound (sometimes)
3. Indications
   Indicated for the following symptoms in patients with medium pattern: Prolonged fever or not feeling refreshed after the temperature has returned to normal, sleep disturbed by frequent coughing or expectoration in convalescent phase of common cold, influenza, pneumonia, etc.

治打撲一方

Jidabokuippo (JDI) Zhì dǎ pū yī fāng
Manifestation

1. Symptoms

- Bruise/sprain: Pain, swelling, muscle stiffness after bruising, arthralgia, numbness, etc. Rhubarb is used for the purpose of eliminating inflammation even if there is no constipation. When there is mild diarrhea after taking this formula, it does not need to be considered a side effect.

2. Signs
   (i) Inspection: Unremarkable.
   (ii) Tongue examination: The tongue body may be dark red. Tongue coating is unremarkable.
   (iii) Pulse examination: Wiry in the acute phase with strong pain. The pulse may be unsmooth when time has passed since the injury.
   (iv) Abdominal examination:
   There is little literature.
   【reference】
   Abdominal strength: Moderate (3/5).
3. Indications
   Indicated for the following symptoms in patients of any pattern who have swelling and pain (from injury): bruises and sprains.

治頭瘡一方

Jizusoippo (JZI) Zhì tóu chuāng yī fāng
Manifestation

1. Symptoms

- Eczema on the head and face: eczema with redness, blisters, scabs, erosions, exudates, and itching. It can be used on parts other than the head and face.
- Constipation: Use for people who are relatively strong and tend to have constipation. Do not use for people who are prone to diarrhea or who have very dry skin.

2. Signs
   (i) Inspection: The face is often flushed. Eczema is often accompanied by erosions and secretions.
   (ii) Tongue examination: The tongue body is often dark red; the tongue coating is unremarkable.
   (iii) Pulse examination: excess (strong).
   (iv) Abdominal examination:
   There is little literature.
   【reference】
   Moderate abdominal strength (3/5).
3. Indications
   Indicated for the following symptoms in patients with medium or excess pattern with skin disease of the face or head that sometimes causes itching and discharge: Eczema/dermatitis and infantile eczema/dermatitis.

調胃承気湯

Choijokito (CJT) Diào wèi chéng qì tāng
Manifestation

1. Symptoms

- Constipation: Accompanied by abdominal pain and bloating.
- Feeling of heat in the torso: During the course of febrile illness, dry mouth and impaired consciousness may occur.

2. Signs
   (i) Inspection: A feverish red complexion characteristic of the middle yang stage and a distracted expression with a lack of focus may be observed.
   (ii) Tongue examination: The tongue body is unremarkable, and tongue coating may be dry and black-brown or yellow (interior heat).
   (iii) Pulse examination: Typically, pulse is deep and excess, but it may be deep and weak (unsmooth).
   (iv) Abdominal examination:
   No specific abdominal manifestations reported.
   Abdominal strength: Moderate to excess (3/5 to 5/5)

Abdominal manifestations
Abdominal distension (sometimes)

3. Indications

Indicated for the following symptoms in patients with medium pattern: constipation, for alleviation of various symptoms associated with constipation, such as a dull headache, hot flashes, eczema, dermatitis, pimples (acne), anorexia (loss of appetite), abdominal distension, abnormal intestinal fermentation, and hemorrhoids.

The primary indication for Choijokito is the following: constipation

釣藤散

Chotosan (CTS) Diào téng sǎn
Manifestation

1. Symptoms

- Headache: May occur in the morning
- Dizziness, hot flashes
- Stiff shoulders and stiff neck
- Irritability
- Insomnia
- Tinnitus

2. Signs
   (i) Inspection: May have red eyes or red face.
   (ii) Tongue examination: The tongue body is pale and often large. Tongue coating may be thick greasy and white.
   (iii) Pulse examination: May be wiry.
   (iv) Abdominal examination:
   There is little literature.
   【reference】
   Abdominal strength: Moderate or less (1/5 to 3/5).
   Abdominal manifestations.
   Occasional epigastric stuffiness and resistance (usual).

3. Indications

Indicated for the following symptoms in patients with medium pattern who have chronic headaches, dizziness, and stiff shoulders: chronic headache, neuralgia, and high blood pressure.

腸癰湯

Choyoto (CYT) Cháng yōng tāng
Manifestation

1. Symptoms

- Lower abdominal pain, abdominal distention: Appendicitis, diverticulitis of the large intestine, inflammatory bowel disease, perianal inflammation, etc.
- Leucorrhea and lower abdominal pain during menstruation: Inflammation in the pelvis, etc.
- Frequent urination/pain during urination: Urinary tract infection, etc.
- Strong-smelling thick sputum: Bronchiectasis, etc.

2. Signs
   (i) Inspection: May have dark complexion and dry skin.
   (ii) Tongue examination: Tongue body may be dark red.
   (iii) Pulse examination: May be wiry and thin.
   (iv) Abdominal examination:
   Abdominal strength: Slightly soft to moderate (2/5 to 3/5)
   Abdominal manifestations
   Tenderness in ileocecal region (usual)
   abdominal distension (often)

3. Indications

Indicated for the following symptoms in patients with medium or slight deficiency pattern who have acute or chronic pain in the lower abdomen, especially in sigmoid region, or the following symptoms accompanied by abdominal bloating and menstrual pain: recovery/chronic period of appendicitis or diverticulitis of the large intestine/inflammatory bowel disease, general abdominal complaints, gynecological diseases/urinary tract inflammation with abdominal pain, respiratory diseases with a lot of sputum, etc.

猪苓湯

Choreito (CRT) Zhū líng tāng
Manifestation

1. Symptoms

- Thirst, dysuria: Feeling of heat and thirst.
- Pain with urination, lower abdominal pain, feeling of residual urine
- Occasional diarrhea
- Hot flashes, psychiatric symptoms: Psychiatric and neurological symptoms such as irritability, insomnia, annoyance, and worrying about trifles.

2. Signs
   (i) Inspection: The face and limbs may be edematous.
   (ii) Tongue examination: The tongue body is crimson. Tongue coating is yellow or yellow and greasy.
   (iii) Pulse examination: Often rapid. It reflects fever.
   (iv) Abdominal examination:
   Abdominal strength: Moderate (3/5)
   Abdominal manifestations
   Tension in lower abdomen (sometimes)
   Chest agitation (sometimes)
3. Indications
   Indicated for the following symptoms in patients of any pattern who have dysuria and thirst: dysuria and thirst, feeling of residual urine, frequent urination, and edema.

猪苓湯合四物湯

Choreitogoshimotsuto (CRTST) Zhū líng tāng hé sì wù tāng
Manifestation

1. Symptoms

- Thirst, dysuria: Feeling of heat and thirst.
- Pain with urination, lower abdominal pain, feeling of residual urine
- Occasional diarrhea
- Hot flashes, psychiatric symptoms: Psychiatric and neurological symptoms such as irritability, insomnia, annoyance, and worrying about trifles.

2. Signs
   (i) Inspection: The face and limbs may be edematous. Dry skin: the skin is drier than choreito pattern, and evidence of blood deficiency (i.e., dull complexion) is more pronounced.
   (ii) Tongue examination: Tongue body is crimson. Tongue coating is yellow moss or yellow and greasy.
   (iii) Pulse examination: Often rapid. It reflects fever.
   (iv) Abdominal examination:
   There is little literature.
   【reference】
   Abdominal strength: Slightly soft to moderate (2/5 to 3/5).
3. Indications
   Indicated for the following symptoms in patients of any pattern who have dry skin and a constitution with an unhealthy complexion without any gastrointestinal disturbance and have dysuria and thirst: dysuria and thirst, feeling of residual urine, frequent urination, and edema.

通導散

Tsudosan (TDS) Tōng dǎo sǎn
Manifestation

1. Symptoms

- Hot flashes.
- Irregular menstruation, menstrual pain, menopausal syndrome.
- Low back pain.
- Abdominal distension, constipation.
- Bruising.
- Symptoms of high blood pressure: Headache, dizziness, stiff shoulders, etc.
- Tinnitus.
- Palpitations.
- Obesity.
- There may be urinary disturbance.

2. Signs
   (i) Inspection: The face is reddish, and the nail color is often dark red.
   (ii) Tongue examination: Tongue body is often dark red or dark purple. Tongue coating is unremarkable.
   (iii) Pulse examination: Often deep, thin, and excess. It can be unsmooth.
   (iv) Abdominal examination:
   Abdominal strength: Moderate to full (4/5 to 5/5)
   Abdominal manifestations
   Tenderness in lower abdomen (often)
   Abdominal distension (especially lower abdomen) "fullness in lower abdomen" (often)
   Epigastric stuffiness and resistance (sometimes)
   Abdominal muscle tension (sometimes)
3. Indications
   Indicated for the following symptoms in patients with medium or excess pattern who have tenderness in the lower abdomen and are likely to have constipation: menstrual irregularity, menstrual pain, climacteric disturbance, low back pain, constipation, bruising (contusion), and symptoms associated with hypertension (headache, dizziness, and shoulder stiffness).

桃核承気湯

Tokakujokito (TJT) Táo hé chéng qì tāng
Manifestation

1. Symptoms

- Menstrual disorders: Irregular menstruation, dysmenorrhea, menstrual pain, etc.
- Menstrual anxiety: Especially before and during menstruation, and after childbirth.
- Constipation
- Hot flashes with cold limbs
- Symptoms of hypertension: Headache, stiff shoulders, dizziness, etc.
- Low back pain
- Overeating

2. Signs
   (i) Inspection: Reddish black complexion.
   (ii) Tongue examination: The tongue body is red or dark purple, and the tongue coating is yellow.
   (iii) Pulse examination: deep, excess, and unsmooth
   (iv) Abdominal examination:
   Abdominal strength: Slightly strong to strong (4/5 to 5/5)
   Abdominal manifestations
   Tenderness around umbilicus, sigmoid colon, and left lower abdomen; lower abdominal cramp (usual)
3. Indications
   Indicated for the following symptoms in patients with medium or excess pattern who have hot flashes and are likely to have constipation: menstrual irregularity, dysmenorrhea, menstrual pain, anxiety during menstruation or after childbirth, low back pain, constipation, symptoms associated with hypertension (headache, dizziness, and shoulder stiffness), hemorrhoid, and bruises.

当帰飲子

Tokiinshi (TKI) Dāng guī yǐn zi
Manifestation

1. Symptoms

- Dry skin.
- Itching: Itching tends to occur especially at night. Often used for senile dry cutaneous pruritus.
- May not be accompanied by a rash.
- Dermatitis without secretions.

2. Signs
   (i) Inspection: The skin is dry, but there are few secretions, and there is little redness. Frail appearance. Rashes are small and few, if any. There may be no rash.
   (ii) Tongue examination: The tongue body is dark red. Tongue coating is minimal and often dry.
   (iii) Pulse examination: Thin/weak.
   (iv) Abdominal examination:
   There is little literature.
   【reference】
   Abdominal strength: Soft to slightly soft (1/5 to 2/5).
3. Indications
   Indicated for the following symptoms in patients with medium or deficiency pattern with sensitivity to cold and dry skin: eczema/dermatitis (with little exudation) and itching.

当帰建中湯

Tokikenchuto (TKT) Dāng guī jiàn zhōng tāng
Manifestation

1. Symptoms

- Abdominal pain, lower back pain: Used for postpartum, abdominal pain, menstrual pain, etc.
- Most suitable for lower abdominal pain that radiates to the lower back; for both men and women with abdominal and lower back pain.
- Postpartum decline in physical fitness: May have low energy and slightly shallow breathing.
- Uterine bleeding/postpartum uterine retrograde insufficiency: Mainly used for those with abdominal pain. Consider using kyukikyogaito for cases with excessive bleeding.
- Irregular menstruation/menorrhagia, headache before and after menstruation.
- Rectal/hemorrhoidal bleeding, anal pain.
- Anorexia.
- Underweight.
- Anemia.
- Sweating tendency.

2. Signs
   (i) Inspection: May have a pale complexion.
   (ii) Tongue examination: The tongue body is pale white or pink; the tongue coating is moist and often absent or slightly white coating.
   (iii) Pulse examination: Often deep and weak, or thin and wiry.

(iv) Abdominal examination:
Abdominal strength: Soft to slightly soft (1/5 to 2/5)
Abdominal manifestations
Tenderness in lower abdomen (usual)
Abdominal muscle tension (often)

3. Indications
Indicated for the following symptoms in patients with deficiency patterns who are easily fatigued and have a poor complexion: Menstrual pain, dysmenorrhea, irregular menstruation, abdominal pain, lower abdominal pain, low back pain, hemorrhoids, pain of anal prolapse, and post-illness/postoperative pain and decline in physical fitness.

当帰四逆加呉茱萸生姜湯

Tokishigyakukagoshuyushokyoto (TSGST) Dāng guī sì nì jiā wú zhūyú sheng jiāng tāng
Manifestation

1. Symptoms

- Cold sensitivity: The extremities, abdomen, and entire lower limbs become cold. May be accompanied by hot flashes.
- Frostbite, Raynaud's disease, skin disease.
- Lower abdominal/inguinal pain: Often accompanied by a feeling of fullness in the abdomen. It becomes worse when it is cold.
- Menstrual pain/ovulation pain.
- Chronic pain: Used for neuralgia, postoperative pain, fibromyalgia, etc.
- Chronic diarrhea: Also used for those with vomiting.

2. Signs
(i) Inspection: Often a thin figure.
(ii) Tongue examination: Tongue body may be pale white. Tongue coating is unremarkable.
(iii) Pulse examination: Often sunken, deficient, and thin. May be wiry with abdominal pain.
(iv) Abdominal examination:
Abdominal strength: Soft to slightly soft (1/5 to 2/5)
Abdominal manifestations
Abdominal pain (often)
Abdominal muscle tension (sometimes)
Tenderness and distention in the lower abdomen (sometimes)
Coldness in lower abdomen or "prolonged cold" (sometimes)

3. Indications
Indicated for the following symptoms in patients with medium deficiency pattern who have a tendency of cold hands and feet, strong cold sensitivity in lower limbs, and are likely to have pain in the legs or lower abdomen when their lower limbs are cold: cold sensitivity, chilblain, headache, lower abdominal pain, low back pain, and menstrual pain.

当帰芍薬散

Tokishakuyakusan (TSS) Dāng guī sháo yào sǎn
Manifestation

1. Symptoms

- Abdominal pain, menstrual pain, premenstrual syndrome.
- Climacteric syndrome.
- Menstrual disorders.
- Pregnancy: Mainly used as a prenatal drug in the latter half of pregnancy. Good for abdominal pain and cough. Use kyukikyogaito when bleeding is the main issue. Poor perinatal physical condition: Use when there is fatigue, uterine bleeding, diarrhea, difficulty urinating, or the following symptoms: anemia and uterine bleeding. For excessive bleeding, use kyukikyogaito or shigyakukaninjinto.
- Dizziness, orthostatic hypotension.
- Heavy headache, tinnitus.
- Stiff shoulders, back pain.
- Cold sensitivity.
- Edema.

2. Signs
(i) Inspection: Often pale with thin figure.
(ii) Tongue examination: The tongue body may be pale white. Tongue coating is often moist.
(iii) Pulse examination: Often deep and weak.
(iv) Abdominal examination:
Abdominal strength: Soft to slightly soft (1/5 to 2/5)
Abdominal manifestations
Splashing sound (often)
Tenderness in lower abdomen (usual)
Abdominal pain (sometimes)

3. Indications
Indicated for the following symptoms in patients with deficiency pattern who are sensitive to cold, tend to be anemic, are easily fatigued, and sometimes complain of lower abdominal pain, dull headaches, dizziness, shoulder stiffness, tinnitus, and palpitation: menstrual irregularity, menstrual abnormality, menstrual pain, climacteric disturbance, prenatal/postnatal or miscarriage disorder (anemia, malaise, dizziness, edema), dizziness/orthostatic hypotension, dull headache, shoulder stiffness, back pain, susceptible to cold of waist and lower limbs, frostbite, edema, skin spots, and tinnitus (Fig. 8.2).

当帰芍薬散加附子

Tokishakuyakusankabushi (TSSB) Dāng guī sháo yào sàn jiā fù zǐ
Manifestation

1. Symptoms

- Chills: For patients with extreme cold.
- Abdominal pain, menstrual pain, premenstrual syndrome.
- Climacteric syndrome.
- Menstrual disorders.
- Pregnancy: Mainly used as a prenatal drug in the latter half of pregnancy. Good for abdominal pain and coughing. Use kyukikyogaito if bleeding is the main issue.
- Poor perinatal physical condition: Use for patients with fatigue, uterine bleeding, diarrhea, difficult urination, or the following symptoms: anemia, uterine bleeding. For excessive bleeding, use kyukikyogaito or shigyakukaninjinto.
- Dizziness, orthostatic hypotension.
- Strong headache, tinnitus.
- Stiff shoulders, back pain.
- Sensitivity to cold.
- Edema.
- Chills: Used for those with severe cold sensitivity.

2. Signs
   (i) Inspection: Often pale and thin figure.
   (ii) Tongue examination: The tongue body may be pale white. Tongue coating is often moist.
   (iii) Pulse examination: Often sunken and weak.
   (iv) Abdominal examination:
   No literature
3. Indications
   Indicated for the following symptoms in patients with deficiency pattern who are extremely cold sensitive, tend to be anemic, are easily fatigued, and sometimes complain of lower abdominal pain, dull headaches, dizziness, shoulder stiffness, tinnitus, and palpitation: menstrual irregularity, menstrual abnormality, menstrual pain, climacteric disturbance, prenatal/postnatal or miscarriage disorder (anemia, malaise, dizziness, edema), dizziness/orthostatic hypotension, dull headache, shoulder stiffness, back pain, tendency to feel cold below the waist, frostbite, edema, skin spots, and tinnitus.

当帰湯

Tokito (TOT) Dāng guī tāng
Manifestation

1. Symptoms

- Chest, back, or abdominal pain: Chest pain syndrome/intercostal neuralgia, etc. Those with abdominal pain also have stomach upset or upper abdominal distension. This formula is often used for angina in the classics, but in modern times, Western medical treatment is prioritized. It is used for intercostal neuralgia and other chest pain syndromes.
- Cold sensitivity: May be accompanied by a feeling of coldness in the back.

2. Signs
   (i) Inspection: Often lacking in vitality. Pain may cause distress.
   (ii) Tongue examination: The tongue body may be pale white. Tongue coating is unremarkable.
   (iii) Pulse examination: Often deep, slow, thin, and weak.
   (iv) Abdominal examination:
   No specific abdominal manifestations are reported.
   Abdominal strength: Soft to slightly soft (1/5 to 2/5)
   Abdominal manifestations
   Mild abdominal distension (often)
   Abdominal pain (sometimes)
3. Indications
   Indicated for the following symptoms in patients with medium or deficiency pattern who have a feeling of coldness in the back and feeling of abdominal distention and abdomen, chest or back pain: chest pain, abdominal pain, and gastritis.

二朮湯

Nijutsuto (NJT) Èr shù tāng
Manifestation

1. Symptoms

- Joint pain, muscle pain, neuralgia: Numbness and pain in muscles and joints such as shoulders and upper arms, accompanied by dullness.
- Movement impairment
- Mild edema
- Gastrointestinal weakness

2. Signs
   (i) Inspection: Due to fluid[TM1] toxicity (fluid[TM1] retention) constitution, muscles may lack tone. Beneficial for obese patients with fluid[TM1] toxicity, but this formula can be used for others.
   (ii) Tongue examination: The tongue body is unremarkable; tongue coating may be white and greasy.
   (iii) Pulse examination: May be slippery

(iv) Abdominal examination:
No specific abdominal manifestations reported
Abdominal strength: Slightly soft (2/5)
Abdominal manifestations
Splashing sound (sometimes)

3. Indications

Indicated for the following symptoms in patients with medium pattern who have pain in shoulders and upper arms, etc.: frozen shoulders

二陳湯

Nichinto (NCT) Èr chén tāng
Manifestation

1. Symptoms

- Nausea, vomiting, morning sickness, sickness: When used for vomiting, it is better to take it cold.
- Stomach discomfort, anorexia.
- Dizziness.
- Palpitations.
- Headache.
- Edema, feeling of heaviness.
- Cough, sputum.
- Shoulder and upper back pain.

2. Signs

(i) Inspection: Many have weak stomachs and do not have a very good complexion.
(ii) Tongue examination: The tongue body is unremarkable; the tongue coating may be slightly white.
(iii) Pulse examination: Unremarkable
(iv) Abdominal examination:
Abdominal strength: Soft to moderate (1/5 to 3/5)
Abdominal manifestations
Splashing sound (usual)
Epigastric stuffiness (usual)
Palpitations (sometimes)

3. Indications

Indicated for the following symptoms in patients with medium pattern who have nausea and vomiting: Nausea, vomiting, stomach discomfort, chronic gastritis, and hangover.

女神散

Nyoshinsan (NSS) Nǚ shén sǎn
Manifestation

1. Symptoms

- Hot flashes.
- Palpitations.
- Dizziness.
- Insomnia.
- Headache, heaviness in the head.
- Low back pain.
- Anxiety, depression.
- Abnormal sweating: The back may burn like fire, and sweat may flow.

2. Signs

(i) Inspection: In many cases, anxiety, depression, and other emotional moods are observed.
(ii) Tongue examination: The tongue body may be red at the tip, and the tongue coating may be white.
(iii) Pulse examination: Deep, thin, and rapid.
(iv) Abdominal examination:
Abdominal strength: Moderate (3/5)
Abdominal manifestations
Tenderness in lower abdomen (sometimes)
Epigastric stuffiness (sometimes)
Abdominal pulsations above and below the navel; palpitation in the supra-umbilical region, palpitation in the infra-umbilical region (sometimes)

3. Indications

Indicated for the following symptoms in patients with medium or excess patterns who have a feeling of flushing and dizziness: neurosis before or after childbirth, menstrual irregularity, autonomic imbalance syndrome related to menstruation, climacteric disturbance, and neurosis.

人参湯

Ninjinto (NT) Rén shēn tāng
Manifestation

1. Symptoms

- Feeling of coldness.
- Gastrointestinal weakness: Diarrhea, abdominal pain, nausea, vomiting, burping, anorexia, and stomach pain.
- Thin spit accumulates in the mouth.
- Frequent urination: Urine is thin and copious.
- Dizziness, dullness in head.

2. Signs

(i) Inspection: In many cases, the patient is lacking in vitality and has a poor complexion. May have pallor of the face and lips.
(ii) Tongue examination: The tongue body is pale; tongue coating may be white and wet.
(iii) Pulse examination: Often deep and thin or deep and slow. It is often slightly weak or weak.
(iv) Abdominal examination:
Abdominal strength: Soft to slightly soft (1/5 to 2/5)
Abdominal manifestations
Epigastric stuffiness and resistance (usual)

Splashing sound (usual)
Upper abdominal stuffiness (sometimes)
Cold epigastrium (sometimes)

3. Indications

Indicated for the following symptoms in patients with deficiency pattern who are easily fatigued and get cold limbs: gastrointestinal weakness, diarrhea, vomiting, gastric pain, abdominal pain, and acute/chronic gastritis.

附子理中湯

Bushirichuto (BRT) Fù zǐ lǐ zhōng tāng
Manifestation

1. Symptoms

- Extreme coldness of limbs
- Insomnia
- Anxiety, nervousness
- Habitual constipation

2. Signs
   (i) Inspection: In many cases, patient is lacking in vitality and has poor complexion. May have pallor of the face and lips.
   (ii) Tongue examination: The tongue body is pale, and tongue coating may be white and wet.
   (iii) Pulse examination: Often sunken and thin or sunken and slow. It is often slightly weak or weak.
   (iv) Abdominal examination:
   There is little literature.
   【reference】
   Abdominal strength: Soft to slightly soft (1/5 to 2/5).
   Epigastric stuffiness and resistance (often).
3. Indications

Indicated for the following symptoms in patients with deficiency pattern who are prone to have extreme coldness of limbs: gastrointestinal weakness, diarrhea, vomiting, gastric pain, abdominal pain, and acute/chronic gastritis.

人参養栄湯

ninjin'yoeito (NYT) Rén shēn yǎng róng tāng
Manifestation

1. Symptoms

- Loss of physical strength: A state in which physical strength does not recover easily after various operations, weak constitution due to pulmonary tuberculosis, atypical mycobacteriosis, congenital heart disease, etc.
- Fatigue
- Anorexia
- Night sweats
- Cold limbs
- Anemia
- Other symptoms: Palpitations, cough, mild fever, tendency of diarrhea or constipation, etc. may also be present.

2. Signs
   (i) Inspection: Fatigue, pale complexion, anemic facial appearance, dry skin, emaciation, etc.
   (ii) Tongue examination: Often tongue body is pale red or normal pink. It may be swollen. Tongue coating is absent or slightly white. May have a mirror tongue.
   (iii) Pulse examination: Sometimes weak and thin
   (iv) Abdominal examination:
   Abdominal strength: Soft to slightly soft (1/5 to 2/5)
   Abdominal manifestations
   Epigastric stuffiness and resistance (sometimes)
3. Indications

Indicated for the following symptoms in patients with deficiency pattern: Decreased physical strength after recovery from disease/operation, etc., fatigue and malaise, anorexia, night sweats, cold limbs, and anemia.

排膿散及湯

Hainosankyuto (HNST) Pái nóng sàn jí tāng
Manifestation

1. Symptoms
   - Suppurative disease of skin and mucous membrane accompanied by pain. Used not only in the early stages but also when suppuration is prolonged or relapses. Use haino-to at onset, or for suppuration that has been drained and becomes open, to promote drainage. Haino-san is effective when the affected area is red and painful, for its anti-inflammatory and analgesic effects. Since this formula is a combination of the above formulas, it can be used for various stages and symptoms of suppuration.
2. Signs
   (i) Inspection: There is a purulent abscess or abscess on the skin/mucous membrane. It can be used for both indurated, non-open and open, pus-producing cases.
   (ii) Tongue examination: The tongue body is unremarkable. The tongue coating tends to be dry and may be white.

(iii) Pulse examination: Unremarkable.
(iv) Abdominal examination:
There is little literature.
【reference】 Abdominal strength: Moderate (3/5).

3. Indications
Indicated for the following symptoms in patients of any pattern who are at an early stage or mild stage of suppurative disease of the skin: gingivitis and tonsillitis.

麦門冬湯

Bakumondoto (BAK) Mài mén dōng tāng
Manifestation

1. Symptoms

- Cough: Coughing with sputum that is small and difficult to expectorate continues persistently. The coughing may not be that persistent, but when it begins, it tends to continue for a long time. The coughing is severe enough to turn the face bright red and produces small amounts of sticky sputum. Therefore, patients may vomit. When this formula is used when there is a lot of sputum and it can be expectorated well, the amount of sputum may increase and the symptoms may worsen.
- Dry throat

2. Signs
(i) Inspection: The face may be flushed and reddish.
(ii) Tongue examination: The tongue body is unremarkable. Tongue coating is slightly white coating, and the tongue and mouth may be dry.
(iii) Pulse examination: Sometimes floating, large, and weak
(iv) Abdominal examination:
Abdominal strength: Soft to slightly soft (1/5 to 2/5)
Abdominal manifestations
Epigastric stuffiness and resistance (often)
Epigastric stuffiness (sometimes)

3. Indications
Indicated for the following symptoms in patients with medium or deficiency pattern who have sputum that is difficult to expectorate, sometimes with severe coughing, or with a dry throat: dry cough, bronchitis, bronchial asthma, pharyngitis, and hoarseness.

八味地黄丸

Hachimijiogan (HJG) Bā wèi dì huáng wán
Manifestation

1. Symptoms

- Lower body decline.
- Low back pain.
- Nocturia.
- Decreased libido.
- Blurred eyes.
- Dry mouth, dry mouth.
- Fever: Although the limbs tend to get cold, unpleasant hot flashes appear in the lower limbs, especially on the soles of the feet.
- Abnormal urine volume: There is a decrease in urine volume and a feeling of residual urine. There is increased urine volume in some cases.

2. Signs
(i) Inspection: Often a slightly frail old person.
(ii) Tongue examination: The tongue body is often dry, and papillae have disappeared and become red. Sometimes it is glossy. There is also a shiny, mirror tongue.
(iii) Pulse examination: The pulse is often deep and small, but it may also be wiry, tight, or surging.
(iv) Abdominal examination:
Abdominal strength: Unremarkable (there is little literature)
Abdominal manifestations
Weakness of the lower abdominal region (usual)
Palpable thin line of linea alba
Contracture below navel (often)

3. Indications
Indicated for the following symptoms in patients with medium or deficiency pattern who tend to fatigue and have cold limbs, decreased urinary output or polyuria, and thirst: pain in lower limbs, low back pain, numbness, senile blurred vision, itching, urinary disturbance, residual urine, nocturnal urine, urinary frequency, edema, improvement of symptoms accompanied with hypertension (shoulder stiffness, dull headache, and tinnitus), and mild urine leakage.

半夏厚朴湯

Hangekobokuto (HKT) Bàn xià hòu pǔ tāng
Manifestation

1. Symptoms

- Gastrointestinal discomfort: Gastrointestinal weakness, mild flatulence, abdominal distention, dysphagia, and gastric stagnation. The feeling of stagnation or nausea in the stomach after eating.

- Bronchitis, bronchial asthma, whooping cough
- Paroxysmal palpitations
- Laryngopharynx discomfort: Globus hystericus (globus syndrome), dizziness
- Hyperemesis gravidarum
- Neurosis, depression, irritability

2. Signs
   (i) Inspection: Appearance of a heavy mood and a depressed affect.
   (ii) Tongue examination: The tongue is slightly thick and has tooth marks (symptoms of fluid retention). The tongue body is light white or light purple-red and moist. The tongue coating is often thin and white.
   (iii) Pulse examination: Slightly wiry and often deep (Pulse disappears when pressure is applied.)
   (iv) Abdominal examination:
   Abdominal strength: Slightly soft (2/5)
   Abdominal manifestations
   Splashing sound (usual)
   Feeling of fullness in the abdomen (often)
   Epigastric stuffiness (sometimes)
   Epigastric aortic pulsation (sometimes)
3. Indications
   Indicated for the following symptoms in patients with medium pattern who have depressed feelings and a sensation of foreign body in the throat and esophagus and who sometimes have palpitations, dizziness, and nausea: anxiety neurosis, nervous gastritis, hyperemesis gravidarum, coughing, hoarseness, and feeling of foreign body in the throat (Fig. 8.4).

半夏瀉心湯

Hangeshashinto (HST) Bàn xià xiè xīn tāng
Manifestation

1. Symptoms

- Obstructive feeling in the epigastrium (epigastric stuffiness)
- Nausea and vomiting
- Anorexia
- Abdominal rumbling, loose stool/diarrhea

2. Signs
   (i) Inspection: Feeling drained for no reason, feeling of obstruction in the epigastric region, and most have diarrhea.
   (ii) Tongue examination: The tongue body is often crimson. Tongue coating is white to yellowish white and greasy.
   (iii) Pulse examination: Slightly tight and slippery
   (iv) Abdominal examination:
   Abdominal strength: Slightly soft (2/5)
   Abdominal manifestations
   Epigastric stuffiness and resistance (usual)
   Abdominal rumbling; borborygmus (usual)
   Feeling of fullness in epigastrium (sometimes)
   Pain in the upper abdomen (sometimes)
3. Indications
   Indicated for the following symptoms in patients with medium pattern who have feeling of obstruction in the epigastrium and occasional nausea, vomiting, anorexia, abdominal rumbling, and a tendency of loose stools or diarrhea: Acute or chronic gastroenteritis, loose stool/diarrhea, dyspepsia, gastroptosis, nervous gastritis, gastro-asthenia, hangover, belching, heartburn, stomatitis, and neurosis.

半夏白朮天麻湯

Hangebyakujutsutemmato (HBT) Bàn xià bái zhú tiān má tāng
Manifestation

1. Symptoms

- Gastrointestinal weakness.
- Headache, dull headache: Headache is persistent but often not very severe.
- Dizziness: Includes various types, from light (floating sensation) to severe (rocking on a ship).
- General malaise.
- Nausea and vomiting.
- Anorexia.
- Postprandial drowsiness: Complaints of strong drowsiness and malaise after eating.
- Cold limbs.
- Palpitations and shortness of breath.

2. Signs
   (i) Inspection: The complexion is pale and often thin, and the appearance lacks vitality.
   (ii) Tongue examination: The tongue body is unremarkable, and tongue coating may be moist and thin white.
   (iii) Pulse examination: Sometimes deep and weak
   (iv) Abdominal examination:
   Abdominal strength: Soft to slightly soft (1/5 to 2/5)

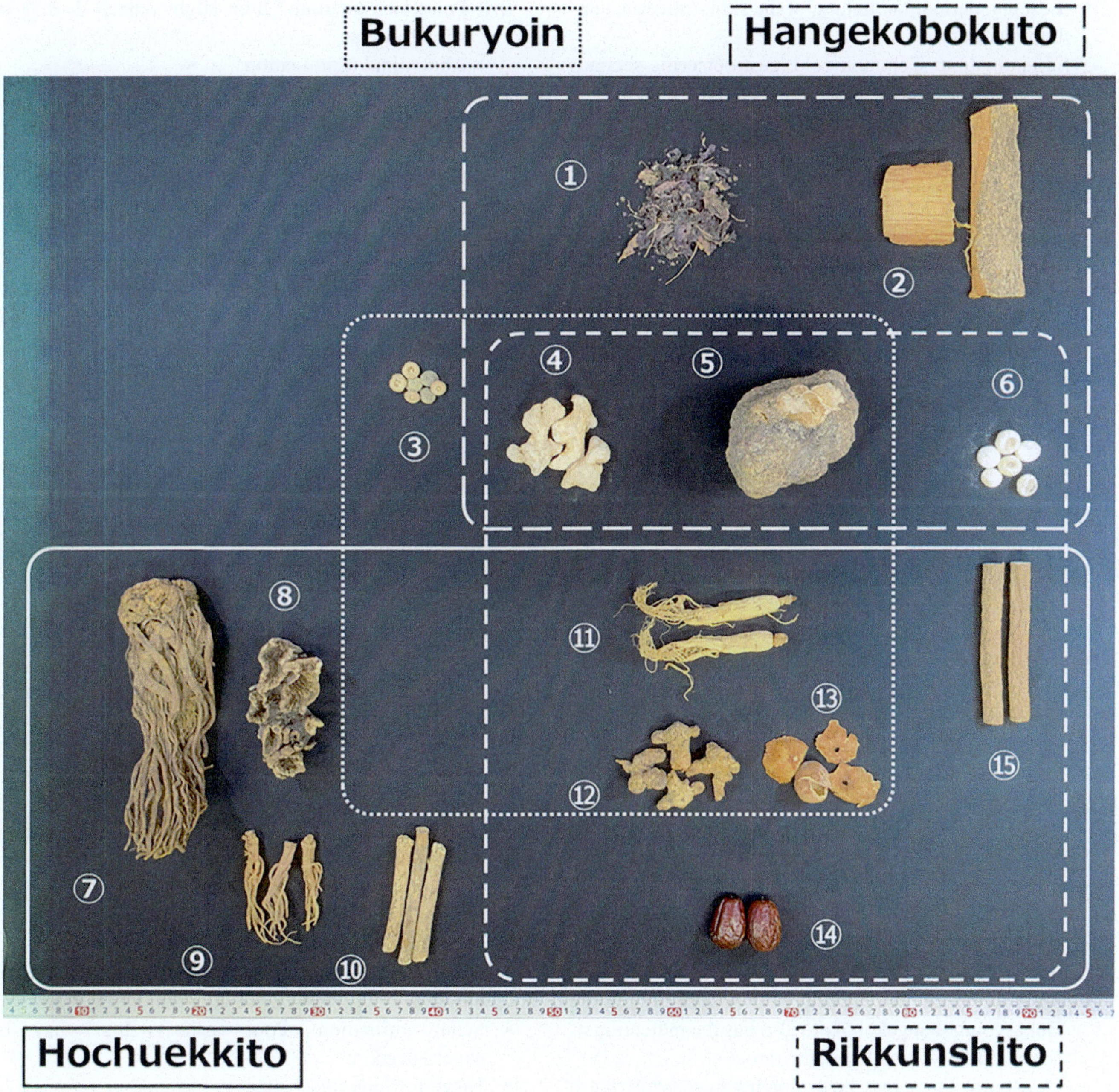

Fig. 8.4 Formulas related to *qi*These are broadly divided into two groups. The former contains Citrus Unshiu Peel, ③ Immature Orange, ② Magnolia Bark, and ① Perilla Herb, which have the effect of relieving qi stagnation (qi regulating formulas). The latter contains Ginseng, Atractylodes Rhizome, and Astragalus Root, etc., which have the effect of improving qi deficiency (qi-tonifying formula)④ ginger, ⑤ Poria Sclerotium, ⑥ Pinellia Tuber, ⑦ Japanese Angelica Root, ⑧ Cimicifuga Rhizome, ⑨ Bupleurum root, Jujube, Glycyrrhiza

Abdominal manifestations
Splashing sound (usual)
Mild epigastric stuffiness and resistance (often)

3. Indications

Indicated for the following symptoms in patients with medium or deficiency pattern who have a weak gastrointestinal tract and cold lower limbs: headache, dull headache, orthostatic hypotension, dizziness, and empyema (sinusitis).

白虎加人参湯

Byakkokaninjinto (BKTN) Bái hǔ jiā rén shēn tāng
Manifestation

1. Symptoms

- Feelings of heat and thirst: Hot flashes, sunstroke, heatstroke

- Eczema, dermatitis: Itching of the skin, urticaria, sunlight dermatitis
- Inflammation: Common cold, gastroenteritis secondary to common cold, and other viral infections
- Symptoms due to diabetes

2. Signs
   (i) Inspection: Severe thirst (prefers cold water), dry mouth and tongue, loss of body fluid due to sweating or polyuria, no constipation.
   (ii) Tongue examination: The tongue body is unremarkable, and tongue coating is often thin and white. Extreme dryness is noticeable.
   (iii) Pulse examination: Slippery pulse or surging pulse.
   (iv) Abdominal examination:
   Abdominal strength: Moderate to slightly hard (3/5 to 4/5)
   Abdominal manifestations
   Epigastric stuffiness and resistance (usual)
   Abdominal distension (sometimes)
3. Indications
   Indicated for the following symptoms in patients with medium or excess pattern who have severe feelings of heat and thirst: thirst, flushing, eczema/dermatitis, and itching of the skin.

茯苓飲

Bukuryoin (BRI) Fú líng yǐn
Manifestation

1. Symptoms

- Fullness in upper abdomen: awareness of fullness in upper abdomen, heartburn, flatulence (belching), feeling of tension and heaviness in epigastric region. Bukuryoingohangekobokuto also has the indication of sensation of obstruction in the throat.
- Heartburn: There may be symptoms such as heartburn and regurgitating sour foods.
- Vomiting: May vomit gastric juice. A characteristic of vomiting often without too much suffering.
- Palpitations: May be accompanied by palpitations.
- Chest pain: May notice pain that makes one feel like the chest is clogged.
- Scanty urination: Poor urine output may be experienced.
- Hiccups: Sometimes used for hiccups.

2. Signs
   (i) Inspection: There may be a slightly depressed facial expression.
   (ii) Tongue examination: The tongue body is often moist; tongue coating is scarce, but it may be slightly white.
   (iii) Pulse examination: Often slightly deep. It may be slightly weak.
   (iv) Abdominal examination:
   Abdominal strength: Slightly soft (2/5)
   Abdominal manifestations
   Splashing sound (usual)
   Feeling of fullness in upper abdomen (usual)
   Epigastric stuffiness and resistance (often)
   Abdominal pulsations (often)
3. Indications
   Indicated for the following symptoms in patients with medium or deficiency pattern who have nausea and heartburn, upper abdominal distention, and scanty urination: gastritis, nervous gastritis, gastrointestinal weakness, and heartburn (Fig. 8.4).

茯苓飲合半夏厚朴湯

Bukuryoingohangekobokuto (BRIHK) Fú líng yǐn hé bàn xià hòu pǔ tāng
Manifestation

1. Symptoms

- Upper abdominal distention: awareness of upper abdominal distention, heartburn, flatulence (belching), tension, and heaviness in the epigastric region. Bukuryoingohangekobokuto also has an indication of obstructive sensation in the throat.
- Heartburn: There may be symptoms such as heartburn and regurgitating sour taste.
- Vomiting: May vomit gastric juice. A characteristic of vomiting often without suffering too much.
- Palpitations: May be accompanied by palpitation.
- Chest pain: May have pain that feels like one's chest is clogged.
- Scanty urination: Poor urine output may be experienced.
- Hiccups: Sometimes used for hiccups.

In addition to the above symptoms (pharmacological indication for bukuryo-in), there are some neurotic symptoms such as depressive tendency, globus hystericus (abnormal sensation in laryngopharynx), dizziness, orthostatic hypotension, and palpitation.

2. Signs
   (i) Inspection: There may be a slightly depressed facial expression.
   (ii) Tongue examination: The tongue body is often moist, tongue coating is scarce, and it may be slightly white.
   (iii) Pulse examination: Often slightly sunken. It may be slightly weak.
   (iv) Abdominal examination:

Abdominal strength: Slightly soft to moderate (2/5 to 3/5)
Abdominal manifestations
Splashing sound (usual)
Epigastric stuffiness and resistance (usual)

3. Indications

Indicated for the following symptoms in patients with medium or deficiency pattern who have depressed feelings, abnormal sensation in the laryngopharynx, occasional palpitations, dizziness, nausea, heartburn, fullness in upper abdomen, and decreased urine volume: Anxiety neurosis, nervous gastritis, hyperemesis gravidarum, heartburn, hoarseness, and feeling of obstruction in throat.

平胃散

Heiisan (HIS) Píng wèi sǎn
Manifestation

1. Symptoms

- Upper abdominal discomfort: Widely used for unremarkable gastrointestinal symptoms such as epigastric stuffiness and fullness, stomach upset, and nausea and vomiting.
- Abdominal pain: May also have abdominal pain.
- Anorexia: Typically appetite loss, but on the contrary, occasionally overeating.
- Stomach rumbling, diarrhea: Especially after eating, the belly may rumble and diarrhea may occur. One may feel rather refreshed after diarrhea.
- Hiccups
- Respiratory symptoms: Shortness of breath, coughing, chest fullness, asthma.

2. Signs
   (i) Inspection: No characteristic findings are known.
   (ii) Tongue examination: The tongue body is unremarkable, and the tongue coating is mostly white.
   (iii) Pulse examination: Often somewhat wiry, but not very deficient (weak).
   (iv) Abdominal examination:
   Abdominal strength: Slightly soft to moderate (2/5 to 3/5) *
   *Strength in indication is different from literature.
   Abdominal manifestations
   Epigastric stuffiness (usual)
   Splashing sound (usual)
   Abdominal distension (often)
   Borborygmus (often)

3. Indications

Indicated for the following symptoms in patients with medium or excess pattern who experience heaviness in the stomach, tendency of dyspepsia, occasional nausea, abdominal sounds after eating, and tendency of diarrhea: Heavy stomach due to overeating, acute or chronic gastritis, dyspepsia, and anorexia.

補中益気湯

Hochuekkito (HET) Bǔ zhōng yì qì tāng

This has similar indications as shosaikoto, but the pulse and abdomen are weak, and discomfort in the flank region and alternating chills and fever are not remarkable. There is anorexia, easy fatigue, lack of energy, and excessive sweating.

Manifestation

1. Symptoms

- Fatigue: Frequent complaints of fatigue in limbs.
- Anorexia.
- Often likes hot foods and drinks.
- There may be a loss of taste.
- Spontaneous sweating and night sweats.
- Sensitivity to cold: The actual coldness of the patient is often slight.
- Tendency of mild fever.
- Tendency of diarrhea.
- May complain of anxiety and insomnia.
- Thin saliva may accumulate in the mouth.
- May complain of mild palpitations and shortness of breath.

2. Signs
   (i) Inspection: In many cases, the complexion is poor with a weak voice and lack of life in the eyes. So the appearance is generally weak.
   (ii) Tongue examination: May be moist and without coating or with a slightly white coating.
   (iii) Pulse examination: Tends to be weak, thin, large, dispersed, and weak.
   (iv) Abdominal examination:
   Abdominal strength: Soft to slightly soft (1/5 to 2/5)
   Abdominal manifestations
   Mild fullness and discomfort in the chest and hypochondrium (often)
   Mild abdominal pulsations in the supra-umbilical region (often)

3. Indications
   Indicated for the following symptoms in patients with deficiency pattern who have no vitality, reduced digestive functions, and easy to fatigue: weak physical strength, fatigability, physical weakness after illness or operation, anorexia, night sweating, and common cold (Fig. 8.4).

防已黄耆湯

boiogito (BOT) Fáng yǐ huáng qí tāng
Manifestation

1. Symptoms

- Tendency to sweat: Although one may sweat like a horse in summer, often there is no thirst.
- Tendency to fatigue: It is a bother to move, because the body feels heavy. Often feels fatigued and tends to tire easily. In addition to these tendencies, they have a hard time in the summer.
- Obesity: This is so-called bloating obesity.
- Arthralgia: There is swelling and pain in the joints; especially common in the knee joints. This formula, however, is usually not indicated for those with strong inflammation.
- Tendency of edema: Edema may be seen especially in the lower body.
- Decreased urine volume: Urine flow may be unsatisfactory.
- Skin disease: May be accompanied by urticaria, skin disease, skin ulcer, and suppuration.
- Irregular menstruation: Irregular menstruation and scanty menstruation may be observed.

2. Signs
   (i) Inspection: Fair-skinned, plump, fat body. Often the skin and muscles are slack.
   (ii) Tongue examination: Tongue body is slightly pale, and tongue coating may be thin and white.
   (iii) Pulse examination: Often, floating and weak.
   (iv) Abdominal examination:
   No specific abdominal manifestations reported
   Abdominal strength: Slightly soft (2/5)
   Abdominal manifestations
   Abdominal distention (often)
   Abdominal distention, "frog belly" (sometimes)
3. Indications
   Indicated for the following symptoms in patients with medium or deficiency pattern who are easily fatigued with a tendency to perspire profusely: swelling and pain of the knee joint with obesity, edema, hyperhidrosis, and obesity (a flabby constitution, so-called bloating obesity).

防風通聖散

Bofutsushosan (BTS) Fáng fēng tōng shèng sǎn
Manifestation

1. Symptoms

- Stiff shoulders and hot flashes: Tends to become irritable sometimes with stiff shoulders, headaches, and hot flashes.
- Obesity: Having ample physical strength, the obesity is often the firm variety, the so-called potbelly.
- Constipation
- Hypertension and hot flashes: Palpitations may occur.
- Skin disease: There may be purulent eczema, especially on the head and face.
- Paralysis and numbness: May be used for paralysis and numbness associated with cerebrovascular accidents.
- Sinusitis.

2. Signs
   (i) Inspection: Typically has a solid physique and tends to be obese. The complexion is relatively white but may have flushing and redness in the face.
   (ii) Tongue examination: Tongue body is crimson; tongue coating is thick, dry, and white or yellow.
   (iii) Pulse examination: Not deficient. Often rapid. It may be wiry or tight.
   (iv) Abdominal examination:
   No specific abdominal manifestations reported
   Abdominal strength: Slightly hard to full (4/5 to 5/5)
   Abdominal manifestations
   Abdominal distension, "potbelly" (usual)
3. Indications
   Indicated for the following symptoms in patients with excess pattern with thick subcutaneous fat in the abdomen and a tendency of constipation: Symptoms associated with hypertension including palpitation, shoulder stiffness, and flushing, obesity, edema, and constipation, empyema (sinusitis), eczema/dermatitis, pimples (acne), and obesity.

麻黄湯

Maoto (MT) Má huáng tāng
Manifestation

1. Symptoms

- Chills/fever: Initially there may be no fever.
- Severe headache: Headache and feeling of stiff neck.
- No sweating: No sweating is observed.

- In the case of acute febrile illness such as influenza, the pulse is floating and tight, and lack of sweating is characteristic. Lack of sweating may be confirmed by touching the back of a patient. This medicine must be stopped once the patient sweats and the fever subsides. Do not use on patients that are sweating from the beginning. For rhinitis, which is not an acute febrile disease, it may be used if the pulse is tight and there is no gastrointestinal disorder, ischemic heart disease, or prostatic hyperplasia.
- Joint pain.
- Panting: Sometimes patient is suffocating and gasping.
- Nasal congestion.

2. Signs
   (i) Inspection: In the case of acute febrile illness, do not use for those with pale faces.
   (ii) Tongue examination: The tongue body is unremarkable, and the tongue coating may be slightly white coating.
   (iii) Pulse examination: Often floating and tight.
   (iv) Abdominal examination:
   No specific abdominal manifestations reported
   Abdominal strength: Moderate to full (3/5 to 5/5)
3. Indications
   Indicated for the following symptoms in patients with excess pattern at the onset of a common cold, with chills and fever, headache, cough, pain in many joints, with no sweating: common cold, rhinorrhea, bronchitis, and stuffy nose (Fig. 8.1).
   Note: Do not use for patients with deficiency pattern.

麻黄附子細辛湯

Maobushisaishinto (MBST)Má huáng fù zǐ xì xīn tāng
Manifestation

1. Symptoms

- Chills: Feeling of cold is strong, but feeling of heat is little. When there is, it is often a mild fever.
- No sweating.
- Headache: Unremarkable.
- Malaise.
- Sore throat.
- Cough.
- Cold limbs.

2. Signs
   (i) Inspection: In cases of the common cold, the complexion is often pale, the sputum is watery and transparent, and nasal discharge is often seen.
   (ii) Tongue examination: The tongue body may be pale, and the tongue coating may be white.
   (iii) Pulse examination: Often deep and thin, but sometimes floating with a common cold.
   (iv) Abdominal examination:
   No specific abdominal manifestations reported
   Abdominal strength: Soft to slightly soft (1/5 to 2/5)
3. Indications
   Indicated for the following symptoms in patients with deficiency pattern who have cold limbs, sometimes with chills: common cold and bronchitis, bronchial asthma, and neuralgia (Fig. 8.1).

麻杏甘石湯

Makyokansekito (MKKS) Má xìng gān shí tāng
Manifestation

1. Symptoms

- Cough, dyspnea, respiratory urgency: Gokoto may cause a severe respiratory condition during an asthma attack.
- Sputum: Viscous sputum, often yellow.
- Fever: Indeterminate. There may be a feeling of heat.
- Spontaneous sweating: There may be no sweat.
- Thirst.
- Hemorrhoid pain.

2. Signs
   (i) Inspection: Often not used for pale complexion. Perspiration may be seen.
   (ii) Tongue examination: The tongue body is unremarkable; tongue coating is slightly dry, and may be yellow or thin white.
   (iii) Pulse examination: Floating, slippery, and rapid.
   (iv) Abdominal examination:
   No specific abdominal manifestations reported
   Abdominal strength: Moderate (3/5)
3. Indications
   Indicated for the following symptoms in patients with medium or excess pattern who have coughing and occasional thirst: coughing, infantile asthma, bronchial asthma, bronchitis, common cold, and hemorrhoid pain (Fig. 8.1).

五虎湯

Gokoto (GT) Wǔ hǔ tāng
Manifestation

1. Symptoms

- Cough, dyspnea, respiratory urgency: May experience severe respiratory distress during an asthma attack.
- Sputum: Viscous sputum, often yellow.
- Fever: Indeterminate. There may be a feeling of heat.
- Spontaneous sweating: There may be no sweat.
- Thirst.
- Hemorrhoid pain.

2. Signs
   (i) Inspection: Often not used for pale complexion. Perspiration may be seen.
   (ii) Tongue examination: The tongue body is unremarkable; tongue coating is slightly dry and may be yellow or thin white.
   (iii) Pulse examination: Floating, slippery, and rapid.
   (iv) Abdominal examination:
   No specific abdominal manifestations reported
   Abdominal strength: Moderate (3/5 to 4/5)
3. Indications
   Indicated for the following symptoms in patients with medium or excess pattern who have severe coughing: coughing, bronchial asthma, bronchitis, infantile asthma, common cold, and hemorrhoid pain.

麻杏薏甘湯

Makyoyokukanto (MKYK) Má xìng yì gān tāng
Manifestation

1. Symptoms

- Fever: Fever occurs in the evening.
- Myalgia/arthralgia: Not acute.
- Dry skin.
- Edema.
- Sweating tendency.

2. Signs
   (i) Inspection: The skin is often dry and dull. There may be a lot of dandruff. Edema can be observed.
   (ii) Tongue examination: The tongue body is unremarkable, and the tongue coating may be thin and white.
   (iii) Pulse examination: It may be deep and tight or floating and tight.
   (iv) Abdominal examination:
   No specific abdominal manifestations reported
   Abdominal strength: Moderate (3/5)
3. Indications
   Indicated for the following symptoms in patients with medium pattern: arthralgia, neuralgia, myalgia, warts, and rough hands and feet (eczema/dermatitis on the hands and feet).

麻子仁丸

Mashiningan (MNG) Mázĭ rén wán
Manifestation

1. Symptoms

- Habitual constipation: The stool may be dry, hard, and lumpy, especially in the elderly and frail.
- Frequent urination/nocturia.
- Hemorrhoids.

2. Signs
   (i) Inspection: Rabbit-like hard stools. The skin may be moistened with sweat.
   (ii) Tongue examination: The tongue body is unremarkable; tongue coating is slightly dry, and may be lacking.
   (iii) Pulse examination: It may be deep and weak or thin.
   (iv) Abdominal examination:
   No specific abdominal manifestations reported
   Abdominal strength: Slightly soft (2/5)
3. Indications
   Indicated for the following symptoms in patients with medium or deficiency pattern: constipation, dull headache, hot flashes, eczema, dermatitis, pimples (acne), anorexia, abdominal distension, abnormal intestinal fermentation, and hemorrhoids associated with constipation.

木防已湯

Mokuboito (MBT) Mù fáng yĭ tāng
Manifestation

1. Symptoms

- Dyspnea
- Respiratory distress
- Palpitations
- Edema
- Reduced urine volume/difficulty with urination
- Thirst
- Do not use it for people who are extremely debilitated or who have a floating and weak pulse. Use for those with fever such as dry mouth, frustration, and fever. For those lacking physical strength, use bukuryoukyouninnkanzoto.

2. Signs
   (i) Inspection: The complexion is dark and dull. Both edema and dyspnea occur, and in severe cases, orthopnea and cyanosis are observed.
   (ii) Tongue examination: The tongue body is unremarkable; the tongue coating is yellow, and it may be slightly dry.
   (iii) Pulse examination: Deep and tight. There may also be arrhythmia.
   (iv) Abdominal examination:
   Abdominal strength: Moderate to strong (3/5 to 5/5)
   Abdominal manifestations
   Strong epigastric stuffiness and resistance (usual)
   Abdominal distension (sometimes)
3. Indications
   Indicated for the following symptoms in patients with medium or excess pattern who have epigastric stuffiness and bad complexion: palpitations, dyspnea, bronchial asthma, and edema.

薏苡仁湯

Yokuininto (YT)Yì yǐ rén tāng
Manifestation

1. Symptoms

   - Numbness, pain, swelling, warmth, and heaviness in the limbs or the whole body: rheumatoid arthritis and arthritis in subacute and chronic stages. Water tends to collect in the affected area, accompanied by a feeling of heat and swelling pain.
   - Movement impairment.

2. Signs
   (i) Inspection: Arthritis with swelling and fluid[TM1] retention may be observed.
   (ii) Tongue examination: Tongue body is unremarkable, and tongue coating may be white or white and greasy.
   (iii) Pulse examination: May be slippery and floating or wiry.
   (iv) Abdominal examination:
   There is little literature.
   Abdominal strength: Slightly soft (2/5).
3. Indications
   Indicated for the following symptoms in patients with medium pattern who have swelling and pain in joints and muscles: joint pain, myalgia, and neuralgia.

抑肝散

Yokukansan (YKS) Yì gān sǎn
Manifestation

1. Symptoms

   - Tendency to get angry, irritated, and lose sleep (nervousness): A sedative effect can be expected, and this formula is indicated widely from children to the elderly. In recent years, it has also been applied to the treatment of behavioral and psychological symptoms of dementia (BPSD) and psychiatric disorders in patients with dementia. In addition, it can be widely used for various symptoms exacerbated by stress.
   - Headache, eye pain, cervical stiffness: It may be effective for eyestrain and headache caused by computer screens (VDT).
   - Eyelid/facial spasm, numbness of limbs, muscle spasm: May be used for sequelae of cerebrovascular accident. In recent years, it has been applied to intractable pain such as neuropathic pain and may also be used for restless legs syndrome (RLS).
   - Nausea, vomiting, and abdominal bloating: If these symptoms are present, consider yokukansankachimpi.

2. Signs
   (i) Inspection: Sometimes patients seem frustrated and restless. On the other hand, they may give the impression of being depressed.
   (ii) Tongue examination: The tongue body is often slightly red, and tongue coating may be white. In cases with white greasy moss, consider yokukansankachimpihange.
   (iii) Pulse examination: Often wiry.
   (iv) Abdominal examination:
   Abdominal strength: * Slightly soft to moderate (2/5 to 3/5)
   Abdominal manifestations
   Muscle tension in upper half of left rectus abdominis muscle (usual)
3. Indications
   Indicated for the following symptoms in patients with medium pattern with nervousness and tendency to get angry and irritable: Neurosis, insomnia, night crying in children, climactic disorder、miscellaneous symptoms associated with menstruation, and bruxism.

抑肝散加陳皮半夏

Yokukansankachimpihange (YKSCH) Yì gān sǎn jiā chén pí bàn xià
Manifestation

1. Symptoms

- Tendency to get angry, irritated, and lose sleep (nerve fogging): A sedative effect can be expected, and this formula is indicated widely from children to the elderly. In recent years, it has also been applied to the treatment of behavioral and psychological symptoms of dementia (BPSD) and psychiatric disorders in patients with dementia. In addition, it can be widely used for various symptoms exacerbated by stress.
- Headache, eye pain, cervical stiffness: It may be effective for eyestrain and headache caused by computer screens (VDT).
- Eyelid/facial spasm, numbness of limbs, muscle spasm: May be used for sequelae of cerebrovascular accident. In recent years, it has been applied to intractable pain such as neuropathic pain and may also be used for restless legs syndrome (RLS).
- Nausea, vomiting, and abdominal bloating

2. Signs
   (i) Inspection: Sometimes patients seem frustrated and restless. On the other hand, they may give the impression of being depressed.
   (ii) Tongue examination: The tongue body is often slightly red, and tongue coating may be white and greasy.
   (iii) Pulse examination: Often wiry.
   (iv) Abdominal examination:
   Abdominal strength: Soft to slightly soft (1/5 to 2/5)
   Abdominal manifestations
   Abdominal pulsations (usual)
   Abdominal muscle tension (usual)
3. Indications
   Indicated for the following symptoms in patients with medium or slight deficiency pattern with slightly weak digestion, nervousness, and a tendency to get angry and irritable: neurosis, insomnia, night crying in children, climactic disorder, miscellaneous symptoms associated with menstruation, and bruxism.

六君子湯

Rikkunshito (RKT) Liù jūn zǐ tāng
Manifestation

1. Symptoms

- Heaviness in stomach, anorexia, nausea/vomiting: Postprandial complaint syndrome including functional dyspepsia, non-erosive reflux disease, proton pump inhibitor-resistant gastroesophageal reflux disease (GERD).
- Abnormal throat sensation, hoarseness, sore throat, chronic cough: laryngopharyngeal reflux disease (LPRD) which presents with otolaryngological symptoms due to GERD

2. Signs
   (i) Inspection: Those with a history of chronic wasting disease may be thin and have a pale complexion and weak eyes. This formula, however, can be used widely regardless of the abovementioned signs.
   (ii) Tongue examination: The tongue body is swollen and has tooth marks. The tongue coating is often moist and white (or thick, white, and greasy).
   (iii) Pulse examination: Often deep and weak in cases of chronic wasting disease.
   (iv) Abdominal examination:
   Abdominal strength: Soft to slightly soft (1/5 to 2/5)
   Abdominal manifestations
   Splashing sound (usual)
   Epigastric stuffiness (usual)
3. Indications
   Indicated for the following symptoms in patients with medium or deficiency pattern who have a weak stomach, anorexia, and obstructive feeling in epigastrium, who are also easily fatigued, anemic, and likely to have cold limbs: gastritis, gastroenterol weakness, gastroptosis, indigestion, anorexia, gastric pain, and vomiting (Fig. 8.4).

立効散

Rikkosan (RS) Lì xiào sàn
Manifestation

1. Symptoms

- Toothache: It is often effective for dental caries-induced tooth pain, pulpitis-induced pain, and post-extraction pain.
- Pain in the oral cavity: Pain caused by the oral mucosa, such as aphthous ulcer, and glossodynia. Trigeminal neuralgia, glossopharyngeal neuralgia, etc.

2. Signs
   (i) Inspection: Unremarkable
   (ii) Tongue examination: Unremarkable

(iii) Pulse examination: Unremarkable
(iv) Abdominal examination:
There is little literature.

3. Indications
Indicated for the following symptoms in patients of any pattern: toothache and pain after tooth extraction.

竜胆瀉肝湯

Ryutanshakanto (RST) Lóng dǎn xiè gān tāng
Manifestation

1. Symptoms

- Headache, tinnitus, dizziness
- Eye conjunctival hyperemia: Conjunctivitis, keratitis, scleritis, uveitis, etc.
- Easy tendency to get angry, frustrated, and lose sleep.
- Chest and abdominal pain: Hepatobiliary disease
- Skin redness/pruritus: Skin diseases such as herpes zoster and psoriasis
- Itching/pain/swelling of the genital area, urinary abnormalities, abnormalities in the thorax: pudendal eczema, urethritis, pelvic inflammatory disease (endometritis/oviductitis/adnexitis), sexually transmitted diseases, Bartholin's gland flame, endometritis, etc.

2. Signs
(i) Inspection: The skin may be dark.
(ii) Tongue examination: The tongue body is often crimson. Tongue coating may be yellow and greasy.
(iii) Pulse examination: May be wiry and rapid.
(iv) Abdominal examination:
Abdominal strength: Slightly strong or strong (4/5 to 5/5)
Abdominal manifestations
Tension/hypersensitivity zone on the lateral margin of the rectus abdominis muscle (sometimes)
Tenderness in lower abdomen (sometimes)

3. Indications
Indicated for the following symptoms in patients with medium or excess pattern who feel heat and pain in the lower abdomen: Micturition pain, a feeling of residual urine, turbid urine, leukorrhea, and frequent urination.

苓甘姜味辛夏仁湯

Ryokankyomishingeninto (RKS) Líng gān jiāng wèi xīn xià rén tāng
Manifestation

1. Symptoms

- Respiratory symptoms such as wheezing, coughing, and shortness of breath. (When formulas with ephedra herb such as shoseiryuto cannot be used due to deficiency pattern.)
- Edema
- Cold sensitivity

2. Signs
(i) Inspection: The face and limbs may be edematous.
(ii) Tongue examination: The tongue body may have teeth marks. Tongue coating is unremarkable.
(iii) Pulse examination: Often deep or small.
(iv) Abdominal examination:
Abdominal strength: Soft to slightly soft (1/5 to 2/5)
Abdominal manifestations
Splashing sound (usual)

3. Indications
Indicated for the following symptoms in patients with medium or deficiency pattern who have gastrointestinal weakness, cold sensitivity, and copious sputum: Bronchitis, bronchial asthma, palpitation, dyspnea, and edema.

苓姜朮甘湯

Ryokyojutsukanto (RKYJK) Líng jiāng shù gān tāng
Manifestation

1. Symptoms

- Cold and painful from the waist down. Waist and hips feel heavy.
- Urine volume increases.

2. Signs
(i) Inspection: Unremarkable
(ii) Tongue examination: Unremarkable
(iii) Pulse examination: Often deep, slow, thin, or faint
(iv) Abdominal examination:
Abdominal strength: Soft to slightly soft (1/5 to 2/5)
Abdominal manifestations
Pulsations in epigastrium (sometimes)
Splashing sound (sometimes)

3. Indications
Indicated for the following symptoms in patients with medium or deficiency pattern who have coldness and pain from the waist down and a high urine output: low back pain, cold lower back, nocturnal enuresis, and neuralgia.

苓桂朮甘湯

Ryokeijutsukanto (RKJK) Líng guì shù gān tāng
Manifestation

1. Symptoms

- Dizziness, orthostatic hypotension, sensation of body swaying
- Shortness of breath, palpitations
- Headache
- Hot flash
- Reduced urine volume

2. Signs
   (i) Inspection: Flushing in the face may be seen.
   (ii) Tongue examination: Tongue body may have teeth marks. Tongue coating is unremarkable.
   (iii) Pulse examination: Deep and tight
   (iv) Abdominal examination:
   Abdominal strength: Soft to slightly soft (1/5 to 2/5)
   Abdominal manifestations
   Splashing sound (usual)
   Epigastric aortic pulsation (usual)
   Distension in epigastrium (sometimes)
   Epigastric stuffiness (sometimes)
3. Indications
   Indicated for the following symptoms in patients with medium or deficiency pattern who have dizziness and light-headed feeling, sometimes hot flashes and palpitations: orthostatic hypotension, dizziness, headache, tinnitus, palpitation, shortness of breath, neurosis, and nervousness (Fig. 8.2).

六味丸

Rokumigan (RJG) Liù wèi wán

Manifestation

1. Symptoms

- Tendency to fatigue, malaise.
- Numbness, especially in lower body.
- Reduced urine volume, polyuria, nocturnal urine, enuresis, feeling of residual urine.
- Erectile dysfunction, nocturnal emission.
- Low back pain.
- Dry mouth.
- Hot flashes in limbs: Even if there is coldness, it is mild.

2. Signs
   (i) Inspection: The complexion and lips are pale, the skin has little redness, and it tends to be dry.
   (ii) Tongue examination: Tongue body is red or dark red, and the tongue coating is often absent or dry and slightly white.
   (iii) Pulse examination: Often deep and rapid or thin and rapid.
   (iv) Abdominal examination:
   Abdominal strength: Soft to moderate (1/5 to 3/5)
   Abdominal manifestations
   Weakness of the lower abdominal region (sometimes)
3. Indications
   Indicated for the following symptoms in patients with medium or deficiency pattern who easily fatigue and have decreased urine volume, or polyuria, occasional hot flashes in limbs, and dry mouth: Dysuria, feeling of residual urine, frequent urination, edema, itching, nocturnal urination, and numbness.

9 List of Crude Drugs

Toshiaki Makino

Below, crude drugs used as the components in 148 ethical Kampo products and OTC Kampo products (approved by Japanese Government) introduced in this book are summarized in the order of alphabet by Japanese pronunciation. The information for each item includes the names, origin, representative constituents, effects and principal Kampo formulas that contain it. The origin is according to the definition in the Japanese Pharmacopoeia Eighteenth Edition (shown as [JP]) or the Japanese standards for non-pharmacopoeial crude drugs 2018 (shown as [non-JP]) [1, 2]. The representative constituents are not pharmacologically active ingredients as described above (see Chap. 4, Sect. 1.4), but these compounds are characteristically contained in the crude drug as the marker constituents. As for the effects, the specific effects are listed after the traditional taste and character [3]. As for the principal Kampo formula, the representative ones approved as ethical Kampo products are shown; the formulas approved only as OTC Kampo products are denoted in "etc."

Effect of Crude Drugs

The effects of crude drugs adopted in this book are expressed as traditional medical terms (*yakuno*) in herbological books published in Edo period, and as modern medical terms (pharmacology, *yakuri*) in textbooks of pharmacognosy after Western medicine was introduced to Japan after Meiji era. The meanings of physiological and pathological terms changed in the Edo period due to the introduction of Western medicine. So, even if the terms for effects appear the same in this book, the meanings of the terms can be distinguished in this book, whether traditional or Western medical sense. For example, "fluid[TM1]-regulating" is a term of traditional medicine for eliminating the stagnation of fluid[TM1] flow, and "diuresis" is the term in Western medicine for promoting the excretion of urine. In traditional medicine, "phlegm[TM]" refers to non-physiological high viscosity turbid secretions resulting from stagnant fluid[TM] flow. In Western medicine, on the other hand, "phlegm" is produced as a result of white blood cells engulfing foreign substances such as bacteria that have invaded the bronchi and lungs. The term "resolving phlegm" literally means to remove "phlegm," but it exclusively means to discharge phlegm in the sense of Western medicine, which is a little different from "resolving phlegm[TM]" in traditional medicine. For this reason, in this text, the term "expectorant" in the Western medical sense and "resolving phlegm[TM]" in the traditional medical sense, so that these two can be distinguished.

Akyo Donkey Glue[Non-JP], アキョウ, 阿膠

Origin: The dried material of fat-removed hot water extract of the skin, bone, sinew or ligament of *Equus asinus* Linné (Equidae), from which the hair has been removed.
Ingredients: Collagen, etc.
Effects: Sweet, neutral. Tonifying blood[TM1], hemostatic, tonifying qi, analgesic (menorrhalgia etc.), antitussive, relieving hematemesis, moistening dryness, stomachic and anti-flatulent
Representative Kampo formula: Choreito, Kyukikyogaito, Unkeito, etc.

Baimo, Fritillaria Bulb[JP], バイモ, 貝母

Origin: The dried bulb of *Fritillaria verticillata* Willdenow var. *thunbergii* Baker (Liliaceae)
Ingredients: Steroid alkaloids, peimine, verticine, etc.
Effects: Bitter, cold. Antitussive, expectorant, resolving phlegm, clearing heat, discharging pus
Representative Kampo formula: Seihaito, Jiinshihoto

T. Makino (✉)
Department of Pharmacognosy, Graduate School of Pharmaceutical Sciences, Nagoya City University, Nagoya, Japan

Kampo Medical Literature Editorial Committee, Narita, Japan
e-mail: office@jsom.or.jp

Kampo Medical Literature Editorial Committee, The Japan Society for Oriental Medicine (ed.), *Complete Japanese Traditional (Kampo) Medicine*, https://doi.org/10.1007/978-981-96-7143-4_9

Bakuga, Malt[JP], バクガ, 麦芽

Origin: The dried ripe cariopsis of *Hordeum vulgare* Linné (Gramineae), after being germinated
Ingredients: Saccharides, maltose, etc.
Effects: Sweet, neutral. Stomachic and anti-flatulent, tonifying qi, resolving phlegm
Representative Kampo formula: Hangebyakujutsutemmato

Bakumondo, Ophiopogon Root[JP], バクモンドウ, 麦門冬

Origin: The dried enlarged part of the root of *Ophiopogon japonicus* Ker-Gawler (Liliaceae)
Ingredients: Steroid-saponins, ophiopogonin A–D, etc.
Effects: Sweet, mild cold. Antitussive, moistening dryness, tonifying qi, expectorant, alleviating lung[TM1] atrophy disorder
Representative Kampo formula: Bakumondoto, Jiinkokato, Chitosan, etc.

Binroji, Areca[JP], ビンロウジ, 檳榔子

Origin: The dried seed of *Areca catechu* Linné (Palmae)
Ingredients: Pyridine alkaloids, arecoline, etc.
Effects: Bitter pungent, warm. Deworming, stomachic and anti-flatulent, regulating fluid[TM1], astringent, resolving phlegm, descending qi, regulating qi, miotic
Representative Kampo formula: Kumibinroto, Nyoshinsan

Biwayo, Loquat Leaf[JP], ビワヨウ, 枇杷葉

Origin: The dried leaf of *Eriobotrya japonica* Lindley (Rosaceae)
Ingredients: Cyanogenic glycosides, amygdalin, etc.
Effects: Pungent, neutral. Antitussive, stomachic and anti-flatulent, moistening dryness, relieving nausea, expectorant, descending qi, relieving skin disease
Representative Kampo formula: Shin'iseihaito

Bofu, Saposhnikovia Root and Rhizome[JP], ボウフウ, 防風

Origin: The dried root and rhizome of *Saposhnikovia divaricata* Schischkin (Umbelliferae)
Ingredients: Chromone derivatives, 4'-*O*-glucosyl-5-*O*-methylvisamminol, etc.
Effects: Pungent, sweet, mild warm. Analgesic (arthralgia, headache, etc.), releasing exterior, eliminating wind, antipyretic, anti-spastic
Representative Kampo formula: Bofutsushosan, Chitosan, Ryutanshakanto, etc.

Boi, Sinomenium Stem and Rhizome[JP], ボウイ, 防已

Origin: The dried climbing stem and rhizome of *Sinomenium acutum* Rehder et Wilson (Menispermaceae); usually cut transversely
Ingredients: Alkaloids, sinomenine, etc.
Effects: Bitter, pungent, cold. Regulating fluid[TM1], diuretic, analgesic (neuralgia, etc.), resolving damp-heat
Representative Kampo formula: Boiogito, Mokuboito, Sokeikakketsuto, etc.

Bokusoku, Quercus Bark[JP], ボクソク, 樸樕

Origin: The dried bark of *Quercus acutissima* Carruthers, *Quercus serrata* Murray, *Quercus mongolica* Fischer ex Ledebour var. *crispula* Ohashi or *Quercus variabilis* Blume (Fagaceae)
Ingredients: Tannins, acutissimin A, etc.
Effects: Bitter, neutral. Astringent
Representative Kampo formula: Jumihaidokuto, Jidabokuippo, etc.

Borei, Oyster Shell[JP], ボレイ, 牡蛎

Origin: The shell of *Ostrea gigas* Thunberg (Ostreidae)
Ingredients: calcium carbonate, etc.
Effects: salty, mild cold. Sedative, anhidrotic, resolving night sweats, sedative, antacid
Representative Kampo formula: Anchusan, Keishikaryukotsuboreito, Saikokaryukotsuboreito

Bosho, Sodium Sulfate[JP], ボウショウ, 芒硝

Origin: The mineral substance, mainly composed of sodium sulfate hydrate ($Na_2SO_4 \cdot 10H_2O$)
Ingredients: Sodium sulfate, etc.
Effects: salty bitter, cold. Purgative, clearing heat, diuretic
Representative Kampo formula: Daijokito, Tokakujokito, daiobotampito, etc.

Botampi, Moutan Bark[JP], ボタンピ, 牡丹皮

Origin: The dried root bark of *Paeonia suffruticosa* Andrews (Paeoniaceae)
Ingredients: Phenols, paeonol, etc.
Effects: Bitter sweet, mild cold. Resolving blood[TM1] stasis, analgesic (headache, etc.), clearing heat, cooling blood[TM1] heat, anti-inflammatory, resolving women's diseases (dysmenorrhea, etc.)

Representative Kampo formula: Unkeito, Kamishoyosan, Keishibukuryogan, etc.

Bukuryo, Poria Sclerotium[JP], ブクリョウ, 茯苓

Origin: The dried sclerotium of *Wolfiporia cocos* Ryvarden et Gilbertson (Polyporaceae), from which usually the external layer has been mostly removed
Ingredients: Sterols, ergosterol, etc.
Effects: Light sweet, neutral. Diuretic, regulating fluid[TM1], resolving fluid[TM1] retention in stomach, purging heart, sedative, stomachic and anti-flatulent, relieving dizziness
Representative Kampo formula: Ryokeijutsukanto, Goreisan, Shimbuto, etc.

Bushi, Processed Aconite Root[JP], ブシ, 附子

Origin: The dried tuberous root of *Aconitum carmichaeli* Debeaux or *Aconitum japonicum* Thunberg (Ranunculaceae) prepared by the following processes. Process 1: Autoclaving. [Processed Aconite Root 1] Process 2: Heating or autoclaving after rinsing in salt or rock salt solution. [Processed Aconite Root 2] Process 3: Treating with calcium hydroxide after rinsing in salt solution. [Processed Aconite root 3]
Ingredients: Alkaloids, aconitine, etc.
Effects: Pungent, hot. Analgesic (arthralgia etc.), dispelling cold, relieving abdominal colic, anti-diarrheic, regulating fluid[TM1], boosting metabolism, relieving impediment disorder, cardiotonic, diuretic
Representative Kampo formula: Shimbuto, Hachimijiogan, Maobushisaishinto, etc.

Byakugo, Lilium Bulb[JP], ビャクゴウ, 百合

Origin: The dried scaly leaves of *Lilium lancifolium* Thunberg, *Lilium brownii* F.E.Brown var. *colchesteri* Wilson, Lilium brownii F.E. Brown or *Lilium pumilum* De Candolle (Liliaceae), usually with the application of steaming
Ingredients: Phenylpropanoid derivatives, regaloside A, etc.
Effects: Sweet, mild cold. Antitussive, sedative, clearing heat, moistening lung[TM1], tonifying qi
Representative Kampo formula: Shin'iseihaito.

Byakyosan, Stiff Silkworm[Non-JP], ビャッキョウサン, 白殭蚕, 白彊蚕, 白姜蚕, 白僵蚕

Origin: The dried rigid larva of *Bombyx mori* Linné Bombycidae) infected by *Beauveria bassiana* Vuillemin (Cordycepitaceae)
Effects: Pungent salty, neutral. Anti-pyretic, analgesic, anti-spastic
Representative Kampo formula: Uyakujunkisan

Byakujutsu, Atractylodes Rhizome[JP], ビャクジュツ, 白朮

Origin: The dried rhizome of *Atractylodes japonica* Koidzumi ex Kitamura (Compositae) (Wa-byakujutsu) or *Atractylodes macrocephala* Koidzumi (Atractylodes ovata De Candolle) (Compositae) (Kara-byakujutsu)
Ingredients: Sesquiterpenoids, atractylone, etc.
Effects: Sweet bitter, warm. Diuretic, regulating fluid[TM1], analgesic (arthralgia etc.), anti-diarrheic, tonifying qi, drying dampness, resolving fluid[TM1] retention in stomach, resolving phlegm, aromatic stomachic, anti-perspirant
Representative Kampo formula: Tokishakuyakusan, Goreisan, Juzentaihoto, etc.

Byakushi, Angelica Dahurica Root[JP], ビャクシ, 白芷

Origin: The dried root of *Angelica dahurica* Bentham et Hooker filius ex Franchet et Savatier (Umbelliferae)
Ingredients: Furanocoumarin derivatives: byakangelicin, etc.
Effects: Pungent, warm. Analgesic (headache, etc.), discharging pus, resolving vaginal discharge, sedative, eliminating wind
Representative e Kampo formula: Keigairengyoto, Goshakusan, Seijobofuto, etc.

Chayo, Green tea leaf[Non-JP], チャヨウ, 茶葉

Origin: The dried leaf of *Cameria sinensis* (Linné) Kuntze (Theaceae), and sometimes accompanied with its branches
Ingredients: Alkaloids, caffeine, etc.
Effects: Bitter, mild sweet, mild cold. Diuretic, analeptic, analgesic
Representative Kampo formula: Senkyuchachosan

Chikujo , Bamboo Culm[Non-JP], チクジョ, 竹筎

Origin: The dried inner culm of *Bambusa tuldoides* Munro, *Phyllostachys nigra* Munro var. *henonis* Stapf ex Rendle or *Phyllostachys bambusoides* Siebold et Zuccarini (Gramineae)
Ingredients: Triterpenoids, friedelin, etc.
Effects: Sweet, mild cold. Resolving hematemesis, antipyretic, cooling, haemostasis, antitussive, preventing miscarriage
Representative Kampo formula: Seihaito, Chikujountanto

Chikuyo, Bamboo Leaf[Non-JP], チクヨウ, 竹葉

Origin: The dried leaf of *Phyllostachys nigra* Munro var. *henonis* Stapf ex Rendle, *P. bambusoides* Siebold et

Zuccarini, *Bambusa textilis* McClure or *B. emeiensis* L. C. Chia et H. L. Fung (Gramineae)
Effects: Sweet, cold. Anti-pyretic, diuretic
Representative Kampo formula: Chikuyosekkoto

Chimo, Anemarrhena Rhizome[JP], チモ, 知母

Origin: The dried rhizome of *Anemarrhena asphodeloides* Bunge (Liliaceae)
Ingredients: Steroid-saponins: timosaponinA-I, A-III, etc.
Effects: Bitter, cold. Clearing heat, moistening dryness, anti-pyretic, diuretic, resolving alternating fever and chills disorder, sedative
Representative Kampo formula: Sansoninto, Jiinkokato, Shofusan, etc.

Chimpi, Citrus Unshiu Peel[JP], チンピ, 陳皮

Origin: The dried pericarp of the ripe fruit of *Citrus unshiu* Marcowicz or *Citrus reticulata* Blanco (Rutaceae)
Ingredients: Flavonoids, hesperidin, etc.
Effects: Pungent bitter, warm. Aromatic and bitter stomachic and anti-flatulent, antitussive, resolving phlegm, expectorant, anti-emesis
Representative Kampo formula: Rikkunshito, Kososan, Heiisan, etc.

Choji, Clove, チョウジ[JP], 丁子

Origin: The dried flowering bud of *Syzygium aromaticum* Merrill et Perry (*Eugenia caryophyllata* Thunberg) (Myrtaceae)
Ingredients: Phenylpropanoids, eugenol, etc.
Effects: Pungent, warm. Aromatic stomachic and anti-flatulent, dispelling cold
Representative Kampo formula: Jidabokuippo, Nyoshinsan

Chorei, Polyporus Sclerotium[JP], チョレイ, 猪苓

Origin: The dried sclerotium of *Polyporus umbellatus* Fries (Polyporaceae)
Ingredients: Sterols, ergosterol, etc.
Effects: Light sweet, neutral. Moistening dryness, diuretic, regulating fluid[TM1], drying dampness, anti-pyretic
Representative Kampo formula: Ireito, Inchingoreisan, Choreito, etc.

Chotoko, Uncaria Hook[JP], チョウトウコウ, 釣藤鈎

Origin: The dried hook or the hook-bearing stem of *Uncaria rhynchophylla* Miquel, Uncaria sinensis Haviland or *Uncaria macrophylla* Wallich (Rubiaceae), sometimes after being passed through hot water or steamed
Ingredients: Indole alkaloids, rhynchophylline, etc.
Effects: Sweet, mild cold. Sedative, anti-spastic, relieving dizziness, calming liver[TM1], purging heart[TM1], analgesic (headache, etc.), relieving hypertension
Representative Kampo formula: Chitosan, Yokukansan, Shichimotsukokato, etc.

Daifukuhi, Areca Pericarp[Non-JP], ダイフクヒ, 大腹皮

Origin: The dried fruit skin of *Areca catechu* Linné or *Areca dicksonii* Roxburgh (Palmae)
Ingredients: Tannins
Effects: Pungent, mild warm. Regulating qi, diuresis, stomachic
Representative Kampo formula: Bunshoto, Kakkoshokisan, Kyososan, etc.

Daio, Rhubarb, ダイオウ, 大黄

Origin: The rhizome of *Rheum palmatum* Linné, *Rheum tanguticum* Maximowicz. *Rheum officinale* Baillon, *Rheum coreanum* Nakai or their interspecific hybrids (Polygonaceae)
Ingredients: Dianthrone glycosides, sennoside A–F, etc.
Effects: Bitter, cold. Purgative, resolving blood[TM1] stasis, clearing heat, stomachic and anti-flatulent, resolving jaundice, resolving sensation of abdominal fullness, anti-inflammatory, relieving abdominal mass, relieving abdominal colic, removing pimples, relieving hot flash and hemorrhoids associated with constipation
Representative Kampo formula: Daiokanzoto, Tokakujokito, Otsujito, etc.

Dokukatsu, Aralia Rhizome[JP], ドクカツ, 独活

Origin: The rhizome of *Aralia cordata* Thunberg (Araliaceae)
Ingredients: Diterpenoids, ent-kaurenoic acid, etc.
Effects: Bitter pungent, mild warm. Analgesic (headache, arthralgia, etc.), relieving impediment disorder, anti-pyretic, releasing exterior, relieving gastroenteritis
Representative Kampo formula: Jumihaidokuto, Sokeikakketsuto

Engosaku, Corydalis Tuber[JP], エンゴサク, 延胡索

Origin: The dried tuber of *Corydalis turtschaninovii* Basser forma *yanhusuo* Y. H. Chou and C. C. Hsu (Papaveraceae), usually after being passed through hot water
Ingredients: Alkaloids, dehydrocorydaline, etc.
Effects: Pungent bitter, warm. Resolving blood[TM1] stasis, analgesic (afterpains, menorrhalgia, headache, abdominal pain, menorrhalgia, etc.), relieving women's diseases (dysmenorrhea, etc.), anti-spastic, regulating qi

Representative Kampo formula: Anchusan

Gaiyo, Artemisia Leaf[JP], ガイヨウ, 艾葉

Origin: The dried leaf and twig of *Artemisia princeps* Pampanini or *Artemisia montana* Pampanini (Compositae)
Ingredients: Monoterpenoids, 1,8-cineole, etc.
Effects: Pungent bitter, warm. Hemostasis, resolving metrorrhafia and metrostaxis, resolving hematemesis, anti-diarrheic, dispelling cold, astringent
Representative Kampo formula: Kyukikyogaito

Genjin, Scrophularia Root[Non-JP], ゲンジン, 玄参

Origin: The dried root of *Scrophularia ningpoensis* Hemsley or *Scrophularia buergeriana* Miquel (Scrophulariaceae)
Ingredients: Iridoids, harpagide, etc.
Effects: Bitter, salty. Nourishing yin, anti-inflammatory, anti-pyretic, sedative
Representative Kampo formula: Kamiuntanto, Shinsentaitsuko, seinetsuhokito, etc.

Goboshi, Burdock Fruit[JP], ゴボウシ, 牛蒡子

Origin: The dried fruit of *Arctium lappa* Linné (Compositae)
Ingredients: Lignans, arctiin, etc.
Effects: Pungent bitter, cold. Anti-pyretic, anti-inflammatory, discharging pus, detoxication, eliminate wind, analgesic (pharyngeal pain, etc.), moistening lung[TM1], resolving serious skin eruption and relieving urticaria
Representative Kampo formula: Saikoseikanto, Shofusan

Goma, Sesame[JP], ゴマ, 胡麻

Origin: The dried seed of *Sesamum indicum* Linné (Pedaliaceae)
Ingredients: Fatty acids: linoleic acid, etc.
Effects: Sweet, neutral. Qi tonifying, detoxication, purgative, nourishing yin
Representative Kampo formula: Shofusan

Goma-abura, Sesame oil[JP], ゴマ油

Origin: The fixed oil obtained from the seeds of *Sesamum indicum* Linneá (Pedaliaceae)成
Ingredients: Triglycerides
Effects: Used as ointment base
Representative Kampo formula: Shiunko, Chuoko

Gomishi, Schisandra Fruit[JP], ゴミシ, 五味子

Origin: The dried fruit of *Schisandra chinensis* Baillon (Schisandraceae)
Ingredients: Lignans, gomisin A, etc.
Effects: sour, warm. Antitussive, expectorant, moistening dryness, tonifying qi, nourishing yin, astringent
Representative Kampo formula: Shoseiryuto, Seishoekkito, seihaito, etc.

Goshitsu, Achyranthes Root[JP], ゴシツ, 牛膝

Origin: The dried root of *Achyranthes fauriei* Leveillé et Vaniot or *Achyranthes bidentata* Blume (Amaranthaceae)
Ingredients: Triterpenoid-saponins: Achyranthoside A–F, etc.
Effects: Bitter sweet, sour neutral. Resolving blood[TM1] stasis, analgesic, relieving stranguria, relieving impediment disorder, tonifying kidney[TM1], diuretic, resolving women's diseases (dysmenorrhea, etc.)
Representative Kampo formula: Goshajinkigan, Sokeikakketsuto, Daibofuto, etc.

Goshuyu, Euodia Fruit[JP], ゴシュユ, 呉茱萸

Origin: The dried fruit of *Euodia ruticarpa* Hooker filius et Thomson, *Euodia officinalis* Dode or *Euodia bodinieri* Dode
Ingredients: Alkaloids; evodiamine, etc.
Effects: Pungent bitter, hot. Analgesic (headache etc.), anti-emesis, stomachic and anti-flatulent, deworming, relieving abdominal colic, dispelling cold, descending qi, regulating qi, drying dampness, resolving phlegm, reducing acid reflux, relieving nausea and reducing sensitivity to cold
Representative Kampo formula: Goshuyuto, Tokishigyakukagoshuyushokyoto, Unkeito, etc.

Hakka, Mentha Herb[JP], ハッカ, 薄荷

Origin: The dried terrestrial part of *Mentha arvensis* Linné var. *piperascens* Malinvaud (Labiatae)
Ingredients: Monoterpenoids, menthol, etc.
Effects: Pungent, cold. Releasing exterior, analgesic (headache, etc.), clearing brain and eyes, clearing heat, aromatic stomachic and anti-flatulent, relieving gastroenteritis
Representative Kampo formula: Kamishoyosan, Keigairengyoto, Bofutsushosan, etc.

Hamabofu, Glehnia Root and Rhizome[JP], ハマボウフウ, 浜防風

Origin: The dried root and rhizome of *Glehnia littoralis* Fr. Schmidt ex Miquel (Umbeliferae)
Ingredients: Furanocoumarins, osthenol-7-*O*-β-gentiobioside, etc.
Effects: Substitute for Saposhnikovia Root and Rhizome
Representative Kampo formula: Seijobofuto, Keigairengyoto

Hange, Pinellia Tuber[JP], ハンゲ, 半夏

Origin: The dried tuber of *Pinellia ternata* Breitenbach (Araceae), from which the cork layer has been removed
Ingredients: Phenols, homogentisic acid, etc.
Effects: Pungent, warm. Anti-emesis, analgesic (angina, etc.), antitussive, regulating fluid[TM1], resolving phlegm, expectorant, resolving fluid[TM1] retention in stomach, descending qi, drying dampnessRepresentative Kampo formula: Hangeshashinto, Rikkunshito, Shosaikoto, etc.

Inchinko, Artemisia Capillaris Flower[JP], インチンコウ, 茵蔯蒿

Origin: The dried capitulum of *Artemisia capillaris* Thunberg (Compositae)
Ingredients: Chromone derivatives, capillarisin, etc.
Effects: Bitter, mild cold. Resolving jaundice, diuretic, resolving damp-heat, choleretic, diuretic, anti-inflammatory
Representative Kampo formula: Inchinkoto, inchingoreisan

Ireisen, Clematis Root[JP], イレイセン, 威霊仙

Origin: The dried root with rhizome of *Clematis chinensis* Osbeck, *Clematis mandshurica* Ruprecht or *Clematis hexapetala* Pallas (Ranunculaceae)
Ingredients: Triterpenoid-saponins, clematis chinenoside A–C, etc.
Effects: Pungent salty, warm. Dispelling wind-damp (relieving rheumatoid arthritis), analgesic (pain in the low back and knee coldness, neuralgia, etc.), diuretic, resolving phlegm
Representative Kampo formula: Sokeikakketsuto, Nijutsuto

Jikoppi, Lycium Bark[JP], ジコッピ, 地骨皮

Origin: The dried root bark of *Lycium chinense* Miller or *Lycium barbarum* Linné (Solanaceae)
Ingredients: Alkaloids, kukoamine A, etc.
Effects: Sweet, cold. Anti-pyretic, clearing heat, tonifying qi, antitussive
Representative Kampo formula: Jiinshihoto, Seishinrenshiin

Jio, Kanjio, Rehmannia Root[JP], ジオウ, 地黄, 乾地黄

Origin: The dried root of *Rehmannia glutinosa* Liboschitz var. *purpurea* Makino or *Rehmania glutinosa* Liboschitz (Scrophulariaceae)
Ingredients: Iridoids, catalpol, etc.
Effects: Sweet bitter, cold. Tonifying blood[TM1], tonifying qi, resolving hematemesis, clearing heat, anti-pyretic, resolving metrorrhagia and metrostaxis
Representative Kampo formula: Shimotsuto, Goshajinkigan, Shichimotsukokato, etc.

Jukujio, Processed Rehmannia Root[JP], ジュクジオウ, 熟地黄

Origin: The dried steamed root of *Rehmannia glutinosa* Liboschitz var. *purpurea* Makino or *Rehmania glutinosa* Liboschitz (Scrophulariaceae)
Ingredients: Iridoids, catalpol, etc.
Effects: Sweet, mild warm. Tonifying blood[TM1], tonifying kidney[TM1], tonifying qi, resolving women's diseases (dysmenorrhea, etc.), resolving alternating chills and fever, anti-pyretic
Representative Kampo formula: Shimotsuto, Goshajinkigan, Shichimotsukokato, etc.

Kakkon, Pueraria Root[JP], カッコン, 葛根

Origin: The dried root of *Pueraria lobata* Ohwi (Leguminosae), from which periderm has been removed
Ingredients: Isoflavonoids, puerarin, etc.
Effects: Sweet pungent, cold. Releasing exterior, moistening dryness, clearing heat, anti-pyretic, anti-spastic
Representative Kampo formula: Kakkonto, Kakkontokasenkyushin'I, Jinsoin, etc.

Kankyo, Processed Ginger[JP], カンキョウ, 乾姜

Origin: The dried rhizome of *Zingiber officinale* Roscoe (Zingiberaceae), after being passed through hot water or being steamed
Ingredients: Phenols, [6]-shogaol, etc.
Effects: Pungent, very hot. Dispelling cold, analgesic (abdominal pain, flank pain, etc.), anti-emesis, antitussive, resolving phlegm, aromatic stomachic
Representative Kampo formula: Shoseiryuto, Ninjinto, daikenchuto, etc.

Karokon, Trichosanthes Root[JP], カロコン, 栝楼根

Origin: The dried root of *Trichosanthes kirilowii* Maximowicz, *Trichosanthes kirilowii* Maximowicz var. *japonica* Kitamura or *Trichosanthes bracteata* Voigt (Cucurbitaceae), from which the cortical layer has been removed
Ingredients: Starches, etc.
Effects: Sweet, mild bitter, sour, mild cold. Moistening dryness, anti-pyretic, antitussive, discharging pus, promoting lactation
Representative Kampo formula: Saikokeishikankyoto, Saikoseikanto

Karonin, Trichosanthes Seed[JP], カロニン, 栝楼仁

Origin: The dried seed of *Trichosanthes kirilowii* Maximowicz, *Trichosanthes kirilowii* Maximowicz var.

japonica Kitamura or *Trichosanthes bracteata* Voigt (Cucurbitaceae)
Ingredients: Fatty acids, etc.
Effects: Sweet, cold. Resolving phlegm, antitussive, expectorant, anti-pyretic, relieving abdominal mass
Representative Kampo formula: Saikanto

Kashu, Polygonum Root[JP], カシュウ, 何首烏

Origin: The dried root of *Polygonum multiflorum* Thunberg (Polygonaceae), often being cut into round slices
Ingredients: Anthraquinones, chrysophanol, etc.
Effects: Bitter sweet, mild warm. Tonifying kidney[TM1], tonifying qi, tonifying blood[TM], tonifying liver[TM1], purgative, darkening hair, resolving serious skin eruption, alleviating lung atrophy disorder
Representative Kampo formula: Tokiinshi

Kanzo, Glycyrrhiza[JP], カンゾウ, 甘草

Origin: The dried root and stolon, with (unpeeled) or without (peeled) the periderm, of *Glycyrrhiza uralensis* Fischer or *Glycyrrhiza glabra* Linné (Leguminosae)
Ingredients: Triterpenoid-saponins, glycyrrhizic acid, etc.
Effects: Sweet, neutral. Analgesic (angina, throat pain, etc.), anti-spastic, antitussive, expectorant, anti-ulcer, harmonizing other drugs
Representative Kampo formula: Kakkonto, Keishito, Maoto, etc.

Kasseki, Aluminum Silicate Hydrate with Silicon Dioxide[JP], カッセキ, 滑石

Origin: A mineral substance, mainly composed of aluminum silicate hydrate and silicon dioxide
Ingredients: Aluminum silicate hydrate with silicon dioxide
Effects: sweet, cold. Diuretic, moistening dryness, anti-inflammatory
Representative Kampo formula: Gorinsan, Choreito, Bofutsushosan, etc.

Keigai, Schizonepeta Spike[JP], ケイガイ, 荊芥穂

Origin: The dried spike of *Schizonepeta tenuifolia* Briquet (Labiatae)
Ingredients: Monoterpenoids, menthone, etc.
Effects: Pungent, warm. Releasing exterior, eliminating wind, anti-pyretic, detoxification, analgesic (headache, etc.), resolving serious skin eruption, resolving skin disease
Representative Kampo formula: Keigairengyoto, Jumihaidokuto, Seijobofuto, etc.

Keihi, Cinnamon Bark[JP], ケイヒ, 桂皮

Origin: The dried bark of the trunk of *Cinnamomum cassia* Blume (Lauraceae), or such bark from which a part of the periderm has been removed
Ingredients: Phenylpropanoids, cinnamaldehyde, etc.
Effects: Pungent sweet, hot. Releasing exterior, tonifying qi, tonifying kidney[TM1], dispelling cold, aromatic stomachic, anti-emesis, anti-pyretic, analgesic (headache, etc.), dryness-moistening, alleviating diabetes
Representative Kampo formula: Kakkonto, Keishibukuryogan, Hachimijiogan, etc.

Keishi, Cinnamon Twig[JP], ケイシ, 桂枝

Origin: The dried twig of *Cinnamomum cassia* Blume (Lauraceae)Ingredients: Phenylpropanoids, cinnamaldehyde, etc.
Effects: Pungent sweet, warm. Releasing exterior, analgesic (headache etc.), descending qi
Representative Kampo formula: Kakkonto, Keishibukuryogan, Saikokeishito, etc.

Kikuka, Chrysanthemum Flower[JP], キクカ, 菊花

Origin: The dried capitulum of *Chrysanthemurn morifolium* Ramatulle or *Chrysanthemum indicum* Linné (Compositae)
Ingredients: Flavonoids, apigenin, etc.
Effects: Sweet mild bitter, mild cold. Relieving eye strain, analgesic (eye swelling pain, headache, etc.), relieving dizziness, eliminate wind, anti-pyretic, detoxification, anti-inflammatory
Representative Kampo formula: Chitosan

Kikyo, Platycodon Root[JP], キキョウ, 桔梗根

Origin: The dried root of *Platycodon grandiflorum* A. De Candolle (Campanulaceae)
Ingredients: Triterpenoid-saponins, platycodin A, etc.
Effects: Bitter pungent, neutral. Expectorant, discharging pus, antitussive, analgesic (angina, pain at the sides of the chest, etc.)
Representative Kampo formula: Kikyoto, Keigairengyoto, Goshakusan, etc.

Kijitsu, Immature Orange[JP], キジツ, 枳実

Origin: The dried immature fruit or the fruit cut crosswise of *Citrus aurantium* Linné var. *daidai* Makino, *Citrus aurantium* Linné or *Citrus natsudaidai* Hayata (Rutaceae)

Ingredients: Flavonoids, hesperidin, etc.

Effects: Bitter, mild cold. Aromatic and bitter stomachic and anti-flatulent, relieving abdominal mass, purging heart[TM1], resolving phlegm

Representative Kampo formula: Daijokito, daisaikoto, Shigyakusan, etc.

Kikoku, Orange Fruit, キコク, 枳殻

Origin: The dried unripe fruit of *Citrus aurantium* Linné (Rutaceae)

Ingredients: Flavonoids hesperidin, etc.

Effects: Bitter, mild cold. Regulating qi, stomachic and anti-flatulent, relieving sensation of abdominal fullness

Representative Kampo formula: Daijokito, daisaikoto, Shigyakusan, etc.

Kippi, Citrus Peel, キッピ[Non-JP], 橘皮

Origin: The dried mature fruit peel of *Citrus tachibana* Tanaka, *Citrus leiocarpa* Tanaka, *Citrus grandis* Osbeck, *Citrus unshiu* Marcowicz or *Citrus reticulata* Blanco (Rutaceae)

Effects: Substitute for ***Chimpi*** (Citrus Unshiu Peel)

Representative Kampo formula: Kumibinroto

Kobei, Brown Rice[JP], コウベイ, 粳米

Origin: The dried caryopsis of *Oryza sativa* Linné (Gramineae)

Ingredients: Starches: amylopectin, etc.

Effects: Sweet, neutral. Dryness-moistening, stomachic and anti-flatulent, tonifying qi, harmonizing other drugs, anti-diarrheic, recovery from exhaustion

Representative Kampo formula: Bakumondoto, byakkokaninjinto

Koboku, Magnolia Bark[JP], コウボク, 厚朴

Origin: The dried bark of the trunk of *Magnolia obovata* Thunberg (Magnolia hypoleuca Siebold et Zuccarini), *Magnolia officinalis* Rehder et Wilson or *Magnolia officinalis* Rehder et Wilson var. *biloba* Rehder et Wilson (Magnoliaceae)

Ingredients: Lignans, magnolol, etc.

Effects: Pungent bitter, warm. Aromatic stomachic and anti-flatulent, descending qi, relieving abdominal colic, resolving phlegm, expectorant, relieving asthma, antitussive, analgesic (abdominal pain, etc.)

Representative Kampo formula: Saibokuto, daijokito, Hangekobokuto, etc.

Kobushi, Cyperus Rhizome[JP], コウブシ, 香附子

Origin: The dried rhizome of *Cyperus rotundus* Linné (Cyperaceae)

Ingredients: Sesquiterpenoids, cyperol, etc.

Effects: Bitter, mild sweet, neutral. Regulating qi, aromatic stomachic and anti-flatulent, analgesic (headache, stomach pain, etc.), resolving women's diseases (dysmenorrhea, etc.), relieving abdominal mass, descending qi

Representative Kampo formula: Kososan, Goshakusan, Nyoshinsan, etc.

Kohon, Ligusticum Sinense Rhizome[Non-JP], コウホン, 藁本

Origin: The dried rhizoma and root of *Ligusticum sinense* Oliver or *Ligusticum jeholense* Nakai et Kitagawa (Umbelliferae)

Ingredients: Phtalides: butylidene phthalide, cnidilide, etc.

Effects: Pungent, warm. Dredging channels, anti-inflammatory

Representative Kampo formula: Jingyokyokatsuto, Seijokentsuto

Koi, Koi[JP], コウイ, 膠飴

Origin: A saccharized substance obtained by hydrolysis of the starch of *Zea mays* Linné (Gramineae), *Manihot esculenta* Crantz (Euphorbiaceae), *Solanum tuberosum* Linné (Solanaceae), *Ipomoea batatas* Poiret (Convolvulaceae) or *Oryza sativa* Linné (Gramineae), or the seed of *Oryza sativa* Linné from which the seed coat is removed

Ingredients: Saccharides, maltose, etc.

Effects: Sweet, mild warm. Tonifying qi, relieving urgency, analgesic, dispelling cold, stomachic and anti-flatulent, harmonizing other drugs

Representative Kampo formula: Ogikenchuto, Shokenchuto, daikenchuto, etc.

Koka, Safflower[JP], コウカ, 紅花

Origin: The dried tubulous flower of *Carthamus tinctorius* Linneá (Compositae) without any treatment or with most of the yellow pigment removed, and sometimes with pressed into a flat slab

Ingredients: Chalcone glycosides, carthamin, etc.

Effects: Pungent, warm. Resolving blood[TM1] stasis, dredging channels, analgesic, moistening dryness, relieving women's diseases (dysmenorrhea, menorrhalgia, etc.)

Representative Kampo formula: Jizusoippo, Tsudosan

Kujin, Sophora Root[JP], クジン, 苦参

Origin: The dried root of *Sophora flavescens* Aiton (Leguminosae) or often such root from which the periderm has been removed
Ingredients: Alkaloids; matrine, etc.
Effects: Bitter, cold. Deworming, stomachic and antiflatulent, anti-pyretic, anti-inflammatory, diuretic, bactericide, clearing heat, tonifying kidney[TM1], anti-diarrheic; (for external use) resolving skin disease
Representative Kampo formula: Sammotsuogonto, Shofusan

Kyokatsu, Notopterygium[JP], キョウカツ, 羌活

Origin: The dried rhizome and root of *Notopterygium incisum* Ting ex H. T. Chang or *Notopterygium forbesii* Boissieu (Umbelliferae)
Ingredients: Coumarins, isoimperatorin, etc.
Effects: Pungent bitter, warm. Dispelling wind-dampness, releasing exterior, analgesic (low back pain, arthralgia, headache, etc.)
Representative Kampo formula: Senkyuchachosan, Sokeikakketsuto, daibofuto, etc.

Kyonin, Apricot Kernel, キョウニン, 杏仁

Origin: The dried seed of *Prunus armeniaca* Linné, *Prunus armeniaca* Linné var. ansu Maximowicz or *Prunus sibirica* Linné (Rosaceae)
Ingredients: Cyanogenic glycosides: amygdalin, etc.
Effects: Pungent bitter, warm. Relieving asthma, antitussive, regulating fluid[TM1], releasing exterior, resolving phlegm, expectorant
Representative Kampo formula: Gokoto, Junchoto, Shimpito, etc.

Mankeishi, Shrub Chaste Tree Fruit[Non-JP], マンケイシ, 蔓荊子 蔓荊子

Origin: The dried fruit of *Vitex rotundifolia* Linné filius or *V. trifolia* Linné (Verbenaceae)
Ingredients: Fatty oils, etc.
Effects: Bitter and pungent, mild cold. Tonifying qi, antipyretic, analgesic, anti-inflammatory
Representative Kampo formula: Jijinmeimokuto, Seijokentsuto, Seikanmeimokuto

Mao, Ephedra Herb[JP], マオウ, 麻黄

Origin: The dried terrestrial stem of *Ephedra sinica* Stapf, *Ephedra intermedia* Schrenk et C.A. Meyer or *Ephedra equisetina* Bunge (Ephedraceae)
Ingredients: Phenethylamine alkaloids, ephedrine, etc.
Effects: Pungent mild bitter, warm. Releasing exterior, analgesic (headache, arthralgia, etc.), relieving asthma, antitussive, anti-pyretic, expectorant
Representative Kampo formula: Maoto, Kakkonto, Shoseiryuto, etc.

Mashinin, Hemp Fruit[JP], マシニン, 麻子仁

Origin: The dried fruit of *Cannabis sativa* Linné (Moraceae)
Ingredients: Fatty oils, linoleic acid, etc.
Effects: Sweet, neutral. Purgative, moistening dryness
Representative Kampo formula: Mashiningan, Junchoto, Shakanzoto

Mitsuro, Yellow Beeswax[JP], ミツロウ, 黄蝋

Origin: The purified wax obtained from honeycombs such as those of *Apis mellifera* Linneá or *Apis cerana* Fabricius (Apidae)
Ingredients: Paraffin, etc.
Effects: Ointment base
Representative Kampo formula: Shiunko, Chuoko

Mokko, Saussurea Root[JP], モッコウ, 木香

Origin: The dried root of *Saussurea lappa* Clarke (Compositae)
Ingredients: Sesquiterpenoids, costunolide, etc.
Effects: Bitter pungent, warm. Aromatic stomachic and antiflatulent, anti-diarrheic, regulating qi
Representative Kampo formula: Kamikihito, Jinsoin, Nyoshinsan, Kumibinroto, etc.

Mokutsu, Akebia Stem[JP], モクツウ, 木通

Origin: The dried climbing stem of *Akebia quinata* Decaisne or *Akebia trifoliata* Koidzumi (Lardizabalaceae), usually cut transversely
Ingredients: Terpenoid-saponins: Akebioside, etc.
Effects: Light sweet, cold. Diuretic, regulating fluid[TM1], anti-inflammatory, promoting lactation, opening blocked orifices, relieving stranguria, relieving women's diseases (dysmenorrhea, etc.)
Representative Kampo formula: Tokishigyakukagosyuyushokyoto, Gorinsan, Shofusan, Ryutanshakanto, etc.

Musui-Bosho, Anhydrous Sodium Sulfate[JP], 無水ボウショウ, 無水芒硝

Origin: The mineral substance, mainly composed of anhydrous sodium sulfate (Na_2SO_4)
Ingredients: Sodium sulfate, etc.

Effects: salty bitter, cold. Purgative, clearing heat, diuretic, moistening dryness
Representative Kampo formula: Daijokito, Tokakujokito, daiobotampito, etc.

Namashokyo, Fresh Ginger, 生ショウキョウ, 生生姜

Origin: The fresh rhizome, with (unpeeled) or without (peeled) the periderm, of *Zingiber officinale* Roscoe (Zingiberaceae)
Ingredients: Phenols, [6]-gingerol, etc.
Effects: Pungent sweet, warm. Anti-emetic, antitussive, aromatic stomachic and anti-flatulent, relieving nausea, regulating fluid[TM1], resolving phlegm, flavor
Representative Kampo formula: Kakkonto, Keishito, Shosaikoto, etc.

Nindo, Lonicera Leaf and Stem[JP], ニンドウ, 忍冬

Origin: The dried leaves and stems of *Lonicera japonica* Thunberg (Caprifoliaceae)
Ingredients: Flavonoids, lonicerin, etc.
Effects: Sweet, cold. Detoxication, relieving serious skin eruption, diuretic, relieving scabies, diuretic, anti-pyretic, anti-inflammatory
Representative Kampo formula: Jizusoippo

Ninjin, Ginseng[JP], ニンジン, 人参

Origin: The dried root of *Panax ginseng* C. A. Meyer (Araliaceae), from which rootlets have been removed, or the root that has been quickly passed through hot water
Ingredients: Triterpenoid-saponins, ginsenoside Ra-Rh, etc.
Effects: Sweet, warm. Qi tonifying, dryness-moistening, nourishing yin, anti-emesis, stomachic and anti-flatulent, anti-diarrheic
Representative Kampo formula: Juzentaihoto, Shosaikoto, Rikkunshito, etc.

Obaku, Phellodendron Bark[JP], オウバク, 黄柏

Origin: The dried bark of *Phellodendron amurense* Ruprecht or *Phellodendron chinense* Schneider (Rutaceae), from which the periderm has been removed
Ingredients: Isoquinoline alkaloids, Berberine, etc.
Effects: Bitter, cold. Clearing heat, anti-inflammatory, bitter stomachic and anti-flatulent, astringent, anti-diarrheic, anti-emesis, deworming, relieving jaundice, relieving red eyes; (for external use) relieving contusions, relieving bruising and sprains, alleviating periodontal disease
Representative Kampo formula: Unseiin, Orengedokuto, Shichimotsukokato, etc.

Ogi, Astragalus Root[JP], オウギ, 黄耆

Origin: The dried root of *Astragalus membranaceus* Bunge or *Astragalus mongholicus* Bunge (Leguminosae)
Ingredients: Triterpenoid-saponins, astragalosideI-VII, etc.
Effects: Sweet, warm. Tonifying qi, anhidrotic, regulating fluid[TM1], diuretic, relieving serious skin eruption, relieving night sweats, relieving hypertension
Representative Kampo formula: Ogikenchuto, Kamikihito, Shichimotsukokato, etc.

Ogon, Scutellaria Root[JP], オウゴン, 黄芩

Origin: The dried root of *Scutellaria baicalensis* Georgi (Labiatae), from which the periderm has been removed
Ingredients: Flavonoids, baicalein, etc.
Effects: Bitter, cold. Clearing heat, anti-inflammatory, purging heart[TM1], anti-pyretic, anti-diarrheic, resolving bloody stools, resolving stranguria, stomachic and anti-flatulent
Representative Kampo formula: Shosaikoto, Orengedokuto, San'oshashinto, etc.

Ohi, Cherry Bark[JP], オウヒ, 桜皮

Origin: The dried bark of *Prunus jamasakura* Siebold ex Koidzumi or *Prunus verecunda* Koehne (Rosaceae)
Ingredients: Flavonoids, sakuranin, etc.
Effects: Astringent, antitussive
Representative Kampo formula: Jumihaidokuto

Onji, Polygala Root[JP], オンジ, 遠志

Origin: The dried root or the root bark of *Polygala tenuifolia* Willdenow (Polygalaceae)
Ingredients: Triterpenoid-saponins, onjisaponin A–G, etc.
Effects: Bitter pungent, warm. Sedative, expectorant, alleviating amnesia, tonifying qi, sedative, tonifying kidney[TM1], alleviating amnesia after middle age
Representative Kampo formula: Ninjin'yoeito, Kamikihito, Kihito, etc.

Oren, Coptis Rhizome[JP], オウレン, 黄連

Origin: The dried rhizome of *Coptis japonica* Makino, *Coptis chinensis* Franchet, *Coptis deltoidea* C.Y. Cheng et Hsiao or *Coptis teeta* Wallich (Ranunculaceae), from which the roots have been removed practically
Ingredients: Isoquinoline alkaloids, berberine, etc.
Effects: Bitter, cold. Purging heart[TM1], anti-diarrheic, hemostasis, anti-inflammatory, bitter stomachic and anti-flatulent, relieving abdominal colic, anti-emesis, sedative

Representative Kampo formula: Orengedokuto, San'oshashinto, Hangeshashinto, etc.

Rengyo, Forsythia Fruit[JP], レンギョウ, 連翹

Origin: The dried fruit of *Forsythia suspensa* Vahl (Oleaceae)
Ingredients: Phenethyl alcohol glycosides, forsythiaside, etc.
Effects: Bitter, mild cold. Discharging pus, analgesic, anti-inflammatory, diuretic, detoxification, relieving serious skin eruption
Representative Kampo formula: Bofutsushosan, Jumihaidokuto, Keigairengyoto, Jizusoippo, etc.

Ren'niku, Nelumbo Seed[JP], レンニク, 蓮肉

Origin: The dried seed of *Nelumbo nucifera* Gaertner (Nymphaeaceae), usually with the endocarp, sometime being removed the embryo
Ingredients: Alkaloids, dimethyl coclaurine, etc.
Effects: Sweet, neutral. Tonifying qi, stomachic and anti-flatulent, anti-diarrheic
Representative Kampo formula: keihito, Seishinrenshiin

Ryokyo, Alpinia Officinarum Rhizome[JP], リョウキョウ, 良姜

Origin: The dried rhizome of *Alpinia officinarum* Hance (Zingiberaceae)
Ingredients: Monoterpenoids: α-cadinene, etc.
Effects: Pungent, hot. Aromatic stomachic and anti-flatulent, dispelling cold, anti-diarrheic, relieving nausea, analgesic (abdominal pain, etc.)
Representative Kampo formula: Anchusan

Ryugan'niku, Longan Aril[JP], リュウガンニク, 竜眼肉

Origin: The dried aril of *Euphoria longana* Lamarck (Sapindaceae)
Ingredients: Saccharides, glucose, etc.
Effects: Sweet, warm. Tonifying qi, tonifying spleen[TM], increasing wisdom, relieving insomnia, sedative
Representative Kampo formula: Kamikihito, Kihito

Ryukotsu, Longgu[JP], リュウコツ, 竜骨

Origin: The dried ossified bone of large mammal, and it is mainly composed of calcium carbonate.
Ingredients: Hydroxyapatite
Effects: Sweet pungent, neutral. Sedative, tonifying kidney[TM1], relieving palpitations and insomnia
Representative Kampo formula: Keishikaryukotsuboreito, Saikokaryukotsuboreito

Ryutan, Japanese Gentian[JP], リュウタン, 竜胆

Origin: The dried root and rhizome of *Gentiana scabra* Bunge, *Gentiana manshurica* Kitagawa or *Gentiana triflora* Pallas (Gentianaceae)
Ingredients: Secoiridoids, gentiopicroside, etc.
Effects: Bitter, cold. Stomachic and anti-flatulent, anti-inflammatory, relieving red eyes, resolving damp-heat, purging fire
Representative Kampo formula: Sokeikakketsuto, Rikkosan, Ryutanshakanto

Saiko, Bupleurum Root[JP], サイコ, 柴胡

Origin: The dried root of *Bupleurum falcatum* Linné (Umbelliferae)
Ingredients: Triterpenoid-saponins; saikosaponin a, etc.
Effects: Bitter pungent, mild cold. Resolving alternating chills and fever, relieving fullness and discomfort in chest and hypochondeium, clearing heat, relieving malaria, anti-pyretic, analgesic (abdominal pain, etc.), sedative, anti-inflammatory, tonifying qi
Representative Kampo formula: Shosaikoto, Otsujito, Kamishoyosan, etc.

Saishin, Asiasarum Root[JP], サイシン, 細辛

Origin: The dried root with rhizome of *Asiasarum sieboldii* F. Maekawa or *Asiasarum heterotropoides* F. Maekawa var. *mandshuricum* F. Maekawa (Aristolochiaceae)
Ingredients: Phenylpropanoids, methyleugenol, etc.
Effects: Pungent, warm. Analgesic (headache, chest pain, etc.), antitussive, expectorant, anti-pyretic
Representative Kampo formula: Shoseiryuto, Maobushisaishinto, Rikkosan, etc.

Sanshishi, Gardenia Fruit[JP], サンシシ, 山梔子

Origin: The dried fruit of *Gardenia jasminoides* Ellis (Rubiaceae)
Ingredients: Iridoid glycosides; genipin, etc.
Effects: Bitter, cold. Purging heart[TM1], clearing heat, anti-pyretic, anti-inflammatory, choleretic, relieving jaundice, relieving hematemesis, sedative, relieving red eyes, hemostasis, relieving stranguria, relieving bruises and sprains

Representative Kampo formula: Orengedokuto, Kamishoyosan, Bofutsushosan, etc.

Sansho, Japanese Zanthoxylum Peel[JP], サンショウ, 山椒

Origin: The dried pericarps of the ripe fruit of *Zanthoxylum piperitum* De Candolle (Rutaceae), from which the seeds separated from the pericarps have been mostly removed
Ingredients: Amide derivatives, α-sanshool, etc.
Effects: Pungent, hot. Aromatic stomachic and anti-flatulent, deworming, anti-diarrheic, dispelling cold
Representative Kampo formula: Daikenchuto, Tokito

Sansonin, Jujube Seed[JP], サンソウニン, 酸棗仁

Origin: The dried seed of *Zizyphus jujuba* Miller var. *spinosa* Hu ex H. F. Chou (Rhamnaceae)
Ingredients: Triterpenoid-saponins, jujuboside A, etc.
Effects: Sweet, neutral. Sedative, relieving insomnia, tonifying qi
Representative Kampo formula: Kamikihito, Kihito, Sansoninto, etc.

Sansyuyu, Cornus Fruit[JP], サンシュユ, 山茱萸

Origin: The dried pulp of the pseudocarp of *Cornus officinalis* Siebold et Zuccarini (Cornaceae)
Ingredients: Iridoid glycosides, loganin, etc.
Effects: sour, mild warm. Tonifying qi, tonifying kidney[TM1], resolving frequent urination, astringent, analgesic (low back pain, etc.), relieving tinnitus, warming liver[TM1], astringent
Representative Kampo formula: Goshajinkigan, Hachimijiogan, Rokumigan, etc.

San'yaku, Dioscorea Rhizome[JP], サンヤク, 山薬

Origin: The dried rhizome (rhizophore) of *Dioscorea japonica* Thunberg or D*ioscorea batatas* Decaisne (Dioscoreaceae), from which the periderm has been removed
Ingredients: Steroid-saponins; diosgenin, etc.
Effects: Sweet, neutral. Tonifying qi, anti-diarrheic, moistening dryness, antitussive
Representative Kampo formula: keihito, Goshajinkigan, Hachimijiogan, etc.

Sanzashi, Crataegus Fruit[JP], サンザシ, 山査子

Origin: The dried pseudocarp of *Crataegus cuneata* Siebold et Zuccarini or *Crataegus pinnatifida* Bunge var. *major* N.E. Brown (Rosaceae) without any treatment or cut crosswise or lengthwiseIngredients: Flavonoids, rutin, etc.
Effects: Sweet, mild warm. Stomachic and anti-flatulent, relieving abdominal colic, resolving blood[TM1] stasis, regulating qi, resolving phlegm
Representative Kampo formula: Kamiheiisan, keihito

Sarashi-mitsuro, White Beeswax[JP], サラシミツロウ, 白蝋

Origin: Bleached Yellow Beeswax
Ingredients: Paraffin, etc.
Effects: Ointment base
Representative Kampo formula: Shiunko, Chuoko

Sekko, Gypsum[JP], セッコウ, 石膏

Origin: Natural hydrous calcium sulfate. It possibly corresponds to the formula $CaSO_4 \bullet 2H_2O$
Ingredients: Calcium sulfate hydrate
Effects: Pungent, cold. Moistening dryness, clearing heat, anti-pyretic, analgesic (headache, etc.), sedative
Representative Kampo formula: Makyokansekito, Gokoto, Shin'iseihaito, etc.

Senkotsu, Nuphar Rhizome[JP], センコツ, 川骨

Origin: The dried longitudinally split rhizome of *Nuphar japonicum* De Candolle (Nymphaeaceae)
Ingredients: Alkaloids, nupharidine, etc.
Effects: Sweet, cold. Resolving blood[TM1] stasis, tonifying qi, hemostasis, relieving women's diseases (dysmenorrhea, etc.)
Representative Kampo formula: Jidabokuippo

Senkyu, Cnidium Rhizome[JP], センキュウ, 川芎

Origin: The dried rhizome of *Cnidium officinale* Makino (Umbelliferae), usually passed through hot water
Ingredients: Phthalides: ligustilide, etc.
Effects: Pungent, warm. Analgesic (headache, etc.), resolving blood[TM1] stasis, tonifying blood[TM1], regulating qi, relieving impediment disorder, sedative, tonifying qi, relieving women's diseases (sensitivity to cold, etc.)
Representative Kampo formula: Tokishakuyakusan, Nyoshinsan, Yokukansan, etc.

Sentai, Cicada Slough[JP], センタイ, 蝉退

Origin: The dried larval exuvia of *Cryptotympana atrata* Stal, *Platylomia pieli* Kato, *Oncotympana maculaticollis* Distant, *Tanna chekiangensis* Ouchi, *Graptopsaltria tienta* Karsch, *Lyristes pekinensis* Haupt, *Lyristes atrofasciatus* Chou et Lei, *Meimuna mongolica* Distant, *Leptosemia sakaii* Matsumura,

Platypleura kaempferi Butler or other species of the same genus (Cicadidae)
Ingredients: Chitin, etc.
Effects: Sweet, cold. Anti-spastic, clearing heat in cold damage, anti-pyretic, reducing night crying in children
Representative Kampo formula: Shofusan

Shakanzo, Processed Glycyrrhiza[JP], シャカンゾウ, 炙甘草

Origin: The product prepared by roasting Glycyrrhiza
Ingredients: Triterpenoid-saponins, glycyrrhizic acid, etc.
Effects: Sweet, neutral. It is said that, compared to Glycyrrhiza, the effects are greater and the side effects are less
Representative Kampo formula: Shakanzoto

Shakuyaku, Peony Root[JP], シャクヤク, 芍薬

Origin: The dried root of *Paeonia lactiflora* Pallas (Paeoniaceae)
Ingredients: Monoterpenoids, paeoniflorin, etc.
Effects: Bitter sour, mild cold. Analgesic (abdominal pain, etc.), astringent, anti-spastic, relieving women's diseases (sensitivity to cold, etc.), relieving abdominal colic, anti-diarrheic, relieving serious skin eruption
Representative Kampo formula: Tokishakuyakusan, Kamishoyosan, Keishibukuryogan, etc.

Shazenshi, Plantago Seed[JP], シャゼンシ, 車前子

Origin: The dried seed of *Plantago asiatica* Linné (Plantaginaceae)
Ingredients: Polysaccharides, plantago-mucilage A, etc.
Effects: Sweet, cold. Diuretic, regulating fluid[TM1], anti-inflammatory, relieving stranguria, analgesic, relieving impediment disorder, antitussive, expectorant, anti-diarrheic
Representative Kampo formula: Goshajinkigan, Gorinsan, Ryutanshakanto, etc.

Shin'i, Magnolia Flower[JP], シンイ, 辛夷

Origin: The dried flower bud of *Magnolia salicifolia* Maximowicz, *Magnolia kobus* De Candolle, *Magnolia biondii* Pampanini, *Magnolia sprengeri* Pampanini or *Magnolia heptapeta* Dandy (Magnoliaceae)
Ingredients: Alkaloids, coclaurine, etc.
Effects: Pungent, warm. Analgesic (headache, etc.), relieving rhinitis, opening blocked orifices
Representative Kampo formula: Shin'iseihaito, Kakkontokasenkyushin'i

Shinkiku, Shinkiku, シンキク, 神麴

Origin: The product from the caryopsis of *Oryza sativa* by fermentation with *Aspergillus oryzae*
Ingredients: Saccharides
Effects: Pungent sweet, warm. Stomachic and anti-flatulent, resolving fluid[TM1] retention in stomach, resolving phlegm, anti-diarrheic, tonifying qi
Representative Kampo formula: Hangebyakujutsutemmato

Shikon, Lithospermum Root[JP], シコン, 紫根

Origin: The dried root of *Lithospermum erythrorhizon* Siebold et Zuccarini (Boraginaceae)
Ingredients: Naphthoquinones, shikonin, etc.
Effects: Bitter, cold. Detoxication, anti-pyretic, cooling blood[TM1] heat, alleviating vaccinia, resolving blood[TM1] stasis, opening blocked orifices, regulating fluid[TM1], resolving skin disease and hemorrhoids, anti-inflammatory
Representative Kampo formula: Shiunko

Shitsurishi, Tribulus Fruit[JP], シツリシ, 蒺藜子

Origin: The dried fruit of *Tribulus terrestris* Linné (Zygophyllaceae)
Ingredients: Phenethylamine derivatives, terrestriamide, etc.
Effects: Bitter pungent, mild warm. Resolving blood[TM1] stasis, tonifying kidney[TM1], alleviating eye disease, anti-inflammatory, dredging channels, sedative, diuretic
Representative Kampo formula: Tokiinshi

Shobaku, Wheat[JP], ショウバク, 小麦

Origin: The dried seed of *Triticum aestivum* Linné (Poaceae)
Ingredients: Starches, etc.
Effects: Sweet, mild cold. Moistening dryness-, anti-inflammatory, relieving heat with agitation, diuretic, sedative, harmonizing other drugs
Representative Kampo formula: Kambakutaisoto

Shokyo, Ginger[JP], ショウキョウ, 生姜

Origin: The dried rhizome, with (unpeeled) or without (peeled) the periderm, of *Zingiber officinale* Roscoe (Zingiberaceae)
Ingredients: Phenols, [6]-gingerol, etc.
Effects: Pungent sweet, warm. Anti-emesis, antitussive, aromatic stomachic and anti-flatulent, relieving nausea, regulating fluid[TM1], resolving phlegm, adjusting flavor
Representative Kampo formula: Kakkonto, Keishito, Shosaikoto, etc.

Shoma, Cimicifuga Rhizome[JP], ショウマ, 升麻

Origin: The dried rhizome of *Cimicifuga simplex* Turczaninow, *Cimicifuga dahurica* Maximowicz, *Cimicifuga foetida* Linné or *Cimicifuga heracleifolia* Komarov (Ranunculaceae)
Ingredients: Triterpenoids, cimigenol, etc.
Effects: Sweet pungent, mild cold. Analgesic (headache, angina, etc.), alleviating oral ulcers, relieving serious skin eruption, clearing heat, anti-pyretic, dispelling wind, detoxification, relieving hemorrhoids
Representative Kampo formula: Otsujito, Hochuekkito, Shpmakakkonto, etc.

Shukusya, Amomum Seed[JP], シュクシャ, 縮砂

Origin: The dried seed mass of *Amomum xanthioides* Wallich (Zingiberaceae)
Ingredients: Monoterpenoids: borneol, etc.
Effects: Pungent, warm. Aromatic stomachic and anti-flatulent, relieving abdominal colic, anti-diarrheic, anti-emesis, preventing abortion, tonifying qi, dislodging food stuck in the throat and esophagus, relieving food stagnation
Representative Kampo formula: Anchusan, Ireito (some ethical Kampo products do not contain it)

Soboku, Sappan Wood[JP], ソボク, 蘇木

Origin: The dried duramen of *Caesalpinia sappan* Linné (Leguminosae)
Ingredients: Homoisoflavonoids, brazilin, etc.
Effects: Sweet salty pungent, neutral. Resolving blood[TM1] stasis, analgesic, hemostasis, anti-inflammatory, clearing bruises, relieving serious skin eruption
Representative Kampo formula: Tsudosan

Sohakuhi, Mulberry Bark[JP], ソウハクヒ, 桑白皮

Origin: The dried root bark of *Morus alba* Linné (Moraceae)
Ingredients: Triterpenoids, α-amyrin, etc.
Effects: Sweet, cold. Antitussive, anti-inflammatory, diuretic, descending qi, expectorant
Representative Kampo formula: Gokoto, Seihaito

Sojutsu, Atractylodes Lancea Rhizome[JP], ソウジュツ, 蒼朮

Origin: The dried rhizome of *Atractylodes lancea* De Candolle, *Atractylodes chinensis* Koidzumi or their inter-specific hybrids (Compositae)
Ingredients: Sesquiterpenoids, hinesol, etc.
Effects: Bitter pungent, warm. Diuretic, regulating fluid[TM1], analgesic (arthralgia, etc.), anti-diarrheic, drying dampness, resolving fluid[TM1] retention in stomach, resolving phlegm, aromatic stomachic, releasing exterior
Representative Kampo formula: Yokuininto, Nijutsuto, Eppikajutsubuto, etc.

Soyo, Perilla Herb[JP], ソヨウ, 蘇葉

Origin: The dried leaves and the tips of branches of *Perilla frutescens* Britton var. *acuta* Kudo or *Perilla frutescens* Britton var. *crispa* Decaisne (Labiatae)
Ingredients: Monoterpenoids, perillaldehyde, etc.
Effects: Pungent, warm. Releasing exterior, regulating qi, descending qi, antitussive, relieving asthma, expectorant, anti-pyretic, detoxifying fish toxin, aromatic stomachic and anti-flatulent, resolving phlegm, relieving beriberi
Representative Kampo formula: Kososan, Saibokuto, Hangekobokuto, etc.

Taiso, Jujube[JP], タイソウ, 大棗

Origin: The dried fruit of *Zizyphus jujuba* Miller var. *inermis* Rehder (Rhamnaceae)
Ingredients: Triterpenoid-saponins, zizyphus saponin I, etc.
Effects: Sweet, mild warm. Tonifying qi, analgesic (abdominal pain, etc.), regulating fluid[TM1], diuretic, sedative, harmonizing other drugs
Representative Kampo formula: Kakkonto, Keishito, Kambakutaisoto, etc.

Tochu, Eucommia Bark[JP], トチュウ, 杜仲

Origin: The dried bark of *Eucommia ulmoides* Oliver (Eucommiaceae)
Ingredients: Iridoid glycosides, aucubin, etc.
Effects: Sweet, warm. Analgesic (pain in the lower back and knee, etc.), tonifying qi, tonifying kidney[TM1], relieving hypertension
Representative Kampo formula: Daibofuto

Toki, Japanese Angelica Root[JP], トウキ, 当帰

Origin: The dried root of *Angelica acutiloba* Kitagawa or *Angelica acutiloba* Kitagawa var. *sugiyamae* Hikino (Umbelliferae), usually after being passed through hot water
Ingredients: Phthalides, ligustilide, etc.
Effects: Sweet pungent, warm. Tonifying blood[TM1], analgesic (abdominal pain, etc.), resolving blood[TM1] stasis, dispelling cold, tonifying qi, relieving women's diseases (dysmenorrhea, etc.), sedative

Representative Kampo formula: Tokishakuyakusan, Bofutsushosan, Hochuekkito, etc.

Takusha, Alisma Tuber[JP], タクシャ, 沢瀉

Origin: The dried tuber of *Alisma orientale* Juzepczuk (Alismataceae), from which periderm has been usually removed
Ingredients: Triterpenoids: Alisol A, B, etc.
Effects: sweet, cold. Diuretic, relieving dizziness, regulating fluid[TM1], moistening dryness, drying dampness, resolving fluid[TM1] retention in stomach, anti-diarrheic
Representative Kampo formula: Goreisan, Tokishakuyakusan, Hachimijiogan, etc.

Temma, Gastrodia Tuber[JP], テンマ, 天麻

Origin: The dried steamed tuber of *Gastrodia elata* Blume (Orchidaceae)
Ingredients: Phenols, gastrodin, etc.
Effects: Sweet, neutral. Sedative, anti-spastic, alleviating epilepsy in children, relieving dizziness, tonifying qi, analgesic (headache, etc.)
Representative Kampo formula: Hangebyakujutsutemmato

Tenmondo, Asparagus Root[JP], テンモンドウ, 天門冬

Origin: The dried root of *Asparagus cochinchinensis* Merrill (Liliaceae), from which most of the cork layer is removed after being passed through hot water or steamed
Ingredients: Steroid-saponins, asparasaponin I, etc.
Effects: Sweet bitter, cold. Moistening dryness, antitussive, tonifying qi, expectorant, tonifying kidney[TM1], resolving phlegm, diuretic
Representative Kampo formula: Jiinkokato, Seihaito

Ten'nansho, Arisaema Tuber[JP], テンナンショウ, 天南星

Origin: The dried tuber of *Arisaema heterophyllum* Blume, *Arisaema erubescens* Schott, *Arisaema amurense* Maximowicz or other species of the same genus (Araceae), from which periderm has been usually removed
Ingredients: Benzoic acid, etc.
Effects: Bitter pungent, warm. Resolving phlegm, expectorant, eliminate wind, antitussive, descending qi, analgesic (angina, etc.), relieving dizziness, anti-spastic in children, alleviating epilepsy
Representative Kampo formula: Nijutsuto

Togashi, Benincasa Seed[JP], トウガシ, 冬瓜子

Origin: The dried seed of *Benincasa cerifera* Savi or *Benincasa cerifera* Savi forma *emarginata* K. Kimura et Sugiyama (Cucurbitaceae)
Ingredients: Fatty oils, oleic acid, etc.
Effects: Sweet, mild cold. Diuretic, anti-inflammatory, discharging pus, antitussive, expectorant, purgative, resolving serious skin eruption
Representative Kampo formula: Daiobotampito, Choyoto

Tonin, Peach Kernel[JP], トウニン, 桃仁

Origin: The dried seed of *Prunus persica* Batsch or *Prunus persica* Batsch var. *davidiana* Maximowicz (Rosaceae)
Ingredients: Cyanogenic glycosides, amygdalin, etc.
Effects: Bitter sweet, neutral. Resolving blood[TM1] stasis, purgative, anti-inflammatory, relieving women's diseases (dysmenorrhea, etc.)
Representative Kampo formula: Tokakujokito, Keishibukuryogan, daiobotampito, etc.

Tonshi, Lard[JP], トンシ, 豚脂

Origin: The fat obtained from *Sus scrofa* Linneá var. *domesticus* Gray (Suidae)
Ingredients: Triglycerides
Effects: Ointment base
Representative Kampo formula: Shiunko

Toshinso, Common Rush[Non-JP], トウシンソウ, 灯心草, 燈心草

Origin: The dried aerial part of *Juncus effusus* Linné (Juncaceae), sometimes used only the pith of the stem
Ingredients: Flavonoids, luteolin, etc.
Effects: Mild sweet, cold. Diuresis, relieving dysphoria, anti-pyretic
Representative Kampo formula: Bunshoto, Kamigedokuto, Jiinmeimokuto

Uikyo, Fennel[JP], ウイキョウ, 茴香

Origin: The dried fruit of *Foeniculum vulgare* Miller (Umbelliferae)
Ingredients: Phenylpropanoids, anethole, etc.
Effects: Pungent, warm. Descending qi, dispelling cold, tonifying kidney[TM1], carminative, aromatic stomachic and

anti-flatulent, alleviating enterogastritis, anti-diarrheic, expectorant

Representative Kampo formula: Anchusan

Ukon, Curcumae Longae Rhizoma[JP], ウコン[局], 鬱金

Origin: The dried rhizome of *Curcuma longa* L (Zingberacear)

Ingredients: Curcuminoids, curcumin, etc.

Effects: Bitter, cold. choleretic, Aromatic stomachic and anti-flatulent, analgesic, hemostasis

Representative Kampo formula: Chuoko

Uyaku, Lindera Root[JP], ウヤク, 烏薬

Origin: The dried root of *Lindera strychnifolia* Fernandez-Villar (Lauraceae)

Ingredients: Monoterpenoids, borneol, etc.

Effects: Pungent, warm. Regulating qi, relieving abdominal colic, eliminate wind wind, tonifying kidney[TM1], analgesic (menorrhalgia, etc.), anti-diarrheic, aromatic stomachic, anti-spastic

Representative Kampo formula: Kyukichoketsuin

Wakyokatsu, Aralia Root[Non-JP], ワキョウカツ, 和羌活

Origin: The root of *Aralia cordata* Thunberg (Araliaceae)

Effects: Substitute for Notopterygium

Representative Kampo formula: Nijutsuto

Yakumoso, Leonurus Herb[JP], ヤクモソウ, 益母草

Origin: The dried aerial part of *Leonurus japonicus* Houttuyn or *Leonurus sibiricus* Linné (Labiatae), collected during the flowering season

Ingredients: Alkaloids, leonurin, etc.

Effects: Pungent mild bitter, mild cold. Resolving blood[TM1] stasis, hemostasis, preventing abortion, alleviating illnesses after childbirth, diuretic, relieving women's diseases (dysmenorrhea, etc.)

Representative Kampo formula: Kyukichoketsuin

Yokuinin, Coix Seed[JP], ヨクイニン, 薏苡仁

Origin: The dried seed of *Coix lachryma-jobi* Linné var. *mayuen* Stapf (Gramineae), from which the seed coat has been removed

Ingredients: Starches, coixenolide, etc.

Effects: Sweet, cold. Regulating fluid[TM1], drying dampness, diuretic, analgesic (arthralgia, neuralgia, etc.), relieving impediment disorder, anti-inflammatory, clearing warts, treating rough skin, tonifying qi, discharging pus

Representative Kampo formula: Yokuininto, makyoyokukanto, Choyoto, etc.

Zenko, Peucedanum Root[JP], ゼンコ, 前胡

Origin: The dried root of *Peucedanum praeruptorum* Dunn or *Angelica decursiva* Franchet et Savatier (Peucedanum decursivum Maximowicz) (Umbelliferae)

Ingredients: Coumarins, praeruptorin A, etc.

Effects: Bitter, pungent, mild cold. Antitussive, expectorant, analgesic (headache, stomach pain, etc.), anti-pyretic, resolving phlegm[TM], descending qi

Representative Kampo formula: Jinsoin

Zerachin, Gelatin[JP], ゼラチン

Origin: The product prepared from aqueous extract of raw collagen by heating. The raw collagen is obtained by acid or alkali treatment of the bone, skin, ligament or tendon of animals

Ingredients: Collagen, etc.

Effects: Substitute for Donkey Glue

Representative Kampo formula: Choreito, Kyukikyogaito, Unkeito, etc.

References

1. Pharmaceutical and Medical Device Regulatory Science Society of Japan. Japanese Pharmacopoeia Eighteenth Edition (JP XVIII). Jiho, Tokyo, 2021.
2. Ministry of Health, Labor and Welfare. The Japanese standards for non-pharmacopeial crude drugs 2018. Ministry of Health, Labor and Welfare, Tokyo, 2018.
3. Makino T, Ishii T, Tobina Y, et al. Draft standardization for crude drug Effects prescribed in ethical Kampo formulation – the Report of Working Group for the standardization of crude drug Effects in the Editorial Committee for Kampo Medical Literature. Kampo Med. 2022;73:146–75.

Index

Kampo Medical Literature Editorial Committee, The Japan Society for Oriental Medicine (ed.), *Complete Japanese Traditional (Kampo) Medicine*, https://doi.org/10.1007/978-981-96-7143-4

F

G

J

K

P

Q

R

S

The manufacturer's authorised representative in the EU is Springer Nature Customer Service Centre GmbH, Europaplatz 3, 69115 Heidelberg, Germany. If you have any concerns regarding our products, please contact ProductSafety@springernature.com

Printed and bound by CPI Group (UK) Ltd, Croydon, CR0 4YY
21/09/2026
02220021-0001